PHYSIOLOGY

The Basis of Clinical Practice

PHYSIOLOGY

The Basis of Clinical Practice

Glenn Irion, PhD, PT, CWS
University of Central Arkansas
Conway, Arkansas

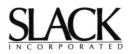

SLACK
INCORPORATED

6900 Grove Road • Thorofare, New Jersey 08086

Publisher: John H. Bond
Editorial Director: Amy E. Drummond
Senior Associate Editor: Jennifer L. Stewart
Illustrations by: Kimberly Taylor

The work SLACK Incorporated publishes is peer reviewed. Prior to publication, recognized leaders in the field, educators, and clinicians provide important feedback on the concepts and content that we publish. We welcome feedback on this work.

Irion, Glenn-
        Physiology : the basis of clinical practice / Glenn Irion.
                p. cm.
        Includes bibliographical references and index.
        ISBN 1-55642-380-2 (alk. paper).
        1. Human physiology. 2. Physical therapy. I. Title.

        QP34.5 .I75 2000
        612--dc21   00-026535

Printed in Canada.
Published by: SLACK Incorporated
                    6900 Grove Road
                    Thorofare, NJ 08086-9447 USA
                    Telephone: 856-848-1000
                    Fax: 856-853-5991
                    www.slackbooks.com

Contact SLACK Incorporated for more information about other books in this field or about the availability of our books from distributors outside the United States.

Last digit is print number: 10 9 8 7 6 5 4 3 2 1

DEDICATION

This book is dedicated to my 24/7 coworker, Jean Irion. We collaborate as faculty in the physical therapy programs at the University of Central Arkansas as well as the Irion family at home. We married as graduate students many years ago and she sat through my dissertation defense 5 months pregnant with our first child, Lindsay. Our second child, Kyle came 2 years later during my postdoctoral fellowship at the Medical College of Virginia, Virginia Commonwealth University, as she continued to work full-time as a physical therapist at Tuckahoe Physical Therapy with Joseph Sutter and Rick Herrod. She has continued to pursue her doctoral degree and work full-time as well as being the mother of our triplets Christina, Phillip, and Connor through the years of development of this project. She is as dedicated to her chosen profession of physical therapy as she is to her own family and has kept the delivery of this newest "child" in the family on track.

I also wish to dedicate this to my mother, Jean Reilly, who supported my academic efforts from early on and made my career possible by encouraging my graduate education.

CONTENTS

UNIT I. HOMEOSTASIS

UNIT II. NEUROMUSCULAR SYSTEM

ACKNOWLEDGMENTS

The author wishes to acknowledge the guidance of several individuals who shaped his understanding of both the art and science of physiology. The physiology faculty of Temple University School of Medicine is gratefully acknowledged, in particular Ronald Tuma, PhD, my advisor. Others instrumental in my development as a physiologist are Alan Freeman, PhD, former chairman, who did a wonderful job of teaching how complex subjects such as electrophysiology can be broken into their simpler components to be presented to others; Michael Wang, PhD, who was kind enough to serve on my dissertation and preliminary exam committees; Steven Houser, PhD; James Heckman, PhD; Thomas Schaefer, PhD; Joan Gault, MD; James Ryan, PhD; Peter Lynch, PhD; and Mary Weideman, PhD, who unfortunately passed away before I finished my program.

The exercise physiology faculty of Temple University is also gratefully acknowledged. Albert Paolone, EdD served as my advisor, my thesis advisor, and served on my dissertation committee. Zebulon Kendrick, PhD was also an important influence, who served on both my thesis and dissertation committees.

My former classmate, William L. Rumsey, PhD and I spent numerous hours together working toward building a basic understanding of physiology. He would never allow us to go into a class or an exam without fully understanding the assigned material. Dr. Rumsey continues to be a very productive scientist to this day.

Chad Lairamore, Kimberly Taylor (also this book's illustrator), and Vicki Pierce Finch contributed greatly to the production of the manuscript in their work as graduate assistants.

I also wish to acknowledge the contributions of my current colleagues. They allow me to place into context my knowledge of physiology with their clinical areas of expertise. They include William Bandy, PhD, PT, SCS, ATC; Staffan Elgelid, MS, PT; James Fletcher, MS, PT; Amy Gross McMillan, PhD, PT; Steven Hearn, MS, PT; Clayton Holmes, EdD, PT, ATC; Jean Irion, EdD, PT, SCS, ATC (also my wife and mother of my children); Loretta Knutson, PhD, PT, PCS; Bruce Mendelson, PhD, PT; Nancy Reese, PhD, PT; and Reta Zabel, PhD, PT, GCS. I certainly could not have completed this textbook without the support and encouragement of my department chair, Venita Lovelace-Chandler, PhD, PT, PCS.

I have also had numerous clinical colleagues who helped me see how my knowledge of physiology could be put to work in patient care. Nathaniel Grubbs, MS, PT, OCS; Lisa Sallings, PT; and Gayla Hearn, OT, PT were particularly helpful mentors in the clinical realm.

I also wish to thank the individuals at SLACK Incorporated for their assistance and patience in developing the "opus magnus." Amy Drummond was particularly important in getting this project from a huge pile of quasi-chapters/classnotes into production as a textbook. I also want to thank John Bond, publisher; Jennifer Stewart, editor; and my two newest best friends, Debra Toulson and Carrie Kotlar.

ABOUT THE AUTHOR

Glenn L. Irion, PhD, PT, CWS is associate professor in the physical therapy programs at the University of Central Arkansas in Conway, Ark and teaches in the professional DPT, postprofessional DPT, and PhD in physical therapy programs. Dr. Irion taught the program's physiology course for his first several years at UCA. He now teaches the cardiopulmonary physical therapy, wound management, pharmacology, and research courses and selected topics of the women's health component of the curriculum. Dr. Irion has served in several positions in physical therapy organizations at the local, state, and national level. He has been treasurer for the Arkansas Physical Therapy Association; editor for Acute Care Perspectives, the publication of the Acute Care Section of the American Physical Therapy Association (APTA); director of research for the Section on Women's Health of the APTA; and has served on the Membership Committee of the Acute Care Section.

Dr. Irion has published in and reviewed articles for prestigious journals including The American Journal of Physiology, Journal of Obstetrics and Gynecology, and Physical Therapy. Published research topics have included environmental physiology, aging and cardiovascular function, maternal-fetal cardiovascular physiology, cardiopulmonary physical therapy, and wound management.

Dr. Irion received his MEd in exercise physiology at Temple University, PhD in physiology at Temple University School of Medicine, and BS in physical therapy at the University of Central Arkansas. He completed a 3-year postdoctoral fellowship in cardiovascular physiology at the Medical College of Virginia and 1 1/2 years in maternal-fetal cardiovascular physiology in the Obstetrics and Gynecology Department at the University of Cincinnati, in conjunction with Children's Hospital of Cincinnati. Dr. Irion is a certified wound specialist, having been recognized by the American Academy of Wound Management in its first year of existence.

Dr. Irion has worked as a physical therapist at Doctor's Hospital in Little Rock, Ark, University Hospital of the University of Arkansas for Medical Sciences, and Arkansas Children's Hospital in the areas of acute care with an emphasis on cardiopulmonary and intensive care physical therapy and wound management, and has provided consultation and part-time assistance at other locations in central Arkansas in the areas of wound management, urinary incontinence, and pelvic pain.

CONTRIBUTING AUTHORS

B. Nathaniel "Nat" Grubbs, MS, PT
Owner, South Arkansas Rehabilitation
Monticello, Arkansas

Sarah N. Jerome, PhD, RRT
Assistant Professor, Department of Health Sciences
University of Central Arkansas
Conway, Arkansas

PREFACE

Physiology is often defined as the branch of biology studying the function of living things, in contradistinction from anatomy, the study of structure. Translated literally from Greek, physiology means the study of nature, implying the involvement of such disciplines as physics and chemistry. Originally, the study of physiology was introduced to the medical curriculum as the scientific basis of medical practice to instill in the future physician a knowledge base to critically examine the treatment provided to the patient. From physiology, several other disciplines have evolved: pharmacology, immunology, biochemistry, and microbiology. All of these disciplines share a common goal—advancement of knowledge through rigorous experimentation so that results can ultimately be applied to patient care.

It is only through the use of the scientific method that the clinician can provide a rational basis for patient treatment. Treatment of patients with specific disorders with "cookbook" therapy simply because "that is what we were taught" will not be tolerated in a discipline seeking acceptance of its practitioners as independent health care providers. Treatment that cannot be shown to be safe and effective must be discarded, and new forms of treatment, based on scientific evidence, rather than unsubstantiated claims or testimonials, must be explored.

Unfortunately, too few students appreciate the benefits of a good scientific basis for clinical practice until they are out of school. This makes the physiologically naive clinician easy prey for sales representatives who make claims for devices that are not supported by research published in peer-reviewed journals. One must maintain a high level of skepticism concerning any treatment for which the only literature available originates with the company that manufactures or distributes the device or from books that are not peer-reviewed. One of the claims often made for interferential therapy is a sympatholytic effect or a stimulation of parasympathetic nerves. The first claim has yet to be demonstrated, and the second cannot exist; the extremities are not innervated by the parasympathetic nervous system. When clinicians use a firm scientific basis to plan treatment, third-party payers and designers of therapeutic modalities will accord them the respect that today's clinicians demand.

The text is divided into six sections by systems. The first six chapters of this book deal with general physiology, the principles underlying the function of all organ systems. This is followed by a systems approach that includes the neuromuscular system, the integumentary system, the musculoskeletal system, and a section dealing with the gastrointestinal and reproductive systems, as these systems may impact or be impacted by the other systems described. A brief description of the renal system is included in the chapter on body fluids to describe how the ionic composition and volume of the internal environment are maintained at fairly constant values. No specific section is included on the endocrine system. The basic concepts of hormonal regulation of physiological processes are included in the chapter on signaling, and specific hormones are included where they control physiological process on a systems basis. A chapter on metabolism, including diabetes mellitus and temperature regulation, is included in the section on general principles.

Within each chapter, concepts of patient/client care are introduced to underscore the importance of physiology in applying a rational approach. Several diseases seen commonly in rehabilitation are discussed within the context of the physiology that has been altered, producing the disease. Each chapter begins with a set of objectives to guide the student in studying the material and ends with questions to allow the student to gain confidence in grasping the material and applying it to a patient situation.

The author has background in physiology as a basic science, with a PhD from a medical school; has authored research articles in high-level publications, such as the *American Journal of Physiology* and the *American Journal of Obstetrics and Gynecology*; has contributed to the journals of the sections of the American Physical Therapy Association (APTA), including the *Cardiopulmonary Physical Therapy Journal* and *Acute Care Perspectives*; and has presented research at the Combined Sections Meeting of the APTA. Moreover, the author has full-time clinical experience as a physical therapist.

The author has taught this material in one of the largest PT programs in the United States and has developed laboratory exercises that complement the textual material. The table of contents is arranged in such a way that the laboratory material can be logically sequenced with the lecture material. Individual instructors may choose to alter the sequence of the textual material to suit their needs.

This textbook was developed because of the lack of a resource that was able to hold the attention of physical therapy students because of the abstractness of principles, variation in the depth of materials, and the lack of integration with clinical principles. For this reason, individual instructors may find that favorite topics have been reduced greatly and topics thought to be of lesser importance have been overemphasized. Examples may include the lack of a chapter on the endocrine system; the endocrine system does not stand alone in physiology. The regulation of body fluid composition and the role of parts of the endocrine system are emphasized greatly. Other parts of the endocrine system are discussed with smooth muscle and the digestive system. The scope of the digestive system has also been reduced greatly compared to classic textbooks, as well as the section on blood. On the other hand, units on skeletal muscle and the nervous system are in comparison much larger than typical physiology texts.

I hope to meet the as-yet unfulfilled needs of clinical students. Physiology is too important an aspect of clinical practice to be perceived as dull, boring, or irrelevant by students. Patients/clients, their families, physicians, and insurers are now demanding clinicians who understand the impairments, functional limitations, and disabilities of their patients and who can devise rational treatment plans. Physiology is the means of reaching that goal.

Homeostasis

Homeostasis refers to the ability to maintain stable conditions in spite of challenges from the external environment. Every organ system plays a role in providing the stability that allows the organism to thrive. All of these systems are interdependent. Loss of function of one system leads to impairments in others, limitations in the ability to function in one's environment, and the potential for disability. Clinicians must understand the physiologic principles that underlie normal and abnormal function in order to remediate impairments and to restore a patient/client from functional limitations and disability or to prevent or minimize functional limitations and disability. A major focus is on the systems of movement. The neuromuscular system controls movement via sensory input, integration of signals, and motor control. The health of the integumentary system is dependent on mobility. A person with impaired mobility is at great risk to injury of the skin. The musculoskeletal system provides both structural stability (posture) and movement. The neuromuscular, integumentary, and musculoskeletal systems are dependent on the cardiopulmonary system to distribute oxygen and other nutrients and to remove wastes to maintain a stable composition of the body chemistry. Just as important, the cardiopulmonary system is dependent on the other systems for normal function. The neuromuscular system controls breathing and modulates the activity of the heart. The integumentary system protects fluid volume and aids in temperature regulation, and the musculoskeletal system provides ventilatory pumping and indirectly influences fluid volume by aiding in the flow of venous blood and lymph from the extremities. The gastrointestinal system provides the interface between the body and the environment to obtain both energy and building blocks of cells, whereas the reproductive system is necessary to perpetuate our species.

In this unit, the basic principles that allow the body to control its composition are described. This unit includes chapters on the regulation of body fluids, metabolic rate, and temperature, which allow the neuromuscular, integumentary, musculoskeletal, and cardiopulmonary systems to perform their tasks.

ONE

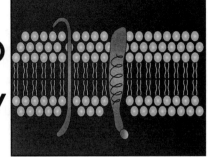

Introduction to Physiology

Glenn Irion, PhD, PT, CWS and Sarah N. Jerome, PhD, RRT

OBJECTIVES

1. Define cell, tissue, organ, and organ system.

2. Define internal environment, homeostasis, interstitial fluid, extracellular fluid, and plasma.

3. Describe the steps involved in exchange of substances from the external environment to the cells.

4. Describe how cells, tissues, organs, and organ systems participate in homeostasis.

5. List seven elements of a negative feedback system.

6. Describe the process of positive feedback, how it is useful, and how it is potentially harmful.

7. Describe feedforward and its role in homeostasis, and provide an example.

LEVELS OF ORGANIZATION

The human body consists of four levels of structural organization: cells, tissues, organs, and systems, all of which offer advantages in terms of illustrating basic principles of physiology. The smallest and most basic unit of the body is the cell. All cells, while very similar in some respects, are also very different. For example, all cells are structurally alike in that they are surrounded by a cell membrane that contains cytoplasmic fluid, a nucleus where the cell's genetic material is located, and other organelles responsible, in part, for producing proteins. However, each cell is different in that it is uniquely adapted to perform one or very few specific functions.

This is partially due to the genetic material within the cell in that, of all the possible genes encoding for different proteins, each cell only expresses a small fraction, thereby creating many possible types of cells.

Cells of similar structure and function are grouped into the second level of organization known as tissues. There are four types of tissue: epithelial, muscle, nerve, and connective tissue.

TISSUES

Cells specialized in the exchange of materials between the cell and its environment are classified as epithelial tissue. Epithelial cells are tightly joined and attached to a basement membrane to form sheets of tissue that line most internal and external surfaces of the body. Because of its variety of locations, epithelial tissue has several diverse functions. For example, the epithelial tissue of the outer layer of the skin performs a protective function, while the epithelial tissue lining the digestive tract helps absorb and secrete substances into body cavities.

Epithelial tissue is subclassified according to the number and arrangement of cell layers and cell shapes. Simple epithelium is formed from a single layer of cells, all of which are in contact with the basement membrane. Two or more layers of cells in which only the deepest layer is in contact with the basement membrane is called stratified epithelium. Epithelial tissue that gives the appearance of consisting of several layers of cells (but all cells are in contact with the basement membrane) forms pseudostratified epithelium. Finally, there are three basic types of cell shape in epithelium. Squamous cells are flat and thin. Cuboidal cells are as high as they are wide, and columnar cells are taller than they are wide.

Muscle tissue is composed of long, thin cells or fibers known as myocytes. These cells, specialized for contraction and force generation, are divided into three subtypes of muscle tissue. Skeletal muscle receives its name because of its role in movement of the skeleton. However, this type of muscle tissue is found attached to tissues other than the skeleton to perform roles such as facial expression. Cardiac muscle pumps blood out of the heart, while smooth muscle controls the movement of substances through tubes and organs. Cardiac and smooth muscle tissue will be described in greater detail in subsequent chapters.

Cells specialized for initiation and transmission of electrical signals are classified as nervous tissue. Nervous tissue is found throughout the body, including the brain, spinal cord, and peripheral nerves that enter muscles, glands, and various organs.

Connective tissue functions as the framework upon which the other types of tissues build functional units. Connective tissue produces what is known as the mesenchymal tissue of organs, whereas other types of cells, such as epithelial cells, make up the functional or parenchymal cells of an organ. For example, the epithelial cells, known as hepatocytes, in the liver cannot function unless they are arranged on the scaffolding produced by the mesenchymal (connective tissue) cells. Connective tissue also forms a framework for tissue that consists of nervous and muscle tissue, which organizes the cells into functional units. In contrast to the other types of tissues, connective tissue is distinguished by having few cells dispersed within an abundant extracellular matrix.

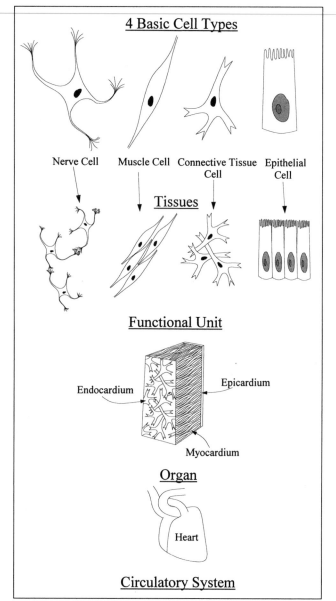

Figure 1-1. Levels of organization of the body: cell types, tissues, functional units, organs, and organ systems.

ORGANS

Organs represent the third level of organization. Each organ is composed of two or more types of tissues consisting of specialized cells along with varying amounts of extracellular material and connective tissue upon which the specialized cells are organized to perform a specific function for the body. Examples include such obvious organs as the heart, lungs, and kidneys and the less obvious organs such as baroreceptors that detect blood pressure.

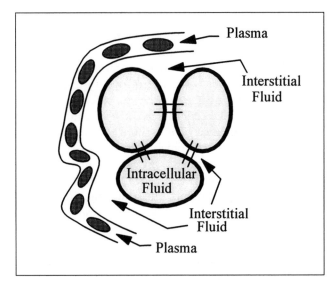

Figure 1-2. Exchange occurs between blood and interstitial fluid and between interstitial fluid and intracellular fluid. Substances obtained from the external environment must then circulate in the blood.

ORGAN SYSTEMS

The fourth level of organization is the **organ system** in which one or more organs collectively perform a related function. For example, the urinary system consists of the kidneys, ureters, bladder, and urethra. While each organ has its own particular job to perform, they together work as a system to remove wastes as well as to conserve needed substances. The different levels of organization are illustrated in Figure 1-1. Eleven major organ systems are typically described. These systems include the nervous system, endocrine system, cardiovascular system, respiratory system, urinary system, muscular system, skeletal system, integumentary system, reproductive system, digestive system, and immune system. While each organ system performs its own special function, they are all interrelated in that they operate together as a unit to keep the whole body healthy and functional.

CONCEPT OF HOMEOSTASIS

INTERNAL ENVIRONMENT

The father of modern physiology, Claude Bernard, once noted that the milieu interieur (internal environment) remains relatively constant despite changes in the external environment. It is this internal environment that directly bathes our body's cells and is under physiologic control (Figure 1-2). Extracellular fluid, while

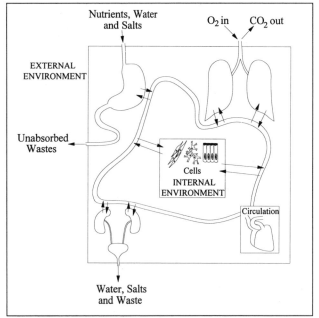

Figure 1-3. Exchanges between blood and the external environment occur in the respiratory, gastrointestinal, and renal systems. The blood then exchanges with the internal environment via the cardiovascular system.

outside the cells but inside the body, includes several components. Among these are plasma, the fluid portion of the blood; interstitial fluid, which directly bathes the cells and fluids of specialized compartments such as pericardial fluid around the heart; pleural fluid around the lung; and cerebrospinal fluid around the brain and spinal cord. It is the interstitial fluid that is considered equivalent to the internal environment. Homeostasis ("keeping the same") describes the body's ability to maintain a relatively constant internal environment (interstitial fluid) in the face of an ever-changing external environment. While every organ system plays a role in the maintenance of this internal environment, a few systems allow for exchanges between the internal and external environments. For example, the respiratory system transfers oxygen into the plasma while the digestive system transfers ingested nutrients into the plasma. It is the important job of the cardiovascular system to then transport these vital substances to the interstitial fluid, which then delivers them to cells, where they are needed for energy production. Wastes produced by the cells are ultimately delivered to the external environment via the urinary system (Figure 1-3).

BASIC PROCESSES TO MAINTAIN HOMEOSTASIS

While the internal environment must be kept relatively stable to maintain homeostasis, this does not mean that certain conditions such as chemical composition

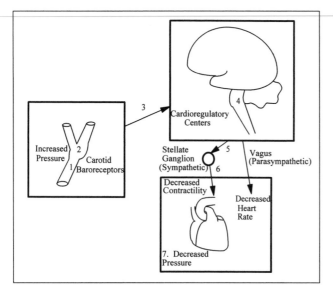

Figure 1-4. Negative feedback. Seven elements make up the negative feedback mechanism. Increased arterial pressure (1) is detected by the carotid baroreceptors (2). Afferent nerves (3) carry an increased number of impulses to integrating centers in the brain stem (4). Efferent nerves (5) carry an increased number of impulses to effectors that decrease arterial pressure (6), while other efferent nerves to effectors that tend to increase arterial pressure carry fewer impulses. Increased impulses from the vagus nerves to the heart decrease heart rate. Decreased impulses from sympathetic nerves to the heart produce both decreased heart rate and a less forceful contraction. Decreased impulses to arterioles decrease peripheral resistance, also contributing to the response (7)—decreased arterial pressure.

and temperature remain absolutely fixed. Rather, a dynamic state exists in which various factors of the internal environment are constantly changing within narrow limits. These factors, such as the concentration of nutrient molecules, water, salt, electrolytes, waste products, and also the body's pH, temperature, pressure, and volume, are constantly being threatened by the internal and external environments. Thus, there is a potential for continual disruption of homeostasis.

To be able to maintain homeostasis, the body must be able to detect alterations of the internal environment that need to be held within a narrow limit. In addition to detection, the body must be able to respond appropriately to these challenges. Two major control systems function to maintain homeostasis: intrinsic and extrinsic. Intrinsic, or local, controls are built into an organ so that the organ itself plays an important role in maintaining its own homeostasis. Extrinsic controls are regulatory mechanisms initiated outside the organ. Many components of the internal environment described in this book are maintained via extrinsic regulation of several organs. Extrinsic control of the various organs and systems is accomplished primarily by the nervous and endocrine systems.

The body's homeostatic control mechanisms, both intrinsic and extrinsic, operate primarily via the **negative feedback** principle. In negative feedback, a change in a **controlled variable**, such as glucose concentration, body temperature, or blood pressure, will trigger a response that opposes the change. For example, if our

The Organism vs. the Organ System

In rehabilitation, one is often tempted to think of a person as a type of patient, such as an orthopedic, a cardiopulmonary, a wound, or a neurologic patient. To some degree, this problem can be alleviated by using "person-first" terminology that does not refer to a person by the primary diagnosis. For example, you might need to provide services to a person with diabetes, not a diabetic. You would be involved in cardiac rehabilitation with the person in room 603, not the MI in room 603. Depersonalized terminology focuses on one aspect and allows the clinician to lose sight of the other aspects of the person that may be important to recovery. Moreover, it is necessary to understand how systems work together to optimize intervention. A person with a primary diagnosis of a knee replacement will have difficulty with rehabilitation with coexisting lung disease that causes the person to fatigue rapidly. An individual with coronary artery disease who requires an assistive device due to musculoskeletal injury will not be able to follow a typical cardiac rehabilitation program because of the greater metabolic cost of ambulating with a walker. A person with a severe musculoskeletal condition may experience a tremendous loss of cardiopulmonary function from lack of activity or upright positioning. An individual with kidney disease may experience significant alterations in body fluid composition causing muscular weakness, cardiac rhythm abnormalities, loss of sensation, and decreased balance leading to deconditioning. A person with bone marrow disease may produce too few red blood cells resulting in weakness, too few platelets leading to bleeding, and too few white cells leading to infection. Each individual brings a unique set of abilities, disabilities, culture, lifestyle, and living arrangements that must be evaluated together to produce a treatment plan meaningful and optimal for each patient or client.

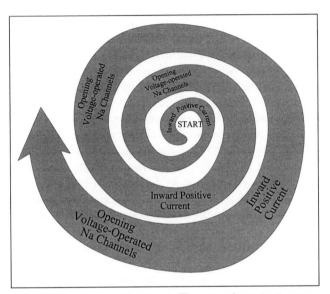

Figure 1-5a. Positive feedback. The most important example is the voltage-operated sodium ion channel that produces the action potential in neurons and muscle cells. Sufficient inward flow of positive charges causes the voltage-operated channels to open. Opening of the channel causes positively charged Na$^+$ to enter the cell, depolarizing the membrane. Either depolarization or opening of the channel causes the other.

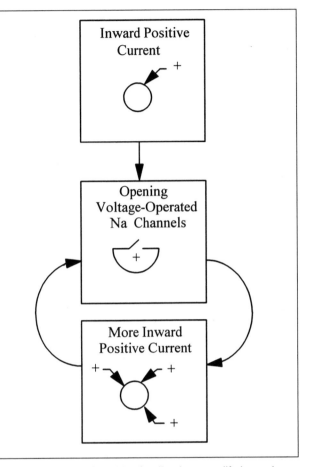

Figure 1-5b. Use of positive feedback to amplify inward current to generate an active potential.

body temperature is too high, the controlling mechanisms in the hypothalamus activate mechanisms to decrease body temperature. In order for this internal homeostasis to be maintained, **sensors**, such as receptors, must monitor the magnitude of the controlled variable. An **integrating center** receives the information via afferent (going toward) pathways where the integrating center then compares the sensor's input with the set point. Finally, efferent (going away from) pathways carry the appropriate signal from the integrating center to the **effector** to bring about the appropriate response; that is, to oppose the deviation from the set point. The brain stem and hypothalamus contain several integrating centers. As discussed later in the text, simple tests such as the knee jerk may be considered as having a simple integrating center in the spinal cord. Negative feedback is illustrated in Figure 1-4.

Another type of regulation is called **feedforward**, in which information of impending change is fed to regulatory systems to allow compensations to be made before the regulated variable changes. For example, a decrease in skin temperature is fed forward to the hypothalamus to increase heat production and decrease heat loss before the internal body temperature falls.

Encountered less frequently in the body, **positive** differs from negative feedback in that the controlled variable is driven in the same direction as the initial change. Thus, rather than counteract the changes, as

was seen in negative feedback, positive feedback enhances the change in the same direction. Because positive feedback moves the controlled variable farther from a steady state, and thus homeostasis, it is not used directly as a regulatory mechanism often in the body; rather it is used as a means to amplify a signal (Figure 1-5a). Positive feedback is also frequently associated with disease processes. One important example of positive feedback control is the voltage-operated Na$^+$ channel, illustrated in Figure 1-5b. This protein structure is found in abundance on muscle and nerve cells and is largely responsible for generation of the action potential, the signal used by most nerves. The protein structures that make up the channel change their shape to allow Na$^+$ to flow into the cell when the cell's membrane potential changes from its resting inside negative value toward zero. When these channels open, Na$^+$ moves rapidly into the cell, thus carrying positive charges with it and further changes from inside negative polarity with respect to the outside of the cell. This loss of polarity, known as depolarization, results in more channels opening and thus more Na+ movement into the cell, thereby causing the cell membrane to depolarize even more. For either good or bad, positive feedback is capable of amplifying a disturbance in the steady state. In the case of the voltage-operated sodium channel, a resting state can be restored by a second process. Another gate on the channel closes shortly after the activation gate opens, which allows a brief, rapid flow of sodium ions into the cell.

An important positive feedback cycle encountered frequently in outpatient clinics is the pain/spasm cycle. Pain causes muscle in the associated area to go into spasm. Muscle spasm causes more pain, which causes more spasm, and therefore even more pain. Many means are available for breaking the pain-spasm cycle. Some are directed at reducing the pain, such as transcutaneous electrical nerve stimulation (TENS), ice, or injection of anesthetic drugs, whereas other techniques, such as massage, stretching, heating, or electrical stimulation, are directed at stopping the muscle spasm.

SUMMARY

Physiological processes are governed by the same laws of chemistry and physics as inanimate objects. A rational treatment must be based on a firm understanding of physiology. Physiology may be studied at many levels from cellular or subcellular to tissue or organ basis. For the most part, this book takes an organ level approach. The concepts of the internal environment and homeostasis are common themes in physiology. Homeostasis refers to the maintenance of the interstitial fluid within narrow limits. Substances from the external environment are exchanged with the blood and between the blood and the internal environment. Cells exchange substances with the interstitial fluid. Each cell must perform basic functions for itself, but also shares some responsibility for homeostasis by performing specialized functions that benefit the entire organism. The most common mechanisms used for homeostasis are negative feedback mechanisms in which the level of some controlled variable is continuously monitored. If the level is too high, it is decreased by mechanisms controlled by an integrating center; if the level is too low, it is increased. Although not straightforward, the positive feedback mechanism, in which a deviation of a controlled variable from its normal value leads to a greater deviation, can be useful. An important example of a positive feedback mechanism is the voltage-operated Na+ channel. In contrast, many problems seen clinically are the result of a positive feedback cycle causing disease or muscle spasm.

BIBLIOGRAPHY

Berne RM, Levy MN. *Physiology*. St. Louis, Mo: Mosby-Year Book; 1998.

Ganong WF. *Review of Medical Physiology*. Norwalk, Conn: Appleton & Lange; 1995.

Guyton AC, Hall JE, Schmitt W. *Human Physiology and Mechanisms of Disease*. Philadelphia, Pa: WB Saunders; 1997.

Hole Jr. JW. *Essentials of Human Anatomy and Physiology*. 4th ed. Dubuque, Ia: Wm C Brown Publishers; 1992.

Schauf C, Moffett D, Moffett S. *Human Physiology: Foundation and Frontiers*. St Louis, Mo: Times Mirror/Mosby College Publishing; 1990.

Solomon EP, Davis PW. *Human Anatomy and Physiology*. Philadelphia, Pa: WB Saunders; 1983.

Treatment of Muscle Spasms

Frequent complaints in the outpatient clinic are muscle spasms in the upper back/cervical region and the lower back/lumbosacral region. Spasm results from either an acute injury, such as whiplash; improper lifting; or chronic insult from poor posture while sitting at a workstation or during sleep, improper carrying, and lifting. Discrepancies in lower extremity length are among a long list of possible causes. Nociceptors carrying pain information to the spinal cord communicate with motor neurons in the spinal cord at the same level that the pain information enters. Activated motor neurons cause abnormal muscle activity that we call spasm. Spasms cause pain; pain causes spasms; and a positive feedback cycle ensues that may lead to complete disability.

Emotion may cause the pain and spasm to spread to areas far beyond the site of the original insult. In one case, a patient was sent directly from the emergency room to the physical therapy clinic because the patient had been immobilized by spasm throughout the spinal musculature. The patient was placed on hot packs on a stretcher while a history was taken and the patient was educated on proper posture at work. The patient's muscles relaxed due to the heat and reassurance. The patient was able to move freely following treatment and did not need to return for any follow-up visits. This case is an illustration of how much the positive feedback cycle of pain and spasm can progress in an individual patient and is rather unusual in how easily the pain/spasm cycle was broken. Other means of breaking the pain/spasm cycle are discussed in subsequent chapters.

STUDY QUESTIONS

1. Provide examples of functions that can be examined at the cellular level, the tissue level, the organ level and the organ system level.

2. Name the components of the respiratory system, gastrointestinal system, the cardiovascular system. How does each component contribute to homeostasis?

3. Why would perforation of the intestine by a nail swallowed by a roofer during a fall cause the roofer to become very ill and possibly die?

4. Why must a mechanism for a positive feedback system have a means of stopping the process? What is the means of stopping the positive feedback process that characterizes the action potential of skeletal muscle cells and neurons?

TWO

Physical and Chemical Bases of Physiology

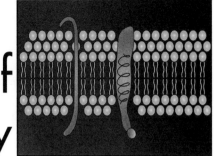

Glenn Irion, PhD, PT, CWS and Sarah N. Jerome, PhD, RRT

OBJECTIVES

1. Describe neutral covalent, polar covalent, and ionic chemical bonds; list common examples of atoms producing these bonds.

2. Describe molecules of each type in terms of solubility in water and ability to carry a current when dissolved in water.

3. For each type of system—electric, thermal, hydraulic, and chemical—name its driving force for flow, its quantity and flow.

4. For each type of system, state the conditions of equilibrium and the name given to the slope of the relationship between driving force and flow, and write an equation describing its flow.

5. Describe the properties associated with elastic materials, such as springs in terms of Hooke's law.

6. Define and contrast the terms equilibrium and steady state.

7. Define balance in terms of a steady state and how a new steady state results when properties of a system are altered.

The purpose of this chapter is not an exhaustive review of chemistry or physics, but to present a physiologist's perspective on a small number of critical principles that are typically part of the prerequisite physics and chemistry. From the domain of physics, the concepts of energy, energy flow, equilibrium, balance, and steady state will be discussed. From chemistry, the ways in which electrons are shared by atoms to form compounds lead to two critical principles of physiology: ionization and the behavior of polar and nonpolar compounds in an aqueous (water) environment.

SHARING OF ELECTRONS

Two basic types of chemical bonds are used in forming compounds—ionic and covalent bonds. In forming an ionic bond, one atom that requires usually only one or two electrons to have a full outer shell captures electrons from an atom that has only one or two electrons in its outer shell. An example of an ionic bond is that which is formed when sodium (Na), which has one electron in its outer shell, combines with chlorine (Cl), which has seven electrons in its outer shell. When Na loses an electron to Cl, Na^+ has one more proton than electrons and, therefore, has a net positive charge. Cl^- then has one more electron than protons and has a net negative charge. The positively charged Na atoms and negatively charged Cl atoms attract each other to form ionic bonds. The attraction also causes NaCl to form a very precise crystal structure. When this crystal structure is placed in water to form an aqueous solution, the individual atoms that had made up the ionic compound are broken apart by water molecules that surround individual atoms that had made up the NaCl crystal. The atoms, thus, become ions that now have an excess of either negative or positive charges. Because ions carry a net charge on them, the solution is capable of producing an electric current if the ion can be forced to move through the solution. The presence of ions in body fluids allows an electric current to be conducted through the body, which permits the use of electric modalities, such as neuromuscular electrical stimulation and transcutaneous electrical nerve stimulation (TENS).

In a covalent bond, the participating atoms have deficiencies of electrons in the outer shell. The involved atoms achieve a more energetically stable arrangement by sharing electrons with neighboring atoms. Part of the time, the shared electrons orbit one atom, and part of the time, they orbit another. Therefore, the involved atoms are attracted to each other in the form of a covalent bond. Examples of covalent bonds include methane, CH_4, in which carbon is short four electrons and four different hydrogen atoms are each short one electron of full outer shell. Hydrogen atoms have only one electron in the outer shell (its only electron shell), but require two electrons for stability. When hydrogen shares its electron with carbon and carbon shares its four outer shell electrons with four hydrogen atoms, all five atoms become more stable. A somewhat different example of covalent bonding is found in the water molecule. Oxygen atoms have only six electrons in an outer shell that needs eight to be stable, and two hydrogen atoms that each need one can share their electrons with one oxygen atom.

POLAR AND NONPOLAR COVALENT BONDS

Although both methane and water are produced by covalent bonds, these two compounds are very differ-

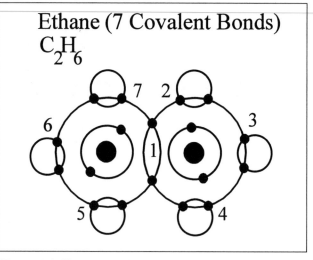

Figure 2-1. Neutral covalent bonds. Each one of six hydrogen atoms shares its one electron with one carbon. Each carbon shares three of its four outer shell electrons with three different hydrogen atoms and the fourth outer shell electron with another carbon, resulting in an energetically favorable state for all eight atoms to form the ethane molecule. Carbon and hydrogen share the electrons on a nearly equal basis; therefore, ethane does not have any partial charges to attract other molecules.

ent. In the case of methane, carbon and hydrogen share the electrons on a nearly equal basis so that, averaged over time, none of the atoms has a significant positive or negative charge. This means that each hydrogen gets the shared electron about 50% of the time and so does carbon. Therefore, no significantly charged areas exist on the methane molecule. Neutral covalent bonds are illustrated in Figure 2-1. In the case of water, oxygen tends to keep the shared electrons more of the time than hydrogen, so that, averaging over time, a slight negative charge exists on the oxygen atom of a water molecule and slight positive charges exist on the hydrogen atoms, creating negative and positive areas, or poles, within the water molecule. This is shown in Figure 2-2. For this reason, we speak of two different types of covalent bonds: neutral covalent, in which the electrons are shared equally, and polar covalent, in which one atom attracts the shared electron more strongly than the other atom. In the case of polar covalent bonds, we often denote this by placing a negative sign in parentheses next to the oxygen atom and positive signs in parentheses next to the hydrogen atoms. This partial charge on oxygen is about 3% of the charge found on an ionized oxygen atom (an oxygen atom that has an extra electron all of the time). Polar covalent bonds are often referred to simply as polar bonds. They occur most often in covalent bonds formed between oxygen and hydrogen or between nitrogen and hydrogen. Neutral covalent bonds are called nonpolar bonds. They are usually the

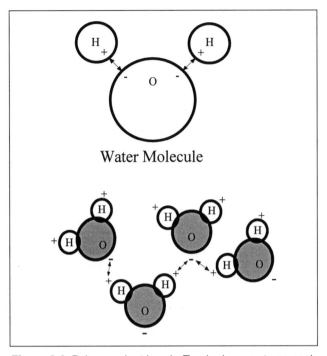

Figure 2-2. Polar covalent bonds. Two hydrogen atoms each share an electron with oxygen, and oxygen shares two of its electrons with two hydrogen atoms, resulting in a stable configuration for all three atoms, forming water. Oxygen attracts the electrons more than hydrogen, resulting in a partial positive charge on the hydrogen atoms and a partial negative charge on the oxygen. These partial charges cause water molecules to attract each other and other charged particles.

result of covalent bonding between carbon and hydrogen.

INTERACTION AMONG IONS AND POLAR AND NONPOLAR MOLECULES IN SOLUTION

Compounds such as lipids that are composed primarily of carbon and hydrogen and, therefore, contain primarily nonpolar bonds are called nonpolar compounds. Compounds such as water that contain primarily polar covalent bonds are called polar compounds. An atom such as Cl^- that has more electrons than protons is called a negative ion or an anion. A positive ion, called a cation, has more protons than electrons. A molecule may contain any one, two, or all three types of bonds. Molecules constructed with ionic bonds typically form crystals called salts. When salts are placed in water, the ionic bond is broken, producing one anion and cation from each molecule. These ions are called electrolytes because they can carry an electric current in

solution. The reason for the formation of ions in solution is related to the presence of polar bonds in water. In a water molecule, the oxygen atom is slightly negative with respect to the hydrogen atoms. When a salt crystal such as NaCl is placed in water (Figure 2-3), the negative oxygen atoms of water molecules are attracted to the positive Na atom of NaCl, and the positive hydrogen atoms are attracted to the negative Cl atom of NaCl. Because of this attraction, the relatively small water molecules move between Na and Cl atoms, surrounding each one so that Na and Cl are no longer attracted to each other, but each becomes surrounded by a cloud of water molecules. The separation of Na from Cl allows the Na and Cl to be evenly and independently dispersed throughout the population of water molecules. The NaCl, which was once a crystal, has been solubilized by the polar water molecules. Other salts are also dissolved easily in water for the same reason.

Just as ions are easily dispersed in water, polar molecules attract water molecules the same way and go easily into solution. Compounds that have ionic and polar bonds are called hydrophilic (water loving) because they attract water molecules to them and, therefore, go into solution. Compounds consisting of nonpolar bonds are called hydrophobic (water fearing). Water fearing is descriptive because the nonpolar atoms tend to cling together as if in fear of the water molecules, resulting in the familiar droplets seen when oil is added to water.

The water molecule's partial charges also cause water molecules to attract each other to form what are called hydrogen bonds. A hydrogen bond exists between the partial positive charge of a hydrogen attached to oxygen (or nitrogen) and an atom with a partial negative charge, such as the oxygen of another water molecule. The attraction of water to itself and to ions, but not to nonpolar compounds, causes hydrophobic compounds to aggregate. Hydrogen bonds are important physiologically for several reasons. They allow water to absorb large quantities of heat without increasing temperature and to lose heat without decreasing temperature, both of which help to maintain a constant body temperature. The polar nature of water allows many of the biologically important molecules to move freely through body compartments without clumping or aggregating, including amino acids, nucleic acids, proteins, and carbohydrates.

AMPHIPATHIC MOLECULES

Special molecules are needed to make nonpolar compounds, such as fatty acids, soluble in body fluids. These molecules are not strictly hydrophilic or

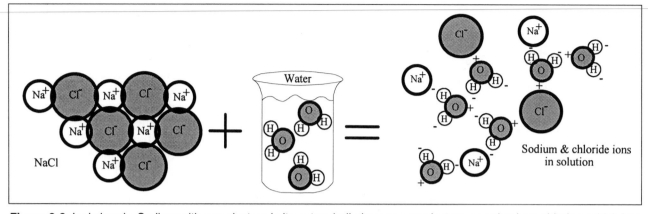

Figure 2-3. Ionic bonds. Sodium with one electron in its outer shell gives up one electron completely to chlorine, which has seven electrons in its outer shell, resulting in stability for both. The positive charge of sodium attracts chlorine with its negative charge, forming a crystalline salt. When placed in water, the partial charges of water cause the relatively small water molecules to move between the sodium and chlorine atoms, producing ionization of sodium chloride in water.

hydrophobic, but have regions of both types within the same molecule. Such compounds are termed amphipathic. Phospholipids that make up cell membranes are examples of amphipathic molecules. Phospholipids have a polar "head" region that is soluble in water and a nonpolar "tail" region that is hydrophobic. Thus, the tail regions tend to clump together away from water, and the head regions face toward the water-phospholipid interface. We will see in the next chapter how the amphipathic nature of phospholipids is used by the cell to create a double layer (lipid bilayer) that acts as the cell's boundary or membrane.

GLANDULAR SECRETIONS AND CYSTIC FIBROSIS

In the genetic disease called cystic fibrosis, the individual has a defective protein for transporting Cl^- ions. The active transport of Cl^- (see Chapter 4) causes water molecules and other ions to follow across the cell membrane. In sweat glands, the lack of active transport of Cl^- prevents the reabsorption of ions from the tubular portion of the sweat gland, resulting in salty sweat. In the airways and digestive ducts, the lack of active transport of Cl^- from the airways increases the susceptibility to lung infection. Recurrent pulmonary infections, in turn, cause more mucus secretion. This is an example of how positive feedback (described in Chapter One) is involved in some diseases. Moreover, thick mucus causes blockage of the ducts that convey digestive enzymes from the pancreas to the duodenum (the first part of the small intestine).

Dietary fat is composed of nonpolar molecules that clump together in the intestine. Bile released from the gall bladder normally allows fat to become soluble in water because one end of the bile salt molecule is nonpolar and dissolves in fat, whereas the other end is polar and dissolves in water. Breaking up or emulsifying fat allows the pancreatic enzyme, lipase, to break dietary fat into molecules that can be absorbed. Without the presence of bile salts from the gall bladder and pancreatic enzymes, a condition called malabsorption results, and fat is allowed to pass through the gastrointestinal tract without much absorption, producing what is called steatorrhea. The signs of malabsorption are often the presenting symptoms of cystic fibrosis due to the blockage of the ducts carrying bile and pancreatic enzymes. Most people with cystic fibrosis take pancreatic enzymes in pill form with meals to reduce malabsorption. Because of malabsorption, many people with cystic fibrosis are very thin.

PHYSICS

Physiology as the scientific basis of clinical practice relies on physical principles that equally apply to inanimate systems. Homeostasis requires exchange of substances and energy; without this exchange, cells eventually die. A review of systems, energy, equilibrium, and steady state will greatly facilitate the learning of physiologic principles. To maintain life, we must expend energy, usually in the form of chemical energy obtained from digesting food, to maintain constant conditions, or a steady state. In contrast to a steady state in which energy is used to maintain a system, equilibrium refers to a condition in which a system stays constant without the expenditure of energy. For cells to survive, we need to use energy to create concentration differences that

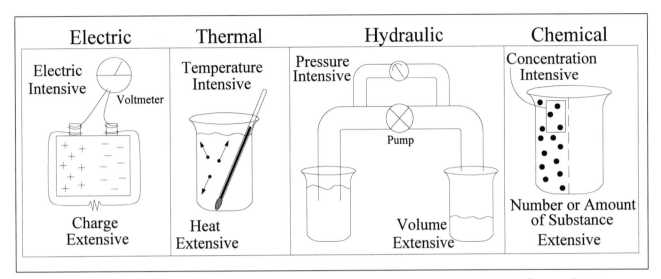

Figure 2-4. Intrinsic and extrinsic properties of electrical, thermal, hydraulic, and chemical systems. Pneumatic systems are similar to hydraulic.

maintain a flow of nutrients into cells and a flow of wastes out. If equilibrium exists with equal concentrations of molecules inside and outside a cell, cells die. Life requires us to expend energy to maintain a steady state; death causes equilibrium to occur.

In physics, types of energy are typically presented in different parts of a course, perhaps over two different semesters of study. The units of each system and the properties that cause storage and flow in the different systems are usually presented separately. In physiology, some very important phenomena occur because of the interaction between two types of energy, which can confuse the person who has never thought of two types of systems co-existing. Four types of energy are typically encountered in physiologic systems: thermal, mechanical, chemical, and electrical.

DRIVING FORCES FOR FLOW

In physiology, we can have systems that can be thought of as strictly thermal, mechanical, chemical, or electrical, or we may need to consider a system that is a combination of two or more. As we have learned in physics, each type of system has a driving force that causes the type of energy to flow from one place to another. This property is termed the intensive property and relates to how much potential exists to make heat, substance, or charge flow to another system. These intensive properties are called temperature, concentration (chemical potential), and electric potential (voltage). Technically speaking, the concept of chemical potential is somewhat more complex than concentration difference between two systems, but, for our purposes, concentration will be sufficient to describe the force that

drives particles in solution to move from one compartment of the body into another.

QUANTITY OF ENERGY OR SUBSTANCE IN A SYSTEM

A second property of a system is the actual quantity of energy contained in the system. This is termed the extensive property. Units in thermal, chemical, and electrical systems are called heat (in joules), n (number of particles in millimoles), and charge (in coulombs), respectively. The flow of energy or material is also given a name in each type of system: heat flow in watts, electric current in amperes, and flux in mM/sec, in thermal, electric, and chemical systems, respectively. What all of these systems have in common is that a difference in the driving force for flow across a cell membrane or within an organ system, whatever its name, causes a quantity of energy or material to flow from an area of high driving force to an area of lower driving force (eg, heat flows from an area of high temperature to an area of low temperature, particles flow from an area of high concentration to an area of low concentration, and charges flow from an area of high electrical potential to low electrical potential). These concepts are illustrated in Figure 2-4.

CONDUCTANCE

The rate at which the flow occurs is not dependent on the driving force alone. A vastly different flow could occur in different systems even if the difference in driving force is identical because of the properties of the individual system. For example, water will flow from a

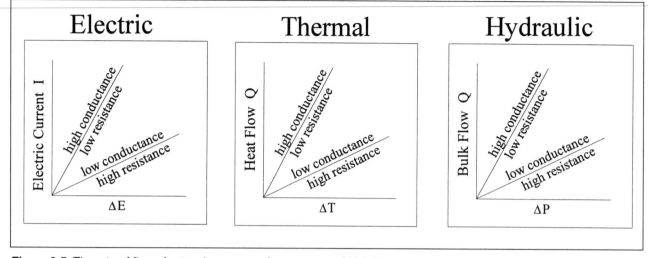

Figure 2-5. The rate of flow of extensive property from an area of high intensive property to low is proportional to the difference in intensive property. Characteristics of the systems also determine the rate of flow. For electrical, thermal, and hydraulic systems, this property—the slope of the relationship between intensive property and flow—is called conductance. In a chemical system, this slope is called the diffusion coefficient. The reciprocal of conductance is called resistance.

large diameter hose faster than through a small diameter hose for the same pressure. If we were to draw a graph of flow vs. driving force, the slope of the graph would demonstrate a second term that determines the rate of flow. In thermal and electrical systems, the term is called **conductance**, which describes how well the energy is conducted from one area to another for a given difference in temperature or electrical potential (Figure 2-5).

Conductance may be the result of physical properties of a particle or a cell membrane, or the result of the presence or absence of specialized channels or carriers for a given molecule or ion. For example, the flow of sodium ions carrying charge into a muscle cell is very slow, even though a tremendous electrical potential exists to drive sodium ions into a cell. This occurs because the conductance of the cell to sodium is very small due to the lack of open channels that allow the movement of sodium into the cell. On the other hand, many channels are available to allow potassium ions to flow out of a cell, but little electric potential exists to drive potassium ions out of a muscle cell, so flow of potassium ions out of muscle cells is very slow. Therefore, we can say the reason for the low flow rate of sodium and potassium across resting muscle cells is that sodium has a high driving force for it into cells, but a low conductance, and potassium has a high conductance for flow of it out of cells, but a low driving force.

EQUILIBRIUM AND STEADY STATE

For equilibrium to occur, the driving force to move flow in one direction must equal the driving force to

move flow in the other direction. A second way of expressing the same idea is that equilibrium occurs when no **net** flow from one direction occurs. In electric systems, we could express that idea of equilibrium as the same driving force in both directions as E1 = E2 (the electric potential or voltage of one compartment equals the electric potential of the other) or perhaps more simply stated as the condition of no net flow as I = 0 (current equals zero). In the case of sodium and potassium ions discussed in the paragraph above, a small flow of sodium into the cell and potassium out of the cell occurs. To maintain a steady concentration of these ions inside the cell, energy is used in the form of the sodium-potassium pump, which actively transports sodium and potassium ions across the cell membrane to maintain a steady state, not equilibrium.

The properties of different systems encountered commonly in physiology are shown in Table 2-1. Hydraulic systems are very common in physiology, notably in the circulatory system, producing what is called bulk flow. Air also moves into and out of the airways and lungs by the same principles of bulk flow. In bulk flow, a difference in pressure produced by muscle work drives the flow of a volume of blood in the circulatory system (or air in the respiratory system) at a rate proportional to the conductance of the tubes (blood vessels or airways) that conduct the flow.

Bulk flow can be contrasted with diffusion, which occurs because of a difference in concentration and which is not produced directly by the use of energy, but usually uses energy indirectly by the creation of a concentration difference. In bulk flow, energy is used direct-

TABLE 2-1

Properties of Systems: Driving Forces, Quantities, Flow, Conditions for Equilibrium, Conductance, and Equation Describing Flow

TYPE OF SYSTEM PROPERTY	ELECTRICAL	THERMAL	HYDRAULIC	CHEMICAL
Driving force for flow	Potential (E)	Temperature (T)	Pressure (P)	Concentration (C)
Units	Volt	°K	mm Hg	millimolar (mM)
Quantity of system	Charge (q)	Heat (S)	Volume (V)	number (n)
Units	Coulomb	Joule	ml or L	millimole (mmol)
Flow	Electric current (I)	Heat flow (Q)	Bulk flow (Q)	Flux (J)
Units	Ampere	Watt	ml/s	mmol/s
Conditions for equilibrium	$E_1 = E_2$ or $I = 0$	$T_1 = T_2$ or $Q = 0$	$P_1 = P_2$ or $Q = 0$	$C_1 = C_2$ or $J = 0$
Slope relating flow to driving force	Conductance (g, 1/R)	Conductance (k)	Conductance (g, 1/R)	Diffusion coefficient (D)
Equation for flow	$I = g\Delta E$	$Q = k\Delta T$	$V = g\Delta P$	Flux $= D\Delta C$
Ohm's law	$\Delta E = IR$	$\Delta T = Q/k$	$\Delta P = QR$	

ly to create a pressure difference, for example by the contraction of the heart or the muscles of inspiration.

SYSTEMS OF MULTIPLE TYPES

In any type of system, equilibrium exists when no net flow in one direction occurs. A second way of expressing equilibrium is that the driving force, such as temperature, of two systems that are in equilibrium are the same. Equilibrium exists when the temperature, pressure, electrical potential, and concentration of all substances are the same in two systems. However, equilibrium also results when the **sum** of these driving forces is equal. Note that all forms of energy that have been discussed have the same units, that of joules. A joule is a unit of either work or energy equal to exerting a force of one Newton (N) over one meter (m). A rate at which work occurs or energy is used per time is called power and is expressed in units of watts (W). All four types of systems can interact with each other and produce important physiological phenomena.

Two important examples for physiology include the equilibrium potential for the flow of an ion across a cell membrane and osmosis. In an equilibrium potential, a difference in concentration of an ion (a charged particle) across a cell membrane can be offset by a difference in electrical potential when the chemical driving force (concentration difference) drives an ion such as potassium out of a cell at the same rate that an electrical potential drives the same ion into the cell, thereby producing equilibrium. In osmosis, the difference in concentration of a particle across a membrane causes water molecules to move from an area of high water (and low particle) concentration to low water (high particle) concentration, thereby increasing pressure in the compartment to which the water moves. Net water movement ceases across the membrane and equilibrium occurs when the difference in pressure that has built up due to net movement of water drives the flow of water molecules at the same rate in the opposite direction that the difference in water concentration drives it. Equilibrium requires only that the sum of all four types of energy be the same in two systems; it does not require that all four be the same (Figure 2-6).

The relationships between flow and driving forces can be expressed mathematically and graphically by plotting the values of a dependent variable along the y-axis and values of the independent variable along the x-axis. Because the rate of flow is dependent on the difference in the driving force, flow is the **dependent variable** (val-

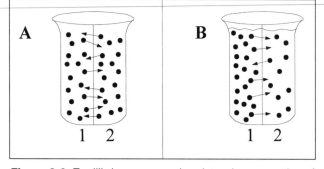

Figure 2-6. Equilibrium occurs when intensive properties of two systems are equal or when no net flow of substance, charge, or heat occurs. If a difference in intensive property exists, net flow occurs from an area of high intensive property to low. In panel A, each side contains 16 molecules. Over time, four molecules pass from side 1 to side 2, and four molecules pass from side 2 to side 1. Concentration 1 equals concentration 2. Net flow equals zero. In panel B, side 1 has 22 molecules, and side 2 has 10 molecules. Over time, five molecules pass from side 1 to side 2, but only one molecule passes from side 2 to side 1. Side 1 has 2.2 times the intensive property (concentration) of side 2; therefore, net flow of extensive property (number of molecules) occurs from the side with high intensive property to the side with low intensive property.

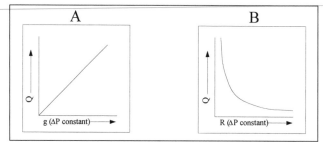

Figure 2-7. Relationship between flow and conductance or flow and resistance. With a constant ΔP, increasing the conductance of a hydraulic, thermal, or electrical system increases flow in a linear manner (panel A). In panel B, we can clearly see that the relationship between flow and resistance is more difficult to describe. At a constant ΔP, increasing resistance does not decrease flow in a linear manner, but fits a hyperbolic curve, because the mathematic product of Q and R equals ΔP in the analogy of the Ohm's law of V = IR (panel B).

ues along y-axis) in this relationship. The difference in driving force (temperature, pressure, voltage, or concentration) between two systems is the **independent variable** and is plotted along the x-axis. The rate of flow for a given difference in the independent variable is the **slope** of the relationship, which is called conductance in thermal, electrical, and hydraulic systems.

APPLYING OHM'S LAW TO PHYSIOLOGIC SYSTEMS

A convenient way of analyzing flow and driving forces in physiology is to generalize Ohm's law to the different types of systems. Ohm's law was originally developed to describe direct current electrical circuits in which the flow of charges (I) occurs in proportion to the difference in electrical potential (E). According to Ohm, the difference in electrical potential across a circuit is equal to the flow of charge (electric current) times the property of the circuit called resistance. In mathematical terms, E = IR. Unfortunately for us, Ohm did not set up his equation in the more intuitive method described above in which dependent variable equals the independent variable times the slope of the relationship. If done this way, flow of not only charge, but also substance and energy, could be more easily visualized (Figure 2-7). A simpler approach is to express the same relationships in terms of the dependent variable equaling the independ-

ent variable times a number describing the slope for a given system. Done this way, I = gΔE, where g is conductance of the electric circuit, I is the electric current, and ΔE is the difference in electric potential. This makes it straightforward to see that the greater the driving force and the greater the conductance of the pathway over which flow occurs, the greater the flow will be.

DETERMINANTS OF CONDUCTANCE

For a given system, conductance is determined by the cross-sectional area available for flow and the length of the pathway over which flow occurs. The greater the cross-sectional area of the pathway, the greater the conductance; and the longer the path over which flow must occur, the lower the conductance. Therefore, a short, thick object conducts more flow for a given driving force than a long, thin one. As the difference in the electrical potential increases between two systems, the rate at which charge flows between two systems increases proportionally. Also, as the conductance increases, the flow increases proportionally. Stated as I = gΔE, the relationship between current and electrical potential is linear. The way Ohm wrote the relationship, the greater the resistance, the lower the electric current produced by a given difference in electrical potential. Moreover, the slope of resistance is not a straight line, and one cannot directly compare the resistance of two different systems by addition or subtraction as one can with conductance. When Ohm's law is stated E = IR, students are often confused when trying to add resistances as $1/R_{total} = 1/R1 + 1/R2 + ... + 1/R_n$. Conductances, on the other hand, add directly as $g_{total} = g1 + g2 + ... + g_n$. It is also obvious that any addition of conductances in parallel yields a greater total conductance, whereas adding resistances in parallel is confusing at best. When analyzing systems, whether electrical, chemical, or hydraulic, the student is best served by thinking in terms of conductance and thinking only of resistance as the reciprocal of conductance. This way, Ohm's law can be applied easily to the flow of not only charge, but also flow of substance and heat.

EXAMPLES OF SYSTEMS IN PHYSIOLOGY

Mechanical energy in the human body is used in hydraulic systems to create blood flow and flow of air into and out of the lungs. The type of flow is called bulk flow with the symbol Q and is measured in units of volume per second, and the driving force is a difference in pressure (P, measured in Pascals, mm Hg, or cm H_2O). Historically, blood pressure has been measured in millimeters of mercury because pressure-measuring devices (manometers) used the upward displacement of a column of mercury in a "U" tube. Pressures in the respiratory system are much smaller and do not cause much movement of a column of mercury. Instead, respiratory pressures are measured in centimeters of H_2O. Because mercury is approximately 13 times as dense as water, the height of a column of water changes 13 times as much. For example, a change in respiratory pressure of 4 mm Hg would be difficult to measure, but a change of 52 mm or 5.2 cm H_2O is easy to measure within a "U" tube. Mercury sphygmomanometers are still used commonly today to measure blood pressure. In bulk flow, a volume of blood or air is moved each second when the heart or muscles of inspiration create a difference in pressure. In analogy to Ohm's law, $\Delta P = QR$ or, expressed in terms of the dependent variable, $Q = g\Delta P$, in which g is the hydraulic conductance of blood vessels or airways.

In discussing muscle function, we use the term distance as the dependent variable (x, in meters) and the driving force is force in Newtons. Equilibrium in terms of an object acted upon by the musculoskeletal system occurs when force produced by the muscle and transmitted to the skeleton equals the external forces placed on the skeleton or force generated by other muscles in the opposite direction (mass of the object times the acceleration due to gravity). Hooke described the same relationship by studying the properties of springs. The relationship between the change in the length of a spring and the force produced by a spring is called Hooke's law. When a force is applied to a spring, its length increases until the spring develops a force equal and opposite to the force that produced the change in

length. This equal and opposite force is called the restoring force and is stored in the lengthened spring just as carrying an object uphill stores potential energy in an object that can be used later when the object is dropped or rolled downhill. If the force that produced the lengthening of the spring is removed, the spring produces a force that can be used to perform work.

The restoring force, or elastic recoil, is also very useful physiologically in systems other than skeletal muscle, especially in the cardiovascular and respiratory systems. Hooke's law is stated as $F = kx$. Force can be either that required to lengthen a spring or the restoring force of the spring; x is the length of the spring, and k is a constant for a given spring. The flow of blood is produced by the heart pumping blood from our veins to our arteries. The left ventricle pumps blood returning from the lungs into the aorta. The heart pumps intermittently at a rate of 60 to 80 beats per minute in most individuals, yet, in small blood vessels, flow appears to be almost constant. The reason for steady flow of blood through our blood vessels is due to an application of Hooke's law. As blood is pumped into the aorta, the pressure produced by moving a volume of blood acts to stretch the aorta, just as the spring in Hooke's law is lengthened. At the end of a beat, the force that stretched the aorta dissipates, allowing the restoring force of the aorta to move blood through the blood vessels, even though the heart is no longer ejecting blood. In the lungs, the energy used to inspire air is stored in the lung's tissues as elastic recoil until the muscles of inspiration relax. The elastic nature of the lungs allows the energy used to inspire to be used for expiration. In emphysema, an individual has difficulty expiring because the lungs lose their elastic recoil. This disease behaves the same way as asthma or chronic bronchitis in which the person has difficulty expiring because of a low conductance of the airways due to bronchospasm or accumulation of secretions in the airways. In the case of emphysema, expiration is difficult because of the lack of elastic recoil to drive air through the airways in the presence of normally conducting airways. In chronic bronchitis and asthma, expiration is difficult because of a decreased conductance of the airways with normal elastic recoil.

The concept of storing energy by performing work is also used in physiologic systems, such as that described earlier in which energy is used to separate charges across the membrane of a skeletal muscle cell. Potassium ions are actively transported into cells, and sodium ions are actively transported out. This energy used in separating charged particles can be used later to produce an electric current when conditions dictate.

STORAGE OF ENERGY OR SUBSTANCE

Two variables determine how much energy or substance can be stored in a system. One is the driving force for flow of energy or substance into a system. The greater the driving force, the greater the storage of energy or substance. For example, the greater the pressure exerted in inflating a balloon, the more air the balloon will hold. However, different systems will not be able to store the same amounts of energy or substance at a given driving force, just as two balloons will hold different volumes for a given pressure if one balloon is stiff and another is more compliant.

In physics, one is taught that the temperature of a system holding a given amount of heat depends on a property called the system's heat capacity (the ratio of heat stored per temperature). A substance with a high heat capacity, such as water, will contain more heat for a given temperature than a substance, such as metal, at the same temperature. A second way to look at heat capacity is to say that, for the same amount of heat present, a block of metal has a higher temperature tending to drive heat out of it than the same quantity of water.

For electrical energy, the amount of charge (q) that can be stored per volt of driving force is called the capacitance. The greater the capacitance, the more charge can be stored for a given electrical potential. The same idea holds for hydraulic systems. The volume for a given amount of pressure is called compliance. A stiff aorta will build up a greater pressure for a given amount of blood ejected into it by the heart than a compliant aorta.

To go one step further with the concept of compliance in physiology, we will see that we can alter the stiffness (or compliance) of certain organs when needed. For example, the bladder can accumulate up to 400 ml of fluid with little change in pressure because the smooth muscle within the wall of the bladder relaxes as the bladder fills. We also alter the compliance of blood vessels through contraction of smooth muscle in the walls of the vessels. To prevent pressure in the great veins that fill the heart from falling during exercise, the smooth muscle in the walls contracts, making them stiffer and increasing pressure for a given volume of blood. On the other hand, anesthesia of the spinal nerves (epidural or spinal anesthesia) or spinal cord injury causes blood pressure to fall because the smooth muscle of blood vessels in the lower extremities relaxes without innervation, causing the vessels to be too compliant and pressure to decrease for a given volume.

In chemical systems, the term that describes how driving force (concentration or, more accurately, chem-

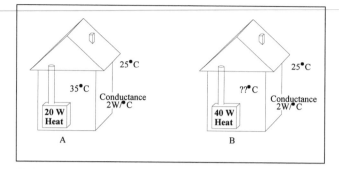

Figure 2-8. Balance of production and loss of extensive properties. Heat generated by a furnace raises temperature in a house. Temperature rises until the difference in temperature (ΔT) is sufficient to cause heat to flow out of the house at the same rate it is generated by the furnace. A change in any of the variables—heat production, outside temperature, and conductances of the house's insulation—will result in a change in indoor temperature unless another variable changes proportionally. In panel A, a steady state occurs when $Q = k\Delta T$ or $20 \text{ W} = (2 \text{ W/°C}) + 25°C = 45°C$.

ical potential) changes with the number of particles is called solubility. A small change in the actual number of oxygen molecules present in the blood plasma can drive a remarkably high number of oxygen molecules into the red blood cells because the intracellular fluid of red blood cells contains hemoglobin. The solubility of oxygen is much greater inside the red cell than in the plasma, and red blood cells can hold a much greater amount of oxygen than an equal volume of plasma.

BALANCE

The concept of balance suggests that the input and output of substance, charge, or energy are equal in a system (Figure 2-8). For example, our bodies produce heat, and our bodies lose heat. If heat production and heat loss are equal, our body temperature remains stable. Therefore, we can maintain a given driving force (temperature) if we produce and lose a quantity of energy (heat) at the same rate. We can increase our heat production to match our rate of heat loss to the environment when it is cold, or, through physiological means, we can increase our rate of heat loss by increasing skin blood flow and sweating to match our rate of production of heat and gain of heat from the environment when we exercise in a hot environment. When the rate of gain and loss are balanced at new level, a new value for the driving force in that system results. For example, if we suddenly increase our rate of heat gain by exercising, we must increase our rate of heat loss to the environment. The rate of heat loss is equal to the difference between temperature of the system and temperature of

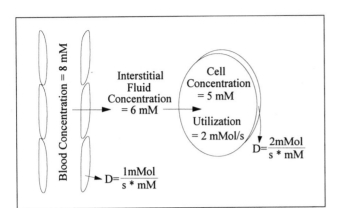

Figure 2-9. Balance of substrates. Steady concentrations can be achieved when substance flows from blood vessels to interstitial fluid and interstitial fluid to intracellular fluid at the same rate that the cells use the substance. If utilization of the substance increases, the intensive properties (concentrations) decrease in the interstitial fluid and intracellular fluid, unless blood flow or concentration in the blood increases in proportion.

the environment times the heat conductance (k): ($Q = k\Delta T$). If we do not change the conductance, we can only drive more heat out of the body by increasing the difference in temperature (ΔT). Temperature of the body would rise until the product $k\Delta T$ (rate of heat loss) equals the rate of heat production (Q).

Fortunately, we can alter conductance (k) of heat from our bodies to the environment physiologically by increasing or decreasing skin blood flow; therefore, our body temperature must rise, but not as much as it would if we could not increase skin blood flow. Another example of balance relates to the concept of wind chill. The wind chill factor takes into account that moving air will carry away heat faster than still air. Comparing an inanimate object to a person, we see that the temperature of an inanimate object will reach equilibrium with the environment because it does not produce its own heat. The wind chill factor does not determine the final temperature of an inanimate object, but determines how fast the object reaches the environmental temperature. In contrast, the wind chill factor does influence our temperature. We produce our own heat; the faster the air speed, the faster we lose heat. Our body temperature reaches balance when our temperature falls low enough that heat production (Q) equals heat loss ($k\Delta T$). The lower the wind chill effective temperature, the lower our body temperature will fall. Because we can increase our heat production and lower the conductance of our skin by decreasing blood flow to the skin, our temperature does not fall much; but it must fall. An example of balance as it relates to substance is illustrated in Figure 2-9.

SUMMARY

Several important concepts for physiology are derived directly from physics and chemistry. Understanding the nature of how electrons are transferred or shared in forming compounds from atoms allows us to understand the behavior of ions and molecules in solution. Ionic bonds are formed when one atom takes an electron from another. When an ionic compound is placed in water, it forms an anion and a cation. Two types of covalent bonds may be formed. Polar covalent bonds are formed between oxygen and hydrogen atoms or nitrogen and hydrogen. Neutral covalent bonds are formed between carbon and hydrogen. The partial charges on oxygen and hydrogen atoms of water interact with ions and molecules with polar bonds to form a solution. Nonpolar compounds aggregate in water. Amphipathic molecules are soluble in water at one place on the molecule and soluble in lipids at another part of the molecule. Generalizing the properties of thermal, electrical, hydraulic, pneumatic, mechanical, and chemical systems allows us to understand how substance, charge, and heat can be exchanged. The different forms of energy may interact to produce equilibrium membrane potentials, osmosis, and other phenomena. Two important laws of physics, Ohm's law and Hooke's law, may be used to understand the movement of blood through the cardiovascular system and air through the respiratory system. Steady state refers to the maintenance of a stable system at the cost of energy. A system may be kept constant if the gain of heat, charge, or substance is balanced with loss of the same quantity. Alteration in the rate of gain or loss is balanced at a new value for the driving force of the system.

BIBLIOGRAPHY

Berne RM, Levy MN. *Physiology*. St. Louis, Mo: Mosby-Year Book; 1998.

Ganong WF. *Review of Medical Physiology*. Norwalk, Conn: Appleton & Lange; 1995.

Guyton AC, Hall JE, Schmitt W. *Human Physiology and Mechanisms of Disease*. Philadelphia: WB Saunders; 1997.

Hole Jr. JW. *Essentials of Human Anatomy and Physiology*. 4th ed. Dubuque, Ia: Wm C Brown Publishers; 1992.

Schauf C, Moffett D, Moffett S. *Human Physiology: Foundation and Frontiers*. St. Louis, Mo: Times Mirror/Mosby College Publishing; 1990.

Solomon EP, Davis PW. *Human Anatomy and Physiology*. Philadelphia: WB Saunders; 1983.

STUDY QUESTIONS

1. What happens to body temperature during exercise? At what point does body temperature stop changing? What advantage is there to altering conductance?

2. What happens to body temperature during cold exposure? At what point does body temperature stop changing? What advantage is there to altering conductance?

3. What is the difference between the effect of wind chill on an inanimate object compared with a person? How does wind speed affect the temperature of an inanimate object at equilibrium? How does wind speed affect the temperature of a person at steady state? Why is an object at equilibrium and a person at steady state?

4. In the equation $Q = g \, \Delta P$, Q is the heart pumping 5000 ml/min, g is the conductance of the systemic circulation and equals 50 ml/(min x mmHg), and ΔP is the difference in pressure between the aorta and the right atrium and is equal to 100 mmHg.

    $$5000 \text{ ml/min} = 50 \text{ ml/(min x mmHg)} \times 100 \text{ mmHg}$$

    If g increases to become 100 ml/(min x mmHg) during light exercise, what would ΔP become if nothing else changed? How could blood pressure be maintained at 100 mm Hg and balance restored? With this in mind, what is the heart's role in responding to local needs for increased muscle blood flow during exercise?

LABORATORY EXERCISES

LABORATORY EXERCISE 2-1

APPLICATION OF HOOKE'S LAW

Objective: Examine relationships between length (extensive property), restoring force (intensive property, and extensibility (slope of the relationship).

Materials: 2.5 lb weight, 5 lb weight, various springs, meter stick, graph paper

Procedures:
1. For each spring, measure its length with no load, a 2.5 lb weight, a 5 lb weight and both the 2.5 and 5 lb weights (7.5 lbs) attached.

2. Plot length (dependent variable, Y axis) as a function of load (independent variable, X axis) for each spring on the same graph.

3. Connect two springs end-to-end (in series). Determine the relationship between load and length. Plot results on same graph.

4. Connect two springs in parallel (both springs directly attached to the load). Plot the relationship between length and load with this arrangement.

5. If we consider the aorta to act as a spring, what happens to the aorta as larger volumes of blood are ejected? What happens to the aorta as the heart stops ejecting blood at the end of each beat? What benefit is there to storing elastic energy in the aorta?

6. Consider the tendons of muscles to have spring-like qualities. If a person lifts 50 lbs with one arm, how much is the biceps tendon stretched compared to how much two biceps tendons are stretched when the load is lifted with two hands?

LABORATORY EXERCISE 2-2

SOLUBILITY AND ELECTRIC CONDUCTIVITY

Objective: Describe the solubility of compounds with different types of chemical bonds in water and the electric conductance of the resultant solution.

Materials: Distilled water, tap water, glucose, NaCl, vegetable oil, multimeter (ohms of resistance)

Procedures:
1. Fill one beaker with tap water and two with distilled water.

2. Using the multimeter, measure the resistance of distilled water and tap water.

3. Add a small amount (approximately one teaspoon) of glucose to one beaker of distilled water and stir. Observe how easily glucose goes into solution. Measure the resistance of the resultant solution.

LABORATORY EXERCISES

4. Add an equal amount of NaCl to the second beaker of distilled water and stir. Observe how easily NaCl goes into solution. Measure the resistance of the resultant solution. Explain any differences in resistance of the solutions.

5. Fill another beaker with tap water. To this, add a few drops of vegetable oil and stir well. Does the oil go into solution?

6. Observe the oil for a time. What happens to the oil? Explain the results.

7. Add soap to the oil and water mixture. What happens to the oil? What special property does soap have to solubilize oil and be soluble in water at the same time?

8. What types of chemical bonds are found in water, glucose, NaCl, and vegetable oil?

9. How does the type of chemical bond influence solubility and electric conductivity?

10. Why are salts in solution called electrolytes?

LABORATORY EXERCISE 2-3

EFFECT OF FLOW ON INTENSIVE PROPERTIES

Objective: Describe the interaction between flowing solvent and rate of addition of the extensive property on the resultant intensive property.

Materials: Funnel, rubber hose, food coloring, four beakers, meter stick

Procedures:
1. Fill a 500 ml beaker with tap water.

2. Fill funnel and rubber hose until water runs out opposite end of rubber hose into a collection beaker. Manually pinch off hose to stop flow. Discard water in collection beaker.

3. Adjust height of the end of hose so that it is 5 cm lower than the top of the funnel.

4. One person must continually add water to the funnel to ensure that the level remains the same throughout the procedure.

5. Release the hose to allow water to flow into the collection beaker for 30 seconds. Pinch off the hose to stop flow.

6. During flow, add one drop of food coloring to the stream of water every 3 seconds (total of 10 drops).

7. Label the first sample "5 cm/10 drops" and replace the collection beaker.

8. Lower the end of hose to 10 cm below the top of the funnel.

LABORATORY EXERCISES

9. Repeat steps 4 through 6. Label the collection beaker "10 cm/10 drops." Compare color of the first and second samples.

10. Consider the flow of water as pulmonary blood flow and the addition of food coloring as oxygen added to the blood due to breathing (ventilation). What would happen to oxygenation of the blood if pulmonary blood flow increased, but ventilation did not change?

11. How could oxygenation (or in our procedure the concentration of food coloring) be maintained in the face of an increased flow rate? If the height difference between the funnel and the other end of the hose is increased from 5 cm to 10 cm, how much does the flow increase? What is the driving force (intensive property) that caused water to flow? What is the formula for determining this intensive property?

12. Design a third experiment to determine if your solution is correct.

LABORATORY EXERCISE 2-4

BALANCE

Objective: Investigate the interactions among intensive properties, extensive properties, and the slope of the relationship between the intensive and extensive properties that allow the loss and gain of extensive properties to balance each other to produce a steady state.

Problem: The heater in a house (a very little house) produces 20 W of heat. The temperature in the house is constant at 35°C and outside the house at 25°C. The insulation of the house yields a conductance of 2W/°C. At these values, heat production exactly balances heat loss: $Q = k\Delta T = k (T_{inside} - T_{outside})$ or 20 W = (2W/°C) x (35°C - 25°C).

1. What does inside temperature become if the outside temperature falls to 15°C and everything else remains constant?

2. What does heat production need to become to keep inside temperature at 35°C if outside temperature is 15°C?

3. What would the conductance of the insulation of the house need to be to maintain the inside temperature at 35°C with an outside temperature of 15°C and a heat production of 20 W?

4. If heat production is increased to 40 W with a conductance of 2W/°C and an outside temperature of 25°C, what would the inside temperature become?

5. If heat production is decreased to 10 W with a conductance of 2W/°C and an outside temperature of 25°C, what would the inside temperature become?

6. For the initial data stated in the problem, the answers obtained in questions 1, 2, 4, and 5 plot Q as a function of ΔT. What does the slope of the graph represent?

THREE

Cell Membrane and Protein Function

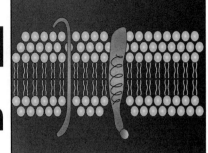

Glenn Irion, PhD, PT, CWS and Sarah N. Jerome, PhD, RRT

OBJECTIVES

1. List four basic functions of the cell membrane.

2. Describe how the cell membrane regulates movement of substances across the membrane based on physical properties of the solute.

3. Define membrane receptor and second messenger; state what binds to receptors.

4. Describe three types of linkages between neighboring cells; describe the physiologic role of each type.

5. Describe the basic structure of the cell membrane; explain how it acts as a barrier to large polar molecules, nonpolar molecules, and ions.

6. List roles performed by integral membrane proteins and by peripheral proteins.

7. Describe how membrane proteins function in the signaling mechanism of norepinephrine binding to β adrenergic receptors and acetylcholine binding to receptors at the neuromuscular junction.

8. Define primary, secondary, and tertiary protein structure.

9. List factors that commonly alter the tertiary structure of a protein.

10. Define ligand; list four properties of protein-ligand binding and define them.

11. List three basic ways of altering the effectiveness of protein-ligand binding.

12. Contrast the mechanisms of allosteric and covalent modulation.

On first inspection, the cell membrane has the obvious function of holding in the cell's contents. The cell membrane, however, is much more than a simple barrier; it has many complex and dynamic functions. Of the many possible functions available to the cell membrane, each type of cell selects a small number from among four broad categories:

1. Regulation of movement of particles into and out of cells
2. Detection of chemical messengers
3. Linking neighboring cells
4. Anchoring of intracellular proteins

REGULATION OF MOVEMENT OF SUBSTANCES ACROSS THE MEMBRANE

The cell membrane is composed almost entirely of phospholipids and cholesterol. The phospholipids, with their polar or hydrophilic head and their two nonpolar or hydrophobic tails, assemble into a lipid bilayer, the basic structure of the cell membrane. This fluid structure determines how well certain substances can cross the membrane. That is, nonpolar, lipid-soluble substances, such as CO_2, O_2, and fatty acids, pass easily through the cell membrane. Small polar molecules, such as water, can also move readily across the membrane. However, ions and larger polar molecules, such as glucose and proteins, are poorly lipid soluble. Therefore, the lipid bilayer serves as an impermeable barrier to these water-soluble substances, and, thus, alternative routes for passage into the cell are provided in the cell membrane.

DETECTION OF CHEMICAL MESSENGERS

Chemical messengers, such as hormones and neurotransmitters, are detected by special membrane structures called receptors. These specialized protein receptors are interspersed along the outside of the plasma membrane. The binding of chemical messengers to these membrane **receptors** triggers a sequence of events that will ultimately alter cell function. For example, the binding of an extracellular chemical messenger to its membrane-bound receptor can open or close specific channels within the membrane, altering the movement of substances into or out of the cell. The binding of a chemical messenger with its membrane receptor can also result in the production of intracellular chemical mes-

sengers called **second messengers**. These second messengers (eg, cyclic AMP, trigger a series of programmed events within the cell).

LINKING ADJACENT CELLS

The cell membrane, in addition to its obvious function of serving as the outer cell boundary, also plays an important role in cell-to-cell adhesion. The linking of cells allows groups of cells to form tissues and organs. However, these linking junctions perform other important functions besides holding tissues together. One type of specialized junction, called a **desmosome**, provides the function of holding cells to their neighbors. This type of junction is compared to a "spot weld" due to the nature of the limited area over which filaments extend from the plasma membrane of two adjacent cells to anchor them together while still allowing interstitial fluid and some substances to flow easily between the adjacent cells. This type of junction is most commonly found in tissues such as the heart and skin, which are subject to considerable stretching.

Other tissues have junctions that hold adjacent cells together more tightly. These **tight junctions** are formed when proteins on the outer surfaces of two adjacent cells are bound tightly, thus preventing materials from simply passing between the adjacent cells. Rather, all substances must pass either through the cell membrane directly or through substance-specific channels and carriers. For example, the tight junction-linked cells that line the digestive tract form a highly selective barrier that separates two very different compartments—the lumen of the digestive tract and the extracellular fluid between the absorptive cells and the vessels that carry nutrients through the body. Thus, movement of many substances across this epithelial surface can be tightly controlled through specific transport mechanisms within the cells of the digestive tract themselves.

A third type of junction is the **gap junction**. Protein complexes form tube-like channels between adjacent cells that allow small molecules and ions to pass from one cell to its neighbor. Cells, such as cardiac and smooth muscle cells, need to communicate rapidly with their neighbors. Rather than using slow chemical messengers, these cells communicate through gap junctions. The signal for cardiac cells and many smooth muscle cells to contract is a change in the cell's membrane potential. This change in membrane potential is caused by the net movement of ions across the cell membrane. The insertion of gap junctions between cardiac muscle cells allows rapid ion movement from one cell to the next, which serves to pass the message for cardiac mus-

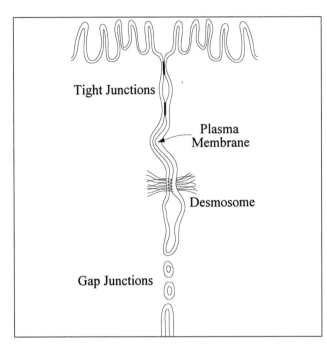

Figure 3-1. Types of cell junctions. A desmosome holds adjacent cells together. Tight junctions create a surface that prevents passage of hydrophilic molecules and ions, especially in the gastrointestinal system and renal tubules. Gap junctions allow movement of ions from one cell to a neighboring cell to produce an electrical signal across adjacent cells.

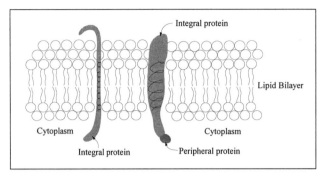

Figure 3-2. Membrane structure, including phospholipids, integral proteins extending through the membrane, and peripheral proteins attached to the inner surface of the membrane.

cell membrane. These filaments are flexible enough to allow red blood cells that may be 10 to 12 μm in diameter to pass through capillaries that are often 8 μm or less in diameter.

MEMBRANE STRUCTURE

Membranes are constructed of two major classes of molecules: lipids and proteins. The lipids comprising most membranes are from the class phospholipids. Phospholipid molecules, as discussed in Chapter 2, are amphipathic. That is, they contain a water-soluble (hydrophilic, meaning water-loving) "head group" and two water-insoluble (hydrophobic, meaning water-fearing or lipophilic, lipid-loving) "tails." When these compounds are associated with two aqueous compartments, they will spontaneously form a lipid bilayer with their water-soluble head groups immersed in the two aqueous phases and their lipid tails forming a hydrophobic surface. No chemical bonds directly hold the phospholipid molecules together. Rather, they are forced into aggregation due to their tails' "fear" of water. The structure is shown in Figure 3-2.

Because of the lack of chemical bonds among phospholipid molecules, the membrane can move easily and is described as being fluid. This allows the membrane to stretch and fold easily. Because the cell membrane is composed primarily of phospholipid molecules, lipid-soluble substances will pass easily through the lipid bilayer by simple diffusion. Water and small water-soluble uncharged molecules (approximately four carbon atoms or smaller) are able to penetrate the membrane through water-filled pores formed by membrane proteins. Larger water-soluble molecules, such as glucose, amino acids, and water-soluble vitamins, require other processes to mediate their entry into the cell.

In addition, particles such as ions do not easily pass

cle cells to contract fairly rapidly throughout the heart to create a heartbeat. The different types of cell linkages are illustrated in Figure 3-1.

ANCHORING OF INTRACELLULAR PROTEINS

Anchoring of intracellular proteins allows for several important functions, including maintenance of cell shape and alteration of cell shape. For example, a muscle cell transmits force by the action of intracellular protein filaments pulling the cell membrane toward its center. In the genetic diseases Duchenne muscular dystrophy and Becker muscular dystrophy, a membrane protein called dystrophin is involved. Dystrophin is not produced in Duchenne muscular dystrophy. The lack of dystrophin in a muscle cell under mechanical stress allows calcium ions to enter muscle membranes, which activates enzymes, damaging the stretched muscle cell membrane and eventually causing muscle cells to die. Becker muscular dystrophy involves an incorrectly produced protein, resulting in later onset with less severity. The red blood cell maintains its biconcave shape due to the presence of intracellular filaments that attach to the through the membrane both because of their charge and their attraction of water. Due to an ion's charge, it carries with it a volume of water molecules, effectively determining the size of the ion. This size is called the ion's hydrated diameter. As an example of the effect of hydrated diameter, the potassium ion, which is larger than the sodium ion, can pass through smaller channels in the membrane than sodium because of the larger "cloud" of water molecules that sodium attracts. Exclusion based on physical properties of solutes allows the concentration of polar and ionized particles to vary substantially between the intracellular and extracellular fluid. Special mechanisms, such as ion channels and transport proteins, regulate the movement of ions and large polar compounds across the cell membrane. The nature of molecules that can cross passively or those that require assistance allows certain molecules to be restricted to one-way traffic across the membrane. For example, a phosphate group is attached to glucose as it crosses the membrane, which prevents the carrier that brought glucose into the cell from carrying it back out.

The second major component of the cell membrane is protein. Cellular regulation of substance movement into and out of the cell depends on the alteration of the shape of and the insertion of new proteins within the membrane. The proportion of proteins to lipids within a cell membrane and the variety of proteins present in the membrane differ among different cell types. As many as 100 different proteins may be present in the membranes of some cells, whereas other cells may only have a few. The expression of different combinations of genes in different cells determines which proteins and how many will be located in a given type of cell.

Most of the lipids and proteins that make up the membrane are free to move within the membrane. This characteristic is described as membrane fluidity. Just as phospholipids are associated because of hydrophobic interaction (exclusion of the nonpolar tails from water), some proteins are held within the membrane solely by this mechanism. Other proteins are held in the membrane by interactions between the partial charges of the polar heads of the phospholipids and certain polar amino groups. Therefore, many lipid and protein molecules are free not only to move within the plane of the membrane, but some proteins function as "molecular machines" by moving within membranes in response to a certain stimulus and flipping from the extracellular surface to the intracellular surface and back again. Other proteins must be anchored in a certain direction to be functional for the cell.

Membrane proteins can be divided into two basic types: integral and peripheral proteins. Integral proteins span the thickness of the cell membrane and, thus, have hydrophobic middles that are surrounded by the hydrophobic, nonpolar tails of phospholipids. Their hydrophilic ends protrude into the intracellular and extracellular aqueous compartments. Peripheral proteins, on the other hand, are electrostatically attached to either the inner or outer surfaces of the lipid bilayer. Integral proteins, because of their position in the membrane, can act as ion channels, receptors, and specialized transport mechanisms. Peripheral proteins have two primary functions: anchoring filaments to the membrane and as enzymes in the process of signal transduction. Some chemical messengers, notably norepinephrine, combine with an integral protein (the β-adrenergic receptor), which in turn interacts with peripheral proteins to activate the enzyme that produces cyclic adenosine monophosphate (cAMP), a second messenger. In addition, some integral proteins may combine functions. The acetylcholine receptor of the neuromuscular junction of skeletal muscle acts as both a receptor and an ion channel. When acetylcholine binds to the receptor, the protein units making up the receptor-ion channel complex change shape to allow Na^+ and K^+ to pass through the channel as long as acetylcholine remains bound to the receptor-ion channel complex.

PROTEINS

Proteins are strings of amino acids that assume complex three-dimensional shapes. The 20 possibilities for amino acids at each location along the string provide an enormous number of possible amino acid sequences. Given a length of only six amino acids, 20^6 or 64 million combinations are possible. Amino acids have various combinations of physical and chemical properties that affect how they interact with each other, with water, and with ions and molecules that may encounter them. Some side chains are nonpolar, and others are polar or ionized. Some amino acids are acidic, and others are neutral. Depending on the different properties, and where in the sequence an amino acid is located, the substitution of one amino acid for another may have little or no effect or may have dramatic results (genetic disease). For example, hemoglobin, a fairly large protein, becomes insoluble in red blood cells at low oxygen levels in the disease sickle cell anemia. Sickle cell anemia is the result of a genetic mutation in which the hydrophilic amino acid glutamic acid is replaced by valine, a hydrophobic amino acid. Genetic disease can also result from the inability of the endoplasmic reticulum to process a sequence of amino acids into a protein. In the most common genetic mutation that produces cystic fibrosis, the cystic fibrosis transmembrane regulator

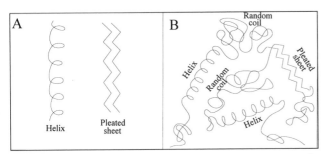

Figure 3-3. Structure of a protein. The primary structure is not shown. (A) The secondary structure is made up of chain segments, such as helices and pleated sheets. (B) The tertiary structure gives the protein its three-dimensional shape and is determined by interactions of physical forces between amino acids within the protein, water molecules surrounding the protein, and other molecules and ions.

(CFTR) protein cannot be processed through the endoplasmic reticulum due to a three amino acid deletion in the protein sequence, though the protein can function normally when placed in the cell membrane.

This string or sequence of amino acids is termed its primary structure. The secondary structure, which often consists of multiple helical segments, is produced largely by the interaction of water surrounding the chain of amino acids. Twists and folds of this secondary structure to form a complex three-dimensional structure produces what is called the tertiary structure (Figure 3-3). The tertiary structure is determined largely by how amino acids within the chain interact with each other and the surrounding medium, including any ions or molecules that may bind to part of the protein. When released to the cell membrane, polar regions of the proteins are most likely to be exposed to water, extending into the water either inside or outside the membrane, whereas nonpolar regions will tend to be pushed toward each other, dissolved in the lipid bilayer itself. This interaction of the protein with the cell membrane and water on either side of the membrane frequently causes proteins to be "woven" in and out of the membrane with several repeating hydrophobic units embedded within the membrane. The shape taken by the protein in the cell after its synthesis and attachment to the membrane, however, is not static, but can be very dynamic and changes as conditions surrounding the protein change.

The dynamic nature of the tertiary structure of proteins is exploited by messengers such as hormones and neurotransmitters, as well as particles as simple as ions by interacting with the structure formed by the protein exposed to outside of the cell. This binding of a chemical messenger to one part of the protein rearranges the chemical and physical forces existing within the protein. Because the protein's shape will take on the most ener-

getically favorable shape, it is likely that introduction of a charged particle, large polar or nonpolar particle, will result in a change in the shape of a protein embedded in a cell membrane.

As the shape of the protein molecule changes in one area, a chain reaction may occur that reaches to areas of the protein that may be on the opposite side of the cell membrane. The shape change in an integral protein that spans the entire thickness of the cell membrane may then affect the shape of a peripheral protein in proximity to the integral protein. Using our previous example of the β-adrenergic receptor, we can now see how the binding of norepinephrine to the outer surface changes the shape of the β receptor. In turn, the shape change of the receptor affects a peripheral protein, which in turn changes the shape of the enzyme that produces cyclic AMP. In the example of the acetylcholine receptor of skeletal muscle cells, acetylcholine changes the shape of the receptor portion of the protein complex. The shape change in one area of the protein causes a shape change for the ion channel portion of the complex that determines what can pass through the channel. When acetylcholine is bound to the receptor, the proteins take on a shape that allows Na^+ and K^+ to pass through the membrane. As soon as acetylcholine comes off the receptor, the ion channel portion changes shape so that Na^+ and K^+ cannot pass through the channel. As soon as another acetylcholine molecule by random movement happens to come in contact with the right part of the receptor protein, the process will repeat itself.

PROTEIN-LIGAND BINDING

A way to communicate to cells to change cellular function is to send chemical messengers that will bind to specific receptors. A chemical messenger interacts with a protein, the protein changes shape, and a cellular function is altered. This process of molecules or ions reversibly binding to proteins is termed protein-ligand binding. A ligand is a molecule or ion that binds to a protein molecule by forces other than covalent bonding. For example, an ion may be attracted to an area of a protein with the opposite charge, or a polar area of a chemical messenger may be attracted to a polar region of a protein. A nonpolar area of a messenger may also be placed in close proximity to a nonpolar region of a protein because of their mutual exclusion from water. The process of protein-ligand binding must be reversible. To regulate a cellular function, we send chemical messengers to bind to specific protein receptors either to increase or decrease a cellular function. If an ion or molecule remains bound permanently to a protein, cell

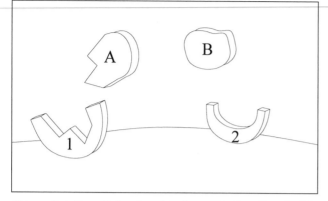

Figure 3-4. Specificity of protein-ligand binding. Protein 1 is more specific than protein 2. Protein 1 will bind ligand A only. Protein 2 will bind either ligand A or B.

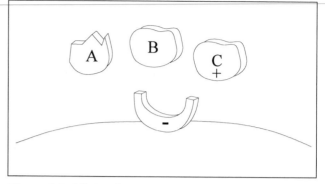

Figure 3-5. Affinity of a protein for different ligands. Ligands A, B, and C will bind to the membrane protein, but not equally well. Ligand B can bind better to the protein than ligand A because of the greater interaction of weak intermolecular forces over a larger area. The presence of a negative charge on the binding site and a positive charge on ligand C causes ligand C to bind better to the protein than ligand B. Note that shape of the ligand is an important determinant of both specificity and affinity.

function cannot be regulated; it is maintained permanently at a different level. By releasing differing amounts of chemical messenger depending on the needs of the cells and allowing the chemical messenger to bind reversibly, we change the probability that at any given moment a ligand is bound to a receptor. When a ligand is bound to a receptor, cell function is altered. In general, the longer the ligand is bound, the greater the change in cellular function.

A binding site is an area within a protein to which a ligand can bind. As discussed previously, proteins are folded into complex three-dimensional structures. These structures may have indentations that allow ligands to fit into specific spaces. These spaces are called binding sites. The presence of ionized or polar groups may aid in retaining ligands that, by chance, come into contact with the binding site. The presence of a ligand in the binding site then redistributes chemical and possibly electrical energy within the protein to which the ligand is bound. The binding of a ligand, therefore, results in a change in the shape of the protein to which the ligand is bound. In turn, the shape change of a protein may then cause the shape of nearby proteins to change. The binding site may be part of a protein that functions as a receptor, an ion channel, a transport mechanism, or an enzyme.

Four properties characterize protein-ligand binding:
1. Specificity
2. Affinity
3. Saturation
4. Competition

Specificity (Figure 3-4) refers to the ability of a protein to bind specific ligand. To control a cell's function precisely, the optimum situation would be one in which the receptor or transport mechanism only functions when one specific ligand binds to the protein. Different proteins vary in their degree of specificity. Specificity is determined in large part by the shape of the binding site. Some shapes will allow several different ligands to bind, whereas others are very specific.

The second property, affinity (Figure 3-5), refers to how well a ligand remains bound or the strength of protein-ligand binding. The greater the affinity of protein for a ligand, the longer the cellular function is altered. A low affinity ligand may simply bounce off the binding site, producing little effect on cell function. Affinity, like specificity, depends upon the shape of the binding site relative to the ligand. The better the fit, the more likely a ligand is to remain bound. Affinity is also determined by the presence of chemical forces that enhance attraction of the ligand, such as polar or ionized groups within the binding site.

Saturation refers to the proportion of existing binding sites occupied by a ligand. If all binding sites are occupied, they are said to be saturated. If half the binding sites are occupied at any given time, we state that the binding sites are 50% saturated. Saturation is dependent on the concentration of ligand in the interstitial fluid surrounding the binding sites. The more ligand that is present, the greater is the probability that ligand will contact the binding site. A second factor determining saturation is the affinity of the binding site for the ligand. The longer the ligand remains bound to the binding site, the less likely a binding site will be unoccupied. Thus, one must consider both concentration and affinity in discussing saturation.

Competition describes the situation in which more than one type of ligand present in the interstitial fluid

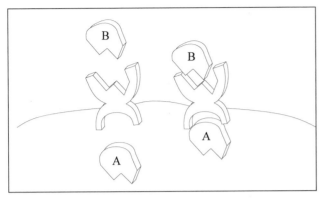

Figure 3-6. Allosteric modulation. The affinity of the membrane protein for ligand B is very low before ligand A binds to the protein. Binding of ligand A changes the shape of the protein, which markedly increases the affinity of the protein for ligand B. The site to which ligand A binds is called the regulatory site. Ligand A is called the regulatory ligand. The functional ligand, B, binds to the functional site, which causes a change in cellular function. Note that allosteric modulation may, in some cases, decrease the affinity of some allosteric proteins for their functional ligand.

may bind to a protein. These ligands compete for binding sites. The relative binding of ligand is determined by the relative concentrations and the affinities of the binding sites for the different ligands. The higher the concentration, the more likely a ligand will contact a binding site. The greater the affinity, the more likely that ligand contacting a binding site will remain on the binding site and the better it will compete. Protein-ligand binding is reversible; ligand continually comes off binding sites. The higher the concentration of a given ligand, the more likely it is that as soon as one comes off a binding site, another of the same type will replace it. The greater the affinity, the less the need is for a ligand to contact the binding sites rapidly, because each ligand remains bound longer.

The physiologic effect of protein-ligand binding is determined by how long ligand is bound to each receptor, how many receptors exist on each cell, and how many cells have receptors. To alter the cellular function, one can alter concentration, affinity, or number of receptors. Concentration of ligand can be altered in several ways. One way is to change the delivery of ligand. Hormone delivery can be increased by either releasing more into the blood or by increasing blood flow to the target tissue. Neurotransmitter delivery can be increased by causing the nerve to release more of its neurotransmitter at a more rapid rate. Other mechanisms for altering ligand concentration include special uptake mechanisms, enzymes that degrade ligand, and by diffusion of ligand away from receptors. Affinity can be altered by the processes of allosteric and covalent modulation of the protein molecule to be described below.

Altering the number of receptors present can also regulate cell function on the target cells. The process of increasing the number of receptors is called up-regulation. Some cells respond to the presence of excess ligand concentration by decreasing the number of receptors, a process called down-regulation. Down-regulation is one explanation for the lack of glucose uptake in type 2 (adult-onset) diabetes mellitus. Chronic overeating in some genetically predisposed individuals may cause excessively high levels of insulin in the blood. Cells then respond by down-regulation of insulin receptors, which in turn causes glucose to accumulate in the blood.

ALLOSTERIC AND COVALENT MODULATION

Allosteric means "different shape." Allosteric modulation refers to the presence of one ligand influencing the affinity of a protein for a second ligand (Figure 3-6). The allosteric protein has two binding sites. One is termed the regulatory site, and the other is termed the functional site. Binding of ligand to the regulatory site alters the affinity of the functional site for the ligand that influences cellular function. The regulatory ligand may either increase or decrease affinity. The change in affinity is due to the "different shape" of the allosteric protein after the regulatory ligand binds to the protein. By having many allosteric proteins of the same type on a cell, the cellular function of interest may be altered by varying the concentration of the regulatory ligand. A common regulatory ligand is Na^+. An example of allosteric modulation is the transport of glucose across the membrane of some cells. When Na^+ binds to the regulatory site, the affinity of the allosteric protein for glucose increases. When glucose binds to the functional site, the transport mechanism changes shape, allowing glucose and Na^+ to enter the cell. Glucose and Na^+ are then released into the intracellular fluid. The protein resumes its previous shape and is ready for a new Na^+ ion to bind to the regulatory site to repeat the process.

Covalent modulation differs from allosteric in that the regulatory ligand does not bind reversibly to the protein, but is covalently bound (Figure 3-7). The covalent modulator is usually phosphate donated from ATP via one of a family of enzymes called protein kinases. Protein kinase is a rather descriptive term. It makes a protein "move." The introduction of a double negative charge can produce a profound effect on protein shape. Covalent binding of a ligand, such as phosphate, is a means of introducing large amounts of chemical energy into a protein to make an otherwise slow process into one sufficiently rapid to perform a useful task. Covalent modulation is one of the major ways in which ATP is used as an energy source for the cell.

As in allosteric modulation, covalent modulation can either increase or decrease the affinity of a protein for a functional ligand. An important example of covalent modulation is the Na-K pump, also known as Na-K ATPase. The use of ATP by this protein allows three Na^+ from the inside of the cell and two K^+ from outside the cell to bind to "the pump" and be transported across the membrane, which allows K^+ to be concentrated within the cell and Na^+ to be concentrated outside the cell. Because phosphate is not reversibly bound to the protein, an enzyme called phosphoprotein phosphatase is required to remove it, so the protein can return to its original shape and its function can be performed again.

Many drugs are exogenous ligands (originated outside the body, in contrast with endogenous ligands produced inside the body) designed to bind to receptor sites on specific proteins. Drugs called competitive blockers may be designed to inhibit a physiologic response by competing for binding sites with endogenous ligand. Competitive blockers do not produce the physiologic effect, but occupy the receptor so the endogenous ligand cannot. A second application for drugs is to enhance a normal response by binding to receptors better than the endogenous ligand. Thirdly, drugs may be useful in producing a more specific response. Some endogenous ligands may bind to more than one type of receptor and produce more than one effect. Synthetic ligands can often be designed to bind effectively to only one type of receptor to produce a more specific response than an endogenous ligand.

SUMMARY

Cell membranes are composed of phospholipids with proteins inserted in the membrane and attached to its inner surface. The physical properties of particles determine their ability to penetrate the membrane. Nonpolar and small polar molecules can pass between phospholipid molecules to enter the cell. Special mechanisms exist to allow the entry of ions and larger polar molecules, such as amino acids and glucose. Proteins in the membrane serve four basic purposes: regulation of movement of particles into and out of cells, detection of chemical messengers, linking neighboring cells, and anchoring of intracellular proteins. Ion channels and transporter mechanisms allow ions and specific substances to enter the cell under physiological regulation. Some proteins act as receptors for chemical messengers such as hormones and neurotransmitters. Cells are linked together for various purposes. Types of junctions

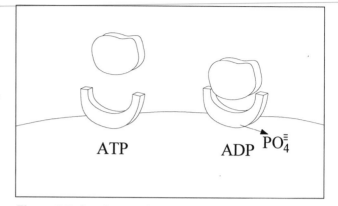

Figure 3-7. Covalent modulation. The affinity of a protein for its functional ligand is increased by covalent (not spontaneously reversible) binding of a regulatory ligand. As in allosteric modulation, covalent modulation may be used to decrease affinity for a functional ligand. To reverse covalent modulation, an enzyme, phosphoprotein phosphatase, is required to remove the covalent modifier.

include desmosomes, tight junctions, and gap junctions. Desmosomes hold adjacent cells together. Tight junctions prevent the movement of particles around epithelial surfaces. Gap junctions allow the movement of ions and small particles between neighboring cells. Proteins take on energetically favorable three-dimensional shapes that are influenced by surrounding ions and molecules. Shape changes of proteins are used to regulate protein function. A molecule or ion that binds to a binding site on a protein is called a ligand. Protein-ligand binding has the properties of specificity, affinity, saturation, and competition. Competition for binding sites on a protein is influenced by relative affinities and concentrations. The effectiveness of protein-ligand binding can be altered by the processes of up- and down-regulation of receptors and allosteric and covalent modulation of protein-ligand binding.

BIBLIOGRAPHY

Berne RM, Levy MN. *Physiology*. St. Louis, Mo: Mosby-Year Book; 1998.

Ganong WF. *Review of Medical Physiology*. Norwalk, Conn: Appleton & Lange; 1995.

Guyton AC, Hall JE, Schmitt W. *Human Physiology and Mechanisms of Disease*. Philadelphia, Pa: WB Saunders; 1997.

Hole Jr. JW. *Essentials of Human Anatomy and Physiology*. 4th ed. Dubuque, Ia: Wm C Brown Publishers; 1992.

Schauf C, Moffett D, Moffett S. *Human Physiology: Foundation and Frontiers*. St. Louis, Mo: Times Mirror/Mosby College Publishing; 1990.

Solomon EP, Davis PW. *Human Anatomy and Physiology*. Philadelphia, Pa: WB Saunders; 1983.

STUDY QUESTIONS

1. Up-regulation is an increased number of receptors in response to a greater concentration of ligand in the extracellular fluid. What advantages and disadvantages might up-regulation produce?

2. Down-regulation is a decreased number of receptors in response to a greater concentration of ligand in the extracellular fluid. What advantages and disadvantages might down-regulation produce? Think of a disease characterized by down-regulation.

3. Allosteric modulation can be used to increase or decrease the affinity of a protein for a particular ligand. Describe allosteric modulation. Members of the group may play the roles of the allosteric protein, the modulating ligand, and the functional ligand to demonstrate to the rest of the class. Describe how allosteric modulation could be useful in a biochemical pathway.

4. Covalent modulation can be used to increase or decrease the affinity of a protein for a particular ligand. Describe covalent modulation. Members of the group may play the roles of the protein, the functional ligand, protein kinase, ATP, and phosphoprotein phosphatase to demonstrate to the rest of the class. What special property does phosphate have that can cause it to make chemical reactions increase in rate?

F O U R

Transport

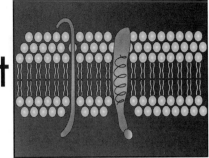

Glenn Irion, PhD, PT, CWS and Sarah N. Jerome, PhD, RRT

OBJECTIVES

1. State two basic principles of transport.

2. Define diffusion; state its driving force and factors influencing its effectiveness.

3. Define convection; explain why convection is necessary; describe where diffusion and convection occur in the respiratory and cardiovascular systems.

4. Describe the relationships among temperature, pressure, and concentration.

5. Define facilitated diffusion; contrast it with simple diffusion.

6. Define active transport; contrast it with simple diffusion and facilitated diffusion.

7. Define secondary active transport; contrast it with primary active transport.

8. Contrast simple diffusion, facilitated diffusion, primary active transport, and secondary active transport in terms of role of concentration gradient, role of membrane proteins, role of ATP, and limiting factors for maximum transport.

9. Define osmosis; describe what must be present for osmosis to occur, how the driving forces of ΔP and ΔC interact to produce equilibrium.

10. Define the unit of osmolarity; state how osmotic pressure is measured and how it can be computed.

11. Define tonicity; describe how two solutions can be isosmotic and not be isotonic.

12. Describe the process of exocytosis.

To maintain function cells require substrates for their chemical reactions, called nutrients, and must rid themselves of waste. Most cells in multicellular organisms are not in a position to obtain needed substances directly from the external environment. Instead, cells obtain nutrients and deposit wastes into the internal environment, the interstitial fluid. This chapter describes the processes by which substances are exchanged between intracellular fluid and interstitial fluid. Because the interstitial fluid is not an infinite reservoir, it must exchange substances with flowing blood to keep its composition constant. The processes to be described include diffusion, a passive mechanism; convection, which transports substances with the help of bulk flow of blood; protein-mediated transport mechanisms of facilitated diffusion and active transport; and osmosis, the movement of water across membranes due to presence of solute that does not penetrate the membrane and movement of molecules without passing directly through the membrane by endocytosis and exocytosis.

Two basic principles that apply to all forms of transport are that transport occurs in both directions across the cell membrane regardless of the direction of net transport and that net movement of substrate occurs from an area in which any given substance has more total energy to an area in which the same substance has a lower total energy (downhill process), unless the cell uses energy in a process called active transport (uphill process). Usually, the difference in energy of the substance is due to a difference in concentration, although mechanical and electrical energy are often used to produce net movement of substance in one direction.

DIFFUSION

Diffusion is a process in which random movement of particles in solution results in the substance becoming dispersed evenly. The biologic significance is that substances used by the cell can diffuse into the cell from the interstitial space to replace what was used (Figure 4-1). In turn, the same substances diffuse from the blood into the interstitial fluid. Wastes diffuse from the cells in which they are generated into the interstitial fluid and from the interstitial fluid into the blood. Using the substance in the chemical reactions prevents the concentration of the substance from becoming equal inside and outside the cell and maintains the concentration difference needed for diffusion to work. Provided that the concentration in the interstitial fluid does not change, the faster a substance is used in the cell, the faster the substance is transported into the cell.

Because random movement can change direction

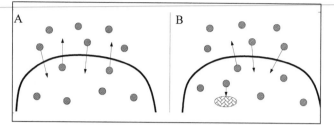

Figure 4-1. At equilibrium (panel A), particles move in and out of a cell at the same rate. Panel B: as a cell uses these particles in chemical reactions, particles continue to enter the cell, but fewer leave, resulting in a net flow into the cell. If the cell is generating particles, the particles continue to enter the cell but exit at a faster rate than they enter, resulting in a net flow out.

from moment to moment (Brownian motion), it is unlikely that random movement of a particle by diffusion will continue in one given direction. Therefore, diffusion can occur rapidly over microscopic distances, such as the thickness of cell membranes, but it is very slow over macroscopic distances. The energy that produces diffusion comes from the thermal energy that produces Brownian motion. Any substance that has a temperature greater than absolute zero has some kinetic energy. This energy causes solute to move throughout a solution. The higher the temperature, the greater the kinetic energy, and, as a result, solutes move more quickly through a solution. As particles move in solution, they strike other particles. As particles collide, they change direction and exchange kinetic energy with particles with which they collide. Therefore, if one adds cold water to hot water, the slow moving (cold) molecules are struck by fast moving (hot) molecules until, after many collisions, the hot molecules have given up enough of their kinetic energy to the cold molecules that all of the molecules have an intermediate level of energy. A second consequence of particle movement is that some particles will, at any given moment, strike the container holding the solution. Collisions by particles of the solution transfer energy into the walls of the container, producing pressure. If temperature is increased, the particles in solution strike the container with greater energy and strike the container more frequently; therefore, increased temperature leads to an increase in pressure in the container if volume is not allowed to change. Conversely, if more pressure is exerted by the container on the solution, the container will exchange energy with the particles in solution, making the particles move more rapidly (ie, increase the temperature of the particles).

One general principle mentioned above is that particles move from an area in which that kind of particle has a higher total energy to an area in which it has a lower total energy. Although it does not matter whether this energy is chemical, thermal, electrical, or mechanical, diffusion is usually described in terms of net movement of particles from an area of high to low concentration. However, net movement of particles will also occur from an area of high temperature to low temperature and from high pressure to low pressure. Any of these forces increase what is called the chemical potential of a given solute. As discussed in Chapter Two, substances will demonstrate a net flow from an area of high chemical potential to low chemical potential. This movement is strictly the result of random movement provided by the energy of the particles. A second principle is that transport occurs in both directions. That is, particles move from an area of high concentration to an area of low concentration, but, at the same time, particles move from an area of low concentration to an area of high concentration. Net movement occurs from the area of high concentration because more particles move out than move in. At the same time, in the area of low concentration, more particles move in than move out. Over time, as the high-concentration area loses particles, the low-concentration area gains particles, and eventually particles will move in and out of both areas at the same rate. This state is termed equilibrium. The rate at which equilibrium results depends on the properties of the particles and any barriers, such as the cell membranes or blood vessel walls. The properties of the particle are incorporated in a term called the diffusion coefficient (D), which is related largely to molecular weight, but also to the physical interaction between solute and the barrier. The movement of some substances is complicated by the process of **solvent drag** in which movement of solute due to bulk flow across a porous surface brings with it molecules of solute that might otherwise diffuse more slowly.

As discussed above, diffusion works well over microscopic distances, but poorly over macroscopic distances. This is shown by the following examples. The equation $d^2 = 2Dt$ describes the distance a particle moves in a given time (t). First, to move O_2 from outside a 100-μm diameter skeletal muscle cell to its center if diffusion coefficient (D) equals 2.0×10^{-5} cm^2/s, distance from outside the cell to its center (d) equals 5×10^{-3} cm, then time (t) would equal 0.625 s. However, if we need to move O_2 1 mm, t would equal $(0.1 \text{ cm}/[2 \times 2.0 \times 10^{-5} \text{ cm}^2\text{s}^{-1}]) = 250$ s. As can be seen from these two examples, diffusion works well over short distances, such as the radius of a cell, but transport is very slow over greater distances. As an example, we could gently place a teaspoon of salt in a glass of water. In the immediate microscopic area, the salt distributes rapidly, but disperses very slowly throughout the rest of the glass. If we wanted the solute to mix rapidly and evenly through the water, we could add mechanical energy in the form of stirring. Near membranes in the body, such as the inner surface of the digestive tract, slow movement of solute may be caused by a region in which no stirring occurs. This area is called an **unstirred layer** and is responsible for a major portion of the transport time because substances must diffuse across this distance.

To make diffusion effective, we must minimize the distance for diffusion. Although a form of stirring occurs in the digestive tract, the process of reducing diffusion distance is accomplished in the body by the cardiovascular system through the process of **convection**. Convection is a term also used in exchange for heat, in which heat exchange by conduction from molecule to molecule is aided by the movement of the fluid with which an object is exchanging heat. The same general idea exists in the exchange of substance. Particles are exchanged by random motion from high concentration to low concentration over short distances from one fluid (the blood) to another fluid (interstitial fluid) aided by bulk flow of the fluid carrying the substance. Convection occurs in both the respiratory and cardiovascular systems to bring oxygen close enough to surfaces to make diffusion effective. Bulk flow of air from outside the mouth and nose to the alveoli brings oxygen to the alveoli where exchange by diffusion occurs, allowing oxygen to enter the arterial blood. Oxygen is then carried by convection to capillaries where oxygen diffuses into the interstitial fluid. Bulk flow also occurs in the gastrointestinal and renal systems to aid diffusion, allowing nutrients to be absorbed and wastes to be excreted.

Unstirred layers of thermal energy occur when a body part is submersed in a tank of water. Transfer of thermal energy (eg, to warm stiff body parts or to cool injured body parts) is facilitated by a turbine to stir the water in what we generally refer to as a whirlpool. The agitation prevents a gradient of temperature that reduces transfer of energy. The agitation is also used to deliver topical medications or to loosen adherent tissue in open wounds.

DIFFUSION OF IONS

Another important factor determining the rate of exchange by diffusion is the interaction between the particle and barriers it must cross. The cell membrane, as described in Chapter Three, consists of phospholipids with proteins inserted throughout. Particles strike the membrane randomly from both sides. How fast particles move across the membrane is determined largely by the interaction of the particle's kinetic energy, physical and chemical properties, and the properties of the cell membrane. Lipid-soluble particles can move easily between phospholipid molecules to cross the membrane. Small polar molecules, such as water and ethanol, can also take this route. Larger polar molecules pass so slowly through the membrane that they require special transport mechanisms that will be described later. Ions do not pass through the phospholipid portion of the membrane to any appreciable extent. Ions must pass through special channels in the membrane. Although ions may be quite small, they attract large numbers of water molecules that move with the ion. The hydrated diameter of ions expresses the effective size of ions. The charge on the ion and its hydrated diameter prevent movement across the phospholipid barrier. For this reason, the rate of ion movement across membranes depends on the availability of ion channels. The number of available channels can be altered physiologically and pharmacologically by changes in membrane potential or binding of ligands, such as neurotransmitters, hormones, and drugs, to membrane receptors. Ion channels typically consist of integral proteins that weave in and out of the membrane several times with portions that can interact with ligands or peripheral proteins or both to regulate their physical appearance, thereby opening or closing the channel to ion flux. Some ion channels (Figure 4-2) are selective for single ions, such as Na^+, others are less selective. The diffusion of ions across the membrane is also complicated by the presence of charge (electrical energy) on the ions. Movement of ions is dependent upon both differences in concentration and differences in charge across the membrane. Later, in Chapter Nine, we will see how differences in concentration and charge interact to produce membrane potentials.

TRANSPORT MECHANISMS OTHER THAN DIFFUSION

Over a given time, many particles strike the cell membrane. Some of these will bounce off and create mechanical pressure; others will pass through the membrane. If conditions are the same on both sides of the membrane, an equal number of particles will pass in both directions. A difference in kinetic energy, charge, or concentration or a differential permeability in one direction will produce net movement in one direction. The cell uses energy to create a differential permeability in the process of active transport. Two types of driving forces, such as electric potential and concentration, may offset each other, but if the sum of these driving forces is greater on one side than the other, net movement of substance will occur. Later in the chapter, we will see

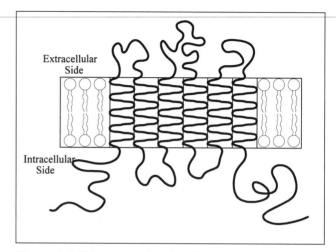

Figure 4-2. Voltage-gated cation channel.

how differences in pressure and concentration across a membrane can offset each other to prevent net movement of water in the process of osmosis. Several special transport mechanisms are available to transport substances that do not move easily by diffusion: mediated transport by facilitated diffusion and active transport and movement of vesicles across the membrane in endocytosis and exocytosis.

FACILITATED DIFFUSION

Although oxygen and carbon dioxide can pass readily through the lipid bilayer of the cell membrane, some important nutrients for cells, such as glucose and amino acids, are larger, polar molecules that are too large to pass through the membrane as easily as water. Because of the physical properties of these molecules, diffusion would be too slow to support life. A process called facilitated diffusion is used to overcome this problem. In this process, transmembrane proteins act as carriers to transport substances across the membrane. The substance to be transported acts as a ligand that binds to specific receptors on the membrane (Figure 4-3). When the molecule binds to the protein on one side of the membrane, the protein changes shape and transports the substance across the membrane. After the protein changes shape, the ligand is released on the other side of the membrane. Release of the ligand allows the protein to return to its original shape. Because the same protein transports the substances equally well in both directions across the membrane, facilitated diffusion, like simple diffusion, produces net transport of substances from an area of high to low concentration only. When the concentration of a substance transported by facilitated diffusion is equal on both sides of a membrane, facilitated diffusion transports the substance across the membrane

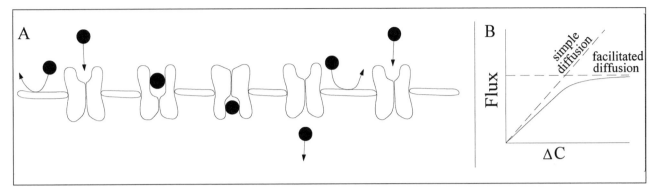

Figure 4-3. Facilitated diffusion. Larger, nonlipid-soluble particles cannot diffuse directly through the cell membrane. Proteins embedded in the cell membrane are used to shuttle these particles from an area of high concentration to an area of low concentration. If concentration is equal across the cell membrane, no net transport occurs by facilitated diffusion. Panel B: the rate of transport by simple diffusion is proportional to the difference in concentration regardless of the magnitude. At low differences in concentration, a linear relationship exists for ΔC and transport by facilitated diffusion. Because facilitated diffusion depends on a finite number of carriers, transport is limited by saturation of the transport proteins.

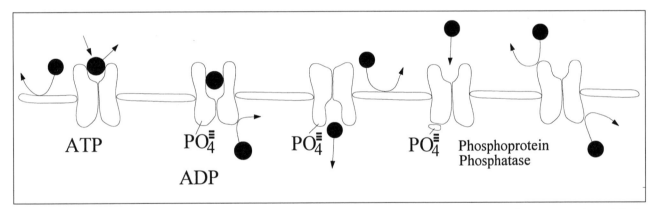

Figure 4-4. Active transport. Use of ATP causes the membrane transport mechanism to carry substances preferentially in one direction. Prior to use of ATP, the transport mechanism has a low affinity for the particle on both sides of the membrane. Covalent modulation of the transporter increases the affinity for the substance on the outside of the cell, but not on the inside. The probability of the transporter moving the particle into the cell becomes 10 to 20 times greater than moving the same substances out of the cell. Active transport is limited to producing a difference in concentration across the membrane that is proportional to the difference in inward and outward transport by the carrier. The cell may then have an inside concentration of a substance that is 10 to 20 times higher than the concentration outside of the cell. As discussed in facilitated diffusion, the rate of transport is also limited by saturation of the carriers. Active transport is also limited if ATP supply is low. Active transport may also be used to transport substances out of the cell.

at the same rate in both directions. This mechanism is often overcome by transforming the molecule into something less likely to be transported back out of the cell. For example, attaching a phosphate group to glucose prevents glucose from binding back onto the carrier.

Because facilitated transport relies on protein-ligand binding, the rate of facilitated diffusion is determined differently from that of simple diffusion. The rate of facilitated diffusion depends on the number of protein carriers and the saturation of carriers. Whereas the rate of diffusion is directly proportional to the difference in concentration across the membrane, this is only true at a low percent saturation in facilitated diffusion.

Transport by facilitated diffusion reaches a maximum value at a concentration that results in membrane carrier saturation. Increasing the difference in concentration further does not increase transport. Therefore, facilitated transport has two possible limits—equal concentrations of the substance across the membrane and saturation of the carriers.

ACTIVE TRANSPORT

Active transport is similar to facilitated transport in that carriers are used and the rate of transport is limited by saturation of the carriers (Figure 4-4). In contrast to facilitated diffusion, active transport can produce net movement of substance from low to high concentration (uphill), but at the cost of ATP utilization. Typically, primary active transport requires a covalently modulated membrane protein. Just as in facilitated diffusion, the carrier moves solute in both directions. Covalent modulation using ATP produces a higher affinity for a ligand on one side of a membrane than on the other; therefore, a solute passes more readily in one direction (usually in the range of 10-fold) than in the other direction. The greater affinity of the carrier for the solute on one side of the membrane causes the carrier to transport more solute in one direction than in the other. The limitation on concentration difference that can be produced across the cell membrane is due to difference in affinity of the carrier protein on the two sides of membrane. As the difference in concentration becomes proportional to the difference in affinity, the difference in concentration drives transport in one direction at the same rate that the difference in affinity drives it in the opposite direction, limiting active transport to concentrate substances to ratios typically in the range of 10:1. As described for facilitated diffusion, active transport is also limited by saturation of carriers.

One of the most important active transport mechanisms is the Na-K pump. This carrier transports two K ions from the outside of the membrane and three Na ions from the inside for each ATP molecule used. The Na-K pump has three major functions in the cell: maintaining cell volume, developing a membrane potential, and producing the concentration gradient for sodium ions necessary to drive secondary active transport. Cells contain a large number of nonpenetrating anions, especially proteins. In addition, cellular metabolism creates an excess number of intracellular particles that must be removed to prevent hyperosmolarity of the intracellular fluid, which in turn leads to cell swelling. This is described after osmosis is discussed below. Because the pump removes three positive charges from the cell and pumps in two positive charges, the net effect of the Na-K pump is to make the inside of the cell negative with respect to the outside of the cell. Usually the Na-K pump makes only a small contribution to the membrane potential relative to the mechanism to be described in Chapter Nine on membrane potentials. The third need for the Na-K pump, which will be described below, is secondary active transport. Active transport of sodium out of the cell is used to drive other substances into the cell.

SECONDARY ACTIVE TRANSPORT

Like primary active transport, secondary active transport can transport substances against a concentra-

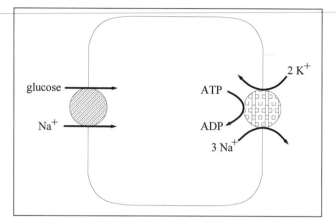

Figure 4-5. Secondary active transport. Na acts as an allosteric modulator to allow glucose, in this example, to be transported into the cell. Glucose and Na are cotransported. The movement of Na from high to low concentration allows glucose to be transported from low concentration to high concentration. The transporter does not use ATP directly. ATP is used to actively transport Na out of the cell, so Na can move down its concentration gradient.

tion gradient. Instead of using ATP directly for covalent modulation of the protein carriers, secondary active transport uses allosteric modulation. The most common allosteric modulator is Na^+. Na^+ binds to a protein carrier, which increases the affinity of the carrier for the substance to be transported on one side of the membrane relative to the other side. Secondary active transport is also limited to the concentration that will drive the substance out at the same rate that the increased affinity on the other side drives the substance in. This type of transport is called secondary active transport because it requires the expenditure of ATP indirectly. The actual transport mechanism itself does not use ATP. Instead, the high concentration of the allosteric modulator (Na^+) on one side of the membrane is produced by active transport. Primary active transport of Na^+ out of the cell causes the Na^+ concentration outside to be higher than on the inside. A greater concentration of allosteric modulator outside the membrane causes ligands, such as glucose or amino acids, to be transported and released inside the cell because the concentration of sodium is higher outside the cell **secondary** to the active transport of sodium out of the cell (Figure 4-5). Therefore, the mechanism of secondary active transport requires ATP indirectly. Secondary active transport can also be used to transport substances out of the cell. One important example is the Na-Ca exchange mechanism in cardiac cells. The high concentration of sodium outside the cell is used to drive transport of calcium out of cardiac cells against a higher concentration of calcium outside the cardiac cell. Like facilitated diffusion, secondary active transport is limited by the number of protein car-

TABLE 4-1

Comparison of Types of Transport Across Cell Membranes

TYPE OF TRANSPORT	DIRECTION	CARRIERS	RATE DETERMINED BY	USES ATP?	CONCENTRATION LIMITED TO
Diffusion	Downhill only	No	ΔC	No	$C_o = C_i$
Facilitated transport	Downhill only	Yes	ΔC, saturation	No	$C_o = C_i$
Primary active transport	Up or downhill	Yes	Saturation	Yes, directly	Relative affinity inside : outside
Secondary active transport	Up or downhill	Yes	Saturation	Yes, indirectly	Relative affinity inside : outside

riers present on the cell membrane. This is the reason glucose appears in the urine of individuals with diabetes mellitus. Because glucose is not taken up normally by cells in diabetes mellitus, glucose accumulates in the blood. Normally, the amount of glucose filtered into the renal tubules produces a concentration that does not saturate the secondary active transport carriers for glucose in the renal tubules, and virtually no glucose appears in the urine. In poorly controlled diabetes, however, the concentration exceeds saturation, glucose cannot be reabsorbed completely from the renal tubules, and some of the filtered glucose passes in the urine. A comparison of the different types of transport is made in Table 4-1.

OSMOSIS

When discussing transport, no mention of water has been made; only the movement of solute has been discussed. If solute moves in one direction across the membrane, other molecules must take the place of the solute particle or pressure will increase on the side to which particles are moving. In a simple situation in which a single solute is in high concentration on one side of a membrane, water concentration must be higher on the opposite side. Net movement of solute occurs in one direction down its concentration gradient; meanwhile, a net movement of water occurs in the opposite direction down its concentration gradient. Diffusion across a membrane occurs because of random motion of solute and water particles. Some particles encounter and cross the membrane; other particles do not pass through, but strike, the membrane, creating pressure on the membrane. If more collisions occur on one side of the membrane than the other, then pressure will be higher on one side. However, transport requires the molecule to pass through the membrane, not just collide with the membrane. If particles on both sides pass through the membrane equally well and pressure is higher on one side, then net transport across the membrane will occur toward the low-pressure side in a process called filtration. Thus, as discussed earlier, both ΔP and ΔC can cause net movement of solute and water across a membrane.

Osmosis refers to the case in which water has a net movement across a semipermeable membrane produced by a difference in water concentration (chemical potential of water) due to the existence of nonpenetrating solute on one side of a semipermeable membrane. Such solutes are called nonpenetrating solutes because they do not "penetrate" the membrane; a semipermeable membrane is one that restricts the movement of some molecules, but not others. In osmosis, water, not solute, moves across the membrane. In simple diffusion, equal volumes of water and solute move across the membrane, so no change in pressure occurs. In osmosis, however, the net movement of water causes pressure to become greater on the side to which water moves. Water moves toward the side on which a higher concentration of nonpenetrating solute exists, because water can move freely across the membrane, but the solute cannot. When pressure is equal on both sides of the membrane, essentially equal numbers of collisions occur on either side of the membrane. On one side of the membrane, all of the molecules that strike or pass through the membrane are water; whereas, on the other side, fewer interactions with the membrane involve water. Because fewer of the interactions on one side of the membrane result in transport, more water crosses the membrane in one direction. Pressure builds with net movement of water until the number of interactions between water molecules on both sides of the membrane becomes equal. At

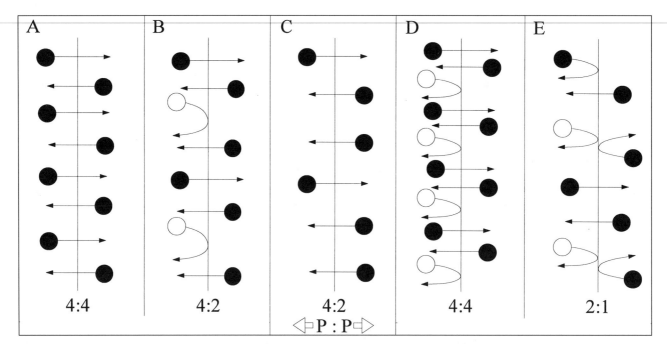

Figure 4-6. Osmosis. Panel A: the same concentration of the same solute exists on both sides of a membrane. Because the solute can penetrate, equal numbers of particles pass in both directions; in panel A, equilibrium exists. Panel B: one-half of the particles on the left of the membrane cannot penetrate the membrane, but all of the particles on the right can. The same number of particles encounter the membrane from both directions, but only one-half of those coming from the left can cross. In this situation, twice as many particles flow from right to left as flow from left to right, producing net flow. The penetrating particles are water. Osmosis is the net movement of water from an area of high water concentration across a barrier due to the presence of nonpenetrating solute. Flow is toward the nonpenetrating solute. Panel C: only water exists on the two sides of the membrane, but the pressure on the right side is twice that of the left side. For this reason, twice as many water molecules move from right to left as from left to right. Hydrostatic pressure produces a net flow of water from right to left. Panel D: 50% of the particles on the left are nonpenetrating solute, so 50% of the particles that encounter the membrane from the left are water. However, because the hydrostatic pressure on the left is twice that of the right, twice as many particles encounter the membrane from the left than from the right. Therefore, the same number of water molecules pass from left to right as from right to left. The difference in water concentration due to the presence of non-penetrating solute is offset by a difference in hydrostatic pressure. Panel E: the actual rate of water movement depends on the relative ease of movement of water and solute across the membrane. The number used to convert difference in osmotic pressure to flow rate is called the reflection coefficient.

this point, the movement of water in one direction due to higher pressure equals the movement in the other direction due to the difference in water concentration, and equilibrium is achieved (Figure 4-6).

The driving force that creates net movement of water is termed osmotic pressure, and the nonpenetrating solute is said to be "osmotically active." In contrast to mechanical pressure, fluid has net movement from a solution with low osmotic pressure to high osmotic pressure because of the way osmotic pressure is defined. Osmotic pressure can be determined by placing mechanical pressure (hydrostatic pressure) on the side of the membrane on which osmotically active solute is present. By applying sufficient hydrostatic pressure (Figure 4-7), the number of water molecules striking and passing the membrane becomes equal on both sides of the membrane, so no net movement of water occurs. The pressure at which no net movement of water occurs

because the gradients of hydrostatic pressure and concentration of water are causing water to move equally in both directions is termed **osmotic pressure**. By definition, the side with a lower water concentration but higher solute concentration has a higher osmotic pressure. Osmotic pressure (with a symbol of π) can be computed for a weak solution by the formula $\pi = CRT$ in which C is the concentration of nonpenetrating solute in milliosmoles/liter (mOsm/l), R is the universal gas constant, and T is absolute temperature in K. At a body temperature of 37°C and taking the universal gas constant into the equation, the equation reduces to $\pi = 19.3 \check{} C$ (mOsm). This equation, however, is only accurate at low concentrations of solute in which the solute particles act independently.

To determine the effect of solute on the process of osmosis, solute concentration is expressed in terms of osmolarity in units of milliosmoles per liter (mOsm).

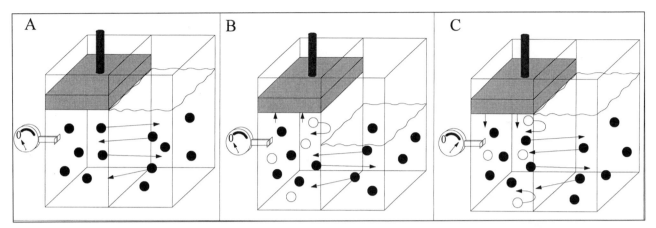

Figure 4-7. Measurement of osmotic pressure. Panel A: only water exists on both sides of a semipermeable membrane. Water molecules move across the membrane in both directions at the same rate. No difference in hydrostatic pressure exists across the membrane. Panel B: half of the molecules on the left of the membrane are nonpenetrating solute. A net movement of water from right to left increases volume and pressure on the left. Panel C: pressure exerted on the solution on the left prevents net movement of water into the compartment on the left. This hydrostatic pressure that prevents net movement is equal to the osmotic pressure generated by the presence of nonpenetrating solute.

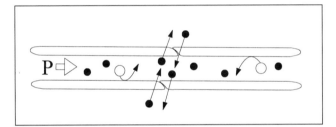

Figure 4-8. Fluid balance across capillaries. In the absence of plasma proteins, the hydrostatic pressure within capillaries would produce net loss of water because of the greater number of collisions inside the capillary than outside. The presence of plasma proteins reduces the number of interactions between capillary walls and water inside so that equal numbers of water molecules move in and out of capillaries.

One milliosmole (mOsm) equals one millimole (mMol) of particles. For substances that remain as a single particle in solution (nonionizing), a 1 mM solution equals a 1-mOsm solution. Because osmotic pressure is generated by the number of particles, and substances that ionize produce more than one particle when in solution (NaCl produces two, $CaCl_2$ produces three), when computing osmolarity, we need to account for the greater number of particles generated by a millimole of an ionizing compound. To convert mMol of NaCl to mOsm, we multiply by two. The osmolarity of a 142 mM NaCl solution, which is similar to interstitial fluid, is 284 mOsm, which generates an osmotic pressure of $19.3 \times 2 \times 142 = 5481$ mmHg.

Osmosis only occurs if the solute does not readily penetrate the barrier readily. In the case of the cell membrane, solute concentration is approximately equal on both sides. The slight excess of particles inside cells is handled by active transport of Na^+ out of the cell, which is useful because Na^+ behaves as a nonpenetrating solute for the cell membrane. Ions, including Na^+, move freely across capillary walls and, therefore, do not produce osmotic pressure. Instead, plasma proteins perform as nonpenetrating solute for capillaries. The osmotic pressure produced by plasma proteins in the blood, which is called oncotic pressure, is $19.3 \times 1.2 = 23$ mmHg. The oncotic pressure driving water into capillaries is approximately equal to the hydrostatic pressure that drives water out of capillaries (Figure 4-8). Because the oncotic and hydrostatic pressures are nearly equal and opposite in direction, only a small amount of filtration results. This fluid is returned to the circulation by lymphatic vessels.

When a difference in concentration of nonpenetrating solute exists across a cell membrane, water will move either into or out of cells. A solution of 290 mOsm is referred to as isosmotic. Any solution with higher solute concentration is called hyperosmotic, and one less concentrated is called hypo-osmotic. To predict the effects of solute concentration on cells, the nature of the solute with respect to the cell membrane must be taken into account. If equal concentrations of nonpenetrating solute exist on both sides of a membrane, no net movement of water across the membrane occurs. A solution that produces no change in cell volume is called isotonic. Solutions with higher concentrations of non-penetrating solute are called hypertonic and cause cells, such as red blood cells, to shrink (crenate) when cells are placed in them. If a red blood cell is placed in a hypotonic solution (a lower concentration of nonpenetrating

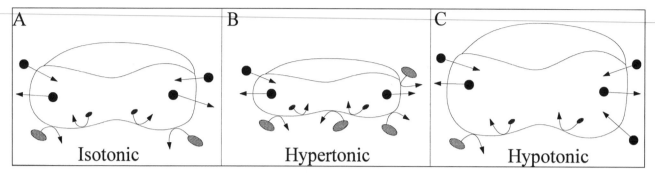

Figure 4-9. Tonicity. Panel A: isotonic solution. Equal concentrations of nonpenetrating solute across the red blood cell (RBC) membrane. Water moves into and out of the cell at the same rate. Panel B: hypertonic solution. A higher concentration of nonpenetrating solute outside of the RBC causes water to move in at a slower rate than it moves out. Cell size decreases (crenation) until concentration of nonpenetrating solute is equal across the membrane. Panel C: hypotonic solution. A lower concentration of nonpenetrating solute outside the cell causes water to move into the cell faster than it moves out. RBC volume increases until nonpenetrating solute concentration becomes equal or the cell bursts (hemolysis).

solute), water is driven into the red cell causing the red cell to swell or even burst (hemolysis). One must always be careful not to confuse tonicity with osmolarity. Osmolarity refers to solute concentration; tonicity refers to the effect of the solution on cell size. Prediction of changes in cell volume can become complex when penetrating and nonpenetrating solutes are mixed. For example, if a cell is placed in a 290 mOsm solution of urea, a penetrating solute, both urea and water can penetrate the cell, but the solutes producing the 290 mOsm solution within the cell do not penetrate. The presence of urea has no osmotic effect because it distributes itself equally across the membrane. As urea diffuses into the cell from the extracellular solution, water becomes driven into the cells, and the cells burst. This isosmotic urea solution is markedly hypotonic. If, instead, a hyperosmotic solution of 290 mOsm NaCl and 100 mOsm urea is used, hemolysis does not result because the urea will be evenly dispersed through the solution and within the cells, with the result that the osmolarity becomes the same inside and outside the cells. In this example, a hyperosmotic solution is isotonic. These phenomena are illustrated in Figure 4-9.

THE DONNAN EFFECT

As previously discussed, the movement of ions across membranes and their distribution across the membrane is influenced by other ions due to the combined effect of electrical and chemical differences. If a membrane is impermeable to a given ion, the distribution of other ions is affected. This is called the Donnan effect. The major consequences are related to the presence of negatively charged proteins inside cells. Because of the Donnan effect, the insides of cells have a greater concentration of osmotically active particles than the outside. An excess of a nonpenetrating solute inside cells will cause water to move into cells and cause them to burst unless another osmotically active particle is removed from the cells. The sodium-potassium pump, using ATP, is responsible for maintaining the volume

Cell Death

Two basic types of cell death have been described: necrosis and apoptosis. Necrosis is a "sloppy" form of cell death in which the membrane is broken down, spilling out the cell's contents. Apoptosis, on the other hand, is a "programmed" cell death in which the contents are destroyed in a neat, orderly manner. Apoptosis is responsible during development for the "sculpting" of body parts, such as the web spaces between fingers and toes and the production of hollow tubes from strands of embryonic tissue. However, apoptosis requires energy in the form of ATP to proceed. Otherwise, severe cell injury will result in necrosis. Necrosis releases potentially harmful particles, including enzymes that break down the membranes of neighboring cells. Release of the contents of dying cells can set up a positive feedback of cell death surrounding the area of most severe injury. Necrosis results in death of neighboring cells that otherwise would have survived an insult, such as lack of blood flow to a small region of heart tissue. Apoptosis can be turned on in the laboratory by manipulating genetic function. The ability to turn apoptosis on in dying cells therapeutically could limit the extension of cell death in myocardial infarction and stroke.

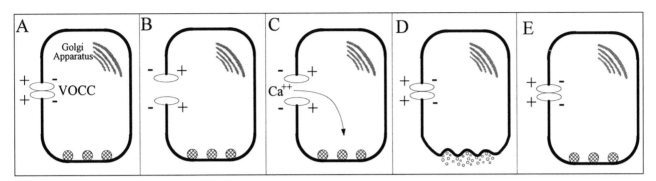

Figure 4-10. Exocytosis. Vesicles containing the substance to be released await near the membrane (panel A). A reversal in membrane potential causes the voltage-operated calcium channel (VOCC) in panel B to open. Ca enters the cell through the VOCC in panel C. Increased intracellular Ca concentration causes the vesicle to fuse with the membrane, releasing the substance into the extracellular space (panel D). Pieces of membrane are recycled, and new vesicles are continually produced by the endoplasmic reticulum and the Golgi apparatus. The number of vesicles released is determined by the amount of Ca that enters the cell.

and, therefore, pressure of the cell. Because this mechanism requires energy, one of the first signs of cell injury and inability to regenerate ATP is cell swelling. The Donnan effect is also responsible for maintaining the oncotic pressure in blood vessels by use of plasma proteins that aid in maintaining the volume of the circulating blood against the hydrostatic pressure generated by the contraction of the heart. A third consequence of the Donnan effect is the generation of an electrical potential across cell membranes. This concept will be developed in greater detail in Chapter Nine.

EXOCYTOSIS

A mechanism that can transport large molecules in large quantities is called exocytosis. Exocytosis is commonly used to place specific cellular products into the interstitial fluid. Examples include neurotransmitters, hormones, and products of exocrine glands, including digestive enzymes of the pancreas. The cellular products usually originate from the endoplasmic reticulum and the

Golgi apparatus, which produce regularly sized packages called vesicles. Vesicles contain the neurotransmitter or other product until release is signaled. Signals include action potentials in nerve cells and chemical signals such as hormones. The signal received by the cell usually causes entry of Ca^{++} into the cell, which in turn causes vesicles of the cellular product to fuse with the membrane and be released. The fragments of cell membrane are recycled, and new vesicles are continually produced (Figure 4-10).

Endocytosis is a process by which large molecules can be taken up by cells and can be thought of as exocytosis in reverse to some degree. Two types of endocytosis are phagocytosis (cell-eating) and pinocytosis (cell-drinking). Larger particles including bacteria can be taken up by phagocytosis. Often, phagocytosis is triggered by binding of specific proteins to receptors. Antibodies and the complement proteins of the immune system are important in triggering phagocytosis when they bind to cells of the immune system. The uptake of small, soluble molecules into vesicles is termed pinocytosis.

Neuromuscular Junction Disease

Several diseases of the neuromuscular junction are related to exocytosis. Of these, myasthenia gravis is the most important. In this disease, antibodies bound to acetylcholine receptors diminish the effect produced by exocytosis of acetylcholine by the motor nerve. Lambert-Eaton myasthenic syndrome (LEMS) is a paraneoplastic syndrome, meaning that it occurs as a complicating factor in cancer, especially small-cell carcinoma of the lung. This disease produces a clinical picture similar to myasthenia gravis by preventing the exocytosis of acetylcholine vesicles. Botulism is a condition in which toxin produced by *Clostridium* botulinum prevents release of acetylcholine. Black widow venom destroys synaptic vesicles of the neuromuscular junction. It produces massive release of acetylcholine followed by paralysis.

One can distinguish between myasthenia gravis and LEMS by the response to repetitive stimulation of motor nerves. An increased amplitude of muscle action potentials occurs with repetitive stimulation in diseases such as Lambert-Eaton myasthenic syndrome in which exocytosis of acetylcholine vesicles is diminished, whereas a decreased amplitude of muscle action potential occurs with repetitive stimulation in diseases such as myasthenia gravis, in which competitive blockade of the neuromuscular junction occurs. In myasthenia gravis, ptosis (drooping eyelid) and weakness of other muscles innervated by cranial nerves are usually first to be observed, along with fatigue with exercise. Untreated myasthenia gravis formerly had a high mortality due to respiratory failure. Today, myasthenia gravis is treated by thymectomy, surgical removal of the thymus, presumably the source of the offending antibodies. Formerly, treatment consisted of drugs such as neostigmine and related anticholinesterases, which permit acetylcholine to remain longer in the synaptic cleft.

In Lambert-Eaton myasthenic syndrome, carcinoma cells express a voltage-operated calcium channel that becomes the antigen against which antibodies are generated. Because the voltage-operated calcium channel is used by neurons as a trigger for exocytosis of neurotransmitter vesicles in motor neurons and autonomic neurons, symptoms of LEMS include proximal muscle weakness, decreased deep tendon reflexes (knee jerk), dry mouth, erectile dysfunction, and constipation.

Botulinum toxin prevents exocytosis of acetylcholine vesicles. It is produced by *Clostridium* botulinum, which is generally found in soil and animal waste. It may be food borne (toxin produced in contaminated food, toxin ingested), develop in open wounds (toxin produced by growing bacteria in infected wound), or be picked up from the environment. Signs and symptoms usually develop 18 to 36 hours after ingestion with bilateral and symmetric neurological signs beginning with cranial nerves, such as dry mouth, diplopia (double vision), loss of accommodation and pupillary light reflexes, dysarthria (difficulty speaking), and dysphagia (difficult swallowing), followed by weakness of the trunk and extremities, but no sensory changes. Infants are particularly susceptible to botulism. Spores may be present in foods, especially honey, but may also be picked up from vacuum cleaner dust and soil. It has been recommended that no raw honey be consumed before the age of one. Today, botulinum toxin is used therapeutically to relieve conditions caused by muscle spasm, such as torticollis ("twisted neck"), and cosmetically to decrease the facial wrinkles caused by fine muscles below the aging skin.

BIBLIOGRAPHY

Garty H, Palmer LG. Epithelium sodium channels: function, structure, and regulation. *Physiological Reviews.* 1997;77:359-396.

Mukherjee S, Ghosh RN, Maxfield FR. Endocytosis. *Physiological Reviews.* 1997;77:759-803.

Palacín M, Estévez R, Bertran J, Zorzano A. Molecular biology of mammalian plasma membrane amino acid transporters. *Physiological Reviews.* 1998;78:969-1054.

Rippe B, Haraldsson B. Transport of macromolecules across microvascular walls. *Physiological Reviews.* 1994;74:163-219.

Wakabayashi S, Shigekawa M, Pouyssegur J. Molecular physiology of vertebrate Na^+/H^+ exchanges. *Physiological Reviews.* 1997;77:51-74.

STUDY QUESTIONS

1. Why does understanding Brownian motion explain why diffusion works well over short distances and poorly over long distances?

2. What role does the circulatory system play in making diffusion useful?

3. Why is facilitated diffusion necessary? What constraint does facilitated diffusion have that diffusion does not?

4. How does secondary active transport differ from primary active transport? Why do you think sodium ions are so commonly used in this process?

5. Why do cells swell when they are depleted of ATP?

LABORATORY EXERCISES

LABORATORY EXERCISE 4-1

GENERATION OF OSMOTIC PRESSURE

Materials:
Osmosis kit (battery jar, thistle tube, dialysis tubing, tubing closure, small rubberbands, thistle tube clamps)
60% sucrose solution or 10% albumin solution
5% NaCL solution
5% starch solution
Meter or yardstick

Objective: Demonstrate how osmotic pressure is generated.

1. Make a tube from dialysis tubing in warm water. Seal one end with a tubing closure. Place the other end on a thistle tube and secure to the thistle tube with rubber bands.

2. Fill the empty battery jar three-fourths full with tap water.

3. Place the clamp around the thistle tube. Leave the screw somewhat loose so it can be adjusted later.

4. Place the thistle tube and attached sac into the battery jar and place the thistle tube in the clamp.

5. Fill the 30 ml syringe with 10% albumin or 60% sucrose solution. Place the needle and attached tubing on the syringe. Gently place the end of the tubing attached to the syringe into the sac at the end of the thistle tube.

6. Fill the sac and continue to fill until the level of the albumin solution is above the clamp. Carefully remove any bubbles from the sac and thistle tube.

7. Measure the height of the fluid above the clamp. If there is no movement during the next 10 minutes, check for air bubbles and ask for help. Measure the height change over the 10 minutes.

8. Carefully remove the thistle tube and clamp and place them into the battery jar containing a 5% NaCl solution. Adjust the height of fluid in the thistle tube to approximately the same level as the first experiment by moving the tube up or down in the clamp. Observe for another 10 minutes. How does the rate of movement of fluid up the thistle tube compare to the first experiment in which the battery jar was filled with tap water?

9. Next place the thistle tube and clamp into the battery jar containing 5% starch solution. Adjust the level of fluid in the thistle tube. Observe for another 10 minutes. How does the rate of movement up the tube compare to the movement when the thistle tube was in the tap water or in the NaCl solution?

LABORATORY EXERCISES

LABORATORY EXERCISE 4-2

MOVEMENT OF SUBSTANCES THROUGH SELECTIVELY PERMEABLE BARRIERS

Materials:
Two large beakers
Dialysis tubing
Tubing closures
Hot plate
Lugol's solution
Fehling's A and B solution
5% glucose solution
5% starch solution

Objective: Demonstrate properties of a semipermeable membrane.

1. Fill two 600 ml beakers with 400 ml of water.
2. Place one beaker on the hot plate and turn the hot plate to its highest setting. Leave the other beaker at room temperature.

3. Add 40 drops of Lugol's solution to the room temperature beaker. Lugol's solution contains iodine and is used as a starch indicator. The solution will change from brown to blue-black in the presence of starch.

4. Add 5 ml of Fehling's A solution and 5 ml of Fehling's B solution to the beaker on the hot plate. Fehling's solution must be handled carefully. Report any spills immediately to the instructor. The Fehling's solution should be blue, indicating the absence of glucose in the beaker. The presence of glucose will turn the solution from blue to green to orange to yellow.

5. Cut a 9-inch length of dialysis tubing. Wet the tubing under running water. The membrane will form a tube when opened by thoroughly wetting one end of the membrane with water and rubbing it between the thumb and forefinger. When opened, it should be thoroughly moistened by allowing water to run through it. Close one end with a dialysis tubing closure.

6. Fill the tube one-fourth with 5% glucose solution and one-fourth with 5% starch solution. Close the tube with another tubing closure.

7. Rinse the tube under running water to remove any glucose or starch on the outside. Gently mix the contents.

8. Place the tube across the room temperature beaker by allowing the tubing closure to hang over the sides of the beaker. Do not spill any of the contents into the beaker.

9. Wait 10 to 15 minutes, then examine the contents of the tube and beaker. Note what you see.

10. Next rinse off the tube again. Now place the tube across the beaker on the hot plate in the same manner as before. Wait several minutes for a reaction to occur. The solution must be hot for Fehling's solution to indicate the presence of glucose.

LABORATORY EXERCISES

Questions:
1. What happened to the iodine, starch, and glucose?

2. How could you tell which substances diffused through the membrane?

3. Did any substances not pass through the membrane?

LABORATORY EXERCISE 4-3

EFFECTS OF TONICITY OF EXTRACELLULAR FLUID ON CELL VOLUME

Materials:
0.9% (normal) saline
Distilled water
0.2%, 0.4%, 1.5% saline

Objective: Demonstrate the effect of isotonic, hypertonic, and hypotonic extracellular fluid on cell volume.
1. Obtain a sample of blood diluted to 20% with 0.9% saline (normal saline). Place on a microscope slide and cover with a coverslip. Observe the shape and size of the red blood cells.

2. Place a drop of 1.5% saline solution next to the coverslip. Place a piece of paper towel on the other side to draw the solution under the coverslip. Observe the red cells. What changes occur?

3. Repeat with 0.9% saline. Then with 0.4%, 0.2%, and 0% (distilled water). Observe what happens to the red cells.

4. Explain your results.

Questions:
Data: Molecular weights: C - 12 g/M, H - 1 g/M, O - 16 g/M, Na - 23 g/M, Cl - 35.5 g/M. Formulas: glucose $C_6H_{12}O_6$, sucrose $C_{12}H_{22}O_{11}$.

1. Compute the osmolarities of each solution (125% sucrose, 0.2%, 0.4%, 0.9%, and 1.5% saline solutions).

2. Determine what an isotonic solution would be for NaCl, $C_6H_{12}O_6$, and $C_{12}H_{22}O_{11}$ in g/dL (%).

3. Compute how much the volume of the red cells would have to change in each of the different saline solutions used in the experiments to become isosmotic with the extracellular fluid.

4. Contrast the effects of NaCl and starch solutions on the outside of the dialysis tubing on the movement of fluid up the thistle tube.

5. Why does NaCl have a different effect on red blood cells than on the dialysis tubing?

6. What is "normal saline?" What is the significance of this solution?

FIVE

Signaling

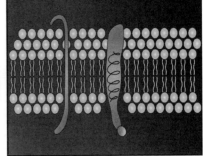

Glenn Irion, PhD, PT, CWS and Sarah N. Jerome, PhD, RRT

OBJECTIVES

1. List two basic types of signals.

2. Describe how neurons use electrical and chemical signals to communicate with other cells.

3. Define synapse; describe how electrical and chemical signals are used at synapses.

4. Contrast directed and nondirected synapses; list advantages and disadvantages of both types and where each type is more efficient than the other.

5. Contrast a neurohormone to a neurotransmitter and to a hormone.

6. Define paracrine, autocrine, and juxtacrine.

7. Describe how messages are sent by the endocrine system. Contrast signaling by the nervous system and endocrine system in terms of speed, duration, and specificity.

8. Describe how signal transduction occurs in opening ion channels.

9. Describe the transduction process involving cAMP and β-adrenergic receptors.

10. Describe the DAG transduction process.

11. Cite examples of ion channel, Ca-calmodulin, cAMP, and DAG transduction processes.

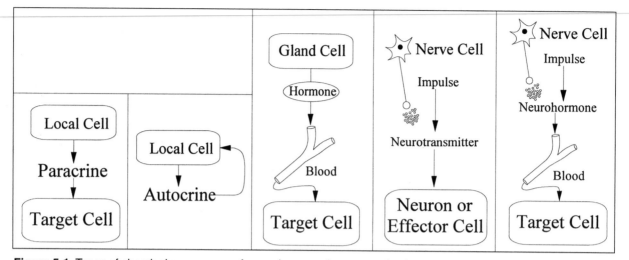

Figure 5-1. Types of chemical messengers. A neurohormone has properties in common with both hormones and neurotransmitters. It is released from a neuron but enters the blood and acts as a hormone.

Signaling mechanisms are very old, both phylogenetically and ontogenetically. Simple chemical messengers are used even by single-celled organisms. Immediately following fertilization, individual cells send chemical signals to each other to ensure proper development. As discussed in Chapter One, cells perform functions for themselves, but also provide specialized functions that benefit the entire organism. To ensure homeostasis, cells must communicate their needs to specialized cells and receive messages from other cells to increase or decrease their own specialized functions. The focus of this chapter is to provide an overview of signaling mechanisms ranging from those used to communicate with neighboring cells to those used to communicate with very distant cells. Factors that influence the speed of communication will also be discussed.

Cells modify their activity in response to information, or signals, received from their environment. These input signals may take several forms, including mechanical, chemical, and electrical. Many cells also respond to light and temperature. Pressure and sheering forces placed on cells may produce a variety of chemical or electrical changes within cells. Electrical signals involve changes in membrane potential. Local, or graded potentials, are localized to a small area of membrane, while the action potential is a stereotyped electrical disturbance of the membrane that propagates along the entire cell membrane in all directions from the site of origin. Electrical signals can also be passed from a cell to its neighbors by the flow of ions through gap junctions. Gap junctions are used by cardiac muscle cells and some types of smooth muscle cells to relay the message to

contract. A minority of neurons also communicate with each other via gap junctions.

Chemical signals are the most common method by which cells communicate with each other. Soluble chemical signals are characterized either according to the cell of origin or the mode of delivery to the recipient cell. Paracrine secretions involve chemicals released from one cell that reach nearby cells via diffusion through the extracellular space, while autocrine secretions act on the cell that produced them. These forms of communication are efficient only when the diffusion distance for the chemical remains short. A recently described mechanism of communication is called juxtacrine, which implies that the signal is sent to a neighboring cell. This type of communication is used by growth factors and does not involve the release of chemicals. Rather, the molecular signal is expressed on the surface of one membrane and binds to a receptor on its neighbor to stimulate development of the neighbor.

Nerve cells are specialized to conduct electrical signals with great speed and over long distances where they ultimately cause the release of chemical signals known as neurotransmitters. These signals then act in a paracrine-type fashion where they diffuse across a short synaptic space to reach the target cell. Some secretory products gain access to the bloodstream, where they are then delivered to distant target organs. This mode of communication is known as endocrine secretion; the secretory product is called a hormone. A final category of cell communication is referred to as neuroendocrine in which the nerve cell releases its secretion, a neurohormone, into the bloodstream to be carried to a distant target cell. These types of signals are depicted in Figure 5-1.

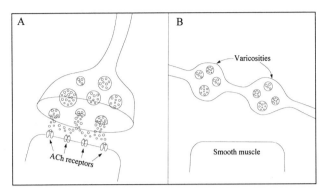

Figure 5-2. Synapse. A: directed synapse of the neuromuscular junction in which a neurotransmitter is released a few nanometers from the receptor across the synaptic cleft. Response is rapid, but many neurons and branches of neurons are required. B: a nondirected synapse of the autonomic nervous system in which norepinephrine is released from varicosities over many smooth muscle cells. The neurotransmitter must diffuse longer distances, but a rapid response is not required for function of this tissue. Binding of neurotransmitter to receptors on some cells leads to depolarization of neighboring cells via gap junctions; therefore, fewer neurons or branches of neurons are required.

NEURONS

Neurons may be a meter or longer in some individuals and can transmit a signal very rapidly. Large neurons propagate their signals at a rate of 60 m/s or faster. A change in the neuron's membrane potential is associated with the exocytosis of vesicles, each containing hundreds of molecules of neurotransmitter. Neurons take very specific courses from the central nervous system to peripheral organs or from peripheral organs to the central nervous system. Neurons originating in the brain or spinal cord receive chemical signals that cause them to depolarize, producing a signal called an action potential, which propagates along neurons. The action potential causes the release of neurotransmitter at the distal end of the neuron. When neurons that originate in the peripheral tissues and enter the central nervous system are depolarized, they release neurotransmitter on other neurons in the brain or spinal cord. A signal from the brain or spinal cord is delivered rapidly to a specific area of tissue by the nervous system. Some neurons, called interneurons, relay information just within the central nervous system.

SYNAPSES

The specificity of the nervous system for its target tissues varies with the type of nerve and target tissue. The junction between a nerve cell and its target tissue is called a synapse Two basic types of synapses are illustrated in Figure 5-2. A neuron may synapse with exocrine glands (cells that release chemicals into ducts, such as tears, pancreatic enzymes, and sweat), endocrine glands, muscle cells (skeletal, cardiac, or smooth muscle), or other neurons. Highly specialized contacts with specific single cells are called directed synapses. An example of a directed synapse is the neuromuscular junction between an α motor neuron and a skeletal muscle cell. The neuron terminates in an indentation in the skeletal muscle (Figure 5-3) cell where receptors for the neurotransmitter acetylcholine are located. The actual release sites on the nerve terminal are lined up directly with the receptors so that the neurotransmitter molecules only need to diffuse a few nanometers to reach the receptors. Neurons may have many branches, ranging from 10 to thousands for α motor neurons, so that many cells can receive the same signal almost simultaneously from the same neuron. Directed synapses are very efficient in terms of producing a response at the target cells rapidly, but are inefficient in terms of the large number of neurons or branches of neurons required to innervate the target cells and the large quantity of neurotransmitter released.

NONDIRECTED SYNAPSES

The nondirected synapse is used by cells that do not require a rapid response of the target cells. Nondirected synapses are often observed in tissues such as smooth muscle on which neurotransmitters of the autonomic nervous system are released into the interstitial fluid around the target cells. Nerves that participate in nondirected synapses have branches that cover the surface of the target cells, but there is no one-to-one relationship between branches of the nerves and the target cells. In contrast to directed synapses that release neurotransmitter at the nerve terminals directly on the target cells, nerves with nondirected synapses have release sites called varicosities along the branches that release neurotransmitters from several locations along the branches that cover the surface of the tissue. Only a few receptors of the target cells need to bind the neurotransmitter to cause a physiologic effect throughout the tissue. Some cells near the varicosities on the autonomic nerve bind the neurotransmitter, which causes the smooth muscle cells to respond. Smooth muscle cells within the tissue then communicate with each other via gap junctions. Nondirected synapses in such tissues are efficient in terms of the number of neurons and amount of neurotransmitter released but are slow to produce a response in the target tissue.

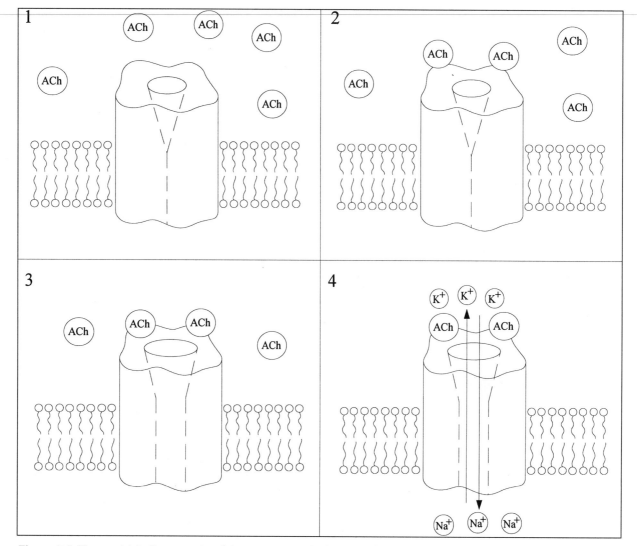

Figure 5-3. The acetylcholine receptor of the neuromuscular junction of skeletal muscle acts as a receptor and ion channel. Binding of acetylcholine causes a change in the shape of proteins making up the receptor/ion channel, resulting in the ability of Na and K ions to pass through the membrane.

NEUROHORMONES

A signaling intermediate between endocrine and neural is called a neurohormone. The endocrine system releases hormones from gland cells. The nervous system has neurons that take very specific paths to pass signals from one location to another that may be very far away. Neurohormones are produced by neurons, but they function as hormones. Neurons release them into the interstitial fluid where they diffuse into blood vessels, circulate in the blood, diffuse out of blood vessels in other parts of the body, and bind to specific receptors on target cells. The difference between hormones and neurohormones is that neurohormones are released by cells that are neurons histologically, not gland cells. The most important neurohormones are oxytocin and antidiuretic hormone, which are released by cells of the posterior pituitary, and release hormones that the hypothalamus produces to signal release of hormones by the anterior pituitary.

PARACRINE AND AUTOCRINE CELLS

The most primitive signaling mechanisms are those that release chemical signals into the interstitial fluid to influence cells within diffusion distance. Two types of signaling methods fall into this category: paracrine and autocrine. The terms paracrine and autocrine are derived from the word endocrine. Whereas the endocrine system distributes chemical messengers throughout the body by secreting hormones that diffuse into the blood, paracrine and autocrine cells release messengers that produce their effects by staying in the interstitial fluid. The messengers released by paracrine cells affect nearby cells. Autocrine cells release chemical messengers that act on the same cells that release them.

ENDOCRINE SYSTEM

A method that allows signals to be sent throughout the body is provided by the endocrine system. The endocrine system consists of specialized organs that release chemical signals called hormones, which diffuse into the blood. The hormones circulate in the blood, diffuse into the interstitial space in distant tissues, and bind to specific receptors on cells called target cells. The hormone is distributed throughout the body, but is only effective when it binds to the receptors for it on the target cells. Although hormones, in general, produce a slower response than release of neurotransmitters by nerves, the effect of endocrine signaling is longer lasting, because the hormone circulates in the blood. In contrast, for a nerve to sustain a signal, it must intermittently release neurotransmitter frequently for a long time. Examples of endocrine glands include the anterior pituitary or adenohypophysis ("gland" part of the pituitary), the thyroid gland, parathyroid glands, adrenal glands, ovaries, and testicles. Other tissues producing hormones include other parts of the brain, stomach, intestines, pancreas, skin, and kidney. Different types of hormones require differing amounts of time to have an effect. Hormones that bind to surface receptors, such as peptides and the catecholamines, may evoke a response rapidly once they bind to a target cell. Thyroid hormones and steroid hormones, such as sex hormones, aldosterone, and cortisol, involve intracellular receptors and interact with DNA. These hormones, therefore, may require minutes to hours to produce their effects. Discussion of specific hormones will await until the specific organ system in which these hormones play a physiologic role is discussed.

Often, the pituitary gland is called the master gland of the endocrine system. It releases hormones that affect other glands, such as the thyroid gland, the adrenal glands, and the gonads, and also releases growth hormone. The pituitary consists of two distinct parts with different functions and embryonic origins. These are the anterior pituitary, which was mentioned above, and the posterior pituitary, which is also called the neurohypophysis, because the posterior pituitary is not a gland, but a collection of nerve cells that secrete neurohormones. These two organs have two things in common: their location and the fact that the hypothalamus controls them both. Although the anterior pituitary does release hormones that control the function of other hormones, the hypothalamus controls the release of the hormones secreted by the anterior pituitary. For example, the release of thyroid hormones is increased by the release of thyroid-stimulating hormone (TSH) by the anterior pituitary, but the hypothalamus controls the release of TSH by secreting thyrotrophin-releasing factor. The posterior pituitary is essentially an extension of the hypothalamus. Neurons originating in the hypothalamus continue into the posterior pituitary and release one of two different hormones: oxytocin, which controls milk ejection and promotes uterine contraction during childbirth, and antidiuretic hormone (ADH), which is also known as vasopressin because of its effect on blood vessels. ADH causes the renal tubules to reabsorb more water, thus preventing diuresis. Because the hypothalamus controls the anterior pituitary and is the origin of the neurons that release the posterior pituitary hormones, the title of "Master Gland of the Endocrine System" should belong to the hypothalamus, not the pituitary gland.

SIGNAL TRANSDUCTION

Dispersed along the outer surface of the plasma membrane of cells are specialized receptors that bind specific chemical messengers that contact the cell. The combination of messenger with specific receptor triggers a sequence of events within the target cell that ultimately controls a particular cellular activity. The sequence of steps between binding of a chemical to a receptor and the response of the target cell is termed signal transduction. For example, an α motor neuron releases acetylcholine onto receptors on skeletal muscle cells, which leads to contraction of skeletal muscle cells. The steps of signal transduction that occur between the binding of acetylcholine and shortening of skeletal muscle cells take place in less than one millisecond. In spite of the numerous possible cellular responses, there are two basic mechanisms by which binding of the extracellular chemical signal (the first messenger) is able to bring about the cellular response. One mechanism involves the opening or closing of specific channels within the membrane, thereby regulating the movement of ions into or out of the cell. A second mechanism involves the transfer of the signal to an intracellular chemical messenger (the second messenger), which in turn produces a series of intracellular events within the target cell.

The example given in Chapter Three of the acetylcholine receptor represents a simple mechanism, in which the receptor at the neuromuscular junction of skeletal muscle is part of the ion channel complex itself. However, many signal transduction processes are much more complex and involve several proteins. For example, binding of ligand to a G-protein-linked receptor or a change in membrane potential may be required to change the shape of several proteins in sequence to cause the proteins of the ion channel to change shape to either open or close specific types of ion channels.

G-protein receptors are commonly involved in the signal transduction process. G-proteins derive their name from the guanine nucleotide-binding protein family that links them to the effector molecule that ultimately causes the cellular response. All members of the G-protein receptor family bind guanine nucleotides and have intrinsic GTPase activity; that is, they convert guanosine triphosphate (GTP) to guanosine diphosphate (GDP). Upon binding its signal molecule, the receptor interacts with the G-protein, producing a conformational change whereby the G-protein exchanges its GDP for a molecule of GTP and then dissociates from the receptor. The free G-protein-GTP complex can then interact with intracellular proteins that will initiate cellular responses. For example, the activated G-protein uses the energy available from the high-energy phosphate of GTP to interact with an ion channel, a peripheral protein such as adenylate cyclase, which in turn generates a second messenger called cyclic AMP (cAMP), or phospholipase C, which in turn generates the second messengers diacylglycerol (DAG) and inositol triphosphate (IP$_3$). Activation of the G-protein may either inhibit or stimulate the next protein in the sequence. Therefore, binding of a ligand to a G-protein-linked receptor may open an ion channel, close an ion channel, increase production of cAMP, DAG, and IP$_3$, or decrease production of cAMP, DAG, and IP$_3$. The general features of second messenger systems are depicted in Figure 5-4.

Calcium ions allowed to enter the cell with opening of certain types of ion channels may themselves be used as second messengers, largely because their concentration within the cytoplasm can undergo rapid and dramatic changes. That is, after stimulation by some agonists, the concentration of free calcium may increase by 10-fold or more. This increase is caused, in part, by release of calcium from within the endoplasmic reticulum and, in part, by an influx of calcium from the extracellular fluid through membrane calcium channels that can be induced to change their configuration and open to allow calcium entry. Increased calcium concentration activates numerous enzymes and triggers events such as muscular contraction. While calcium can act alone, it generally binds reversibly with a protein called calmodulin. The calcium-calmodulin complex is then able to bind to certain enzymes, usually protein kinases, thus activating or inactivating them. One important use of calcium-calmodulin is activation of smooth muscle contraction. Of particular importance is the α-adrenergic receptor. Binding of norepinephrine or related ligands to the α receptor opens specific calcium ion channels in the membrane that lead to smooth muscle cell contraction via the calcium-calmodulin system. Calcium ion channels may also be opened by changes in membrane potential, which causes calcium to bind to calmodulin and smooth muscle contraction to occur.

Another important second messenger mentioned already is cyclic adenosine monophosphate (cyclic AMP, cAMP). Cyclic AMP is formed from ATP by the enzyme adenylyl cyclase, which is located near G-protein receptors within the plasma membrane. Cyclic AMP then produces many of its effects on cellular processes via activation of the enzyme, protein kinase A, which catalyzes the transfer of a phosphate group of ATP to other cellular proteins to increase or decrease their activity. For example, production of cAMP in some types of smooth muscle activates a protein kinase that causes calcium ions to be actively transported out of cells and causes them to relax. In contrast, in ventricular heart cells, cAMP causes the amount of calcium in the cells to increase and increases the force of contraction of these cells. In cells that initiate the heart beat, cAMP causes the cells to initiate heart beats more frequently. The second messenger, cyclic AMP, is produced in many different cells, always functioning to mediate the intracellular action of many different agents, each of which produces a uniquely different pattern of cellular response because of different protein kinases expressed inside the cell. Thus, the same second messenger mediates both hepatic cell glucose production, smooth muscle cell relaxation, and many other functions.

Although physiological functions may be altered by increasing or decreasing the amount of ligand that leads to production of cAMP, such as epinephrine, norepinephrine, ADH, and glucagon, a second method for altering cAMP exists. An enzyme called phosphodiesterase is used in the cell to turn off cell functions by breaking down cAMP in cells. Certain drugs may either block the effect of phosphodiesterase or mimic its effect, changing the quantity of cAMP. Aminophylline is a drug used to treat bronchospasm in diseases such as asthma by inhibiting phosphodiesterase. Inhibition of phosphodiesterase allows cAMP to accumulate in the bronchial smooth muscle cell, which, in turn, causes calcium to be actively transported out of the cell. Removal of calcium allows the smooth muscle cells to relax and free breathing to be restored. Alternatively, bronchospasm can be treated by drugs such as epinephrine and synthetic

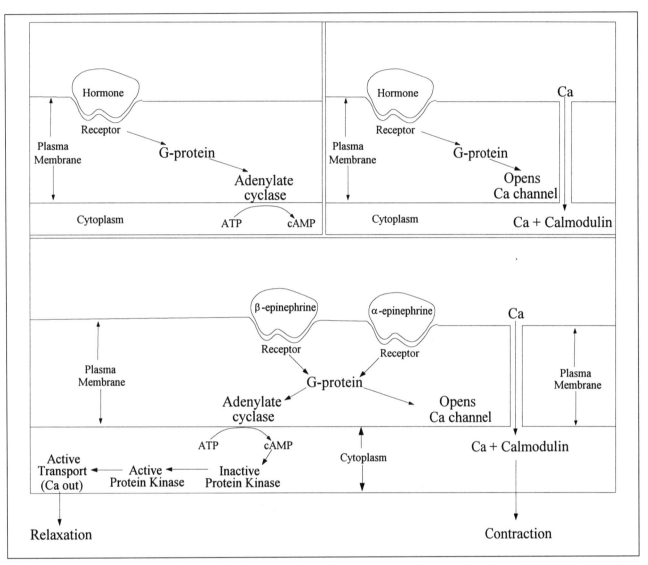

Figure 5-4. Second messenger systems. A: Binding of a ligand to a receptor activates a G-protein, which in turn may either inhibit or stimulate adenylate cyclase, resulting in a change in cAMP production. B: Binding of a ligand to a receptor activates a G-protein, which, in turn, opens a Ca channel. Ca binds to calmodulin, altering cell function. C: Both α and β receptors may be occupied by epinephrine with possibly different effects. Binding to the α receptor results in opening of a Ca ion channel and smooth muscle contraction, whereas binding to a β receptor causes production of cAMP, transport of Ca out of the cell, and smooth muscle cell relaxation.

analogs that bind to β-receptors. Cyclic AMP, via activation of protein kinase A, can also be used to activate proteins, which, in turn, cause messenger RNA transcription of specific areas of DNA to be stimulated or inhibited, resulting in increased or decreased protein synthesis by the cell.

Instead of being linked to adenylyl cyclase, some G-protein receptors are coupled with another enzyme known as phospholipase C (PLC). Interaction of G-proteins with their agonists activates the membrane-bound phospholipase C. Phospholipase C then hydrolyzes the membrane phospholipid phosphatidylinositol 4,5-

triphosphate into diacylglycerol (DAG) and inositol 1,4,5-triphosphate (IP_3) (Figure 5-5). Both compounds function as second messengers. DAG plays two important roles as a second messenger. DAG activates protein kinase C, which, like protein kinase A, catalyzes the phosphorylation of certain enzymes, thus activating or inactivating them. A second role involves the conversion of DAG into arachidonic acid, which is then converted into two families of chemical signals called prostaglandins and leukotrienes. Corticosteroids, used as anti-inflammatory drugs, prevent the conversion of phosphatidylinositol to DAG; aspirin is useful as an anti-inflammatory drug by preventing the conversion of arachidonic acid into prostaglandins. Recently, new drugs have been developed to treat the inflammation underlying asthma by preventing the synthesis of leukotrienes or blocking their receptors.

Inositol triphosphate, which is released into the cytosol along with DAG, binds with plasma membrane receptors within the endoplasmic reticulum to bring about the release of stored calcium. This resulting increase in free cytosolic calcium complements the effects of DAG in activating protein kinase C. The increased concentration of free cytosolic calcium can then cause a variety of cellular responses.

Numerous other types of signaling mechanisms exist. While its role is less well understood than that of cyclic AMP, cyclic 3',5'-guanosine monophosphate (cGMP) functions as a second messenger. Many cells have been shown to express guanylyl cyclase activity and cGMP-dependent protein kinase. For example, cGMP is the intracellular mediator of the effects of nitric oxide on smooth muscle relaxation. Many agents, including hormones, cytokines, and growth factors, stimulate their target cells by interacting with membrane-bound receptors that use another mechanism involving enzymes called tyrosine kinases. Cyclic GMP is also broken down by a form of phosphodiesterase. The popular drug Viagra inhibits a specific type of phosphodiesterase, allowing cGMP to accumulate and produce Viagra's intended effect.

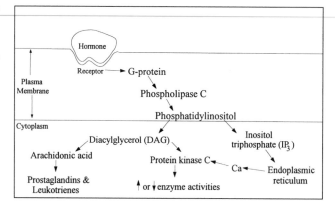

Figure 5-5. DAG/IP$_3$ mechanism. Binding of a ligand to a G-protein-linked receptor causes activation of phospholipase C, which in turn converts phosphatidylinositol to DAG and IP$_3$. DAG may be converted to arachidonic acid, which then gives rise to prostaglandins and leukotrienes, or it may activate protein kinase C. IP$_3$ causes release of Ca needed for protein kinase C activity.

requires many neurons and branches of neurons and large amounts of neurotransmitter. A nondirected synapse is effective for signals that may be received more slowly. The series of steps between detection of a chemical messenger and a physiologic response is called signal transduction. Signal transduction usually involves either ion channels or the production of a second messenger. The commonly used mechanisms of cyclic AMP, DAG/IP$_3$, and Ca-calmodulin are described.

SUMMARY

Two basic forms of signaling mechanisms exist: electrical and chemical. Electrical signaling occurs across gap junctions of cardiac and smooth muscle cells and a small number of neurons. Endocrine, paracrine, autocrine, and nervous systems use chemical messengers. Endocrine signaling involves the release of a hormone that diffuses into the blood and is carried throughout the body in the circulatory system. The hormone diffuses out of the blood and binds to receptors on target tissues to produce an effect. Hormonal mechanisms are generally slower, but are longer lasting than the nervous system. Paracrine mechanisms release chemicals into the interstitial space and influence nearby cells only. Autocrine cells release chemicals that affect themselves only. Nerve cells release chemicals called neurotransmitters onto fairly specific targets. At a directed synapse, a nerve cell releases neurotransmitter onto a specific site on a single cell. At a nondirected synapse, neurotransmitter is released onto a wider area. A directed synapse is required to produce a rapid response but

BIBLIOGRAPHY

Aguilar-Bryan L, Clement JP IV, Gonzalez G, Kunjilwar K, Babenko A, Bryan J. Toward understanding the assembly and structure on K+ATP channels. *Physiological Reviews.* 1998;78:227-245.

Argetsinger LS, Carter-Su C. Mechanism of signaling by growth hormone receptor. *Physiological Reviews.* 1996;76:1089-1107.

Dockray GJ, Varro A, Dimaline R. Gastric endocrine cells: gene expression, processing, and targeting of active products. *Physiological Reviews.* 1996;76:767-798.

Holder JR, Klinshin A, Sedoua M, Hüser J, Blatter LA. Capacitative calcium entry. *News in Physiological Sciences.* 1998;13:157-163.

Janmey PA. The cytoskeleton and cell signaling component, localization, and mechanical coupling. *Physiological Reviews.* 1998;78:763-781.

Latone R. The intimacies of potassium channels revealed. *News in Physiological Sciences.* 1993;8:1-2.

Lee HC. A signaling pathway involving cyclic ADP-ribose, cGMP, and nitric oxide. *News in Physiological Sciences.* 1994;9:134-137.

Lee HC. Mechanism of calcium signaling by cyclic ADP-ribose and NAADP. *Physiological Reviews.* 1997;77:1133-1164.

Metcalfe DD, Baram D, Mekori YA. Mast cells. *Physiological Reviews*. 1997;77:1033-1079.

Navar LG, Inscho EW, Majid DSA, Imig JD, Harrison-Bernard LM, Mitchell KD. Paracrine regulation of the renal microcirculation. *Physiological Reviews*. 1996;76:425-536.

Nemeth EF. Calcium receptor-dependent regulation of cellular function. *News in Physiological Sciences*. 1995;10:1-5.

Palmer LG. Epithelial sodium channels and their kin. *News in Physiological Sciences*. 1995;10:61-67.

Pozzan T, Rizzuto R, Volpe P, Meldolesi J. Molecular and cellular physiology of intracellular calcium stores. *Physiological Reviews*. 1994;74:595-636.

Pusch M, Jentsch TJ. Molecular physiology of voltage-gated chloride channels. *Physiological Reviews*. 1994;74:813-827.

Rehfeld JF. The new biology of gastrointestinal hormones. *Physiological Reviews*. 1998;78:1087-1108.

Reneman RS. Endothelial cells as mechanoreceptors. *News in Physiological Sciences*. 1993;8:55-56.

Robinson JD. Steps to the sodium-potassium pump and sodium-potassium ATPase. *News in Physiological Sciences*. 1995;10:184-188.

Sims SM, Janssen LJ. Cholinergic excitation of smooth muscle. *News in Physiological Sciences*. 1993;8:207-212.

Somlyo A. Modulation of the calcium switch by G proteins, kinase, and phosphate. *News in Physiological Sciences*. 1993;8:2.

Taglialatela M, Brown AM. Structural correlates of potassium channel function. *News in Physiological Sciences*. 1994;9:169-173.

STUDY QUESTIONS

1. Compare the signaling mechanisms of the endocrine and nervous system in terms of speed of response, specificity, and duration. What is the benefit of nervous system control of skeletal muscle? What is the benefit of endocrine control of body fluid volume and composition?

2. Contrast the directed and non-directed synapse. What is the benefit of using a directed synapse for skeletal muscle? What is the benefit of using a non-directed synapse on the smooth muscle of the gastrointestinal system?

3. Signal transduction at the neuromuscular junction is very simple. What benefit is derived from its simplicity in terms of the function of skeletal muscle?

4. Signal transduction in smooth muscle cells is very complex, involving ligand, electrical signals, and several intracellular second messengers. How does this benefit the function of smooth muscle cells in the gastrointestinal tract that require a degree of tone that must change gradually with events such as feeding?

S I X

Fluid Regulation

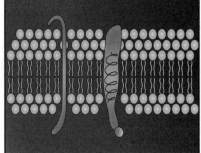

1. Describe the distribution of body fluids between intracellular and extracellular fluid, interstitial fluid, and plasma.

2. Describe how balance of fluid between intra- and extracellular fluid spaces is determined.

3. Describe how relative volumes of plasma and interstitial fluid are balanced; cite factors causing plasma volume to be lost to interstitial volume.

4. Define edema, ascites, joint, pericardial and pleural effusion, and hydrocephalus.

5. Contrast the composition of plasma, interstitial fluid, and intracellular fluid in terms of concentrations of sodium, potassium, chlorine ions, and protein.

6. Name the functional regions of the nephron; state the primary function of each region.

7. List three basic processes of the nephron and how they relate to the function of excretion.

8. Describe the roles of ADH and aldosterone in renal function.

9. Describe the stimuli for release of ADH and mechanisms by which ADH conserves water.

10. Describe stimuli for release of aldosterone and how it participates in negative feedback control of blood pressure and sodium content of extracellular fluid.

11. Describe how extracellular potassium ion concentration is regulated and the result of conflict with sodium ion regulation.

12. Describe how calcium ion concentration is regulated and the effect on bones and the nervous system.

13. Describe the roles of magnesium ion and how it is regulated.

14. Describe the process of micturition in terms of the bladder reflex, cortical influence modulating the reflex, and the role of voluntary muscles in micturition.

The chemical reactions necessary for life occur within an aqueous environment; molecules and ions diffusing through water encounter other molecules and ions, producing the chemical reactions necessary for homeostasis. As discussed in Chapter Four, nutrients are transported from the blood to the interstitial fluid and from the interstitial fluid to the intracellular fluid. To ensure normal function, many substances must exist in different concentrations in different body fluids. For example, the concentration of sodium ions in the interstitial fluid and blood is much higher than in the intracellular fluid, and the concentration of potassium is much higher in the intracellular fluid than in the blood or interstitial fluid. If these differences are not maintained, cells become very sick or die. This chapter describes the normal composition of body fluids and how the composition is regulated.

The importance of regulating water volume becomes obvious when we appreciate that water accounts for approximately 70% of our mass other than fat tissue (lean body mass). Almost the whole of the volume of the adipocytes (fat cells) consists of fatty acids with very little water. Taking fat mass into account, 50% of body mass of women and 60% of the body mass of men consists of water. For convenience in discussing regulation of body fluids, we discuss different "compartments." We can compare the volume and composition of fluid that is within cells (intracellular) to that outside cells (extracellular). Approximately two-thirds of the body water is intracellular, and one-third is extracellular. For the sake of simplicity, the intracellular fluid is discussed as a single compartment, rather than considering 75 billion separate compartments, one for each cell. To refine our discussion of body fluids further, we make the distinction between the fluid that directly bathes individual cells, called interstitial fluid, and the fluid part of the blood that transports nutrients and wastes via the circulation, which we call plasma. We also have several minor compartments that are typically associated with particular organs that will be discussed below. Of the extracellular fluid, approximately three-quarters is interstitial fluid, and one-quarter is plasma. For example, the average 70 kg individual would have 42 L of total body water divided into 28 L of intracellular water and 14 L of extracellular fluid. The extracellular fluid is then divided into 11 L of interstitial fluid and 3 L of plasma. As a percentage of body weight, total body water is 60%, intracellular fluid is 40%, extracellular fluid is 20%, interstitial fluid is 15%, and plasma is 5%. These volumes are summarized in Figure 6-1.

Added, large amounts of fluids are located in spe-

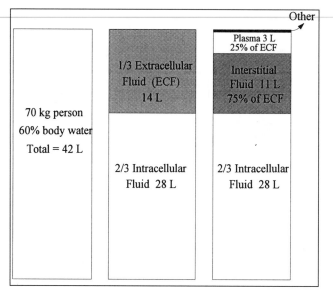

Figure 6-1. Distribution of body fluids. Body water constitutes approximately 60% of body mass. In a 70 kg person, total body water is 70 kg ˇ 0.60 = 42 L. Two-thirds of body water exists in the intracellular space; one-third is extracellular. Of the extracellular fluid, 25% is plasma, and 75% is interstitial fluid. Other compartments normally make up a small percentage but may increase markedly in disease.

cialized compartments, and the size of these compartments can increase greatly with disease. The cerebral ventricles and spinal canal contain about 150 ml of specialized fluid called cerebrospinal fluid (CSF). In terms of protecting the central nervous system (CNS) from trauma, maintaining the volume of this fluid is particularly important. Because the CSF is contained in a closed area, excessive pressure could damage the brain or spinal cord. Low pressure, on the other hand, reduces the cushioning effect of the CSF on the brain and spinal cord. The gastrointestinal tract varies tremendously in the quantity of fluid. Following a meal, as much as 6 L of fluid may enter the gastrointestinal tract. Failure to reabsorb this fluid, as occurs in various forms of diarrhea, can produce profound changes in the volume and composition of the body fluids. Small amounts of fluid are located in the pericardium, peritoneum, and intrapleural space. Disease states can greatly increase the volume of these spaces and interfere with filling of the heart and expansion of the lungs. Pathologic volumes of fluid in the pericardial and pleural spaces are called pericardial and pleural effusions, respectively. Injuries to synovial joints cause them to fill with fluid, producing a joint effusion. Accumulation of fluid in the abdomen is called ascites. A general term for excess interstitial fluid due to upset of fluid balance is called edema.

TABLE 6-1

Ionic Composition of Body Fluids

ION FLUID	PLASMA	INTERSTITIAL FLUID	INTRACELLULAR
Na^+	142	145	12
K^+	4	4	135
Cl^-	104	117	4
$HCO3^-$	24	27	12
Proteins	14	0	25

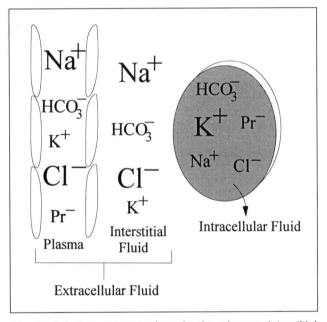

Figure 6-2. Ion concentrations in the plasma, interstitial fluid, and intracellular fluid. Interstitial fluid may be approximated as an NaCl solution. Plasma varies from interstitial fluid by the presence of plasma proteins. Intracellular fluid is characterized by its low Na and high K concentration.

COMPOSITION OF BODY FLUIDS

The major differences between intra- and extracellular fluid are the concentrations of sodium and potassium. Intracellular fluid has a much greater concentration of potassium and a much lower concentration of sodium (Figure 6-2). Maintaining these concentration differences, as we will see in this and subsequent chapters, is critically important. Plasma differs from interstitial fluid by the presence of plasma proteins. These proteins have several functions, but, in terms of the regulation of fluid volume, plasma proteins play a vital role in maintaining the plasma volume relative to the interstitial volume. Because of factors discussed in Chapter Four (the Donnan effect), the fluid compartments also differ in their anion concentrations. Because of the negatively

charged proteins present inside cells, the concentrations of chloride and bicarbonate ions are lower than those found in extracellular fluid and, because of plasma proteins, are slightly lower in the plasma compared with interstitial fluid.

DISTRIBUTION OF WATER AMONG FLUID SPACES

In general, water is free to move between the intracellular fluid and the interstitial fluid and is free to move between the interstitial fluid and plasma. Specific exceptions will be discussed below. The factors that determine the relative amounts of fluid among the different compartments are related to osmotic pressure, which is determined by the distribution of osmotically active particles. For the cells, sodium is the major solute responsible for movement of water between intracellular and extracellular compartments by osmosis. Therefore, the major factor determining how fluid is divided into intracellular fluid and extracellular fluid is the **amount**, not **concentration**, of sodium in the extracellular fluid. When sodium and water are ingested, they move across the intestine into the blood and equilibrate with the interstitial fluid. Water is free to move into either the intracellular or extracellular compartment based on osmotic pressure, whereas sodium is confined to the extracellular compartment due to the Na/K pump. Because sodium represents such a large proportion of the extracellular solute, the amount of sodium in the extracellular fluid chiefly determines its osmolarity. One may reasonably estimate extracellular osmolarity as double the concentration of sodium in the interstitial fluid. Normally, the interstitial fluid concentration of sodium is 145 mM, which gives us the estimate of an interstitial fluid osmolarity of approximately 290 mOsm. If the concentration of sodium increases due to an increase in the amount of sodium in the body (eg, by consuming table salt), interstitial osmolarity increases, and water is driven out of cells until the osmolarities of the intracellular and extracellular fluids become equal, and extracellular fluid volume increases at the expense of intracellular volume. Conversely, if water is consumed with a lower concentration of sodium than body fluids, the amount of sodium in the body becomes diluted, reducing extracellular osmolarity and driving proportionally more water into cells than the amount of ingested fluid that remains in the extracellular space, increasing both intracellular and extracellular fluid volumes with a greater increase in the intracellular volume.

Regulation of body fluid volume and composition is described later in this chapter. For now, we can say that the osmolarity of the extracellular fluid can be increased by a loss of water from the body due to the lack of water conservation by the renal system or due to profuse sweating (sweat is hypotonic). These situations can be life-threatening by altering the concentrations of particular ions in the body fluids and by reducing the volume of the intracellular space. If large amounts of water are lost from the intracellular space, cells can be severely damaged, especially those that are anchored in specific locations. For example, cerebral blood vessels can be torn when the brain shrinks secondary to loss of fluid. Consumption of sodium increases extracellular osmolarity and extracellular fluid volume at the expense of intracellular fluid volume.

Osmolarity of fluids is decreased by the excessive consumption of water or the loss of sodium conservation by the kidney. When water only is ingested, it is absorbed from the gastrointestinal fluid, rendering the extracellular fluid hypotonic. Water is driven by osmotic pressure into the intracellular fluid until osmolarity becomes equal. If large quantities of water are ingested faster than the kidney can excrete the excess water, cerebral swelling will occur, resulting in a state called water intoxication. This syndrome is characterized by headaches, drowsiness, convulsions, and possibly permanent brain damage.

In some individuals, the volume of extracellular fluid is pathologically excessive. This occurs in congestive heart failure and in some individuals with high blood pressure. In these individuals, a therapeutic decrease in the amount of sodium in the body is desired to reduce extracellular fluid volume. Decreased sodium intake and an increased renal excretion of sodium accomplish this goal.

The osmolarity of plasma is slightly greater than that of the interstitial fluid due to the presence of proteins in the plasma. Water and other solutes move freely across capillaries, so the high osmotic pressure of the interstitial fluid of 5400 mmHg produces no net movement of fluid across capillaries. Plasma proteins, however, do not normally pass easily across capillaries in most tissues.

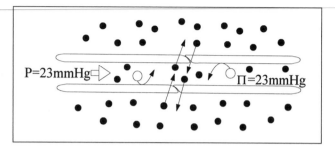

Figure 6-3. Hydrostatic pressure and oncotic pressure are approximately equal in capillaries. The tendency of hydrostatic pressure to drive water and solute into the interstitial fluid is offset by the presence of the nonpenetrating plasma proteins, which decrease the number of interactions of water inside the capillary to approximately the same extent that the hydrostatic pressure increases the number of interactions. This results in a small net loss of fluid from capillaries in general, although some capillaries may lose fluid, while others gain fluid from the interstitial space.

Only in tissues such as the liver and spleen, where large molecules must be able to pass into and out of blood vessels, or following injury to a blood vessel and during inflammation, do proteins cross capillaries to any extent. This small concentration of nonpenetrating solute would produce net movement of water into capillaries in the absence of any other forces. However, a mechanical force, blood pressure inside capillaries, is approximately equal to the 23 mmHg osmotic pressure generated by plasma proteins (Figure 6-3). Therefore, the relative volumes of the interstitial fluid and plasma are maintained by the presence of nonpenetrating proteins within the blood vessels and the hydrostatic pressure of blood within vessels. Loss of fluid from the plasma, causing excessive fluid volume of the interstitial space and swelling, is called edema. Circulatory factors causing edema will be discussed in Chapter Twenty-Two. Decreases in the amount of plasma protein in the blood can produce tremendous edema. The amount of plasma protein can be reduced either by decreased synthesis or loss of proteins in the urine. The liver produces plasma proteins from ingested amino acids; malnutrition or liver disease results in decreased synthesis. Plasma proteins are normally not filtered or excreted in the urine, but kidney disease can cause proteins to be excreted in tremendous quantities.

Fluid balance among the three major compartments is attained by both neural and hormonal regulation of fluid volume and osmolarity. In emergencies, plasma volume can be expanded by replacing lost blood, infusing plasma, or a plasma substitute such as dextran, which contains non-penetrating solute. If isotonic saline only is used to replace blood volume, only 25% of it will remain in the blood, and 75% of it will go into the interstitial

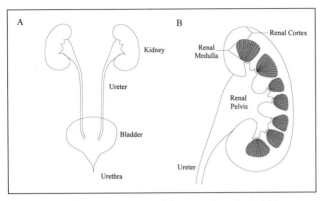

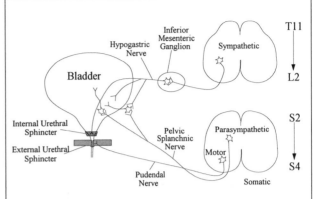

Figure 6-4. A: components of the renal system. Urine produced in the kidneys moves by bulk flow through the ureters to the bladder, from which it is intermittently voided via the urethra. B: Cross-section of the human kidney.

Figure 6-5. The micturition reflex.

space for reasons discussed above. The kidney is largely responsible for maintaining fluid volume and concentration. The mechanisms will be described later in this chapter. When the kidney fails to perform these functions adequately, hemodialysis or peritoneal dialysis is used to maintain fluid composition.

THE KIDNEY

The kidney performs its function of regulating body fluids by receiving a large portion of the cardiac output and actively adjusting its composition. The renal arteries combined carry approximately 20% of the cardiac output. As described below, a large fraction of the plasma entering the kidney will be subjected to renal functions. The kidney has several functions related to maintenance of fluid composition. They include the obvious function of excretion, but also some endocrine functions that maintain fluid ion composition, volume, osmolarity, and red blood cell production. The parts of the kidney are shown in Figure 6-4. Each kidney is an encapsulated organ that consists of approximately 1 million units called nephrons. The nephrons (renal tubules) are long coiled tubules that produce the fluid called urine and drain into the renal pelvis. The kidney consists of an outer layer called the cortex and an inner layer called the medulla. Within the cortex, the extracellular fluid surrounding the renal tubules is approximately isotonic with the rest of the body fluid. Extracellular fluid surrounding the renal tubules that extend into the medulla is markedly hypertonic and becomes increasingly hypertonic as one moves from the cortex toward the innermost area called the renal pelvis. Certain parts of the nephron are located in either the cortex or medulla, which impacts the function performed by the area of the tubule. The renal pelvis contains no tubules; it serves

only a storage function. The renal pelvis drains into the ureter, which is capable of a rhythmic muscular action called peristalsis that moves urine from the kidney into the bladder, regardless of posture. The bladder stores urine until micturition occurs.

MICTURITION

Micturition, also known as urination and many less precise names, is the process by which the remaining filtered fluid leaving the collecting duct is voided into the external environment. Urine is formed continually by the renal tubules at a rate of approximately 1 ml per minute and is stored in the renal pelvis. Urine is moved by peristalsis through the ureters from the pelvis into the bladder. Gravity is not required for this movement to occur. Urine is stored in the bladder, until it is excreted at a convenient time and location. Under normal circumstances, no alteration in the composition of urine occurs once the fluid enters the renal pelvis. Obstruction or infection of the urinary tract may result in altered composition.

The process of micturition involves several reflexes. The major reflex consists of stretching of the bladder walls leading to emptying of the bladder. As children, we learn to control the reflex. When this learning is accomplished, we are said to be "potty-trained." Stretch receptors in the wall of the bladder send impulses via nerves to the spinal cord. When sufficient input reaches the spinal cord, parasympathetic nerves from the sacral area of the spinal cord send the message to the bladder smooth muscle to contract to cause emptying of the bladder (Figure 6-5). Information received from the stretch receptors is also sent up the spinal cord to the cortex to allow us to be aware of bladder fullness. Signals sent to the spinal cord from the cortex allow us to delay bladder emptying until a convenient time within limits of bladder fullness. This is possible for two reasons. First, the bladder smooth muscle relaxes with increasing volume to keep pressure low. The bladder can hold approximately 400 ml (a bit more than 12 oz) before reflex contraction occurs. At the typical rate of urine formation of 1 ml/min, this allows us to avoid micturition for more than 6 hours. Secondly, to prevent emptying of the bladder, skeletal muscle surrounding the urethra (external urethral sphincter) contracts when necessary. The reflex to void is extinguished for a time as the bladder continues to fill. With increasing stretch, the strength of the reflex contraction increases. One can usually comfortably maintain bladder volume up to 600 ml or so (Figure 6-6). Although this volume would seem to allow a period of 10 hours of bladder filling, most individuals tend to void on a 4-hour schedule during the day. This occurs for two major reasons. We tend to drink large quantities of fluid intermittently during waking hours and will fill our bladders more frequently than an average urine production figure might suggest. Moreover, we tend to void at certain convenient times during the day. We can usually delay voiding overnight due to the lack of fluid intake while asleep. Beyond a volume of 600 ml, most people become quite uncomfortable. In the absence of the nervous pathway over which the reflex occurs, as happens in some spinal cord or peripheral nerve injuries, the denervated bladder is capable of holding up to 1000 ml. In infants and some individuals with spinal cord injuries, micturition is controlled strictly by reflex. Eventually, infants learn to control micturition voluntarily (become potty-trained), and some people with spinal cord injuries can also learn to void at specific times or with specific stimuli by what is called bladder training.

Voluntary micturition involves several steps. First, one usually has a conscious awareness of bladder fullness or knows that another opportunity may not occur at a convenient time. The bladder is supported in the pelvis by muscles called the pelvic diaphragm. When the pelvic diaphragm is contracted, the bottom of the bladder is held higher in the pelvis. This reduces the stretch of the walls of the bladder and acts to keep the neck of the bladder closed. Voluntary micturition is facilitated by relaxation of the pelvic diaphragm. Some individuals have difficulty initiating micturition in public due to the inability to relax the pelvic floor muscles (shy kidney). When these muscles relax, the bottom of the bladder moves away from the top of the bladder, thereby stretching the bladder walls and enhancing its stretch reflex. In addition, lowering the bladder opens the neck of the bladder, which decreases the resistance to flow into the urethra. Stimulation of the parasympathetic

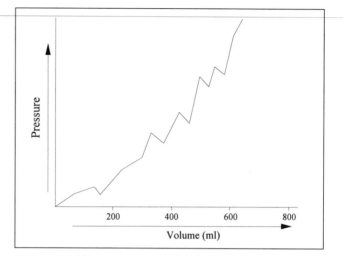

Figure 6-6. Effect of volume on bladder pressure. At low volumes, the bladder is able to relax to accommodate increasing volume. At approximately 400 ml of volume, the micturition reflex is stimulated, resulting in the spikes in pressure. Voluntary effort to contract the external urethral sphincter can prevent micturition until 600 to 700 ml has accumulated in the normally innervated bladder. A denervated bladder is capable of holding about 1000 ml due to the absence of the reflex.

nerves to the bladder causes the smooth muscle in the walls of the bladder to contract and also pulls the neck of the bladder open even wider. Under normal circumstances, the urinary tract does not become infected due to the "flushing" action performed by complete voiding of the bladder. Incomplete voiding, leading to urinary tract infection and potentially to a life-threatening infection of the kidney called pyelonephritis, can occur due to several conditions. Neurologic disease, such as multiple sclerosis, and spinal cord and peripheral nerve injury can weaken the bladder. Obstruction of the urinary tract due to pregnancy or a neoplasm impinging on the urinary tract can prevent the bladder from emptying. Individuals may need to be trained in self-catheterization or maneuvers to increase abdominal pressure to empty the bladder.

PROCESSES OF THE RENAL TUBULE

Renal tubules (nephrons) have three basic processes: filtration, secretion, and reabsorption. The net result of the three processes is excretion. Approximately 20% of the plasma that enters the kidneys is filtered into the renal tubules. In addition to substances filtered into the tubules, tubular cells can transport substances from the interstitial space outside the tubules into the tubules, thereby providing a second pathway for solute to enter the tubule; this process is called secretion. Reabsorption is the transport of solute from the lumen, or inside, of the tubule into the interstitial space surrounding the tubules. Blood vessels called peritubular capillaries transport substances to the interstitial space surrounding the renal tubules to be secreted by the tubules and transport reabsorbed solute back to the circulation. Excretion is the algebraic sum of the three processes described. The solute and water filtered plus that secreted minus that reabsorbed is the quantity of water and solute that is excreted (Figure 6-7).

THE NEPHRON

The nephron is the functional unit of the kidney. It consists of a long coiled tubule that has several important functional segments (Figure 6-8). The most proximal part of the nephron is the glomerulus. The glomerulus is the site at which plasma is filtered from the glomerular capillaries into the tubule. Renal arteries divide into smaller arteries that in turn give rise to vessels called afferent arterioles. One afferent arteriole supplies each glomerulus. The network of capillaries arising

Incontinence

Incontinence is the unwanted leakage of urine. Many women and some men experience this problem, but few seek help for this condition. Several interventions are available to rehab professionals with specialized training to reduce incontinence. These techniques include pelvic floor muscle exercises, which may be used along with biofeedback, vaginal cone retention, and electrical stimulation. If these techniques are used in isolation without regard to other aspects, such as general conditioning, abdominal muscle strength, posture, and work and home environment, success is likely to be limited. Successful interventions require a thorough evaluation of the entire individual, lifestyle, and modification of the treatment plan as progress occurs.

Therapeutic interventions are most useful for the types of incontinence called stress incontinence and urge incontinence. Stress incontinence is a condition in which leakage of urine occurs when abdominal pressure increases during coughing, sneezing, exercising, heavy lifting, climbing stairs, or similar maneuvers. Urge incontinence results from an overly sensitive bladder that empties before it should. Some individuals have mixed incontinence, which is usually a combination of stress and urge incontinence.

The pelvic floor consists of layers of muscle that connect the bones of the pelvis. These muscles normally support the pelvic organs—the bladder, rectum, and vagina—and allow these organs to function normally. These muscles also act to help the bladder contain urine until emptying is desirable and to hold back strong urges. Interventions include improving the function of the pelvic floor muscles by addressing strength and coordination of the pelvic floor muscles, strengthening and coordinating abdominal muscles, and improving posture. The major types of treatment are

- Vaginal cones: A series of progressively increasing weighted plastic cones is used to gradually strengthen and help coordinate the pelvic floor. An individual is progressed in terms of posture from lying supine to sitting and standing and by introducing functional activities. This intervention will not work well unless the individual already has some muscle strength.
- EMG biofeedback: The activity of pelvic floor muscles is measured by sensors that detect electrical activity produced by muscles. This technique has the greatest potential for restoring good pelvic floor function because it teaches the individual how to contract, relax, and grade pelvic floor muscle activity.
- Neuromuscular electrical stimulation: An electric current is used to assist the pelvic floor muscles to strengthen and coordinate them to regain normal pelvic floor function. Electrical stimulation is a good way to start an individual who is too weak to benefit from vaginal cones or EMG biofeedback. Once a person develops some muscle strength, the person is more likely to benefit from EMG biofeedback.

The type of treatment that will most effectively reduce urine leakage depends on several factors unique to each individual. A thorough examination, including an internal examination of the pelvic floor muscles, is performed to isolate specific problems causing urine to leak. Each person has an individual treatment plan developed based on specific findings and preference of each individual. Many individuals can expect complete dryness or nearly so. Those with severe weakness and nerve damage to the pelvic floor may not respond as well to treatment.

from each afferent arteriole is surrounded by a capsule (Bowman's capsule) that directs the filtered plasma into the first part of the tubule, the proximal **convoluted** tubule. In contrast to most capillary networks in the circulation, the glomerular capillaries converge to form an efferent arteriole instead of a venule. The efferent arteriole then branches into the peritubular capillaries that surround each nephron and participate in the functions of secretion and reabsorption described above. The peritubular capillaries then converge to form venules that drain blood from the kidney.

The proximal convoluted tubule is sometimes simply called the proximal tubule. The word convoluted refers the coiling of the proximal tubule within the cortex of the kidney, near the glomerulus. The proximal tubule performs most of the reabsorption, roughly two-thirds of the water and sodium filtered into the tubule. Following the proximal tubule is the loop of Henle. As the name implies, this segment forms a loop. This loop extends a variable distance into the medulla. The greater the distance into the medulla that the loop extends, the more solute can be concentrated in the tubule. The loop of Henle provides, in part, the mechanism necessary to allow us to excrete solute in a higher concentration than that of the plasma to conserve water by concentrating urine. You may have noticed that when you are dehydrated, your urine appears darker, and when you are overhydrated, the urine appears clear. Functions performed by the loop of Henle and the distal part of the nephron allow the concentration of urine to be varied. Although most of the reabsorption of fluid and solute occurs in the proximal tubule, the distal convoluted tubule and collecting duct perform the physiologic regulation of water, sodium, potassium, and pH, using mechanisms that will be described below. The collecting duct is a common tubule into which several distal convoluted tubules drain. A special area of the tubule where the ascending portion of the loop of Henle has doubled back in close proximity to the glomerulus is called the juxtaglomerular apparatus. At this point, the distal tubule also passes between the afferent and efferent arterioles. The juxtaglomerular apparatus consists of the macula densa, which is part of the distal tubule, and granular cells located within the wall of the afferent arteriole. These specialized areas of the nephron are responsible, to a large degree, for detecting the status of fluid volume and composition and initiating corrective action.

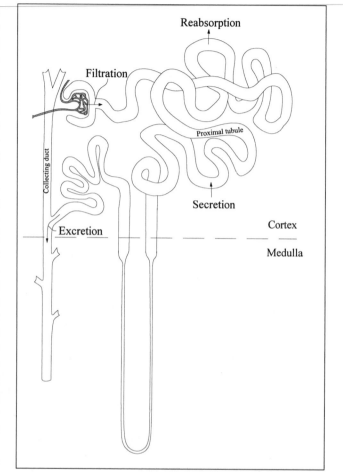

Figure 6-7. Four basic processes of the renal tubules.

FILTRATION

The glomerular capillaries arise from an afferent arteriole and are drained by an efferent arteriole. These capillaries receive a high blood flow under greater pressure than most capillaries in the circulation. Renal blood flow is about 20% of cardiac output at rest, and renal arterial vessels are wide and short. Because these vessels have little resistance to flow, the pressure within the glomerular capillaries is much greater than most capillaries. Moreover, compared with most capillaries, the spaces between endothelial cells lining the glomerular capillaries are greater, resulting in greater net movement of water and solute out of glomerular capillaries than others in the body. Approximately 20% of the plasma that enters the afferent arteriole is filtered into the prox-

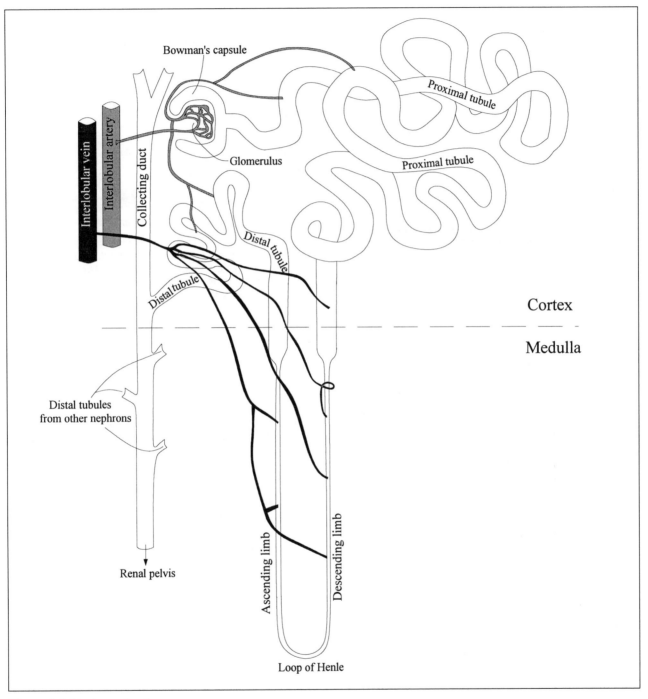

Figure 6-8. Nephron structure.

imal tubule. The fraction of plasma filtered is called the filtration fraction. The amount of fluid filtered into the proximal tubule from the glomeruli is called the glomerular filtration rate and can be computed as renal plasma flow times filtration fraction. We use the term plasma flow instead of blood flow because only the fluid part of blood, the plasma, can be normally filtered into

the renal tubules. In men, 45% of the blood consists of red blood cells, only 55% of the blood flow is plasma (in women, approximately 40% of the blood consists of red cells). Assuming that cardiac output is 5 L/min and that 20% of the cardiac output going to the kidneys, renal blood flow is 1 L/min. If renal plasma flow equals 55% of renal blood flow, then renal plasma flow would be equal to 550 ml/min. With a typical filtration fraction of 20%, the glomerular filtration rate is approximately 110 ml/min (Figure 6-9). Because only about 1 ml/min of urine is produced, we can see that more than 99% of the fluid filtered into the proximal tubule is reabsorbed. Proteins are normally not filtered into the renal tubules for two reasons. Plasma proteins are large, and the slits that perform the filtration have a negative charge that prevents passage of the negatively charged plasma proteins. In some forms of kidney diseases, the renal tubular cells lose their negative charge, and large quantities of plasma protein are lost in the urine.

PROXIMAL TUBULE FUNCTION

In a given day, approximately 180 L of water, 26,000 mMol of sodium, 19,000 mMol of chloride, 4300 mMol of bicarbonate, and 180 grams of glucose are filtered into the renal tubules. Yet, we only excrete about 2.5 L of water, 100 to 250 mMol of sodium and chloride, 2 mMol of bicarbonate, and virtually no glucose. Our renal tubules, by allowing large volumes of plasma to filter into the renal tubules, have the potential to rid the body of large amounts of some solutes and, at the same time, fine tune the composition of body fluids. The major function of the proximal tubule is reabsorption; almost all of the glucose and amino acids and about two-thirds of the NaCl are reabsorbed by the proximal tubule. Glucose is reabsorbed by secondary active transport using sodium as the allosteric modulator. Because glucose transport by the proximal tubule cells requires a carrier, it is subject to saturation. For the entire mass of renal tubules, the limit on glucose transport (denoted TM) is about 375 mg/min. If glucose is filtered into the renal tubules at a rate faster than 375 mg/min, glucose will appear in the urine. Given the normal renal blood flow and filtration fraction, a plasma concentration above 200 mg/dl is the usual threshold value before glucose appears in the urine. In addition, the glucose remaining in the renal tubules acts as a non-penetrating solute for the remainder of the tubule and, therefore, decreases water reabsorption from the renal tubules. As a result, a greater than normal production of urine occurs in the disease diabetes mellitus (mellitus means "sweet"). Diabetes mellitus will be distinguished from diabetes insipidus later in this chapter.

The reabsorption of salt and water from within the proximal tubule is driven indirectly by active transport of sodium ions from the basolateral surface of the proximal tubular cells into the interstitial space. Sodium from inside the lumen then can diffuse into the tubule cells through specialized channels on the apical surface of the

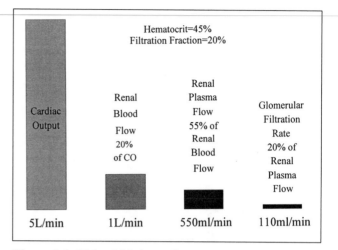

Figure 6-9. Of the 5 L/min cardiac output, 110 ml of fluid filters into the renal tubules each minute. Twenty percent of the cardiac output is received by the kidney, and 20% of the fluid part of the blood (the plasma) is filtered.

cells and then can be transported out of the tubule by the Na/K pump. The presence of the Na/K pump on the basolateral surface of the tubule instead of on the apical (luminal side) allows the concentration of sodium to remain low inside the renal tubular cells. The indirect use of the Na/K pump to remove Na from the tubule by lowering the concentration of sodium inside the cell allows the concentration of sodium inside the tubule cells to be lower than it would be if sodium ions were pumped into the apical side of the proximal tubule cells. Water and other ions, including potassium, chloride, and bicarbonate, follow an osmotic gradient caused by the active transport of sodium out of the tubule. Throughout the proximal tubule, equal reabsorption of salt and water keeps the tubular fluid isotonic.

LOOP OF HENLE

The loop of Henle is responsible for setting up the conditions that allow the kidney to concentrate urine. Because of the loop, the kidney can excrete a greater proportion of some of solutes present in the plasma than the water excreted. The concentration of solute is due to a mechanism called the countercurrent multiplier. A countercurrent multiplier requires the inflow of the system to run parallel to and in the opposite direction (countercurrent) of the outflow. In terms of a heater, as the bottom of the loop is heated in a flowing system, the cooler fluid coming down is heated by the warmer fluid coming up the ascending limb, which adds to the heat produced at the bottom of the loop. As fluid runs through the system, a gradient of temperature exists such that the tip of the loop is the hottest and the loop is progressively cooler at the top. Multiplication of the quantity at the bottom of the loop occurs as the energy is added to the descending loop from the ascending loop. By analogy, in the kidney, a solute gradient is established by osmoles being added at the tip of the loop and osmoles from the ascending limb being transferred to the descending limb. This process concentrates tubular fluid as it descends the loop of Henle and dilutes as it ascends. This is accomplished by selective permeabilities of different regions of the nephron. The descending loop is permeable to water, but does not actively transport salt out of the tubule, and the ascending part of the loop is impermeable to water, but actively transports salt into the medulla of the kidney. As fluid descends the loop of Henle, water readily moves out due to the presence of salt and urea in the interstitial fluid, which makes the tubular fluid progressively more concentrated as it approaches the bottom of the loop. In the ascending part of the loop, salt is actively transported into the interstitial fluid, which creates the osmotic gradient for the movement of water from the descending part of the loop. In a way, one can envision that osmoles from the ascending limb are being transferred to the descending limb of the loop of Henle. The osmotically active particles are trapped in the medulla of the kidney due to the presence of blood vessels called vasa recta that parallel the loops of Henle and recirculate the solute between the tubules and vasa recta. A more comprehensive description of the countercurrent multiplier mechanism can be found in any of several medical physiology textbooks. Because the loop of Henle reabsorbs 25% of the filtered sodium, but only 15% of the filtered water, the fluid that reaches the distal tubule is hypo-osmotic. The greater removal of salt than water from the loop of Henle is one reason for the increasing osmolarity of interstitial fluid moving from cortex to medulla and explains why loops that extend more deeply into the medulla can concentrate urine more. In humans, this mechanism can produce an osmolarity of about 1200 mOsm, but is more effective in other animals, especially those living in environments such as deserts.

DISTAL TUBULE

In the proximal tubule, fluid is isotonic with the interstitial fluid surrounding the tubule in the cortex. The loop of Henle deposits salt in the medulla, making the medullary interstitial fluid hypertonic, and the tubular fluid that enters the distal tubule is hypotonic compared with the interstitial fluid of the cortical interstitial fluid that surrounds it. The distal tubule is impermeable to water, but can reabsorb about 5% of the filtered sodium by active transport of sodium across the basolateral

(outer) surface of the distal tubule cells, further diluting the tubular fluid.

COLLECTING DUCT

At this point, we begin to see actual regulation of fluid composition. To make diluted urine so that extracellular fluid volume can be decreased and body fluid osmolarity can be increased, all we need to do is let the hypotonic tubular fluid pass into the renal pelvis as urine. To make urine more concentrated so we may conserve water and decrease osmolarity, we allow water to be reabsorbed from the collecting ducts as they pass through the medulla where osmolarity is high. The osmolarity of the tip of the medulla just before the tubule empties into the renal pelvis can be as high as 1200 to 1400 mOsm compared with a normal body fluid osmolarity of 290 mOsm. This difference in osmolarity drives water out of the collecting duct until the urine osmolarity approaches that of the renal medullary interstitial fluid if we allow water to leave the collecting ducts by physiologic regulation of their permeability (Figure 6-10). The functions of the collecting duct can be described better by examining separately events in the cortical and medullary portions of the collecting duct. In the cortical region, interstitial fluid is isotonic, and tubular fluid is hypotonic. Water can be conserved by release from the posterior pituitary of the hormone antidiuretic hormone (ADH), which is also known as vasopressin because of its effect on blood vessels. In the absence of ADH, the collecting duct is impermeable to water, and massive quantities of water are lost and may lead to death if ADH is not replaced. ADH binds to receptors on collecting duct cells, which leads to the opening of water channels in the collecting duct cells. The greater the amount of ADH released by the posterior pituitary, the more pores are produced, and the greater the water reabsorption. In the presence of ADH, water can move out of the tubule, and tubular fluid in the cortical portion of the collecting duct becomes isotonic. As fluid continues through the medullary part of the collecting duct, it becomes hypertonic as water moves into the increasingly hyperosmotic medulla. The greater the concentration of ADH in the blood, the closer urine osmolarity approximates that of the medullary interstitium. At very high levels of ADH, the urine osmolarity can reach as high as 1200 mOsm. At very low levels of ADH, the osmolarity may be as low as 50 mOsm. A lack of ADH in the disease diabetes insipidus ("nonsweet" diabetes) leads to production of massive quantities of urine that may become fatal in a short time.

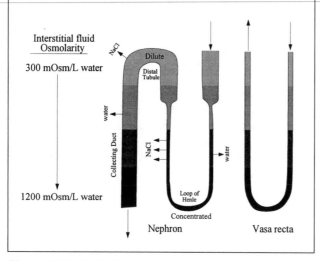

Figure 6-10. Production of concentrated urine.

CONTROL OF SODIUM

Physiological control varies the reabsorption of sodium between 95% when sodium needs to be excreted to 99.5% reabsorption when sodium needs to be conserved. This regulation is achieved by the steroid hormone aldosterone. Aldosterone binds to specific receptors on cells of the collecting duct. Binding of this hormone leads to a complex series of intracellular events. Both the number of sodium channels on the apical membrane and the number of Na/K pumps on the basolateral membrane are increased (Figure 6-11). These changes produce greater reabsorption of sodium but cause increased potassium excretion. Because aldosterone is a hormone that causes production of proteins inside the cell, approximately 30 minutes is required for aldosterone to affect sodium reabsorption.

REGULATION OF POTASSIUM

Normal extracellular potassium concentration is 4 to 5 mM. Because of the role of potassium in cell membrane potentials, the concentration must be regulated carefully. If it falls below 2.5 mM, membranes hyperpolarize, which makes production of action potentials more difficult. This results in muscle weakness and cardiac arrhythmias. A potassium concentration greater than 5.5 mM produces depolarization of membranes, which causes muscle weakness and cardiac arrest. Normally, extracellular potassium concentration is low and does not increase much with ingestion of potassium because potassium is pumped into the intracellular space by the Na/K pump. Although 90% of the filtered potas-

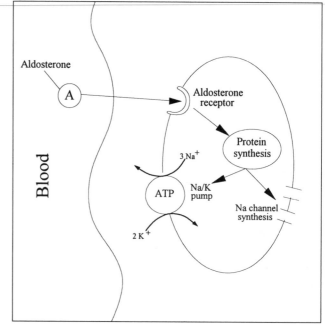

Figure 6-11. Cellular actions of aldosterone on the collecting duct.

sium is reabsorbed by the time it reaches the collecting duct, secretion of potassium from the interstitial fluid surrounding the collecting duct into the collecting duct is the mechanism that regulates potassium concentration of the extracellular fluid. Two major factors determine the rate of potassium secretion; both are controlled by aldosterone. An increased level of plasma potassium causes the adrenal cortex to secrete aldosterone. One mechanism is passive transport; the greater the amount of potassium in the body, the higher intracellular potassium becomes. Aldosterone increases the number of open potassium channels on the apical membrane, causing more potassium to diffuse out of tubular cells into the lumen, which, in turn, causes potassium to diffuse more rapidly into the tubular cells from the interstitial space. In addition, aldosterone increases the number of Na/K pumps available to pump potassium into the collecting tubule cells. As intracellular potassium rises because of an increased amount of potassium in the body and increased active transport into the collecting duct cells, more potassium diffuses into the lumen to be secreted.

INTERACTION BETWEEN NA AND K REGULATION

Aldosterone controls both sodium reabsorption and potassium secretion. A decreased interstitial sodium

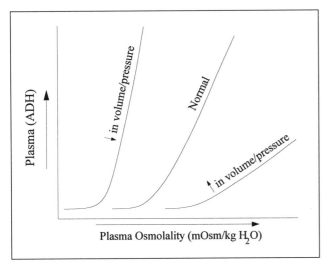

Figure 6-12. Stimuli for ADH secretion.

concentration indirectly increases aldosterone secretion by the adrenal cortex (discussed later in this chapter). An increased potassium concentration directly increases the amount of aldosterone secreted. Some popular diuretic agents work by decreasing reabsorption of sodium. These agents cause loss of both water, the desired effect, and sodium. Loss of sodium stimulates production of aldosterone, which, in turn, stimulates both reabsorption of sodium and secretion of potassium, resulting in hypokalemia.

CONTROL OF EXTRACELLULAR FLUID VOLUME

As discussed earlier, sodium concentration of extracellular fluid (ECF) normally determines the osmolarity of the ECF. When sodium concentration changes, the relative proportions of ECF and intracellular fluid (ICF) change to maintain osmolarity. Because of this, the total sodium content of the ECF determines ECF volume. When sodium content increases, ECF volume increases at the expense of ICF volume. ECF osmolality and volume can be controlled in two ways: by mechanisms that alter the amount of water in the body and those that control the amount of sodium in the body. Water volume is controlled by either conservation or excretion of water under the control of ADH and is also controlled by the development of thirst. The amount of sodium in the body is controlled by mechanisms to be described later. ADH is produced in the hypothalamus and is stored in neurons in the posterior pituitary. An increase in the osmolarity of cells in the hypothalamus, called osmoreceptors, causes ADH to be released into the blood (Figure 6-12). Under normal circumstances (an

osmolarity of 290 mOsm), some ADH is released; the threshold for ADH release is 280 mOsm. Following overhydration, ICF osmolarity may fall below 290 mOsm, leading to a decrease in ADH release. Very large increases in water volume may cause ADH release to cease and may allow almost all of the water entering the distal renal tubules (approximately 12 ml/min) to be excreted. Therefore, the maximum urine output of a person with normal kidney function is limited to about 12 ml/min. The increased urine production, called diuresis, requires 15 to 30 minutes to occur because of the time required to perform the hormonal and second messenger mechanisms. A greater degree of diuresis can be obtained by preventing the removal of solute, usually sodium, from the tubular fluid. This increases the osmolarity of the tubular fluid and decreases the osmotic gradient between the collecting duct and renal medullary fluid. These drugs can produce tremendous quantities of fluid and may be necessary to save the life of a person with pulmonary edema. ADH is also regulated by baroreceptors (receptors that respond to increased stretch due to pressure). Low pressure stretch receptors are located in the left atrium. A blood volume increase of 10% to 15% inhibits and a blood volume decrease of 10% or more increases ADH production via these baroreceptors. Drinking alcohol is counterproductive to increasing ECF volume. Alcohol inhibits the release of ADH, causing the kidney to excrete more volume than that taken in. Dehydration secondary to alcohol consumption appears to account, in part, for what is commonly known as a hangover.

THIRST

A desire to drink fluids is necessary to maintain body fluid volume. Thirst is stimulated by binding of the hormone angiotensin II (discussed later in this chapter) to receptors in the hypothalamus. Other stimuli for thirst include osmoreceptors in the hypothalamus and the baroreceptors in the left atrium. Increased plasma osmolarity and decreased blood volume stimulate the desire to drink.

ROLE OF THE JUXTAGLOMERULAR APPARATUS

The juxtaglomerular apparatus (JGA) includes parts of the distal tubule and the afferent arteriole. The JGA is located next to the glomerulus, where the afferent arterioles and efferent arteriole pass next to the distal

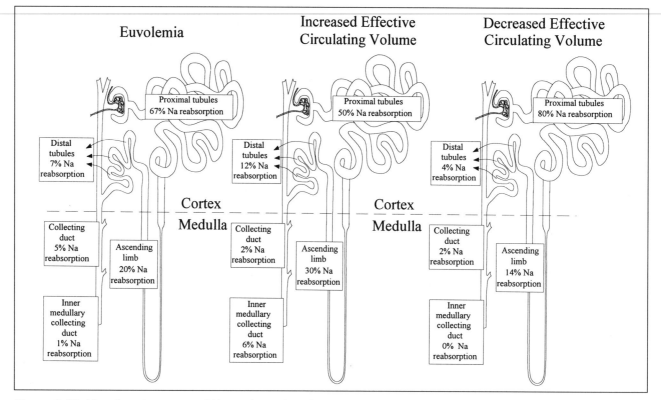

Figure 6-13. Alterations in segmental Na⁺ reabsorption with changes in blood volume.

tubule. The JGA has two functional parts: granular cells and the macula densa. Granular cells located within the walls of the afferent arteriole secrete a hormone called renin, whereas the macula densa is a sensor for sodium. When sodium content of the distal tubule decreases, the macula densa stimulates the granular cells to secrete renin. Other stimuli for the granular cells include reduced stretch of the afferent arteriole due to decreased pressure in the afferent arteriole or decreased renal blood flow and sympathetic stimulation. Therefore, renin secretion is stimulated when either blood pressure is decreased or the content of sodium within the distal tubule is decreased. The secretion of renin initiates a series of events that corrects these two problems (Figure 6-13). Within the blood is an inactive peptide called angiotensin, which is produced by the liver. Renin acts as an enzyme to remove two amino acids from the peptide to form angiotensin I. Angiotensin I is a decapeptide that has a weak physiological effect compared with angiotensin II. Angiotensin II, the active form of angiotensin, is formed by converting enzyme, which is located primarily on the endothelium of the lung. As blood flows through the lungs, converting enzyme removes two more amino acids to form an octapeptide. Angiotensin II has two functions: it stimulates the adre-

nal cortex to secrete aldosterone and it increases blood pressure. Aldosterone, secreted by the adrenal cortex upon stimulation by angiotensin II, stimulates reabsorption of sodium. Production of renin in response to low pressure or decreased sodium content leads to aldosterone secretion to conserve sodium and angiotensin II production to elevate blood pressure. These are depicted in Figure 6-14. Several anti-hypertensive drugs operate by either blocking angiotensin II receptors or conversion of angiotensin I to angiotensin II.

Another mechanism useful in controlling ECF volume is atrial natriuretic factor (ANF), which is also called atrial natriuretic peptide (ANP) and atriopeptin. ANF is produced by cells in the atria in response to increased stretch. Secretion of ANF leads to loss of sodium in the urine (natriuresis). Diagrams summarizing renal control of fluid are shown in Figures 6-15 and 6-16.

REGULATION OF CALCIUM

Ionized calcium is critically important to the function of nerve and muscle cells. It maintains voltage-operated sodium channels in the closed position. A low calcium concentration increases the excitability of nerve and muscle cells (brings them closer to threshold). Low

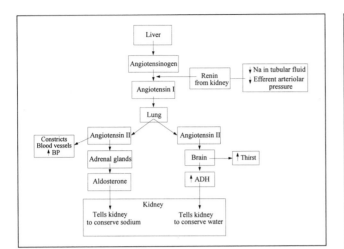

Figure 6-14. The renin-angiotensin-aldosterone-ADH system.

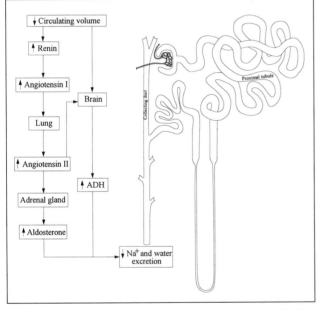

Figure 6-16. Renal response to a decrease in the effective circulating volume.

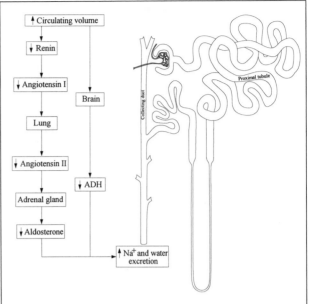

Figure 6-15. Renal response to expansion of the effective circulating volume.

cium from the gastrointestinal system and the excretion of calcium by the kidney. Parathyroid hormone also acts on the bone. Bone is a large store for calcium. With increased levels of parathyroid hormone, Ca^{++} is released by bones. Secretion of parathyroid hormone is controlled by calcium concentration in the plasma. As calcium concentration falls, parathyroid hormone secretion is stimulated. Parathyroid hormone has four functions that increase plasma calcium:

1. Release of calcium from bone
2. Increased reabsorption of calcium from the renal tubules
3. Conversion of vitamin D to its active form by renal cells
4. Decreased reabsorption of phosphate by the renal tubules

Calcium concentration is increased by conversion of vitamin D to its active form because vitamin D increases the absorption of calcium from the gastrointestinal tract. Loss of phosphate in the urine decreases the amount of plasma calcium that can be incorporated in the bone. Both calcium and phosphate are necessary to produce the bone-forming salt hydroxyapatite $[(Ca_3PO_4)_2]_3Ca(OH)_2$. Magnesium, like calcium, is a divalent cation and has some functions similar to calcium. Decreased magnesium can cause numbness, arrhythmias of the heart, and increased excitability rather than decreased excitability of skeletal muscle. Magnesium absorption is also regulated by parathyroid hormone and vitamin D.

extracellular calcium concentration causes more voltage-gated channels to open, which produces hypocalcemic tetany of small muscles, especially in the hand and wrist, and causes numbness of the fingers, toes, and around the mouth. Hypocalcemia can be functionally produced by alkalosis, which reduces the concentration of ionized calcium in the interstitial fluid. Hyperventilation due to anxiety is frequently a cause of these symptoms. High levels of calcium increase the threshold for membrane depolarization and can cause fatal heart arrhythmias.

Calcium concentration is regulated by both the kidneys and the gastrointestinal system via the parathyroid glands. Parathyroid hormone controls absorption of cal-

SUMMARY

Body fluids are the medium in which the chemical reactions and transport to support the chemical reactions take place. Both the volume and composition of the body fluids must be regulated. Extracellular fluid is characterized by a high concentration of sodium and low concentration of potassium. Because sodium acts as a nonpenetrating solute at the cell membrane, the total amount of sodium in the body determines extracellular volume relative to intracellular volume. Plasma proteins act as a nonpenetrating solute in blood vessels and determine the volume of the plasma. Decreased plasma protein concentration because of kidney disease, liver disease, or malnutrition allows large volumes of fluid to leak from blood vessels into the interstitial space. Collection of fluid in the abdomen is called ascites. Normally, small volumes of fluid exist in specialized compartments: cerebrospinal fluid, pericardial fluid, pleural fluid, and synovial fluid. Disease or injury can cause increased volume of these spaces called hydrocephalus, pericardial effusion, pleural effusion, and joint effusion, respectively.

The renal tubule, called a nephron, consists of regions with specialized functions. Filtration of plasma into the proximal tubule occurs in the glomerulus. The proximal tubule performs the bulk of reabsorption, the removal of substances from the lumen of the tubule. Secretion is the addition of substances from the interstitial space surrounding the tubule into its lumen. The loop of Henle sets up conditions for reabsorption of water and concentration of urine by concentrating salt and urea in the medulla of the kidney and removes more solute than water. The distal tubule further dilutes urine by removing salt, but not water.

Water conservation is controlled in the collecting duct by release of ADH, which stimulates production of water channels, allowing water to diffuse out of the collecting duct into the hyperosmotic medulla. Aldosterone is released to conserve salt by increasing the active transport of sodium out of the collecting duct. Juxtaglomerular cells release renin when a decreased amount of sodium or decreased tubular pressure is detected. Renin stimulates the production of angiotensin I, which is converted to angiotensin II. Angiotensin II stimulates release of ADH to conserve water and aldosterone to conserve sodium. Several other mechanisms contribute to the control of ADH and aldosterone, including osmoreceptors and baroreceptors. Excretion is the sum of filtration, less reabsorption plus secretion. The volume excreted is transported by peristalsis by the ureter to the bladder where it is stored until micturition. Micturition is based on a stretch reflex in which stretch receptors signal the state of bladder fullness to the micturition center in the sacral spinal cord. Voluntary control is superimposed on the bladder reflexes to allow socially acceptable timing of micturition. Skeletal muscle of the pelvic floor supports the bladder and maintains, to a large extent, continence. Relaxation of the pelvic floor muscles stretches the walls of the bladder and opens the bladder neck, decreasing the resistance to outflow. Stress incontinence can result from weakness or lack of coordination of these muscles.

BIBLIOGRAPHY

Aukland K, Reed RK. Interstitial-lymphatic mechanism in the control of extracellular fluid volume. *Physiological Reviews*. 1993;73:1-78.

Brown D, Stow JL. Protein trafficking and polarity in kidney epithelium: from cell biology to physiology. *Physiological Reviews*. 1996;76:245-297.

DiBona GF. Role of renal nerves in edema formation. *News in Physiological Sciences*. 1994;9:183-188.

DiBona GF, Kopp UC. Neural control of renal function. *Physiological Reviews*. 1997;77:75-197.

Gekle M. Renal proximal tubular albumin reabsorption: daily prevention of albuminuria. *News in Physiological Sciences*. 1998;13:5-11.

Koepsell H, Busch A, Gorboulev V, Arndt D. Structure and function of renal organic cation transporters. *News in Physiological Sciences*. 1998;13:11-16.

Lang F, Busch GL, Ritter M, et al. Functional significance of cell volume regulatory mechanisms. *Physiological Reviews*. 1998;78:247-306.

Lang F, Busch GL, Völk H, Häussinger D. Cell volume: a second message in regulation of cellular function. *News in Physiological Sciences*. 1995;10:18-22.

Lang F, Rehwald W. Potassium channels in renal epithelial transport regulation. *Physiological Reviews*. 1992;72:1-32.

McCarty NA, O'Neil RG. Calcium signaling in cell volume regulation. *Physiological Reviews*. 1992;72:1037-1061.

Pritchard JB, Miller DS. Mechanism mediating renal secretion of organic anions and cations. *Physiological Reviews*. 1993;73:765-796.

Reed RK, Woie K, Rubin K. Integrins and control of interstitial fluid pressure. *News in Physiological Sciences*. 1997;12:42-48.

Saboli I, Brown D. Water channels in renal and nonrenal tissue. *News in Physiological Sciences*. 1995;10:12-17.

Share L. Control of vasopressin release: an old but continuing story. *News in Physiological Sciences*. 1996;11:7-13.

STUDY QUESTIONS

1. Describe what happens to the distribution of intracellular and extracellular volume when a person sweats profusely. What type of fluid does the average person need to replace fluid volume after exercise?

2. In cystic fibrosis, the sweat has a salt content similar to that of plasma. How does fluid replacement during exercise differ if a person has cystic fibrosis?

3. Explain how the presence of plasma proteins prevents plasma from leaking out of blood vessels. How does the negative charge of the tubular cells in the glomerulus help maintain fluid volume?

4. Explain why the collecting duct is the site of regulation of water and sodium reabsorption even though the vast majority of salt and water are reabsorbed in the proximal tubule.

5. Explain how angiotensin II corrects the stimuli that resulted in its production.

6. Contrast the process of micturition in a baby and an adult.

7. Explain how weakness of the pelvic floor muscles following difficult deliveries leads to stress incontinence.

LABORATORY EXERCISE 6-1

URINALYSIS

Urinalysis is the qualitative evaluation of the presence of protein, glucose, bile pigments, ketones, pH determination, microscopic examination of the sediment, and determination of solute concentration (specific gravity).

Objective: Use urine dipsticks to determine the presence of leukocytes, urobilinogen, protein, determine pH, presence of blood (actually either hemoglobin or myoglobin), check specific gravity (we will also use a urinometer), presence of ketones, bilirubin, or glucose. Note that each test may require a different incubation period before reading the dipstick.

Urinary sediment may include crystals and casts. Casts, as the name implies, are material in the shape of renal tubules. Various types of materials may become deposited in the renal tubules. Although a small number of some types of casts may be normal, an analysis of the casts may suggest the presence of renal disease.

A major function of the kidney is to rid the body of excess solutes while conserving water. The greater the concentration of solute in the urine, the greater its density. Specific gravity is the density compared to that of water. Urine with no solute in it has a specific gravity of 1.0. If we drink an excessive amount of water, specific gravity will be close to 1.0. If we are dehydrated, specific gravity will approach 1.04. Normal specific gravity is about 1.02.

Materials:
Urine collection cups
Multistix 10 SG dipsticks
Urine hydrometer

Methods:
1. Using the control sample from Laboratory Exercise 6.2, place dipstick in urine. Be sure to wet all 10 patches. Hold dipstick so that the patches are up and hold near the dipstick bottle. Compare the color of all 10 patches with those on the sample colors on the bottle. Record your findings below. Compare specific gravity obtained using the urine hydrometer to that given by the dipstick color.

Results:

Leukocytes	_____	Negative
Nitrite	_____	Negative
Urobilinogen	_____	(0.1 to 1.0 Ehrlich units/dL)
Protein	_____	Negative
pH	_____	(4.6 to 8.0)
Blood	_____	Negative
Specific gravity	_____(d/s)/_____	(direct) (1.003 to 1.030)
Ketones	_____	Negative
Bilirubin	_____	Negative
Glucose	_____	Negative

LABORATORY EXERCISES

Interpretation of urinalysis:

Leukocytes

Presence of leukocytes indicates infection or other inflammatory disease of the urinary system.

Nitrites

Nitrates can be converted to nitrites by bacteria in the urine. Normally there is no nitrite in the urine. Presence of nitrite generally requires a 4-hour incubation in the bladder.

Urobilinogen

Normally there are trace amounts of urobilinogen in the urine. Urobilinogen is formed from bilirubin excreted from the gall bladder into the intestine. Bacteria synthesize urobilinogen from bilirubin in the intestine. Urobilinogen is then reabsorbed and excreted in the urine. Elevated urobilinogen indicates hemolytic anemia, pernicious anemia, or malaria.

Protein

Proteinuria can be caused by elevated protein concentration, increased secretion of protein, decreased reabsorption, or increased filtration due to increased glomerular permeability. Daily total of <1 g considered normal with a urine protein/creatinine ratio of <0.1. Proteinuria >2 g/day or protein : creatinine ratio of >3.0 indicates nephrotic syndrome. Orthostatic and exertional proteinuria are not considered abnormal. Exercise proteinuria is usually accompanied by hemoglobinuria, hematuria, and myoglobinuria and is observed in distance runners and boxers.

pH

Useful in identifying crystals in urine. In renal tubular disease, the kidney is unable to decrease pH below 5.5 with an acid load. Normal values: 4.5 to 8.0; urine <6.0 considered acid, >6.0, considered alkaline. In renal tubular acidosis due to proximal tubule disease: low serum HCO_3^-, normal urine pH; distal tubule disease: normal serum HCO_3^-, urine pH > 6.0. pH > 8.4 indicates bacterial contamination.

Blood

Test indicates positive result in presence of either hemoglobin or myoglobin. Color of urine will help distinguish. Smokey color indicates red blood cells (RBCs); red color indicates hemoglobin. RBC in urine indicates glomerular injury, neoplasm, or stones. Hemoglobinuria or myoglobinuria indicates acute renal failure

Specific gravity

Indicative of urine solute concentration. May simply indicate state of hydration—we will see a dramatic demonstration of this in Laboratory Exercise 6-2. Loss of urine concentrating ability indicates renal dysfunction.

Ketones

Ketonuria (not specific of any one type of ketone) indicates metabolic acidosis, starvation, uncontrolled diabetes mellitus, or even ethanol intoxication. It is not specific for any intrinsic urinary system disease

Bilirubin

Normally no bilirubin should be detected in the urine. Bilirubinuria indicates hepatobiliary disease, such as hepatitis, cirrhosis, or biliary obstruction.

LABORATORY EXERCISES

Glucose

Usually glucosuria indicates diabetes mellitus with normal renal glucose transport. It may, however, be due to normal blood glucose and renal tubular dysfunction. Blood glucose levels will differentiate between these possibilities.

Urine appearance:

Normal:	light yellow color
Yellow:	bilirubin
Blue:	vegetable dyes
Orange:	antibiotics, urinary tract anesthetic
White, milky:	obstruction
Red:	hemoglobin, requires immediate medical attention
Brown, green, or black:	can be due to old hemoglobin
Smokey:	RBCs

Sediment:

From the *Atlas of Urinary Sediment* review pages 3, 4, 8 (fatty casts only), 11, 12, 13, and 23 about casts; pages 32 to 37 about crystals.

Normal urine contains small numbers of cells and formed elements shed from the urinary system; elevated number of cells suggest urinary system disease.

RBCs:	infection, tumor, stones, inflammation
WBCs:	infection or other inflammatory disease
Crystals:	oxalate, phosphate, urate; depending on urine pH and concentration, salts lose solubility
RBC cast:	glomerulonephritis
WBC cast:	pyelonephritis
Waxy and broad casts:	advanced renal failure

Collection:

AM:	Most concentrated, indicates renal function over last 8 hours; more likely to detect pus and mucus indicative of infection
Clean catch:	Prevent contamination with urethral bacteria; disinfection of external urethral area and midstream catch
Within 1 hour:	pH changes, bacterial growth, disintegration of cells and casts occur

Urine volume and strength:

Anuria:	<100 ml/day, total loss of kidney function; end-stage kidney failure
Oliguria:	<600 ml/day, <300 ml/day is dangerous; causes: nephritis, urinary obstruction, fluid loss
Eu-uria:	1500 ml/day
Polyuria:	>2000 ml/day; causes polydipsia, diabetes mellitus or insipidus, end-stage failure
Isosthenuria:	"same strength"—isosthenuria is not normal, specific gravity should vary; causes renal damage—kidney cannot change composition of urine. Normal situation specific gravity of 1.012, individual drinks water, specific gravity >1.002, concentrated urine specific gravity of 1.02.

LABORATORY EXERCISES

Renal syndromes:

Azotemia: Nitrogen in the blood, elevated blood urea nitrogen (BUN) and creatinine. Prerenal azotemia may be caused by gastrointestinal bleeding. Renal azotemia results when fewer than 500,000 glomeruli are left. Postrenal azotemia is caused by obstruction of the urinary tract.

Uremia: Clinical signs and symptoms associated with development of azotemia. Uremia is a clinical syndrome, whereas azotemia is a biochemical abnormality.

LABORATORY EXERCISE 6-2

REGULATION OF BODY FLUIDS

Objective: Demonstrate how water and sodium chloride reabsorption are regulated physiologically.

Materials:
Urine collection cups
Water cups
Medicine droppers
2.9% silver nitrate solution
20% potassium chromate solution

1. Void bladder 1 to 2 hours before laboratory session. It is important that the bladder is completely empty and that you note the time at which this is done. You will be determining the rate of urine formation. For this, you will take urine collections at certain times and will need to know both the volume excreted and the time during which the bladder was filling.

2. Collect a control sample at the very beginning of the laboratory session. Save this sample for Laboratory Exercise 6.1, Urinalysis.

3. The class will be divided into two groups:
    Group A: Drink 800 ml of water. Do not drink anything else for the remainder of the laboratory session.
    Group B: Walk up and down 10 flights of stairs. Do not drink anything else for the remainder of the laboratory session unless necessary.

4. Every 30 minutes collect another sample. If you cannot obtain a sample, or must void before the 30-minute time period, make sure you keep track of the amount of time during which urine was collected in the bladder.

For each sample, including the control sample at the beginning of the laboratory session, but excluding the urine voided 1 to 2 hours before the laboratory session; make the following three measurements and write the results for the appropriate time and group on the chalkboard.

Volume: Pour the collected sample into an appropriately sized graduated cylinder. Measure the volume and return the urine to the collection cup. Thoroughly rinse the graduated cylinder when finished. Divide volume in ml by the number of minutes during which urine collected in the bladder. Express in ml/min. Write your results on the chalkboard for the appropriate time and group.
Chloride concentration: Using a medicine dropper, place 10 drops of the urine sample into a

LABORATORY EXERCISES

culture tube. Add one drop of potassium chromate and swirl. At this point, add single drops of silver nitrate to determine the chloride concentration. As each drop is added to the culture tube, a small reaction occurs in which a brown color is seen. As the tube is swirled the brown color should go away. Count the drops until the brown color remains despite swirling. The number of drops represent the concentration of sodium chloride in the urine sample in units of mg/ml.

NaCl excretion: Multiply the volume output of urine in ml/min by the sodium chloride concentration in mg/ml in the sample to obtain a result of mg/min of NaCl excretion.

Specific gravity: Using the appropriately sized urine hydrometer, fill to about 1 inch from the top. Place the float into the hydrometer and spin the float to ensure that it does not adhere to the side. Make sure enough volume exists in the hydrometer so that the float does not rest on the bottom. Wait for the urine to cool to room temperature. The density of urine increases as it cools to room temperature. Most urine hydrometers are calibrated for refrigerated samples.

For each group and each time period, determine the group average for urine output, NaCl excretion, and specific gravity. Plot the results of the four groups.

Questions:
1. Compare the results from the overhydrated (800 ml of water) to the exercising group. How did these two groups differ in urine output, NaCl excretion, and specific gravity?

2. How long did physiological mechanisms for excreting excess water take? Why did it take this long? How long did the kidney continue to void excess water? Why does it take so long to void excess water?

3. How long did physiological mechanisms for excreting NaCl take? Why did it take this long?

SEVEN

Metabolic Rate and Temperature Regulation

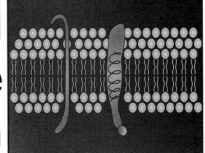

As homeotherms, we are required to maintain internal temperature within narrow limits for survival. We generate heat through metabolism, and we can either gain heat or lose heat to the environment passively, as do inanimate objects. Several physiologic processes are described in this chapter either to aid or minimize the passive heat exchange mechanisms through control of cutaneous circulation and sweating. A review of how metabolism affects body temperature precedes the discussion of temperature regulation.

METABOLIC RATE

Nearly all metabolism results in either external work or heat; some of this heat is then transformed to infrared radiation to the environment. The energy produced by chemical reactions may produce work as defined in physics as a force applied to move an object a distance. Otherwise, the chemical energy is dissipated as heat. Because of this phenomenon, metabolic rate can be measured as the heat produced by a body if the physical work is taken into account. Calorimetry is the term applied to measurement of metabolic rate by measuring heat production. Two types of calorimetry are available. Direct calorimetry is the measurement of heat produced by an individual while in a special chamber with adiabatic walls to prevent heat from being transferred to the environment. Heat produced by an individual warms water circulated through the chamber. Metabolic rate is computed based upon the idea that heat produced by metabolism is equal to total volume of water passing through chamber times the change in temperature times the heat capacity of water. Direct calorimetry is not practical for most applications because using it is expensive and the equipment is not readily available. A more practical method is called indirect calorimetry, which is performed by measuring oxygen consumption. It is assumed that metabolism is totally supported by oxidative phosphorylation when metabolic rate is computed this way. Historically, the unit used in calorimetry is the calorie, which is the heat required to raise temperature of 1 g of water by 1°C. The acceptable unit in physics is the watt, which is 1 Newton-meter per 1 second, or force applied over a distance per time. When metabolic rate causes body temperature to increase, we can say that more heat is stored in the body. Heat storage of an individual is computed as the person's mass times the change in temperature times the body's heat capacity, which is near that of water. External work per time (power) also needs to be taken into account to balance heat production with heat loss and heat storage. External work is quantified easily using a device, such as a treadmill or bicycle ergometer, on which a person's power output can be monitored and kept at a steady rate and the device can be calibrated accurately. Many commercially available exercise bicycles are not suitable for this task because there is no way to measure how much actual work is performed.

One may need to convert from one type of unit to another because of the way the device is calibrated, because values in published literature are in a certain unit, or because the patient's record may contain values in different units. The kilocalorie (kcal or Cal) is often used as a unit of heat production. For a person with average mechanical efficiency, 1 W of external work requires 3.5 kcal per hour. Commonly used power outputs for patients are in 50 W increments. Some older bicycle ergometers use a unit called kpm per minute, which means that the individual moves a mass of 1 kg 1 meter in 1 minute. This unit ignores the acceleration due to gravity and uses 1 minute instead of 1 second. Therefore, to convert kpm/min to watts, we need to divide by 60 to convert to seconds and multiply by the acceleration due to gravity, 9.8 m/sec². Usually, we simply divide the number of kpm by 6 to obtain watts. An individual's metabolic rate can also be expressed in terms of the quantity of oxygen that a person consumes to support metabolism per minute in liters per minute or relative to body size in milliliters per minute per kg of body weight. We can estimate oxygen consumption and energy expenditure with simple equations, assuming everyone has the same mechanical efficiency. Examples for the average person are given below:

$$50 \text{ W} = 300 \text{ kpm/min requires } 900 \text{ ml O}_2/\text{min} = 260 \text{ kcal/hour}$$
$$100 \text{ W} = 600 \text{ kpm/min requires } 1500 \text{ ml/min} = 434 \text{ kcal/hour}$$

From oxygen consumed for support of metabolism, one can estimate metabolic rate, because the variability in efficiency among individuals is low. We can predict the required oxygen consumption for a given task rapidly using a simple, linear relationship if we take into account the individual's resting metabolic rate of approximately 300 ml/min or 86 kcal/hr: oxygen consumption $(VO_2) = 12 \times W + 300$ ml/min or, using kpm/min instead of watts, the equation becomes $2 \times$ kpm/min $+ 300$ ml/min. For example, the numbers above can be derived as 50 W $\times$ 12 ml O_2/min per W + 300 ml O_2 for resting metabolism = 900 ml O_2/min. Instead of estimating oxygen consumption based on intensity of work, we can get a better idea of metabolic rate by actually measuring oxygen consumption by collecting the subject's expired gas and measuring its vol-

TABLE 7-1

Metabolic Rate Per Oxygen Consumption

	CARBOHYDRATE	FAT	PROTEIN
kcal/gram	4.1	9.3	4.3
L of O_2/gram	0.75	2.03	0.97
kcal/L of O_2	5.0	4.7	4.5

kcal/gram is the content of energy in each gram or the energy-density of the substrate, L/gram is oxygen required to completely reduce the substrate to its simplest form to extract the maximum energy from it, kcal/L is the energy derived from using 1 L of oxygen for a given type of substrate.

ume and fraction of O_2. Another method is to allow the person to breathe 100% O_2 from a calibrated container (spirometer), remove the expired CO_2, and determine how much oxygen was removed from the spirometer.

To convert oxygen consumption to metabolic rate, we need to know how much heat is produced from how much oxygen consumed. Use of different types of fuel alters the relationship between VO_2 and metabolic rate. One gram of a different type of fuel results in production of a different amount of heat as shown in Table 7-1. Each type of fuel (carbohydrate, protein, and fat) requires a different amount of oxygen to reduce it to simplest form. Because more energy-dense fuel requires more oxygen to metabolize it, each type of fuel produces a similar amount of heat per liter of oxygen consumed. The typical mixture of fuels produces an average of 4.825 kcal per liter of oxygen consumed.

BASAL METABOLIC RATE

The minimum metabolic rate required to sustain vital functions while awake is called the basal metabolic rate (BMR). During sleep, metabolic rate may be less than BMR, but while awake, metabolic rate is usually greater than BMR. We usually do not measure BMR, but resting metabolic rate. The reason for measuring resting metabolic rate instead is the list of the requirements for measuring BMR, which are:

1. Twelve hours or more have elapsed since food was last ingested.
2. Measurement is preceded by a restful night's sleep.
3. The person is awake and has been at rest for 30 to 60 minutes.
4. The person is in a reclining position.
5. There is an ambient (surrounding) temperature between 62° and 87°F.

Metabolic rate is influenced by many factors, the most obvious of which is size. The dimension of size

that best correlates with metabolic rate is body surface area (BSA). BSA is also important to metabolic rate and heat balance because heat is lost to the environment in proportion to BSA exposed to the environment. Other factors influencing metabolic rate include growth, age, gender, sleep, emotional state, activity, and other calorigenic effects, such as ingestion of food and circulating levels of hormones, especially thyroid hormones and epinephrine. Growth is an important consideration because metabolic rate must sustain activity plus growth; metabolic rate declines with age after growth is complete. For a given BSA and all other factors being equal, metabolic rate is higher in males. The effect of eating on the metabolic rate is called food-induced calorigenesis. Ingestion of food can increase metabolic rate 10% to 20%. Protein appears to have the greatest effect. The increased metabolic rate is believed to be due to processing of nutrients by the liver. Metabolic rate is also influenced by environmental temperature. The increase in metabolic rate with increases in temperature is called the Q_{10} effect, which refers to the increased metabolic rate for each 10° increase in temperature. Infection with its accompanying fever and wound healing, especially with burns of large areas of skin, also increases metabolic rate. Although it is generally the role of the dietician to determine the nutritional needs of a patient, situations may arise in which other health care professionals should, at least qualitatively, understand the changing nutritional needs with factors that influence metabolic rate. By far, the greatest effect on metabolic rate is produced by muscular activity, which can increase metabolic rate 15 times or more. For example, a normal metabolic rate for the average size person is 1500 kcal/day, but a lumberjack may produce 7000 kcal/day.

HORMONAL INFLUENCES

Two major thyroid hormones influence the metabolic rate. Both are simple molecules consisting of two amino acids (tyrosine) with either three iodine atoms (triiodothyronine, T_3) or four (thyroxine, T_4). Approximately 90% of the circulating thyroid hormone is T_4, and 10% is T_3. Most of the biological effects are due to T_3, however. An excess of thyroid hormone is called hyperthyroidism and is associated with increased food intake, decreased body weight, sweating, skin vasodilation, and heat intolerance due to excessive metabolic rate. In contrast, a person with hypothyroidism displays cold intolerance and shivering in temperatures that would be considered comfortable to most people.

Epinephrine released by the adrenal medulla also has a calorigenic effect. It stimulates glycogen and triglyceride metabolism and is thought to produce what are called futile cycles in which ATP is used for both breakdown and resynthesis of substrates, which produces heat. During physical or emotional stress, stimulation of the adrenal medulla causes secretion of epinephrine.

TEMPERATURE REGULATION

Thermoregulation is the set of physiologic processes that act to produce a balance between heat loss and heat production. As homeotherms, we must maintain temperature within narrow limits to maintain biochemical reactions at a normal rate. As discussed above, all heat produced in the body is from chemical reactions. Although we use the same mechanisms to exchange heat with the environment as inanimate objects, we are capable of either enhancing or reducing heat exchange through physiologic mechanisms (described later in this chapter) (Figure 7-1). Two types of regulation can be described. These are called behavioral and physiologic temperature regulation.

Behavioral regulation is conscious, voluntary maintenance of comfort through such behaviors as changes in surface area, use of clothing and other insulation, changing surroundings, including using protective structures, and climate controls (heaters, fans, and air conditioners). The change in surface area can be readily observed as a person curls up to decrease exposed surface area in the cold or spreads out the extremities in a hot environment. A related concept is that of habituation, in which one no longer responds to a condition that formerly elicited a response. Habituation is observed in certain populations, such as Australian aborigines, in response to chronic exposure to cold.

Physiologic regulation is the collection of involuntary responses to maintain "core" temperature at a "set point" determined by the hypothalamus. The core refers to the central area of the body, including the brain and

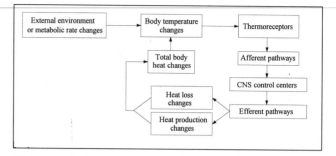

Figure 7-1. Temperature regulation. Negative feedback mechanisms compensate for changes detected by thermoreceptors. Effector mechanisms (discussed later in this chapter) produce changes in either heat production or heat loss.

viscera, which are maintained at a constant temperature. The set point is the temperature about which heat loss and gain are controlled to maintain temperature. The shell is the area of the body allowed to vary in temperature as needed for thermoregulation. The relative sizes of the core and shell vary with thermoregulatory needs. Stated briefly, the core becomes larger in a hot environment and smaller in a cold environment as the temperatures of peripheral tissues are sacrificed to maintain the temperature of the vital organs.

When thermal balance occurs to maintain temperature at a given set point, heat production plus any heat gained from the environment equals heat loss to the environment. This idea can be expressed mathematically as:

$$M - (W + R + K + C + E) = 0$$

where M = heat of metabolism, W = external work performed, R = heat loss to the environment by infrared radiation, K = heat loss by conduction of heat directly to another object, C = heat loss by convection (heat conducted to a flowing medium), and E = heat loss by evaporation of sweat. The difference between body temperatures integrated from thermoreceptors throughout the body and the set point of hypothalamus drives physiologic thermoregulatory responses. As temperature increases above set point, heat loss increases to equal heat production. Temperature becomes steady, but must be elevated to continue to drive heat loss mechanisms. As temperature decreases below set point, heat loss decreases, and heat production may increase to balance heat loss and heat gain at a temperature lower than the set point.

In a thermoneutral environment (25° to 30°C or 75° to 86°F), temperature is maintained without any noticeable regulation, such as sweating or shivering. Regulation of skin blood flow influences passive heat exchange with the environment to maintain core tem-

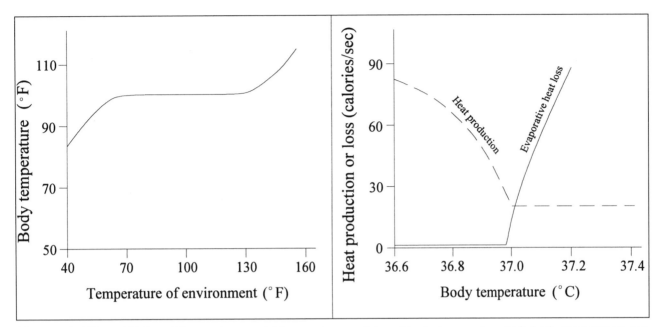

Figure 7-2. Effect of high and low environmental temperature on internal body temperature. Left: body temperature can remain stable despite a wide variation in environmental temperature. Right: changes in heat production and evaporative heat loss with changes in body temperature.

perature. As temperature rises, more heat is brought to the body surface through convection, using skin blood flow, and heat is lost to the environment by convection and infrared radiation. A decrease in temperature causes skin blood flow to decrease, thereby decreasing the body heat carried to the body surface. When ambient temperature falls below the point that decreased skin blood flow can maintain body temperature, shivering occurs. Sweating results when ambient temperature rises high enough that increasing the delivery of heat to the skin is no longer sufficient to maintain body temperature. The temperature considered thermoneutral is dependent on activity, also. A range of 75° to 86°F would be considered above thermoneutral during exercise (Figure 7-2).

As discussed above, the central core temperature changes very little under normal circumstances compared with the extremes in temperature to which the body is exposed. The volume of the core is greatly influenced by environmental temperature, but the periphery or shell is subject to wide variation in temperature. This change in the size of the core is produced by alterations in peripheral blood flow. The shell temperature and, therefore, the average temperature throughout the body may increase or decrease, but altering the size of the core acts to keep core temperature fairly constant. In a warm environment, or during increased metabolic activity, peripheral tissue is allowed to increase toward core temperature by pumping more warm blood through the

shell. In a cold environment, peripheral tissues are allowed to decrease toward environmental temperature by decreasing blood flow to the periphery, which reduces the removal of heat and, therefore, the fall in core temperature (Figure 7-3). In addition to negative feedback mechanisms that have been discussed previously, the thermoregulatory system also uses feedforward mechanisms, in which a potential disturbance is detected before a change occurs. Temperature receptors in the skin feed information of impending heat loss or gain to the hypothalamus, which can activate the appropriate physiologic response before a change in core temperature occurs.

TEMPERATURE VARIATIONS (RECTAL READINGS)

Temperature varies normally throughout the day within a range of 96.6°F (35.9°C) to 99.1°F (37.3°C). In a cold environment, the range is somewhat lower (96° to 97°F). Temperature may increase with emotional experiences or mild exercise to a range of 100° to 101°F and may increase during heavy exercise to a range of 101° to 105°F (Figure 7-4). As described more fully in Chapter 29, the female hormone progesterone increases body temperature. The increase in progesterone following ovulation produces an increase of about 0.5°F. With pregnancy, progesterone secretion is elevated, causing temperature to be greater than pre-pregnancy temperature (Figure 7-5).

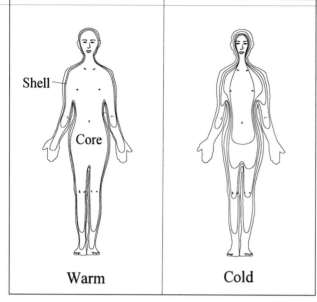

Figure 7-3. The concepts of a shell and a core. The core temperature is maintained by physiologic mechanisms, whereas the temperature of the shell is allowed to vary as needed. In a warm environment, the core is expanded as peripheral blood flow carries warm blood toward the periphery. In a cold environment, the shell is expanded due to peripheral vasoconstriction, which diminishes loss of heat to the environment.

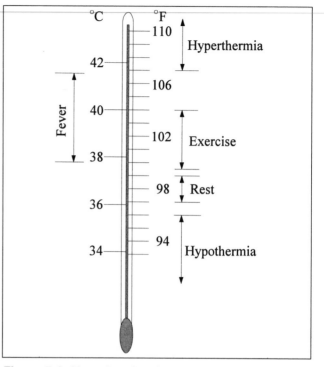

Figure 7-4. Normal and pathologic variations in internal temperature.

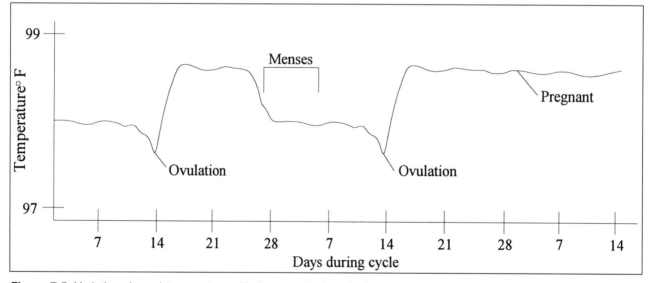

Figure 7-5. Variations in oral temperature with the menstrual cycle. Increased progesterone following ovulation increases temperature. During the second cycle, pregnancy occurs, and temperature remains elevated.

During exercise, an increased body temperature drives thermoregulatory mechanisms in proportion to the increased metabolic rate. Temperature rises until heat loss again balances heat production. A more fit athlete can support a greater blood flow to the skin and higher sweat rate than an untrained individual. The rise in body temperature is, therefore, not proportional to the absolute increase in metabolic rate, but is increased in proportion to the percentage of maximum VO_2. A trained athlete will have a lower body temperature and heart rate and a higher sweat rate at any given power output than an untrained individual (Figure 7-6).

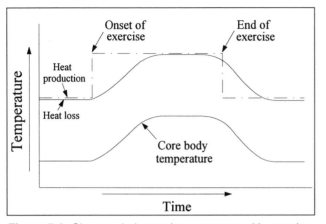

Figure 7-6. Changes in internal temperature with exercise. Core temperature increases in proportion to the percentage of maximum oxygen consumption elicited by the exercise.

ABNORMAL VARIATIONS

Temperature is expected to rise during exposure to a hot environment and exercise; however, systemic disease states can produce a rise in temperature not related to metabolic rate or ambient temperature, called fever. Temperature may increase to dangerous levels, producing an internal temperature of 100° to 105°F. The source of fever should be investigated, if necessary, by a physician. Fever can be a sign of infection, autoimmune disease, or cancer. During fever, the set point around which thermoregulation is controlled is increased by substances called cytokines that include tumor necrosis factor (TNF), interleukin-1, and interleukin-6. Macrophages activated by infection appear to be one major source of cytokines that reset the hypothalamic set point to a higher temperature. These cytokines (TNF, IL-1, and IL-6) may operate through prostaglandin synthesis. One piece of supporting evidence is that aspirin, which inhibits prostaglandin synthesis, is effective at reducing fever.

A fever can be described in three phases (Figure 7-7). In the first phase, body temperature is below the new set point, chills are present, and the patient feels cold and outwardly appears cold with vasoconstriction and shivering. The second phase is a plateau temperature at which the person feels thermal comfort, in spite of an elevated temperature. During the third phase (crisis, breaking of the fever), the person feels warm, and intense sweating and vasodilation occur as body temperature is greater than the now normal set point. Although fever may be beneficial in destroying hostile invaders, if temperature increases too much, central nervous system (CNS) damage may result.

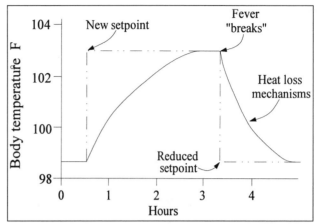

Figure 7-7. Changes in internal temperature before, during, and following fever. Fever is heralded by a change in set point and thermoregulatory responses appropriate for decreased internal temperature (chills, shivering) until temperature reaches the new set point. As fever breaks, set point returns to normal, and thermoregulatory responses (sweating, vasodilation) appropriate for an elevated temperature are observed.

HEAT EXHAUSTION

Hypotension resulting from exercise in a hot environment is called heat exhaustion. Plasma volume is decreased due to sweating, and combined with extreme vasodilation and a decreased cardiac output, arterial pressure falls. In heat exhaustion, body temperature does not become excessively high because the situation is partially self-correcting; heat exhaustion stops work in heat due to fainting. Thermoregulatory mechanisms are still functional, and the person's skin is red, clammy, and cold due to sweat. Fluid needs to be restored, and the person should be removed from the hot environment.

HEAT STROKE

A more ominous problem with thermoregulation is heat stroke, which is a loss of the ability to dissipate heat. During heat stroke, body temperature rises to dangerous levels and may lead to collapse, delirium, seizures, and prolonged unconsciousness or death. Heat stroke is caused by exposure and overexertion in a hot environment. Heat stroke may follow prolonged heat exhaustion, particularly in the elderly and those with cardiovascular disease. Heat stroke is characterized by failure to sweat; therefore, the skin is dry and hot, compared with the cold, clammy skin of an individual in heat exhaustion. These individuals need to be cooled off as soon as possible and taken for emergency care.

Temperature may also rise secondary to brain

lesions and heat stroke to 105° to 110°F. A life-threatening condition, which elicits a positive feedback mechanism of increased temperature with destruction of tissue, is called malignant hyperthermia, which may also increase core temperature to 105° to 110°F. Malignant hyperthermia is usually a reaction to general anesthetics and can be treated by paralytic agents. Lethal temperatures are considered above 40.5°C or 105°F or below 27°C or 80.6°F. Although many individuals have been resuscitated at temperatures below this range, expert medical care is required to do so.

PASSIVE MECHANISMS OF HEAT LOSS

Conduction, convection, and infrared radiation are mechanisms used to exchange heat by inanimate objects (Figure 7-8). Thermoregulation can be thought of as the sum of physiologic mechanisms that optimize these processes to achieve thermal balance. Conduction is the flow of heat from one object to another with which it is in contact. Energy is lost by the direct transfer of energy from one molecule to another. Heat loss is a function of the difference in temperature between the two bodies, the amount of surface in contact, and the respective thermal conductivities in analogy to Ohm's law (conductance = 1/resistance). The conductivity of substances that may contact the body varies greatly. The conductivity of water is 0.0014 cal/cm/sec/°C, brass is 0.225 cal/cm/sec/°C, air is 0.000056 cal/cm/sec/°C, and muscle is 0.001 cal/cm/sec/°C. Conduction has a tremendous ability to exchange per degree difference in temperature, but because we are usually in contact with air and wear clothes that have low conductivity, conduction is usually an unimportant mechanism for heat exchange. Moreover, we learn to avoid contact with substances of high conductivity during extremes in temperature. For example, we learn that sitting on a hot wooden bench or cloth seat will not cause much exchange of heat, but sitting on a nail in the bench or on a vinyl seat will cause an uncomfortable amount of heat to be exchanged. Another consequence of differences in conductivity is that we lose heat much more rapidly in water than in air at the same temperature. Although we may be quite comfortable at a room temperature of 70°F, we feel very cold in water of the same temperature.

Convection is the transfer of energy through a fluid medium in which moving molecules that collide with the surface of an object absorb heat and then move away (conduction aided by flow of the medium). Heat loss depends on both the difference in temperature and the rate of movement of the fluid medium. Free convection occurs when fluid surrounding the body is warmed,

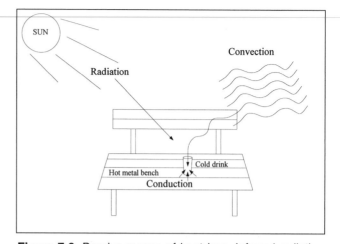

Figure 7-8. Passive means of heat loss. Infrared radiation transfers heat via sunlight and from warmer objects to cooler objects. Conduction transfers heat by direct contact from a warmer object to a cooler object and normally is responsible for little exchange of heat between the body and the environment. Convection uses a flowing medium (air or water) to carry heat to or from the body.

rises, and is replaced by cooler fluid. Forced convection occurs when energy is used to cause flow of a medium across the body. Examples of forced convection used for heat loss in the human body include air flowing through the respiratory tract (panting is used to a great degree in non-sweating homeotherms) and blood flow through the body carrying heat from the core of the body to the skin due to the pumping of the heart. The use of a turbine in a whirlpool is another example of forced convection. In still water, the convection current is so slow that the temperature of the water in contact with the body approaches that of the skin. Agitation of the water maintains the temperature at a uniform level throughout the whirlpool to maintain the exchange of heat with the body.

Radiation is the exchange of heat between the body and the environment in the form of electromagnetic waves. The amount of heat lost is a function of the difference in skin temperature and the temperature of the object to which energy is radiating and the surface area exposed. One can increase or decrease heat loss or gain by altering posture to change the body surface area exposed to the environment. Because of radiation, one can lose a substantial amount of heat through closed windows to the colder outdoor environment and feel cold even if the temperature in the room is normal. Heat exchange is also dependent on the nature of the surface. Objects with dark colors and rough surfaces exchange more heat than those with light colors and smooth textures.

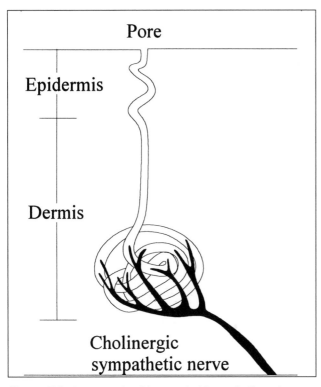

Pore

Epidermis

Dermis

Cholinergic
sympathetic nerve

Figure 7-9. A sweat gland innervated by a cholinergic sympathetic nerve. Fluid with the same electrolyte concentration as blood is produced, but much of the electrolyte content is removed as the fluid travels through the duct, leaving a dilute salt solution on the surface of the skin.

EVAPORATIVE HEAT LOSS

Passive mechanisms are sources of heat loss or heat gain depending on the difference between the temperature of the body and the environment, whereas evaporation produces only heat loss. When liquid water enters the gas phase, it carries 0.6 kcal of heat with it for each gram of water evaporated. Loss of heat through evaporation is dependent upon an unequal distribution of thermal energy in the water. As water molecules reach a certain energy level, they can break free from hydrogen bonds with other water molecules and escape into the air (ie, evaporate). As the highest energy water molecules leave the body surface, the average kinetic energy of water on the surface of the skin is decreased, resulting in a decreased temperature. This loss of heat then allows more heat to flow from the warm blood to the skin and from the skin to the sweat. Therefore, sweat must evaporate to produce heat loss. Dripping of sweat is wasteful; it produces no heat loss, but produces a loss of body fluid. In addition to the amount of sweat produced, a second factor determining heat loss by evaporation is humidity. Water is in equilibrium between liquid and gas phases. How much water goes into the gas

phase relative to the liquid phase and thereby causing heat loss is determined by both air temperature and the concentration of water vapor in the air, which is called the absolute humidity. Warmer air is capable of holding more water vapor than cold air. As temperature of the air increases, the equilibrium between liquid and gas phases is shifted to more water in the gas phase. Relative humidity is the percent saturation of the air. At different temperatures, a given water vapor concentration will produce a higher relative humidity if the air is cold and lower if the air is warm. Therefore, the water vapor expired on a cold day will condense, allowing one to see one's breath.

To be effective, evaporation must be aided by convection on both surfaces of the skin. Skin is warmed by skin blood flow, and flow of air across the skin brings cooler air with low water concentration air into contact with skin. When humidity is high, sweat drips off before it can evaporate. Therefore, a hot, humid environment is more stressful than a hot, dry environment. A healthy individual can withstand extremely high temperatures if humidity is low (130°C if dry), but 40°C is very uncomfortable if the air is humid. If sweat is not allowed to evaporate, skin temperature rises and causes sweat to be produced at a higher rate. Some people use this concept to try to lose weight rapidly. Wearing a watertight suit during exercise or while sitting in the sauna can cause a tremendous loss of fluid and, therefore, weight. However, this weight loss is temporary until water is replaced. Moreover, this practice is dangerous and has led to the deaths of several wrestlers attempting to lose weight. The inability to evaporate sweat causes body temperature to increase to a dangerous level that may lead to heat stroke and alters electrolyte composition.

When heat loss by passive means (radiation, conduction, and convection) is no longer adequate to prevent a rise in body temperature, sweat glands are activated. Two types of sweat glands have been described in humans. Eccrine glands are primarily involved in heat loss, whereas apocrine glands are involved in emotional stress, as antiperspirant manufacturers let us know in their commercial advertisements. Insensible evaporative heat loss occurs through the respiratory system and skin, is not regulated, and contributes a small amount to heat loss before sweat glands are activated. Our sweat glands, which number about 2.5 million, are innervated by cholinergic postganglionic sympathetic fibers (Figure 7-9). Maximum sweat rate is approximately 4 L/hour, which, if all evaporated, could rid the body of 2400 kcal/hour. Sweat is essentially a weak solution of NaCl. Similar to fluid of the distal tubule of the nephron, the composition of sweat is under control of aldosterone. In addition, the composition of sweat is also determined by the rate of sweating. At low rates, much of the solute is removed, but at a high sweat rate, composition approaches that of plasma as less time is available for solute removal. Because sweat is so dilute, most individuals can replace the fluid lost simply through drinking tap water. Athletes who sweat at a high rate for a long time may need to replace electrolytes and water with a dilute salt solution. People with cystic fibrosis (CF) need to replace nearly isotonic fluid due to the inability of the sweat glands to reabsorb solutes. Many people with CF take pretzels with them when they exercise to replace this salt.

Thermoregulatory Responses to Cold

Thermogenesis is the additional production of heat to maintain a balance between heat lost to the environment and heat production. Heat can be gained through metabolism by the breakdown of food and hormonal effects, especially thyroid hormones and epinephrine. Shivering uses ATP, but produces no external work, therefore, increasing temperature. Vasoconstriction of cutaneous blood vessels conserves heat by bringing less heat to the skin, and because skin temperature is decreased, less heat is lost by radiation and convection to the environment. However, decreased blood flow to the extremities also decreases the delivery of nutrients and risks thermal injury to these parts. Most peripheral tissues can withstand low blood flow for a relatively long time (30 to 60 minutes), but blood flow is needed to provide nutrients and to periodically rewarm skin to avoid damage (frostbite). The Lewis hunting reaction is a cyclic change in skin blood flow during exposure to cold. Periodic increases in blood flow temporarily elevate skin blood flow, especially to fingers to maintain the integrity of the skin (Figure 7-10).

The response of the extremities is exaggerated in a condition called Raynaud's disease and Raynaud's phenomenon. In both conditions, blood vessels, particularly in the fingers, go into spasm when exposed to cold or emotional stress. The affected fingers, toes, and sometimes ears and nose become white due to the lack of blood flow and, if prolonged, turn blue. After several minutes or longer, the affected area turns red due to a compensatory increased blood flow, or hyperemia. People with these conditions need to protect their hands when the weather becomes cold. Raynaud's disease differs from Raynaud's phenomenon in that the disease has no known cause (idiopathic), whereas the phenomenon is related to an underlying disease such as atherosclerosis, Buerger's disease, lupus, and especially scleroderma. Any person in whom this response to cold is observed

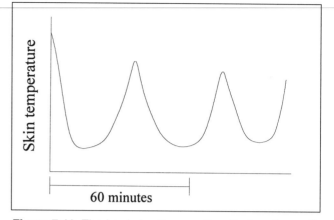

Figure 7-10. The Lewis hunting reaction. Cycles of vasodilation during cold exposure periodically rewarms the skin and prevents skin injury.

should be worked up for the possibility of one of these underlying diseases.

Other circulatory responses to cold involve countercurrent blood flow between paired arterial and venous vessels. The paired arteries and veins run parallel to each other and exchange heat. Deep veins are paired with arteries, but more veins exist than corresponding arteries. In addition, many superficial veins return blood to the central circulation. In a cold environment, the veins running along arteries can carry almost all of the blood back to the heart, and superficial veins carry little of the returning blood. As venous blood becomes colder, more heat is transferred from the deep arteries to their paired veins, which warms the venous blood returning to the central circulation and reduces the heat carried to the skin. This mechanism works in the opposite way to help dissipate heat. As skin temperature increases, superficial veins carry more of the venous blood so less heat is transferred from artery to vein. The arterial blood reaching skin is warmer, and blood as it runs through superficial veins can continue to dissipate heat. The forearm, in particular, has a large number of superficial veins and is involved in what is probably a learned but unconscious behavior of rolling up sleeves to dissipate heat.

Nervous Control of Temperature Regulation

Under resting conditions, in a comfortable environment, most heat loss (~60%) occurs by radiation with small contributions by insensible evaporation (~20%) and convection (~15%). However, when ambient temperature exceeds skin temperature, passive heat loss mechanisms become heat gain mechanisms, and all heat loss occurs via evaporation of sweat. When skin loses

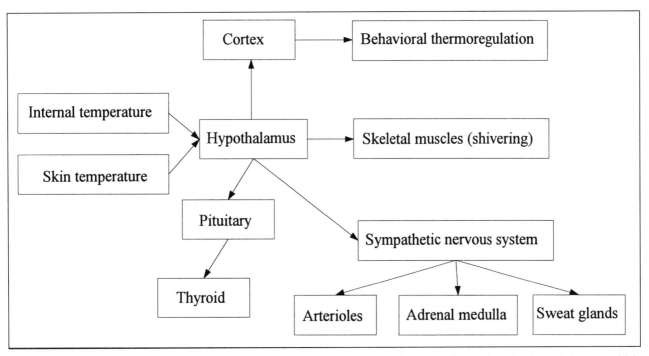

Figure 7-11. Thermoregulatory processes. Temperature receptors feed information forward to the hypothalamus, which directs output to effectors, including the cortex for behavioral thermoregulation, the pituitary for endocrine responses, the skeletal muscles to promote shivering as needed, and through the sympathetic nervous system to constrict blood vessels in the periphery as needed, to promote heat production via the adrenal glands, and to activate the sweat glands as needed to dissipate heat.

more heat to the environment than metabolism produces, the thermoregulatory system reduces heat loss by the skin and may increase heat production via nervous control of temperature regulation.

Thermal receptors are located throughout the body: on the skin and within viscera, muscles, spinal cord, and the hypothalamus. This information is integrated within the hypothalamus where heat loss and gain mechanisms are controlled to produce thermal balance (Figure 7-11). Spinal cord injuries and other injuries or diseases affecting the relay of temperature information to the hypothalamus may interfere with temperature regulation. Effectors for the thermoregulatory system include sympathetic nerves to sweat glands, skin arterioles, and the adrenal medulla. Other effectors include hypothalamic input to produce thyroid-stimulating hormone-releasing factor from hypothalamus to stimulate the anterior pituitary to release thyroid-stimulating hormone (TSH), which in turn increases release of thyroid hormone, somatic nerves to produce shivering, and the cerebral cortex to produce thermoregulatory behavior. Sympathetic nerves to the adrenal medulla produce epinephrine, and the thyroid produces and secretes its hormones. Brown adipose tissue (BAT), found in neonates, rats, and other species, increases metabolic activity in cold. BAT is important because neonates have poor thermoregulation, which is compounded by their rela-

tively large surface area for their body mass. Sympathetic stimulation causes heat production by this tissue. Nervous control of thermoregulation during increased temperature produces increased skin blood flow and activation of sweat glands if necessary, whereas decreased temperature results in inhibition of sweating, vasoconstriction of the skin, activation of piloerector muscles, and the hormonal changes described above.

ACCLIMATIZATION TO EXERCISE IN HEAT

Training in a hot environment produces characteristic, reversible adaptations in thermoregulation called acclimatization. It is characterized by changes in sweating onset, volume, and composition. The acute response to exercise in a hot environment is a rapid increase in core temperature and heart rate. After 7 to 10 days of exposure to heat, exercise produces less of an increase in core temperature and heart rate, sweating begins earlier, and sweat rate (ml/hour) increases. These changes include regulating plasma volume at a higher level, an improved retention of plasma volume during exercise, and a decreased NaCl level in sweat due to aldosterone. These changes are similar to adaptations that occur from exercise alone. The combination of exercise and heat produces more pronounced adaptations than passive exposure to heat or exercise alone.

ACCLIMATIZATION TO EXERCISE IN COLD

Exercise in the cold is less of a problem than in heat, because we can wear clothes for insulation. The usual problem during work is dissipating heat, not generating it. The dangers in exercising in a cold environment include frostbite on body parts with a large surface area to volume ratio, including the ears, nose, fingers, toes, nipples, and penis. Another danger is the possibility of an injury by running long distances alone in the wilderness resulting in hypothermia if the individual cannot reach shelter. Much of the research on exercise in a cold environment comes from studying pearl divers who stay in cold water for a long time. Adaptations to exercise in the cold include increased metabolic rate, increased insulation, an ability to withstand cold without shivering, and increased blood flow to the periphery.

REGULATION OF GLUCOSE

The processing of nutrients is required to maintain cellular functions. One of the most important nutrients is glucose. Glucose metabolism is adjusted throughout the day to maintain a steady concentration in the blood. The metabolism of glucose includes events that lower blood glucose after eating and while glucose is being absorbed from the gastrointestinal tract and events that prevent blood glucose from falling after it has been absorbed. These two conditions are referred to as the absorptive state and the postabsorptive state. During the absorptive state, ingested nutrients are entering the blood. The postabsorptive state occurs when the gastrointestinal tract has emptied, and we must use stored nutrients. A meal takes approximately 4 hours, depending on its composition, for complete absorption. We are usually in the postabsorptive state during late morning, late afternoon, and most of the night.

During the absorptive state, ingested materials are used as energy, and the remainder is put into stores. Amino acids and monosaccharides are transported from the intestine to the blood and to the liver via the portal circulation. The venous drainage of the intestine is routed through the liver to allow a large fraction of absorbed amino acids and monosaccharides to be taken up by the liver before circulating through the rest of the body. Products of fat digestion are transported via the lymphatic system to the systemic venous circulation.

During the absorptive state, glucose is used in several ways. First, it becomes the preferential substrate for metabolism in most tissues. In muscle tissue and liver, it is stored as glycogen. Some of the glucose is also transformed into triacylglycerols for storage in the liver and adipose tissue. Amino acids may be used by cells to form proteins or may be deaminated to be used in other ways. The NH_3 produced by deamination is converted to urea to be excreted in the urine. Once deaminated, amino acids may be converted to keto acids to be used for energy or may be converted to fatty acids and then triacylglycerols to be stored as fat. The excess proteins, carbohydrates, and fats ingested are stored in the forms of protein, glycogen, or fat and may be mobilized for energy production during the postabsorptive state. These processes allow us to eat intermittently and use excess nutrients later as needed.

During the postabsorptive state, synthesis of glycogen, fat, and protein decreases, and net catabolism begins. Because no glucose is absorbed from the intestine at this time, we require mechanisms to maintain plasma glucose levels. In particular, the cells of the nervous system require glucose to maintain their integrity. Blood glucose is maintained by releasing glucose into the blood by the liver and by glucose sparing. Glucose sparing refers to the ability of other tissues to generate energy by using fuels other than glucose, such as fatty acids and keto acids. Sources of blood glucose include glycogenolysis, the breakdown of liver glycogen into glucose, and gluconeogenesis, the synthesis of glucose from molecules other than glycogen, such as pyruvate, lactate, glycerol, and amino acids. Although muscle cells have glycogen, they can only reduce glycogen to glucose-6-phosphate. Muscle cells lack the enzyme to remove phosphate from glucose to allow glucose to exit the cell and be used elsewhere. Liver glycogen can be used for energy by any cell in the body; muscle glycogen can only be used by the cell that stores it. A second source of energy during the postabsorptive state is lipolysis. Triacylglycerols are broken down into glycerol and free fatty acids. Glycerol can be transformed into glucose, and fatty acids can be metabolized to be used in the Krebs cycle. Some fatty acids can also be metabolized into ketones that may be used for energy in some cells.

The metabolism of fatty acids during the postabsorptive state leads to formation of acetyl CoA. Acetyl CoA combines with oxaloacetic acid to form citrate in the Krebs cycle. The ability of acetyl CoA to enter the Krebs cycle depends upon the availability of oxaloacetate. If fat breakdown predominates during the postabsorptive state, not enough oxaloacetate exists for the acetyl CoA generated from fat metabolism to be used in that pathway. Instead, two acetyl CoA molecules are converted into acetoacetate, a ketone body. In the presence of high levels of H^+, acetoacetate is converted in acetone, which can be smelled on the breath of an individual with severe ketoacidosis. If acetoacetate can be reduced (a hydrogen ion is picked up by NAD), D-3-hydroxybutyrate is formed, which can be used for energy by some tissues.

Acetoacetate can be used by tissues such as heart muscle, renal cortex, and the nervous system. Because humans lack the enzymes necessary to convert fatty acids into glucose, fatty acids must be converted into ketones to be used for catabolism. The inability to metabolize glucose due to starvation or diabetes mellitus leads to the use of fatty acids as the primary fuel, thereby producing ketoacidosis, a potentially life-threatening condition.

REGULATION OF BLOOD GLUCOSE

Blood glucose level is controlled primarily by two hormones from the pancreas. The pancreas is both an exocrine and an endocrine gland. The pancreas produces digestive enzymes and secretes a fluid rich in bicarbonate to neutralize the acid that enters the intestine from the stomach. In addition to the exocrine cells, the pancreas has islands of endocrine cells nestled between the ducts with their exocrine cell lining. These cells, totaling approximately 1 million with a combined mass of 1.0 to 1.5 grams, are called the islets of Langerhans. Four types of islet cells may be observed. They are called α cells, β cells, D cells, and PP cells. The α cells constitute 20% of the islet cells and produce the hormone glucagon. The β cells constitute 70% of the islet cells and produce the hormone insulin. D cells (5 to 10% of islet cells) produce somatostatin, and PP cells produce pancreatic polypeptide.

Insulin affects both transport and enzymes involved in metabolism. It binds to specific insulin receptors, which leads to a decrease in cAMP by inhibiting adenylate cyclase. Binding of insulin to target cells increases transport of glucose into skeletal muscle and adipose cells by increasing the number of glucose transport proteins. In addition, insulin promotes glycogen synthesis and inhibits glycogenolysis. In the liver, insulin decreases gluconeogenesis and increases glycogen synthesis. The effects of insulin on adipose cells include stimulating the facilitated diffusion of glucose into adipocytes, promoting the conversion of glucose into triglycerides for storage and uptake of fatty acids by adipocytes. Summarized simply, insulin leads to decreased concentrations of substrates of metabolism in the blood by increasing uptake and promoting conversion of substrates into appropriate storage forms (glycogen and triacylglycerols). Insulin acts as part of a negative feedback mechanism for regulating blood glucose levels. The events of the absorptive state are largely those of the effects of insulin. Increased plasma glucose following a meal (during the absorptive state) stimulates the release of insulin from β cells. Increased levels of insulin lead to increased glucose uptake by cells and inhibition of glucose output by the liver, which then results in returning blood glucose levels to normal. In addition to the effect of blood glucose on insulin release, other factors are involved in insulin regulation. Increased levels of amino acids promote insulin release, whereas sympathetic stimulation and circulating epinephrine both inhibit release of insulin.

Glucagon, the hormone released by α cells, opposes the effects of insulin. Glucagon binds to its receptors, but also binds to β adrenergic receptors. Binding of glucagon to receptors leads to production of cAMP. Cyclic AMP-dependent protein kinases then produce effects opposing those of insulin. Events of the postabsorptive state are produced by the decreased release of insulin and the increased level of glucagon. Glucagon, like insulin, also is central to a negative feedback mechanism. In the face of decreased glucose concentration in the blood, α cells release glucagon. Glucagon then results in increased levels of energy substrates. In the liver, glucagon produces increased glycogenolysis (break down of glycogen to glucose), gluconeogenesis (formation of glucose from other molecules), and ketone synthesis. Glucagon also causes lipolysis in adipocytes. The result of glucagon secretion is increased glucose, fatty acids, glycerol, and ketones in the blood. Many of the same controlling factors for insulin also affect the secretion of glucagon, but usually in the opposite direction. Glucagon secretion by α cells is stimulated by decreased blood glucose concentration, increased sympathetic stimulation to the pancreas, circulating epinephrine, and increased levels of plasma amino acids. Note that increased amino acid levels in the blood stimulate both insulin and glucagon secretion. This produces a margin of safety following ingestion of a protein meal. If amino acids stimulated insulin secretion alone, blood glucose level would be driven downward by insulin, even if glucose is not absorbed during the meal. The secretion of glucagon also during a protein-rich meal offsets insulin's effect and prevents a large decrease in blood glucose concentration following the ingestion of a protein-rich meal.

OTHER CONTROLS ON PLASMA GLUCOSE CONCENTRATION

Epinephrine, the hormone released by the adrenal medulla, and norepinephrine, the neurotransmitter released by postganglionic sympathetic neurons, have an effect that opposes insulin. During periods of stress, the sympathetic nervous system makes increased blood glucose concentration available through direct and indirect means. First, catecholamines inhibit the release of insulin by β cells. Sympathetic nerves to the liver and adipocytes lead to increased glycogenolysis and gluconeogenesis by the liver and lipolysis by adipocytes. In addition, epinephrine increases glycogenolysis and decreases glucose uptake by skeletal muscle. Circulating epinephrine has the same effect on the liver and adipocytes as stimulation of sympathetic nerves to the liver and adipocytes. Another mechanism involving the sympathetic nervous system is a reflex mediated by glucose receptors in the brain. When plasma glucose decreases, sympathetic nerves to the adrenal medulla are stimulated to cause release of epinephrine, and sympathetic nerves to the liver and adipocytes are stimulated to release fatty acids into the blood. This increase in sympathetic activity explains some of the characteristics of hypoglycemia, including increased heart rate, palpitations, shaking, and a feeling of anxiety.

Cortisol is a glucocorticoid released by the adrenal cortex in response to stress through a negative feedback mechanism. During stress, the hypothalamus is stimulated to secrete corticotropin releasing factor (CRF). CRF stimulates the anterior pituitary to release adrenocorticotrophic hormone (ACTH). ACTH, in turn, stimulates the adrenal cortex to secrete corticosteroids. Two classes of corticosteroids are produced by the adrenal cortex. Mineralocorticoids, of which aldosterone is the primary one, affect the handling of sodium and potassium. Although ACTH affects the secretion of aldosterone, the major determinant of aldosterone secretion is the level of angiotensin II in the blood. The second category of corticosteroids is the glucocorticoids. The primary glucocorticoid is cortisol, also known as hydrocortisone. Ninety-five percent of the glucocorticoid activity is due to cortisol, with a small contribution by corticosterone.

Cortisol is necessary for the events of the postabsorptive state. Although not directly responsible for them, a lack of cortisol diminishes the effect of decreased insulin, increased glucagon, and the effects of catecholamines. During stress, increased levels of cortisol oppose the effects of insulin, leading to an increased blood glucose concentration. High levels of cortisol can result in a phenomenon called adrenal or steroid diabetes due to the high blood glucose level that can be attained due to cortisol. Cortisol has four major functions. It stimulates gluconeogenesis, it mobilizes protein for fuel substrate, it mobilizes fatty acids from adipocytes, and it has an anti-inflammatory effect. Due to these effects of cortisol, treatment of patients with corticosteroid medications has important side effects:

1. Breakdown of protein—excessive use of corticosteroids as an anti-inflammatory can cause destruction of structures.
2. Opposition of insulin—people with diabetes treated with corticosteroids may require an increased dose of insulin.
3. Retardation of growth and wound healing—corticosteroids must be used carefully in youngsters and in patients with healing wounds.
4. Immune suppression—although corticosteroids may be used primarily for this effect in several autoimmune diseases. Immune suppression can be fatal in youngsters exposed to otherwise benign infections, such as chickenpox.

GLUCOSE REGULATION DURING EXERCISE

During exercise, several fuels are available to regenerate ATP, including blood glucose, fatty acids, and muscle glycogen. Although muscle glycogen can only be used within the cell in which it is stored, liver glycogen and triacylglycerides may be mobilized from the liver and adipocytes for all cells to use. Sources of blood glucose include liver glycogenolysis, gluconeogenesis, pyruvate, lactate and glycerol as metabolic byproducts, and glycerol from lipolysis in adipocytes.

During exercise of moderate intensity, blood glucose changes little initially. With prolonged exercise of 30 minutes or so, however, blood glucose may fall as supplies of glycogen become depleted. This appears to account for the phenomenon of "hitting the wall." The primary difference between aerobic athletes training for long distances, such as the 10,000 meters and longer, and those running shorter distances, such as the mile, is the ability to manage carbohydrate resources. Whereas success in the mile run depends on the maximum rate at which oxygen can be used for a time less than 4 minutes, much longer races depend more on the ability to sustain blood glucose levels and to a lesser extent on a high level of oxygen consumption. Long-distance runners accomplish this by having a greater storage of glycogen and decreasing the proportion of aerobic metabolism derived from carbohydrate metabolism (glycogen sparing).

During exercise, a decrease in insulin secretion occurs. The stimulus may be the high rate of sympathetic stimulation during exercise. The question then becomes how cells can take up sufficient quantities of glucose during exercise if insulin levels fall. Fortunately, muscle contraction by itself has a stronger effect on glucose uptake than insulin. In animal experiments, it has been shown that glucose uptake occurs at a greater rate during muscle contraction than the maximum level that can be obtained with insulin stimulation.

SUMMARY

Metabolic rate leads to either external work or production of heat. Metabolic rate can be measured either by direct or indirect calorimetry. Indirect calorimetry relies on measurement of oxygen consumption. Oxygen consumption is directly related to external work and can be estimated if the work rate (power) is known. Basal metabolic rate is different from resting metabolic rate, in which several conditions apply. Several factors that determine metabolic rate are discussed; the most important is exercise. Thyroid hormone and epinephrine can increase metabolic rate and generate heat in a cold environment. Temperature regulation depends on feedforward mechanisms to detect changes in the ambient temperature before core temperature falls and on negative feedback mechanisms to minimize the increase or decrease in the core temperature. Physiologic mecha-

---

Diabetes Mellitus

Two major types of diabetes mellitus (DM) exist. People with type 1, also known as insulin-dependent diabetes, juvenile-onset diabetes, or ketosis-prone diabetes, tend to be younger at the onset of disease, and the symptoms are more severe. Without treatment, type 1 diabetes can be fatal within a period of days. Those with type 2, known also as noninsulin-dependent or adult-onset diabetes, tend to be middle-aged or older at onset and tend to be obese. Type 1 diabetes is an autoimmune disease, typically following an upper respiratory infection or a viral infection. Antibodies made due to the human leukocyte antigen of the individual lead to destruction of β cells. In these individuals, insulin must be replaced by injection. Type 2 diabetes appears to be caused by an interaction between chronic overeating and the person's genetic makeup. Chronic overeating in susceptible individuals leads to a down-regulation of insulin receptors, rendering a person with type 2 diabetes insensitive to the insulin produced during the absorptive state. Many people with type 2 diabetes can be treated by a regimen of exercise and diet. Acute manifestations of the disease are particularly severe in the person with type 1 diabetes. The inability to take up glucose leads to elevation of blood glucose. The glucose filtered into the renal tubules exceeds the transport maximum and acts as a nonpenetrating solute in the rest of the renal tubule. The presence of high levels of nonpenetrating solutes prevents the normal reabsorption of water in the distal tubule and collecting duct, thereby producing diuresis. In addition, the inability to use sufficient glucose causes reliance upon fatty acid metabolism, leading to ketoacidosis. The combination of acidosis and dehydration can cause death over a short time. The absolute need for exogenous insulin to prevent death is the basis of the terms "insulin-dependent" for type 1 and "noninsulin-dependent" for type 2. Many individuals with type 2 diabetes mellitus depend on insulin to be healthy, but will not die in a matter of days without it.

Pathologies Secondary to DM

Poorly controlled DM leads to several secondary pathologies. These include blood vessel, nerve, eye, and kidney disease. Of primary importance to health care professionals are the effects on blood vessels and nerves. DM is a major risk factor for the development of atherosclerosis. Atherosclerosis leads to coronary artery disease, peripheral vascular disease, and cerebrovascular disease (stroke). Peripheral vascular disease often leads to arterial insufficiency that produces open wounds on the most distal parts of the lower extremities and even gangrene requiring amputation. To compound problems, DM reduces the ability of the immune system and slows wound healing. Therefore, a disproportionate number of people with diabetes are seen for cardiac rehabilitation, stroke rehabilitation, amputee care, prosthetic training, and wound care. Kidney disease occurs secondary to damage to renal blood vessels and accumulation of sorbitol, a byproduct of glucose in cells. Diabetic retinopathy can be caused by proliferation and hemorrhaging of capillaries on the retina.

Diabetic neuropathy produces what is known as a "glove and stocking" distribution of decreased sensation. The nerves are affected on the basis of length. The longest nerves (those in the feet) are usually the first affected. Demyelination and vascular sclerosis appear to cause the neuropathy. The person with diabetes poses tremendous problems related to wound care. Decreased sensation allows the feet to be injured without the person with diabetes knowing it. The decreased immune competence allows wounds to become infected. Reduced blood flow to the distal extremity slows healing and presents the need for amputation of slowly healing, infected, or gangrenous foot wounds. Individuals with diabetes need to be trained in foot care and must conscientiously control blood glucose levels to minimize the secondary pathologies. Loss of motor neurons can produce muscle imbalance in the foot leading to deformities and injury to the foot, and loss of autonomic neurons may exacerbate the condition by causing dry skin on the foot.

nisms sacrifice the shell temperature to keep the core temperature from changing. Behavioral thermoregulation is a change in behavior to prevent temperature changes. Heat is exchanged passively with the environment through conduction, convection, and infrared radiation. Most of our heat loss at room temperature occurs by infrared radiation. Evaporation of sweat becomes more important as we increase exercise intensity. In a hot environment, these mechanisms can cause the body to gain heat, and only sweating can dissipate heat. In a cold environment, skin blood flow is decreased to minimize heat loss, and shivering may occur. A countercurrent of blood flow in arteries and veins diminishes heat loss in the cold and improves heat loss in the heat. Body temperature is expected to increase in a hot environment, during exercise, and with increases in progesterone. Fever is a response to release of cytokines in response to infection or other systemic disease. Heat exhaustion causes decreased blood pressure and fainting. Heat stroke is a life-threatening condition in which thermoregulation ceases. The skin is hot and dry. Gradual exposure to exercise in the heat causes adaptations in fluid regulation and circulation that increase the safety of exercise in the heat. We can also adapt to cold exposure.

BIBLIOGRAPHY

Horowitz M. Do cellular heat acclimation responses modulate central thermoregulatory activity? *News in Physiological Sciences.* 1998;13:218-225.

Jansk" L. Humoral thermogenesis and its role in maintaining energy balance. *Physiological Reviews.* 1995;75:237-259.

Pagliaro L. Glycolysis revisited—a funny thing happened on the way to the Krebs cycle. *News in Physiological Sciences.* 1993;8:219-223.

Rolfe DFS, Brown GC. Cellular energy utilization: molecular origin of standard metabolic rate in mammals. *Physiological Reviews.* 1997;77:731-758.

STUDY QUESTIONS

1. What happens to the energy in kilocalories that are ingested as food?

2. If you perform isometric contraction and no work is performed as defined in physics, is energy used? If so, where does the energy go?

3. Why do you think that using a treadmill or a bicycle on which work can be quantified for a person with cardiac disease to exercise is important?

4. Explain how the "core" of the body changes during exercise. How does it change in the cold?

5. Trace thermal energy from the body core to the skin and to a molecule of water (sweat).

6. Based on the large number of veins present in the forearm, explain how rolling up sleeves aids in dissipating heat.

7. How is measuring temperature useful in becoming pregnant?

8. Contrast the exchange of body heat in still water and turbulent water.

9. Explain the color changes in the fingers of a person with Raynaud's phenomenon (or disease).

10. Explain the danger of wearing a watertight suit during exercise or while sitting in a sauna.

11. What outward signs (other than temperature) indicate the onset of fever and the breaking of fever?

12. Contrast the outward signs of heat stroke and heat exhaustion. Why is heat stroke life-threatening?

LABORATORY EXERCISE

LABORATORY EXERCISE 7-1

GLUCOSE TOLERANCE TEST

Glucose tolerance tests are typically performed after a 12 to 18 hour fast. For this lab, one person will skip the previous meal. We will also perform the test on one individual who ingests a large carbohydrate meal. Following measurement of control levels of blood glucose using a glucometer, the two subjects will ingest 1 gram of glucose per kilogram of body weight in the form of a refrigerated beverage. Every 30 minutes following ingestion another blood glucose measurement will be made.

Questions:

1. Why does diuresis occur in diabetes mellitus (DM)?

2. What changes could be detected in a routine urinalysis to screen for DM?

3. Define gluconeogenesis.

Neuromuscular System

The neuromuscular system includes the central nervous system and the peripheral nerves that innervate skeletal muscle, cardiac muscle, smooth muscle, and glands. The central and peripheral nervous systems are unique in their degree of specialization. As such, very localized injury to the central or peripheral nervous systems can produce profound impairments. The nervous system uses membrane potentials (small voltages on the surface of the cell) to communicate in ways that allow information to be received by the central nervous system, to be interpreted, and to signal appropriate responses. The process that allows signals to be propagated from one cell to another is called synaptic transmission. The input of information to the central nervous system is termed sensation, which occurs at the conscious level (eg, taste, touch, sight, hearing, and smell) or at the unconscious level (eg, blood pressure and the chemical composition of body fluids). Pain is a complex concept involving the sensation called nociception (reception of noxious stimuli) and the interpretation in the brain. It is a common reason for a patient/client to seek a rehabilitation professional. Sleep is a complex and necessary process for the long-term function of the neuromuscular system. Sleep deprivation results in poor function of all systems, not just the neuromuscular system. Sleep/wakefulness can be deranged by insult to the brain, including trauma and anoxia. Control of motor function at the level of the spinal cord and muscle is discussed in the musculoskeletal unit to cap discussion of motor function.

EIGHT

Organization of the Nervous System

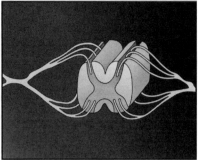

OBJECTIVES

1. List the four basic functions of neurons: input, integration, conduction, and output.

2. List the components and locations of the peripheral nervous system: somatic sensory and motor neurons, autonomic neurons, and ganglia.

3. Describe the functions of neurons: somatic sensory, motor, autonomic, and interneurons.

4. Describe the functions of cell bodies, axons, and dendrites.

5. Describe the processes of convergence and divergence in the nervous system.

6. Describe the functions of microglia compared with macrophages outside the CNS.

7. Compare the functions of oligodendrocytes in the CNS and Schwann cells in the PNS.

8. List four functions of astrocytes.

9. List components of the dorsal and ventral roots.

10. Describe the nomenclature of the spinal nerves.

11. Describe the structure of the autonomic nervous system in terms of where sympathetic and parasympathetic preganglionic cell bodies are located and the relationships of pre- and post-ganglionic autonomic neurons and the location of autonomic ganglia.

12. List the effects of the autonomic nervous system on the heart, airways, gastrointestinal system, eyes, bladder, male reproductive system, liver, kidneys, blood vessels, sweat glands, and adrenal medulla.

13. Compare the effects of the neurotransmitter norepinephrine to the hormone epinephrine.

In Chapter Five, signaling mechanisms were discussed. The most rapid and specific signaling mechanism is the nervous system. The nervous system receives information from the periphery, relays it to the central nervous system (afferent pathways), gathers information to "make decisions" (integration), and sends information to the periphery (efferent pathways). The nervous system uses separate afferent nerves and efferent nerves and synapses to ensure one-way conduction of messages. Afferent (sensory) pathways send information from cells designed to gather information about mechanical, thermal, and chemical events and light. Efferent (motor) pathways send information to effectors. Effectors include muscle cells of different types and glands. Interneurons function to relay messages from one neuron to another. Table 8-1 summarizes the inputs, outputs, and roles of interneurons and motor and sensory neurons.

In this chapter, the organization of the nervous system is described. Properties of the central and peripheral nervous systems and the autonomic and somatic nervous systems are described. Researchers have found classification of neurons into different types to be useful. Classifications are based on the size (diameter) of neurons, the presence or absence of a coating material called myelin, and how fast a neuron conducts an impulse. To understand fully how nerve classification and function are related, a review of basic electrical phenomena is also provided with the classification of neurons in Chapter Ten. Neurons communicate with each other and with other tissues due to their ability to maintain a steady electrical difference across their membranes, called a resting potential, and due to their ability to rapidly reverse the electric potential across their membranes in a stereotypical manner, called an action potential. These and other forms of membrane potentials are described in Chapter Nine. Most neurons communicate by release of chemicals called neurotransmitters onto a specific location. The location at which a neuron interacts with another cell is called a synapse. The communication process, synaptic transmission, is described in Chapter Ten. In Chapter Eleven, sensory processes commonly encountered in rehabilitation—touch, temperature, vibration, proprioception, kinesthesia, and equilibrium—are discussed.

Pain is more than a sensation; it carries with it strong emotional and motivational aspects. Pain is probably the most common reason other than very obvious loss of function that causes people to seek therapeutic intervention. Pain is the subject of Chapter Twelve. Sleep patterns can be disturbed severely during long-term hospitalization or following an injury to the central nervous system, which can impact negatively on a patient's ability to participate in rehabilitation. Sleep is the subject of Chapter Thirteen.

CENTRAL VS. PERIPHERAL NERVOUS SYSTEM

The nervous system is often divided, for the sake of discussion, into the central nervous system (CNS) and the peripheral nervous system (PNS). In general, the CNS consists of the cells of the brain and spinal cord, whereas the PNS consists of neurons outside the brain and spinal cord. The PNS may be further divided into the somatic and autonomic nervous system. The somatic nervous system consists of motor nerves to skeletal muscle and sensory neurons of the dorsal root ganglia and cranial ganglia. Ganglia are clusters of cell bodies of neurons within the PNS, producing a knot-like structure, thus the name ganglion. Collections of cell bodies of neurons within the CNS are called nuclei. The somatic sensory cells innervate skin, muscle, joints, and the surfaces of internal organs, producing the sensations of touch, vibration, temperature, pain, muscle length and tension, trunk, head and limb position, and movement. The somatic nervous system also includes cells that innervate skeletal muscle, called motor neurons. Although the somatic motor system is considered part of the peripheral nervous system, the cell bodies of these neurons are located within the spinal cord.

PARTS OF THE NEURON

The neuron is the functional unit of the nervous system. Each cell has a cell body in which the nucleus is located and in which protein synthesis occurs under the direction of the genetic material. A healthy cell body is necessary for proper cell function. Proteins synthesized in the cell body must be transported to even the most distant parts of the cell, which may be 3 feet or more away. Specialized transport processes are required to perform these functions, called fast axonal and slow axonal transport. Diffusion is too slow to transport substances over these distances adequately. When neurons become sick, as can occur in diabetes mellitus and other conditions, the longest neurons innervating the feet and toes are the first to be affected.

Projections from the cell body on to which other cells release neurotransmitters are called dendrites. The dendrites serve as receptive areas for neurotransmitters, although some neurons may also synapse with the cell body directly. Electrical changes produced by synaptic transmission are conducted from the dendrites to the

TABLE 8-1

Characteristics of Neurons by Direction of Information

TYPE	INPUT	OUTPUT	NUMBER OF AXONS	ROLE
Motor	CNS	Muscle or gland	One	↑tone of skeletal muscle ↑ or ↓tone of smooth muscle ↑ or ↓HR, contractility of heart ↑ or ↓exocrine gland secretion
Sensory	Mechanical, chemical, thermal, or light energy	Dorsal root ganglion or trigeminal nerve ganglion	Two	Reception of sensory stimuli
Interneuron	Neuron	Neuron	One	Transmission of converging or diverging signals

HR = heart rate

cell body. If a strong enough signal is received by the neuron, it produces an electrical event called an action potential that is propagated along another type of process called an axon. In sensory neurons, two axons exist; one axon conducts action potentials from the periphery to the cell body in the dorsal root ganglion and the second axon continues the conduction of the action potential from the dorsal root ganglion along its bifurcated axon and into the spinal cord where the sensory nerve may have synapses with many other cells. Sensory neurons convert various types of stimuli to signals when appropriate and relay the signal to the CNS. This is accomplished through either specialized receptors or free nerve endings; therefore, these cells do not have dendrites to receive information from other neurons. In motor neurons, the action potential travels away from the cell body along a single axon peripherally to the effector. Interneurons may be part of a sensory or motor chain of neurons or may transmit information from a sensory neuron to a motor neuron as occurs in some reflexes. Interneurons, like motor neurons, receive information from dendrites, integrate a signal along the cell body, and transmit the signal along an axon to another cell, in this case, another neuron. Interneurons may transmit information locally (local interneurons) or at great distances within the CNS (projection interneurons).

CLASSIFICATION SCHEMES FOR NEURONS

Neurons may be classified based on other characteristics in addition to the division by function into motor, sensory, and interneuron. Neurons that carry information toward the CNS are termed afferent. Afferent and sensory are synonymous. Efferent or motor neurons carry information from the CNS toward effectors. In some cases, a chain of a sensory or motor neuron and one or more transmission interneurons is required to relay the information to or from the CNS. For motor systems, we use the terms upper and lower motor neurons. The upper motor neuron originates in the brain and travels to the ventral horn of the spinal cord to synapse with the lower motor neuron, which has its cell body in the ventral horn, but its axon runs through the peripheral nervous system. Neurons of the autonomic nervous system are divided into preganglionic neurons carrying information from the CNS to autonomic ganglia. Preganglionic autonomic neurons synapse with postganglionic neurons within the autonomic ganglia. Many important sensory systems have three neuron chains. The neuron with the sensory function in the periphery is termed the first order neuron. Its cell body is located in the dorsal root ganglion, and a second axon extends into the spinal cord to synapse with a second-order neuron. Second-order neurons run up the spinal cord into the brain where they synapse with third-order neurons either in the thalamus or the reticular formation. Third-order neurons typically carry sensory information from the thalamus to the cortex to provide conscious perception of the sensory event.

Neurons are also classified by the targets of the motor neurons or source of sensation of the sensory neurons into visceral and somatic. Visceral neurons innervate internal organs (viscera) and body segments developed from the branchial arches. Somatic neurons innervate areas other than viscera, including skin, bone,

TABLE 8-2

Types of Neurons Based on Direction of Information, Anatomic, and Embryologic Origin

	SOMATIC		VISCERAL	
GENERAL	**Afferent (GSA)** Sensation of face, tongue, mouth (other than taste) and body	**Efferent (GSE)** Eye, tongue, skeletal muscle movement	**Afferent (GVA)** Visceral sensation, baroreception, chemoreception	**Efferent (GVE)** Pupillary constriction, lens accommodation, lacrimation, salivation, regulation of digestive system, and regulation of heart
SPECIAL	**Afferent (SSA)** Vision, equilibrium, hearing	**Efferent (SSE)** Regulation of tone of muscles regulating vestibular and auditory function*	**Afferent (SVA)** Olfaction, taste	**Efferent (SVE)** Muscles of mastication (chewing), facial expression, soft palate, trapezius**, sternocleidomastoid**

*Various authors classify the neurons regulating the muscles that control inner ear and tympanic membrane function in various ways.
**The neurons of cranial nerve XI that innervate these muscles are sometimes classified as GSE by some authors, depending on the interpretation of the origin of the neurons' nucleus.

and associated structures and skeletal muscle. A third classification divides neurons into special and general. Special refers to neurons that either carry information to or from structures derived from the branchial arches or carry information from organs of special senses. Within the category of special neurons, special visceral afferent neurons carry information about taste and smell (branchial arch origin), and special somatic neurons carry visual, auditory, and equilibrium information. Special visceral efferent neurons innervate muscles derived from the branchial arch, including muscles of mastication (chewing muscles) and muscles of facial expression. Some authors include the motor neurons of the trapezius and sternocleidomastoid muscles in this category, whereas others argue that the neurons belong in the general somatic efferent category. General neurons are those that do not belong in the special category.

Based on these three dichotomous divisions, eight categories result. Many authors actually only describe seven categories, leaving out the special somatic efferent. As defined, special somatic neurons are only sensory (or afferent). Some, however, classify the neurons that control the muscles that regulate inner ear function as special somatic efferent. General somatic afferent neurons are responsible for the sensations of the body, face, and mouth other than taste, whereas general visceral afferent neurons are responsible for sensation originat-

ing in the viscera, including chemoreception and baroreception (pressure receptors). General somatic efferents are the motor neurons of skeletal muscle, muscles that control eye movement, and movement of the tongue.

General visceral efferent neurons control the pupils and lens of the eyes, salivation, tear production, and regulate digestive organs. Special neurons innervate special sensory organs and structures derived from the branchial arches. Special somatic afferents relay visual, auditory, and equilibrium information, whereas special visceral afferents carry olfactory and taste information. The classification scheme into these eight categories is usually of greatest interest in the study of cranial nerves and the brain stem. Certain cranial nerves carry certain types of neurons, which you will be expected to learn in a neuroanatomy class. Moreover, specific classes of neurons are segregated as they travel through the brain stem either entering or leaving nuclei of the cranial nerves or passing through the brain stem into higher centers. The types of neurons and their functions are summarized in Table 8-2.

FUNCTIONS OF NEURONS

Neurons have four basic functions: input, integration, conduction, and output. The **input** function is provided by dendrites and sometimes the cell body com-

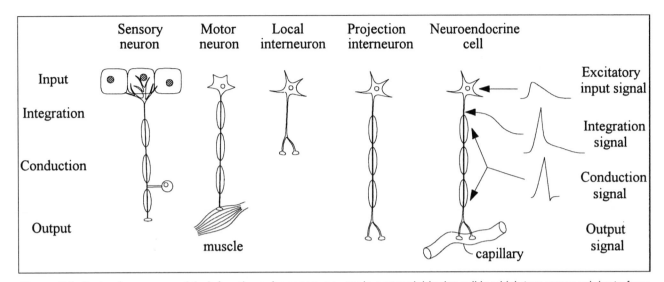

Figure 8-1. Parts of neurons and their functions. A sensory neuron is a pseudobipolar cell in which two axons originate from the cell body. It is not a true bipolar cell, because the initial part of the axon is a single projection that splits into peripheral and central neurons. No dendrites appear on these neurons; instead, information is received by receptor potentials from specialized sensory receptors or free nerve endings. Beyond the receptors, integration of input determines if an action potential will be generated. The action potential provides the conductive function of all types of neurons shown here. The output function is the release of neurotransmitter on an interneuron in the spinal cord or higher centers with which the sensory neuron synapses. Motor neurons have dendrites with which central (upper) motor neurons synapse and release neurotransmitter. The cell body integrates the input, and an action potential is generated at the axon hillock if threshold is reached. The output function of the motor neuron is release of the neurotransmitter acetylcholine onto the motor end plate of skeletal muscle. Interneurons receive input at the dendrites and cell bodies, use the cell body to integrate the signal and action potential propagated along the axon for the conductive function, and release neurotransmitter onto another neuron for the output function.

municating by the use of synapses to receive either inhibitory or facilitatory messages. In the case of sensory neurons, a sensory stimulus is translated by the cell, rather than receiving input from another neuron. The cell body, up to the junction between the cell body and axon, called the axon hillock, sums the messages received by the dendrites. The **integration** function is produced by the electrical summation of excitatory and inhibitory signals. These processes are depicted in Figure 8-1. Due to the process by which membrane potentials are generated (Chapter Ten), the value must be between –90 and +40 mV. As discussed previously, the resting membrane potential of neurons is approximately –70 mV in contrast to muscle cells that have a resting membrane potential close to the maximum value of –90 mV. Skeletal muscle receives only stimulatory signals and functions well at that membrane potential. The membrane potential of neurons is slightly depolarized compared with skeletal muscle, which allows the membrane to become either more negative (hyperpolarizing), which decreases the possibility of producing a signal, or to depolarize and increase the possibility of sending a signal to the next neuron(s) along the network. If strong enough stimulatory signals are received, an action potential is conducted along the axon (function

of **conduction**). Arrival of the action potential at axon terminals results in release of neurotransmitter, the **output** function of a neuron. The neurotransmitter may be released on an effector by a motor neuron or on the dendrites or cell body of another neuron, producing the input function of the next neuron in a chain.

CONVERGENCE AND DIVERGENCE

Neurons do not simply pass information from one cell to the next. One cell may receive information from several different cells. This situation is called convergence. Moreover, a neuron may send information to more than one other neuron; this is called divergence (Figure 8-2). In a simple reflex, such as a knee jerk, sensory neurons signal motor neurons from the same muscle that was stretched to produce a muscle contraction that occurs before we even become aware that the quadriceps tendon was struck. During the knee jerk, interneurons relay the sensory information about the quadriceps being stretched to the brain and, at the same time, to the neurons innervating the hamstring muscles. The quadriceps muscles contract, the hamstrings relax,

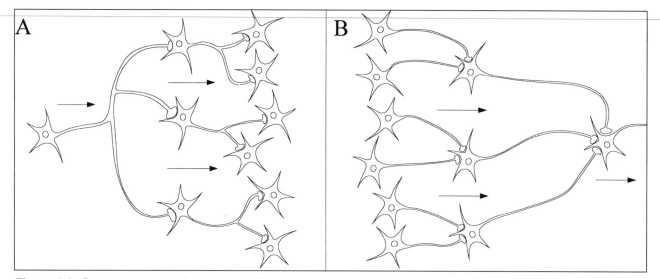

Figure 8-2. Convergence and divergence. A: Divergence provides many neurons with information from one neuron. B: Convergence allows a neuron to receive information from several neurons and to act as a decision maker dependent upon the information received.

and shortly thereafter we realize that the quadriceps tendon has been struck. This is an example of divergence. The signals may be excitatory (quadriceps muscle) or inhibitory (hamstring muscles). In convergence, the signals may also be either excitatory or inhibitory. The neuron receiving large numbers of messages electrically adds up the excitatory and inhibitory messages. The sum of the signals determines if the neuron generates an action potential to send a message elsewhere. Having both excitatory and inhibitory messages allows certain neurons to act as "decision makers."

GLIAL CELLS

The word glia comes from Greek for glue. Glial cells provide supporting functions that allow neurons to perform their tasks. There are many times more glial cells than neurons. Estimates vary from 10 to 50 times more glia than neurons. Without glial cells, the nervous system would consist of a clump of unorganized cells that could not function in any meaningful way. Glial cells may be divided into two types: microglia and macroglia. Microglia are found in the CNS, but are not actually nervous system cells; they are derived from cells of the immune system. Microglia act as garbage collectors to remove unwanted substances including dead cells. Microglia, however, are not as effective as the related cell, the macrophage that performs the same function in the PNS. This is one possible reason why regeneration of damaged cells is possible in the PNS, but does not occur naturally in the CNS. Moreover, macrophages produce growth factors that microglia do not.

Macroglia consist of Schwann cells, astrocytes, and oligodendrocytes. These cells provide physical support for neurons, may provide nutritional support for neurons, and contribute to the formation of the blood-brain barrier. Macroglia also have the ability to take up relatively large quantities of potassium ions to minimize changes in extracellular $[K^+]$ that might otherwise occur during high levels of nervous system activity. Oligodendrocytes in the CNS and Schwann cells in the PNS produce myelin, a substance that insulates axons. In a later chapter, we will see how myelin decreases the build up of charge on the membrane, thereby allowing axons to conduct action potentials more rapidly. In addition to their different locations, oligodendrocytes and Schwann cells have other differences. Oligodendrocytes form myelin sheaths around an average of 15 different axons at once, whereas a series of individual Schwann cells is found along individual axons. Schwann cells also appear to aid in the regeneration of damaged peripheral axons, whereas oligodendrocytes may actually inhibit regeneration of central neurons.

Astrocytes have several functions related to their ability to take up various substances. They maintain the extracellular concentration of potassium ions, remove neurotransmitter from the extracellular fluid to end signaling mechanisms, and may deliver nutrients from capillaries to neurons. Astrocytes also seal the gaps in capillaries to form the blood-brain barrier to prevent harmful substances from simply leaking into the extracellular fluid of the brain (Figure 8-3).

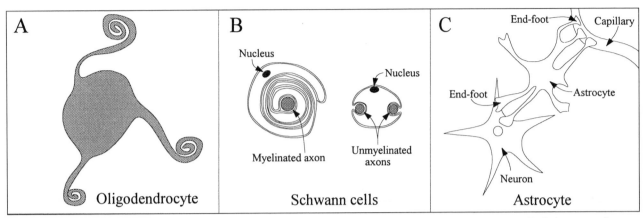

Figure 8-3. Glial cells. A: Oligodendrocytes form myelin sheaths around several central axons at once. B: Schwann cells perform a similar function in the peripheral nervous system, but individual Schwann cells myelinate only one axon. Many Schwann cells line up along peripheral axons with bare spots between them called nodes of Ranvier. The myelin sheath is due to the wrapping of Schwann cells around the cells several times, forming concentric layers of myelin. C: The star-shaped astrocyte making contact with both a capillary and a neuron, providing a nutritive role and sealing the space between endothelial cells of capillaries to form the blood-brain barrier.

CENTRAL NERVOUS SYSTEM

A number of different ways exist to divide the central nervous system, depending on the reasons of the author. Brief descriptions of the following functional parts will follow: 1) spinal cord, 2) medulla oblongata (often simply referred to as the medulla), 3) pons and cerebellum, 4) midbrain, 5) diencephalon, 6) cerebral hemispheres.

The spinal cord extends from the base of the skull to the first lumbar vertebra. The spinal cord receives information from skin, joints, muscles of the trunk and limbs, and the internal organs. The spinal cord also contains the cell bodies of the motor neurons that produce voluntary and reflex muscle activity. The spinal cord appears to be able to produce primitive stance and rhythmic muscle activity sufficient for locomotion without connection to the rest of the CNS. Sensory and motor activity of the head is largely controlled by the brain stem. Some overlap does exist. For example, sensation from skin on the back of the head is routed to the spinal cord; two muscles controlling the neck and shoulders are innervated by the eleventh cranial nerves.

Within the spinal cord, and throughout the CNS, neurons are organized according to function and into gray and white matter. The gray matter contains cell bodies of neurons, and white matter consists of myelinated axons. The dorsal (posterior) part of the cord consists of sensory neurons. Cell bodies of motor neurons are found in the anterior (ventral) part of the spinal cord. Projecting from the spinal cord are dorsal and ventral roots. Bulges on the dorsal roots are the dorsal root ganglia where cell bodies of sensory neurons are located. The central branch of the sensory neuron communicates with extensive networks of neurons in the posterior horn gray matter. The peripheral branch of the sensory neuron ends in some type of sensory apparatus. This may be a specific sensory end organ, or it may be a free nerve ending. Motor neurons, with their cell bodies in the anterior cord, travel through the ventral root along with neurons of the autonomic nervous system.

Small bundles of axons, called rootlets, combine to form either a dorsal or ventral root. The length of spinal cord that gives rise to a given dorsal and ventral root is called a spinal cord level. A short distance from the cord, the dorsal and ventral roots unite to form 31 pairs of spinal nerves that exit between the 30 vertebrae for which they are named (Figure 8-4). Because there is one more pair of spinal nerves than vertebrae, an adjustment must be made in the naming of the spinal nerves. This is done at the cervical level. In the cervical cord, spinal nerve C1 exits above vertebra C1, C7 exits above vertebra C7, and spinal nerve C8 exits below vertebra C7 and above T1. From T1 to the coccygeal nerve, the spinal nerves are named for the vertebra above the spinal nerve as it exits (Figure 8-5). As each spinal nerve exits, it often combines with other nerves to form plexuses, and from plexuses, peripheral nerve trunks arise. This mixing of neurons from different spinal nerves into various peripheral nerve trunks complicates evaluation of neurologic injury. Neurons from specific spinal nerves tend to provide sensation to broad areas of skin called dermatomes ("skin slices") (Figure 8-6). Areas of skin, however, are innervated by specific peripheral nerves with a distribution that is somewhat different from that

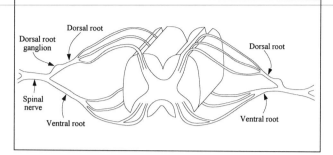

Figure 8-4. Ventral and dorsal roots unite to form spinal nerves between each pair of adjacent vertebrae. Axons of motor neurons in the anterior (ventral) horn of the gray matter form the ventral root. Central axons of pseudobipolar cells of the dorsal root ganglion form the dorsal root. Many of these cells synapse with cell bodies or dendrites within the posterior (dorsal) gray matter. Ventral roots, dorsal roots, and spinal nerves are bilateral.

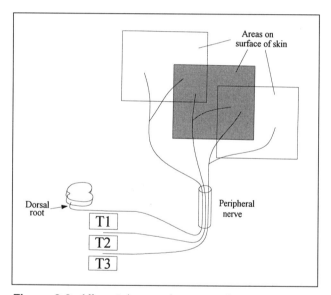

Figure 8-6. Afferent (sensory) neurons from one area of skin tend to be incorporated within the same spinal nerve and dorsal root ganglion. This slice of skin is called a dermatome. Dermatomes are distributed in a head-to-tail direction with rotation around the extremities. Placing the body in a quadruped position and externally rotating the extremities places the dermatomes in a more understandable position. Because spinal nerves contribute to several peripheral nerves, some overlapping of dermatomes occurs. Loss of a dorsal root will severely diminish sensation in a dermatome, but will not produce anesthesia.

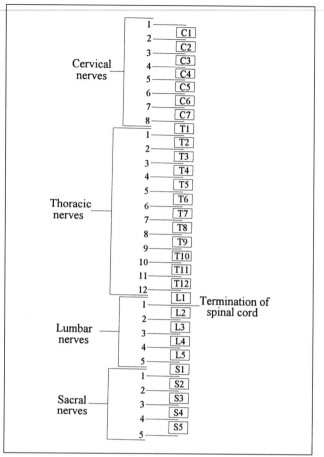

Figure 8-5. Relationship of spinal nerves to vertebra. Note C8 exits between C7 and T1 vertebrae. Above C8, spinal nerves exit above vertebrae for which they are named. Below C8, spinal nerves exit below vertebrae for which they are named. Also note that the spinal cord ends at L1. Below this, only spinal nerves are found.

of the dermatomes. Distinguishing between sensory deficits within a dermatomal distribution (Figure 8-7) or a peripheral nerve distribution often aids in determining whether damage has occurred to a peripheral nerve or a nerve root or the spinal cord. Evaluation becomes particularly difficult when part of a plexus is damaged; the deficits do not completely fit spinal nerve or peripheral nerve distributions. Specific muscles are innervated by specific peripheral nerves that consist of neurons that come from typically two to four spinal nerves, although some muscles have contributions from fewer or more. Severing a spinal nerve results only in weakness of a number of muscles, in contrast to the paralysis that results if a peripheral nerve is severed.

For the face, head, and neck, the brain stem serves many of the same functions that the spinal cord does for the rest of the body. It receives its sensory input and produces motor output through cranial nerves. In addition, the brain stem is largely responsible for special senses located in the head. The brain stem also consists of pathways between the spinal cord and higher centers of the brain. Within the brain stem, a primitive network of neurons, called the reticular formation, exists. This network appears to be related to the state of arousal.

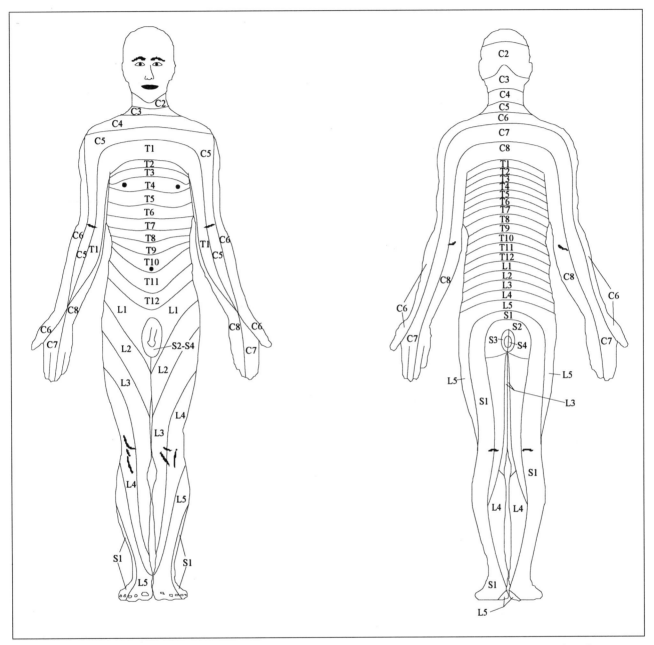

Figure 8-7. Dermatome maps used to infer which spinal nerves or dorsal roots are involved in sensory dysfunction.

The medulla is the part of the brain stem immediately adjacent to the spinal cord. Within the medulla are several vital centers responsible for regulation of breathing, swallowing, and the cardiovascular system. The pons is located between the medulla and midbrain and primarily is a pathway ("bridge") between the cerebral hemispheres or spinal cord and the cerebellum. The cerebellum is involved in the learning of motor skills and has a modifying effect on muscle activity. It receives information from the cerebral cortex, the vestibular sys-

tem, and neurons carrying information on body position and is largely responsible for maintenance of posture and coordination of head and eye movement. The midbrain controls several functions, in particular, those related to vision and hearing, including eye movements.

The diencephalon consists primarily of the thalamus and hypothalamus. The diencephalon is found between the cerebrum and midbrain. The thalamus processes and distributes almost all sensory and motor information going to the cerebral cortex. The hypothalamus regu-

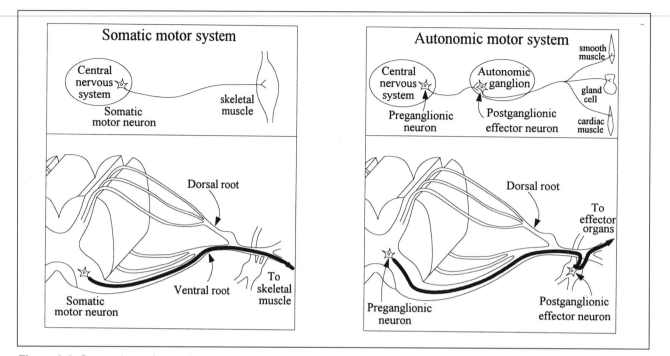

Figure 8-8. Comparison of somatic motor system to autonomic system. A: Somatic motor; cell body of motor neuron is within anterior horn of gray matter of the spinal cord. The axon travels through the ventral root to innervate skeletal muscle. B: In the autonomic system, the cell body is found in the intermediolateral gray matter; the axon travels through the ventral root to an autonomic ganglion. A sympathetic ganglion is depicted here. Within the ganglion, the presynaptic neuron synapses with post-synaptic neurons. Postsynaptic neurons innervate smooth muscle, glands, and cardiac muscle.

lates autonomic nervous system activity and hormonal secretion of the pituitary gland.

The cerebral hemispheres are the largest region of the brain. They consist of cortex, white matter, basal ganglia, the hippocampus, and amygdala. The cerebral hemispheres are responsible for perception, cognition, higher motor functions, emotion, and memory. The basal ganglia are involved in the planning of movement. Deficits in areas of the basal ganglia may result in either too much or too little movement and are manifested in diseases such as Parkinsonism and Huntington's disease. The hippocampus and amygdala and associated areas of the cerebral cortex comprise the limbic system. The amygdala modulates activity of the autonomic nervous system and release of hypothalamic hormones in response to motivational state and emotion. The hippocampus is involved in the processing of memory storage and is damaged in Alzheimer's disease.

AUTONOMIC NERVOUS SYSTEM

The autonomic nervous system has three divisions: sympathetic, parasympathetic, and enteric nervous systems. These systems are physically and usually functionally separate. The sympathetic nerves arise from the tho-

racic and lumbar spinal cord, and, in general, sympathetic nervous system function can be related to the response to stress. The parasympathetic nervous system arises from the brain stem and sacral spinal cord. Cell bodies of both the sympathetic and parasympathetic, as are the somatic motor neurons, are physically located within the CNS. An anatomic comparison of the somatic motor system and autonomic motor system is depicted in Figure 8-8. Many parasympathetic functions are considered to be related to restoration of homeostasis, although we will see that the sympathetic and parasympathetic nervous systems have functions that are not related simply to stress and restoration. A comparison of features of the two systems is depicted in Figure 8-9 and Table 8-3. The enteric nervous system is the "brain" of the gastrointestinal tract. The enteric nervous system interacts with the sympathetic and parasympathetic systems to coordinate gastrointestinal activity. However, the enteric nervous system is capable of functioning independently of the other divisions of the autonomic nervous system. The autonomic nerves do not directly send messages from the central nervous system. Instead, we have a two-neuron "relay" system consisting of what are called preganglionic and postganglionic autonomic nerves. The cell bodies of the preganglionic neurons reside in the central nervous system and synapse with

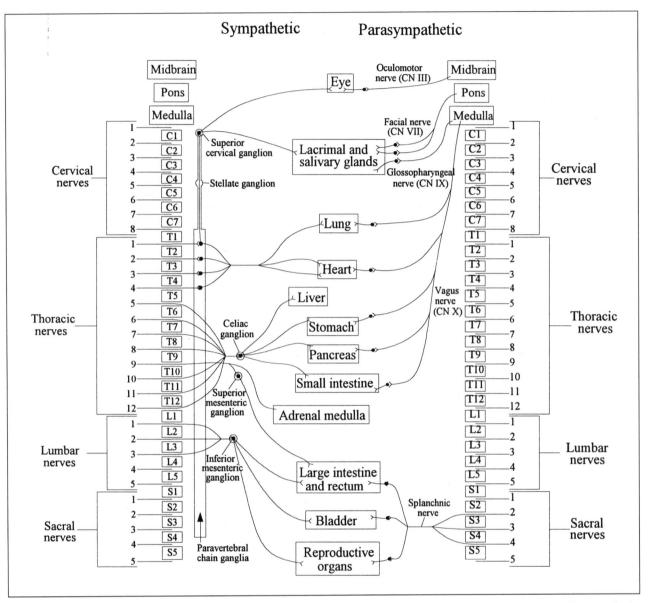

Figure 8-9. Comparison of the sympathetic and parasympathetic divisions of the autonomic nervous system. Preganglionic neurons originate from the thoracic and lumbar spine and travel short distances to ganglia, many of which terminate in the paravertebral sympathetic chain. Postganglionic neurons travel long distances to effectors. Parasympathetic neurons originate in the brain stem and sacral spine and travel long distances to ganglia in or near the effector. Postganglionic neurons travel very short distances to the effector.

other neurons, called postganglionic neurons, within autonomic ganglia. The postganglionic autonomic nerves have their cell bodies in ganglia and extend axons from the ganglia to the tissue of interest.

The autonomic nervous system (as in autonomous) is primarily a motor system of organs such as the eye, heart, liver, and kidneys, but also innervates other tissues and organs, such as blood vessels and sweat glands. The autonomic nervous system controls functions over which we have little voluntary control. Most of the func-

tions of the autonomic nervous system are automatic and are not perceived. Examples include control of blood pressure and skin temperature. However, these functions can be controlled with practice and the use of biofeedback. In many cases, the sympathetic nervous system and parasympathetic systems have opposite effects on organs. An example of this is the heart. The sympathetic nervous system increases heart rate, rate of conduction of the action potential through the heart, and force of contraction. The bilateral vagus nerves

TABLE 8-3

Characteristics and Functions of the Autonomic Divisions

	SYMPATHETIC	PARASYMPATHETIC
Location of preganglionic cell bodies	Thoracic/lumbar spinal cord	Brain stem and sacral spinal cord
Location of ganglia	Close to CNS, distant from target organ	Distant from CNS, on or close to target organ
Neurotransmitter released by preganglionic neurons	Acetylcholine onto nicotinic receptors on postganglionic neurons	Acetylcholine onto nicotinic receptors on postganglionic neurons
Neurotransmitter released by postganglionic neurons	Norepinephrine onto adrenergic receptors on target organ*	Acetylcholine onto muscarinic receptors on target organ
Heart	Increased heart rate, increased force of contraction, and faster spread of the action potential from the atria into the ventricles	Decreased heart rate and slower spread of the action potential from the atria into the ventricles
Airways	Dilation of airways by relaxation of smooth muscle	Constriction of airways
Gastrointestinal system	In general, sympathetic stimulation slows processes	In general, parasympathetic stimulation facilitates processes
Eye	Dilation of the pupil	Narrows the aperture and rounds the lens by producing contraction of the ciliary muscle Decreasing the size of the pupil increases depth of field; rounding the lens allows us to focus on near objects
Bladder	Increases tone of the internal urethral sphincter, inhibiting micturition	Increases tone of the smooth muscle of the bladder wall, thereby facilitating micturition
Male reproductive system	Ejaculation	Erection
Liver	Glycogenolysis, increasing blood glucose level	
Kidney	Decreased renal blood flow, increased renin secretion, and conservation of salt and water	
Blood vessels	Vasoconstriction	Vasodilation of reproductive organs with engorgement of erectile tissues
Sweat glands	Production of sweat	
Adrenal medulla	Release of epinephrine and norepinephrine	

*sweat glands are innervated by cholinergic postganglionic sympathetic neurons.

(parasympathetic innervation of the heart and most of the body other than the head and pelvis) decrease heart rate, slow conduction of the action potential, and decrease force of contraction. In some other cases, the two systems may have complementary roles; the parasympathetic nerves produce erection, and the sympathetic nerves produce ejaculation. In other cases, only one division innervates a type of structure. Blood vessels and sweat glands are innervated by the sympathetic nervous system, but not by the parasympathetic nervous system.

Other differences between the sympathetic and parasympathetic nervous systems include the location of the neurons and the neurotransmitters released by the neurons. Both the sympathetic and parasympathetic nervous systems have two neuron chains between the CNS and the effector. The preganglionic neuron that exits the spinal cord has its cell body in the spinal cord and terminates in a ganglion. Both the sympathetic and parasympathetic nervous systems have these "knots" (ganglia) of cells in which the cell bodies of the second neurons in the pathway are found. In the case of the sympathetic nervous system, the ganglia are a short distance from the spinal cord and originate from the thoracic and lumbar spinal cord. The sympathetic preganglionic nerves are short compared with the long postganglionic sympathetic nerves. The sympathetic ganglia are interconnected at each spinal level and form a chain along the thoracic and lumbar spine. Parasympathetic neurons are found in certain cranial nerves and in preganglionic nerves originating from the sacral portion of the spinal cord. The pair of vagus nerves carry the preponderance of the parasympathetic innervation to the trunk, including organs such as the heart, liver, stomach, and intestines. The extremities do not receive parasympathetic nerves. The parasympathetic nerves from the sacral spinal cord innervate the distal colon, bladder, and reproductive structures. Preganglionic nerves either approach or reach the target organs, and the postganglionic parasympathetic nerves are very short. The usual neurotransmitter of postganglionic sympathetic neurons is norepinephrine, and that of postganglionic parasympathetic neurons is acetylcholine. Acetylcholine is also released by the preganglionic sympathetic and parasympathetic neurons onto their respective postganglionic neurons. However, the type of acetylcholine receptors located within the autonomic ganglia (nicotinic) is different from the type of receptor located on the target organs of the postganglionic parasympathetic neurons, which is muscarinic. The receptors located on the postganglionic neurons of both the sympathetic and parasympathetic neurons that receive acetylcholine from the preganglionic neurons are structurally more similar to the receptors for acetylcholine on the surface of skeletal muscle cells. Neurotransmitters of the autonomic nervous system will be discussed in greater detail in Chapter Ten.

As described above, many of the functions of the sympathetic and parasympathetic nervous systems oppose each other. In the case of the male reproductive system, the functions are complementary. Successful reproduction under normal circumstances requires the function of both. Parasympathetic stimulation produces erection; sympathetic stimulation produces ejaculation. Under unusual circumstances, however, they may occur independently. Some spinal cord or peripheral nerve injuries may produce loss of either erection or ejaculation or both, depending on the level of the injury. Loss of the ability to achieve erection does not produce infertility. Various methods exist to solve the problems of erectile dysfunction. Moreover, the loss of the ability to ejaculate does not necessarily preclude fertility. Research

Thermal Biofeedback

Two basic types of biofeedback are used in rehabilitation. Thermal biofeedback monitors temperature, and electromyographic biofeedback monitors muscle activity and will be described separately in a later chapter. The purpose of biofeedback is to allow control of a physiologic function that cannot normally be controlled voluntarily by providing feedback. Thermal biofeedback devices measure skin temperature, usually the middle finger, with a sensor called a thermistor. A visual or auditory display of skin temperature is provided using numeric displays, bar graphs, deflecting needles, and various tones, beeps, or buzzes to allow the person to know how the temperature of the skin is changing. Skin temperature is chiefly a product of blood flow to the skin, which is controlled by sympathetic activity. Reducing the sympathetic input to the blood vessels of the skin increases skin temperature. Therefore, as one learns to increase temperature of the monitored skin, one is also learning to decrease sympathetic activity to the skin. Thermal biofeedback is used primarily for producing relaxation. When one is relaxed, the activity of the sympathetic nervous system is, in general, decreased, and the activity of the parasympathetic system is increased. Many individuals can learn in one or two 20-minute sessions how to accomplish relaxation this way.

Differential Diagnosis of
Neuromuscular Disease

Knowledge of the organization of the nervous system aids greatly in performing differential diagnosis of neuromuscular disease. Injury to a nerve is expected to cause both decreased strength and sensation. Weakness without sensory disturbance suggests a number of possibilities based on onset, location, and progression. A rapid onset of weakness is usually a sign of Guillain-Barré syndrome in which the myelin of peripheral motor nerves is damaged to a much greater extent than sensory nerves. Myasthenia gravis may also appear to develop over several days, but muscles innervated by cranial nerves tend to be affected first. As a general rule, diseases of muscles, called myopathies, tend to affect proximal muscles first, whereas diseases of neurons, called neuropathies, tend to affect distal muscles. Inflammatory muscle diseases, such as polymyositis/dermatomyositis, are also associated with pain, which is indicative of inflammatory disease. The muscular dystrophies produce gradual weakness over a longer time frame as does amyotrophic lateral sclerosis, in which the motor neurons in the anterior horn of the spinal cord are progressively damaged causing muscle weakness and atrophy (amyotrophy) and hardening of the lateral spinal cord (lateral sclerosis). When both sensory and motor losses occur, the distribution of loss can help identify the cause. Peripheral nerves (eg, radial, ulnar, and median) innervate an area of skin that encompasses pieces of several dermatomes for which several "maps" are available in anatomy textbooks. The weakness is also limited to certain muscles that the particular nerve innervates. Compression of a spinal nerve, which may occur with a bulging disc in the spinal column, will cause sensory changes limited to the spinal nerve or dorsal root that is being compressed. Muscle weakness will occur over a number of muscles innervated by different peripheral nerves, but all receive some contribution to their peripheral nerves from the same spinal nerve. Plexus injuries, most commonly to the brachial plexus, are more difficult to diagnose, because based on what part of the brachial plexus is injured, sensory loss and weakness may occur over the distribution of more than one peripheral nerve and several spinal cord levels. Often, one needs to rule out all the peripheral nerves and dermatomes and, combined with a history of the injury, determine its site as the brachial plexus.

Case Study

A right-handed 60-year-old farmer is referred for therapy with progressive weakness and sensory loss in the right upper extremity. His medical history includes lung cancer for which he is receiving intermittent rounds of chemotherapy. Otherwise, he has no other health problems and had been working until the weakness in the right upper extremity became severe. He reports having a large mass in the upper lobe of his right lung, but no evidence of metastasis. He is no longer able to dress himself and requires some assistance for eating with his left hand. The man presented with tremendous wasting of the muscles of the hand and the forearm and sensory loss of the anterior forearm, fingertips, the backs of the fourth and fifth fingers, and the entire palm of the right hand. Carpal tunnel syndrome and ulnar nerve entrapment had been ruled out by a neurologist.

How could lung cancer affect the strength and sensation of the right arm?

Why was this man tested for carpal tunnel syndrome and ulnar nerve entrapment?

What is the anatomic relationship between the apex of the lung and the innervation of the upper extremity?

What finding should immediately raise the suspicion of a plexus injury as opposed to a peripheral nerve injury or compression of the spine in this case?

What medical/surgical treatment might potentially restore some of his lost upper extremity function?

currently underway is greatly improving fertility in patients with this problem.

The parasympathetic nervous system does not innervate extremities. Blood vessels and sweat glands are innervated only by the sympathetic nervous system. In several organs, only sympathetic modulation of function occurs. These include the liver, kidneys, and adrenal medulla in addition to sweat glands and blood vessels. One exception to autonomic control of blood vessels is the parasympathetic innervation of the reproductive organs. Parasympathetic stimulation increases blood flow to the entire region, resulting in engorgement of erectile tissues.

Innervation of sweat glands is another exception to the general rules of autonomic innervation. In general, postganglionic sympathetic nerves release norepinephrine on their target organs. Sweat glands, on the other hand, are stimulated by cholinergic sympathetic nerves, meaning that the postganglionic sympathetic nerves of sweat glands release acetylcholine instead of norepinephrine.

Sympathetic stimulation of both small arterial vessels, called arterioles, and larger arteries results in vasoconstriction. Blood vessels have a tonic state of partial contraction due to sympathetic stimulation. By increasing the rate of stimulation, both arteries and arterioles constrict more, leading to increased blood pressure. By decreasing the rate of sympathetic stimulation, blood vessels dilate leading to decreased blood pressure. At the local level, many tissues produce vasodilator substances as needed to overcome the effect of sympathetic stimulation, which provides an appropriate level of blood flow for the tissue's needs. Sympathetic blockade by drugs or surgery causes loss of the ability to constrict blood vessels. If a large number of blood vessels are dilated, a person has difficulty adjusting to changes in posture. Standing rapidly results in postural hypotension due to the lack of reflex mechanisms to stimulate the effectors (blood vessels).

Sympathetic stimulation of the adrenal medulla results in the release of epinephrine and norepinephrine. Epinephrine, although similar in structure and function to that of the sympathetic neurotransmitter norepinephrine, binds better to β adrenergic receptors, whereas norepinephrine binds better to α adrenergic receptors. Epinephrine released by the adrenal medulla increases metabolic rate, increases alertness, and causes blood vessels of skeletal muscle to vasodilate via stimulation of β receptors. Table 8-3 summarizes important differences between the sympathetic and parasympathetic divisions of autonomic functions.

SUMMARY

Organization of the nervous system is described. The nervous system is divided into the central nervous system and the peripheral nervous system. The CNS consists of the brain and spinal cord. The PNS consists of sensory nerves with cells bodies in the dorsal root ganglia, somatic motor nerves with cell bodies in the anterior horn of the spinal cord, and the autonomic nervous system. The autonomic nervous system consists of the sympathetic, parasympathetic, and enteric nervous systems. The autonomic nervous systems control functions over which we have no conscious perception and little ability to control. The hypothalamus exerts control over the autonomic nervous system. Important functions provided by the autonomic nervous system are described.

BIBLIOGRAPHY

Berne RM, Levy MN. *Physiology*. St. Louis, Mo: Mosby-Year Book; 1998.

Ganong WF. *Review of Medical Physiology*. Norwalk, Conn: Appleton & Lange; 1995.

Guyton AC, Hall JE, Schmitt W. *Human Physiology and Mechanisms of Disease*. Philadelphia, Pa: WB Saunders; 1997.

Lüscher HR, Clamman HP. Relationship between structure and function in information transfer in spinal monosynaptic reflexes. *Physiological Reviews*. 1992;72:71-99.

STUDY QUESTIONS

1. Describe the roles of the four basic functions of neurons.

2. Contrast the structure of sensory neurons to motor neurons, and relate the structural differences to their differences in function.

3. Two people pick up hot cups of coffee. One person is holding a prized heirloom cup over a rare Oriental rug. The other is holding a hot paper cup over a sink. Explain why one person holds the cup until it can be put down gently and the other person drops the paper cup in the sink immediately. Base your response on the concepts of divergence of the hot/pain sensory signals and convergence of neural signals on the motor neurons responsible for holding the cup.

4. Contrast the structure and functions of Schwann cells in the PNS and oligodendrocytes in the CNS. Discuss how these differences allow regeneration of neurons in the PNS, but not in the CNS.

5. A person develops weakness of the flexor muscles of the wrist and all of the hand muscles after being dragged by the upper extremity in an altercation. What is the cause? How do you develop this conclusion?

6. Following a fracture of the humerus, a person develops numbness of the posterior surface of the forearm and hand and cannot extend the wrist. What is the cause?

7. Describe a situation in which sympathetic input functions are counter to parasympathetic function. Describe a situation in which the functions of these complement each other and a situation in which only one system is active.

8. Based on the principles of signaling by the endocrine system compared with the nervous system, contrast the results of epinephrine release by the adrenal medulla to sympathetic stimulation.

NINE

Membrane Potentials

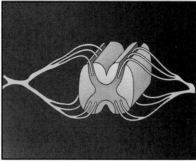

OBJECTIVES

1. List the four basic functions of neurons and the processes that produce them:
   a. Input—receptor or synaptic potential
   b. Integration—summation of receptor or synaptic potentials
   c. Conduction—action potential
   d. Output—release of neurotransmitter

2. Compare action potentials with receptor and synaptic potentials in magnitude, conduction, hyperpolarizing, or depolarizing.

3. Define depolarization, hyperpolarization, overshoot, and undershoot.

4. State the convention for measuring membrane potential.

5. Explain the need for ion channels.

6. List stimuli for opening gated channels.

7. Describe how an equilibrium potential for potassium can exist and the properties of glial cells that allow their membrane potential to exist at the potassium equilibrium potential.

8. List equilibrium potentials for sodium, potassium, and chloride ions.

9. Describe the relative permeability of sodium and potassium under resting conditions in a neuron.

10. Explain how the Goldman equation can be used to estimate membrane potential at any given condition of relative permeability of different ions.

11. Describe the actions of the sodium activation gate, sodium inactivation gate, and potassium activation gate during an action potential, including how relative permeabilities change with time during an action potential.

12. Explain the needs for the sodium inactivation gate and the potassium activation gate.

13. Explain the role of the sodium inactivation gate in the absolute refractory period.

14. Explain the role of the potassium activation gate in the relative refractory period.

In Chapter Eight, four basic functions of neurons were discussed: input, integration, conduction, and output. These four functions depend on the ability of the membrane potentials to change. These types of membrane potentials include the receptor potential, synaptic potential, and the action potential in addition to an electric potential that exists across the membrane of a neuron at rest, called the resting potential.

The resting potential is a stable condition maintained until the membrane is stimulated to produce one of the other types of potentials mentioned above. In this chapter, only the neuron and skeletal muscle cells are discussed. Other tissues will be considered in later chapters. The resting potential is a steady value until the cell is perturbed in some way. In later chapters, however, we will see examples of cells that do not have a steady "resting" potential. In neurons, the resting potential is on the order of –70 mV, whereas this value is about –90 mV in skeletal muscle cells. The direction given to the membrane potential indicates that the inside of the membrane has a negative charge relative to the extracellular fluid. This convention is used because of the way membrane potentials are measured. One electrode is placed in the extracellular fluid, and a second electrode is placed inside the cell. Therefore, one is measuring the difference in electric potential between the extracellular fluid and the inside of the cell. Extracellular fluid is considered the reference point, or 0 mV. In the resting state, potential exists for positively charged particles (cations) to enter the cell.

Receptor and synaptic potentials have three features in common: 1) they are small and graded, 2) they are local potentials that are passively conducted and dissipate with distance, and 3) they may be either depolarizing or hyperpolarizing. Receptor and synaptic potentials are smaller in magnitude than action potentials, and both are proportional to the size of the stimulus. Receptor potentials and synaptic potentials are sometimes called **graded** potentials for this reason; they are graded to the size of the stimulus. Action potentials are all-or-none events with no variation in magnitude unless the ionic concentrations responsible for the action potential are altered. Both the receptor and synaptic potentials are local potentials that are not regenerated. Local potentials dissipate with distance. In contrast, action potentials, which serve the conductive function of the neuron, are regenerative, and under normal conditions, they do not change in magnitude to any appreciable extent as they are conducted along the membrane. Thirdly, receptor and synaptic potentials may be either depolarizing or hyperpolarizing. Depolarization refers to the loss of membrane polarity; the membrane potential goes toward zero. Hyperpolarization means that the

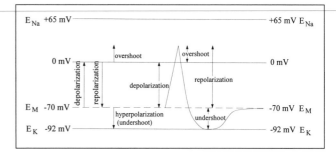

Figure 9-1. Definitions of depolarization, repolarization, hyperpolarization, undershoot, and overshoot, and these events labeled on an action potential.

membrane potential moves farther away from zero, which means the inside of the cell becomes more negative with respect to the extracellular fluid. A third possibility, in addition to hyperpolarization and depolarization, is an overshoot. An overshoot refers to a membrane potential that not only depolarizes, but, instead of stopping at zero, the membrane reverses polarity to become positive inside. Action potentials are depolarizing events only; they do not hyperpolarize a cell. In nerve and skeletal muscle cells, an overshoot can be observed during the action potential. The terms undershoot and hyperrepolarization are used to describe a repolarization that exceeds the resting potential. These terms are shown graphically in Figure 9-1.

Synaptic potentials are commonly the result of many incoming signals, which may be either excitatory or inhibitory. Synaptic potentials are used to make decisions based on information sent by many other neurons converging on a neuron. Excitatory signals cause a slight depolarization, whereas inhibitory signals may produce hyperpolarization or use some other mechanism to render depolarization of the neuron more difficult. If sufficient depolarization of the neuron occurs, the neuron receiving the signals will develop an action potential at the axon hillock that will be conducted along the axon leading to the output response of the neuron.

Receptor potentials are used to input information to the nervous system. Examples include touch and other types of receptors. The greater the magnitude of the stimulus, the greater the receptor potential becomes. If the receptor potential becomes great enough, the integrating portion of the neuron produces an action potential, which is then conducted along the axon to signal the output response of the neuron. In the more frequent case, as the receptor potential becomes greater, action potentials are generated and conducted along the axon more frequently, resulting in more frequent release of neurotransmitter onto cells in the spinal cord or brain stem. It should be noted, however, that receptor potentials may be either depolarizing or hyperpolarizing. One

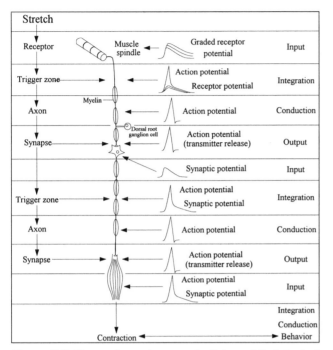

Figure 9-2. Types of membrane potentials and their typical uses. In this case, the tendon reflex is used to demonstrate receptor potential in the sensory structure, a synaptic potential in the lower motor neuron, and action potentials used to conduct the signal along both axons.

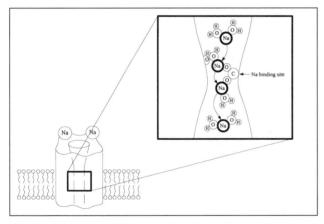

Figure 9-4. Proposed mechanism for making an ion channel selective for sodium and exclude potassium.

example of a hyperpolarizing receptor potential is that of retinal cells exposed to greater intensities of light. The types of membrane potentials are illustrated in Figure 9-2.

ION CHANNELS

Alterations in membrane potential are used for signaling by the neuron. To change membrane potential,

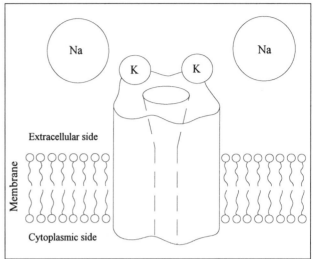

Figure 9-3. An ion channel can selectively allow potassium but not sodium through, based solely on hydrated diameter.

ions must move across the membrane. Ions do not penetrate the cell membrane easily because of the effects of charge and hydrated diameter. For ions to flow across the membrane, special protein-lined ion channels must be present. The different qualities of the types of membrane potentials (resting potential, synaptic potential, receptor potential, and action potential) are due to differences in the magnitude and timing of ion flux and the types of ions that cross the membrane. Membrane potentials, therefore, require selectivity of ion channels. Membrane potentials of cardiac and smooth muscle will be described in later chapters.

A simple way of producing selectivity is based on size. Although potassium is a bigger atom than sodium, sodium ions attract more water molecules to them and, therefore, have a larger hydrated diameter than potassium ions. Small ion channels will selectively allow potassium, but not sodium, through (Figure 9-3). Selectivity for sodium over potassium requires a filtering mechanism to prevent potassium ions from passing through the sodium channel (Figure 9-4). In the resting neuron and skeletal muscle cell, non-gated channels are always available for movement of potassium and sodium ions. The ratio of nongated monovalent cation (Na^+ and K^+) flux through these channels is approximately 25 K^+ for every Na^+. Other channels have mechanisms for gating the channels. That is, the channels remain closed until the appropriate signal opens them. Stimuli for opening gated channels include depolarization of the cell, hyperpolarization of the cell, binding of ligand to the ion channel, production of a second messenger, such as cAMP or Ca^{++}, and stretching the cell membrane. The types of membrane potentials involved in this chapter

TABLE 9-1

Features of the Different Types of Membrane Potentials Observed in Neurons and Skeletal Muscle

POTENTIAL	AMPLITUDE	DURATION	PROPAGATION
Receptor potential	A fraction to a few mV Graded to stimulus	5 to 100 ms	Decays with distance
Synaptic potential	A fraction to a few mV Graded to stimulus	A few ms to minutes	Decays with distance
Action potential	Over 100 mV	About 1 ms	Self-propagating

are either voltage-operated or ligand-operated. Some receptor potentials are stretch-operated. Membrane potentials in cardiac and smooth muscle involve several types of gating mechanisms and a multiplicity of different types of channels for different ions. The characteristics of different types of membrane potentials are summarized in Table 9-1.

THE RESTING POTENTIAL

To have an electric potential across a surface, charge must be separated across the membrane. Separating charged particles requires work. This amount of work is quantified by the term zFE in which z is the valence of the ion (number of charges per particle), F is Faraday's constant, and E is the electric potential. One way to separate charge is to use the Na-K pump, which transports three sodium ions out of the cell for two potassium ions pumped into the cell, producing a net negative charge inside the cell relative to the outside. A small contribution to the resting membrane potential is made by the electrogenic nature of the Na-K pump, but this usually only accounts for approximately –10 mV of the –70 to –90 mV membrane potential. Another mechanism is analogous to the development of osmotic pressure, in which the selective permeability of a membrane to water, but not solute particles, creates the condition in which a concentration difference can be offset by a difference in pressure, allowing equilibrium to occur.

A good example to illustrate the generation of the resting potential is the glial cell in which virtually all of the nongated channels are specific for potassium. Because this membrane is selectively permeable for potassium, very little sodium is allowed to cross it. These cells use a chemical gradient, not to develop osmotic pressure, but to develop electric potential. Just as osmosis uses a chemical gradient to create pressure, the work done to separate charge in glial cells comes from the sep-

aration of a chemical, the potassium ion in the presence of nonpenetrating ions. The energy to create a concentration difference for potassium ions across the glial cell membrane comes from transport of K$^+$ into the cell against the concentration gradient via the Na-K pump. The work done to create a difference in concentration of K$^+$ across the membrane is quantified as RT ln [K$^+$]$_{out}$/[K$^+$]$_{in}$, where R is the universal gas constant, T is absolute temperature in degrees Kelvin, and ln is natural log.

Because the only charged particle that is free to flow across the glial cell membrane is K$^+$, the movement of the positive particles (K$^+$) out of the cell from high concentration to low concentration results in the net movement of positive charge out of the cell. If other ions were free to cross the membrane, the movement of K$^+$ out of the cell would be accompanied by either movement of positive ions, such as sodium into the cell, or negative ions, such as chlorine or bicarbonate out of the cell, to create electrical equilibrium. Just as with osmosis, water and solute particles would move in equal numbers across the membrane to prevent pressure if solute particles were free to move. In osmosis, a difference in concentration results in a net flow of particles until pressure increases on the other side so that ΔC drives water in one direction at the same rate that ΔP drives it in the other. In osmosis, a difference in pressure could offset a difference in concentration to produce equilibrium (provided the system could develop sufficient pressure). Also, recall that we could stop the net movement of water by using energy to create a ΔP sufficient to offset the ΔC, which is described as a steady state rather than equilibrium due to the use of energy.

The resting potential of glial cells is the membrane potential that occurs when K$^+$ is in equilibrium across the cell. ΔC is a driving force to cause net flux of K$^+$ out of the glial cell; ΔE is a driving force to cause net flux of K$^+$ into the cell (Figure 9-5). When equilibrium is achieved, the concentration difference for potassium

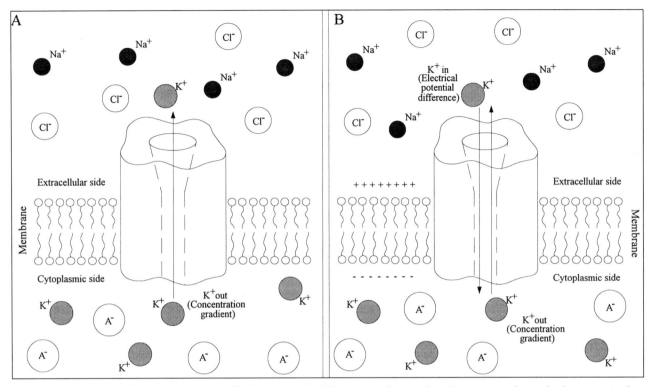

Figure 9-5. Creation of the potassium equilibrium potential. Movement of potassium ions occurs due to both concentration difference and electric potential across the membrane. In panel A, net movement of potassium across the membrane in an absence of membrane potential occurs due to a concentration difference for potassium across the membrane. In panel B, equilibrium results at a membrane potential that drives potassium into the cell at the same rate that the concentration difference drives potassium out of the cell.

across the membrane will drive potassium out of the cell at the same rate that the membrane potential drives potassium into the cell, and no net flux of potassium will be present. The work done to separate charge across the membrane is accomplished by, and therefore equal to, the work done to create a concentration difference across the membrane. In 1888, Walter Nernst developed the equation to describe this situation. Stated mathematically, $zFE = RT \ln [K^+]_{out}/[K^+]_{in}$. The intra- and extracellular concentrations at which K^+ will be in equilibrium are essentially equal to those of body fluids in general. The equation above can be rearranged to solve for the membrane potential (Em) that will exist at equilibrium: $E = (RT \ln [K^+]_{out}/[K^+]_{in})/zF$. This equation is referred to as the Nernst equation. The Nernst equation can be used to compute the membrane potential for any ion in equilibrium across the membrane. In our example, we would call this potential the potassium equilibrium potential (E_K). By substituting the values for R, z, and F and using 37°C (310°K) in the equation and converting from natural log (ln) to base 10 (log), the equation simplifies to $E_K = 60 \log [K^+]_{out}/[K^+]_{in}$. In glial cells, $E_m = 60 \log 4/135 = -92$ mV. Only K^+ can pass through the glial cell membrane when $E_m = E_K$, the

potassium equilibrium potential. At a difference in concentration of potassium of 4/135 and a membrane potential of –92 mV, no net movement of K^+ will occur; K^+ will be in equilibrium. If we artificially change the membrane potential in the laboratory, K^+ will move across the cell to produce a concentration ratio that again satisfies the equation. Conversely, if the ratio of ion concentrations across a membrane changes, the membrane potential will change to reestablish equilibrium. This is one of the dangers of drugs, such as diuretics, that alter the ion concentrations of body fluids.

RESTING POTENTIAL IN NEURONS

The Nernst equation applies equally to any ion that can equilibrate across the membrane. If only Na^+ can cross the membrane, the equilibrium potential for Na^+ is $E_{Na} = 60 \log 145/12 = +65$ mV. What happens in neurons in which more than one ion can flow across the membrane? If both K^+ and Na^+ can cross the membrane down their respective concentration gradients, and they have different equilibrium potentials (–92 mV and +65

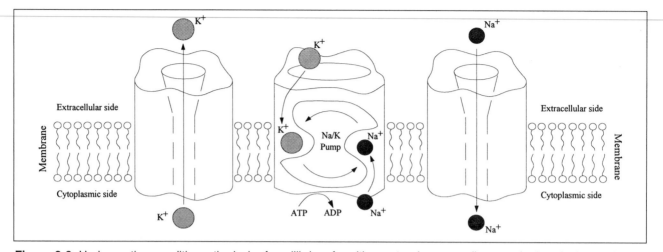

Figure 9-6. Under resting conditions, the lack of equilibrium for either potassium or sodium results in a leakage of both, which is corrected by continuous pumping of potassium in and sodium out by the Na-K pump.

mV, respectively), neither of the ions can be in equilibrium across the cell membrane. If more than one type of ion can cross the membrane, the movement of positive charges out will allow equal numbers of positive charges to go in. In this case, we will have cations leaking out (K^+) at the same rate that they leak in (Na^+) and net flux of K^+ out with net flux of Na^+ in. The rate at which potassium leaks out is determined by the difference between E_m and E_K, of 20 mV and the permeability of the membrane to K^+, whereas the rate that sodium leaks into the cell is determined by the difference between E_m and E_{Na} of +135 mV and ΔC, both driving Na^+ into the cell, and the permeability of the membrane to this ion. As stated above, the permeability of the membrane to K^+ is 25 times that of Na^+.

The combination of low permeability and the high driving force for Na^+ flux into the cell causes approximately equal leakage in as the combination of high permeability and low driving force for K^+ out of the cell. The leakage of potassium out and sodium in is corrected by the Na-K pump, which maintains E_m constant. Because energy is used, a steady state, rather than equilibrium, results as shown in Figure 9-6.

The steady-state membrane potential in the presence of multiple permeable ions can be computed with the Goldman equation, which states that the membrane potential at any time is the average of the equilibrium potentials of the ions that can penetrate the membrane weighted by the permeabilities. This equation expresses the idea that the ion that dominates in terms of permeability largely determines resting membrane potential. The Goldman equation is stated as

$$E_m = (RT/F) \ln \frac{P_K[K^+]_o + P_{Na}[Na^+]_o + Pcl[Cl^-]_i}{P_K[K^+]_i + P_{Na}[Na^+]_i + P_{Cl}[Cl^-]_o}$$

where P is the permeability of the membrane to the individual ions, i is inside the cell, and o is outside the cell. In glial cells in which the cell is permeable only to K^+, the Goldman equation reduces to the Nernst equation. In resting neurons, typical relative values of permeability are P_K:P_{Na}:P_{Cl} = 1:0.04:0.45. Because the permeability of the cell to K^+ is about 25 times greater than it is to Na^+, the resting membrane potential of neurons is close to the K^+ equilibrium potential. Application of the Goldman equation using the concentrations given in Table 6-1 yields a membrane potential of –72 mV, a value close to that measured in the laboratory for neurons and about –90mV for skeletal muscle cells. The equilibrium potential of Cl^- is approximately equal to –88 mV and, therefore, contributes little to the resting potential of skeletal muscle cells, but as we will see, increasing a neuron's permeability to Cl^- can diminish the ability of the cell membrane to vary from –88 mV due to the relationship explained by the Goldman equation.

If the permeability of the membrane to Na^+ should become much greater than the permeability to K^+, E_m will become close to +65 mV. This is what happens during the peak of the action potential. The resting potential is close to the K^+ equilibrium potential because, at rest, the preponderance of available channels are specific for K^+ and, at the peak of the action potential, the preponderance of open channels are sodium channels. Production of different potentials (synaptic, receptor, and action potentials) is the result of altering the relative numbers of channels through which different ions can flow, resulting in a membrane potential that can be computed using the Goldman equation.

THE ACTION POTENTIAL

The action potential provides the conductive function of neurons. Depending on the diameter and degree of myelination of a neuron, the action potential is propagated at a rate of approximately 6 m/s for every μm of axon diameter. Synaptic and receptor potentials are local potentials that die out with distance from the site of initiation, whereas action potentials are propagated without significant loss of potential along the entire axon. The difference between local potentials and action potentials lies in the channels responsible for their production. Local potentials are produced in localized areas of the membrane by channels that are ligand-gated. The opening of one channel due to the presence of neurotransmitter or other ligand does not cause adjacent channels to open. Action potentials, on the other hand, are regenerative due to the positive feedback mechanism described in Chapter One. The opening of one channel responsible for the production of the action potential promotes opening of neighboring channels of the same type.

Action potentials are primarily the result of a positive feedback between inward current of Na^+ carrying positive charges and opening the channels through which the inward current travels. The issues to be discussed are 1.) what initiates the positive feedback, 2.) what stops the positive feedback cycle, 3.) how we can return membrane potential back to the resting potential rapidly enough for neurons to depolarize as frequently as 100 times per second, and 4.) absolute and relative refractory periods.

In nerve cells and skeletal muscle cells, the positive feedback of opening voltage-operated sodium channels is initiated by either receptor potentials generated by sensory neurons or by synaptic potentials produced by ligand-operated channels. If the graded synaptic or receptor potentials produced by their respective stimuli are great enough to produce enough inward movement of positive charge, voltage-operated sodium channels will open. If sufficient numbers of voltage-operated sodium channels open quickly enough, the inward current will result in the opening of adjacent voltage-operated sodium channels, thereby initiating the positive feedback mechanism of inward current and open sodium channels. The presence of voltage-operated sodium channels all along the length of the axon is what produces the regenerative aspect of the action potential. On myelinated peripheral nerves, the Schwann cells produce an insulatory layer of myelin. Between each cell, an uninsulated spot called the node of Ranvier exists. The presence of myelin allows the current carried by inward flow of Na^+ to travel quickly from one node of Ranvier to the next. Because production of the action potential requires the presence of "bare" membrane to exchange ions between the intra- and extracellular fluid, the only place along a myelinated axon at which an action potential can occur is at the node of Ranvier. This allows the action potential to be regenerated rapidly at a distance, hastening the conduction of action potential along the axon. This gives the appearance of the action potential jumping from node-to-node, a phenomenon termed saltatory conduction (*L.* saltare, to leap). Therefore, the nodes must be placed closely enough that the Na^+ current can reach the next node, but placed far enough apart to maximize conduction velocity.

OTHER GATING MECHANISMS REQUIRED FOR THE ACTION POTENTIAL

Two of the factors addressed above, stopping the positive feedback cycle of voltage-operated sodium

Carpal Tunnel Syndrome

The carpal tunnel is an anatomic tunnel from the forearm into the hand formed by a bony arch of carpal bones covered with a tough connective tissue. The functional significance lies in the passage of the median nerve and finger flexor tendons. Damage to myelin slows the conduction of the action potential through the carpal tunnel. Inflammation of the tendons from overuse (such as typing this book), fluid retention, or trauma, from activities such as operating a jack-hammer, can compress the median nerve, resulting in tingling or numbness and weakness of the portion of the hand innervated by the median nerve. Another condition, thoracic outlet syndrome, can produce signs similar to carpal tunnel syndrome. In thoracic outlet syndrome, the brachial plexus is stretched as it crosses from the neck into the upper extremity. Thoracic outlet syndrome has several causes: one of them is poor posture with a forward head, protracted scapulae, and internally rotated upper extremities. Carpal tunnel syndrome occurs frequently in pregnancy due to fluid retention and swelling in the carpal tunnel; however, the postural changes that produce thoracic outlet syndrome can also occur in pregnancy. A good evaluation will reveal sensory and motor loss related to compression of the brachial plexus, rather than the median nerve alone.

channels and returning E_m as rapidly as possible to resting potential, require two other voltage-operated gating mechanisms. One operates on the sodium channel; another is a voltage-operated potassium channel. This voltage-operated potassium channel is not the same channel (the nongated potassium channel) that is responsible for the resting membrane potential. The voltage-operated sodium channel has two gating mechanisms with different time-dependence. One gating mechanism remains closed at the resting potential and opens as the membrane depolarizes. The second mechanism is slower to operate than the first. The slower gating mechanism is open and available for Na$^+$ flow at resting potential, but closes as the membrane depolarizes. The faster "gate," which is closed at rest, is called the activation gate. The slower "gate," which is open at rest, is called the inactivation gate. Sodium ions are capable of flowing into the cell only about 1 millisecond between opening of the activation gate and closing of the inactivation gate.

The inactivation gate will keep the channel closed until the membrane potential returns to near resting potential. Therefore, a new action potential cannot occur until the inactivation gate returns to its open position. The action of the activation and inactivation gates of the voltage-operated sodium channel appear to be linked. When the activation gate is opened, the inactivation gate closes within a prescribed time, and when the activation gate closes, the inactivation gate opens after a prescribed time.

The voltage-operated potassium channel serves the role of returning E_m to resting potential more rapidly. Although E_m would return on its own to the resting potential without it, the opening of voltage-operated K$^+$ channels drives E_m toward the potassium equilibrium potential faster by increasing permeability of the membrane to K$^+$. The opening of the voltage-operated potassium channel results in an outward positive current of K$^+$, which is rapid because the membrane potential is far from the potassium equilibrium potential at the peak of the action potential. This rapid outward current quickly ends the action potential. This voltage-operated K$^+$ channel opens even more slowly following membrane depolarization than the inactivation channel of the voltage-operated sodium closes. The sequence of the three gating mechanisms is sodium activation gate, followed by the sodium inactivation gate, and then the potassium gate. Note that there is no inactivation gate on the potassium channel. As E_m returns to resting potential and even undershoots it, the voltage-operated potassium channels close. At the time that all voltage-operated gating mechanisms are returned to their resting configurations, resting potential is achieved again. These actions are depicted in Figure 9-7.

The changes in membrane potential during the action potential can be explained solely on the basis of the Goldman equation. At rest, membrane permeability to potassium is 25 times greater than that for sodium; therefore, at rest, the membrane potential is near the equilibrium potential of potassium. As voltage-operated sodium channels begin to open, many more sodium channels are opening than there are available channels for potassium. At the peak of the action potential, there are 20 times as many channels carrying sodium inward as there are channels carrying potassium outward. Based on the Goldman equation, membrane potential at the peak of the action potential should be approximately +50 mV. At the peak of the action potential, inactivation gates on the voltage-operated sodium channels begin to close gradually, returning the ratio of open potassium channels to open sodium channels to the same as the resting condition and back toward E_k. The individual components creating the action potential are illustrated in Figures 9-8 and 9-9. Eventually, enough K$^+$ would leak out to return E_m to the resting potential to allow the voltage-operated sodium channels to become functional again. The advantage of the slowly opening, voltage-dependent potassium channel is to hasten the process of leaking potassium out of the cell. The undershoot of the action potential is due to the even greater ratio of open potassium to open sodium channels, bringing E_m even closer to E_k than resting potential as both nongated and voltage-gated channels are open for potassium while the only sodium movement is through nongated channels. The more rapid depolarization caused by voltage-operated potassium channels allows a second action potential to be elicited more rapidly.

The ionic basis of the action potential requires movement of Na$^+$ into the cell and K$^+$ out of the cell. Eventually, this ionic movement would result in changes in the concentrations of these ions and, therefore, resting potential. However, a relatively small number of ions actually crosses the membrane. The number is so small that more than 100 action potentials could be generated without significantly altering Na$^+$ and K$^+$ concentrations. The slight change is managed by continuous operation of the Na/K pump. As Na$^+$ leaks into the cell and K+ leaks out, the activity of Na/K pumping increases. This pumping activity is not directly linked to the action potential, but along with synthesis and active transport of neurotransmitters requires continual utilization of ATP to maintain neuron health.

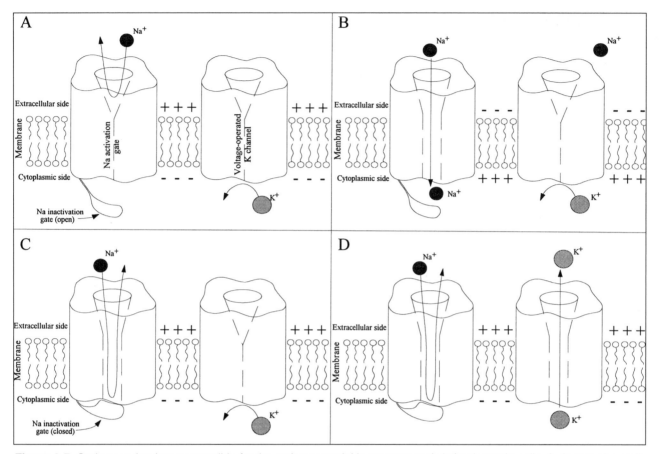

Figure 9-7. Gating mechanism responsible for the action potential in neurons and skeletal muscle cells. A: At rest, the sodium activation gate is closed, the sodium inactivation gate is open, and the voltage-operated potassium channels are closed. B: When the cell is depolarized, the sodium activation gate opens, the sodium inactivation gate remains open for approximately 1 millisecond, and the voltage-operated potassium channels remain closed, causing membrane potential to approach the sodium equilibrium potential. C: Inward sodium flux is halted as the sodium inactivation gate closes, the sodium activation gate is still open, and voltage-operated potassium channels are beginning to open. This results in membrane potential beginning to repolarize. D: To increase the rate of repolarization, voltage-operated potassium channels open to allow outward flux of potassium, bringing membrane potential back toward the potassium equilibrium potential, while the voltage-operated sodium channels remain closed. The sequence of events ends with the configuration shown in A as membrane potential is restored.

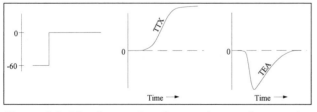

Figure 9-8. The fluxes of sodium and potassium can be viewed separately by blocking these channels during electrical stimulation of a neuron's membrane. Tetrodotoxin (TTX) blocks the sodium channel, allowing the action of the potassium channel to be seen by itself. Tetraethylammonium (TEA) blocks the voltage-operated potassium channels, allowing the flux of sodium to be seen by itself.

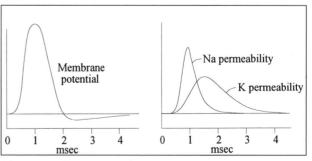

Figure 9-9. The shape of an action potential is the result of the components of permeability of the membrane to sodium early to produce a membrane potential close to the equilibrium potential for sodium, followed by a rapid decline in permeability of sodium to produce the initial repolarization, followed by an increase in permeability to potassium, which results in a more rapid repolarization and the undershoot.

REFRACTORY PERIODS

Earlier in this chapter, it was mentioned that the size of the action potential does not vary. Every time an action potential is elicited, the magnitude and time course are identical, unless the ion concentrations used in the Goldman equation are altered. This can occur when body fluid composition is not maintained or ATP concentration falls. The new magnitude of the action potential can then be computed with the Goldman equation. Because the magnitude of the action potential cannot be varied under normal circumstances, the only method for the neurons to vary the message sent is to alter the rate at which action potentials are produced. After initiating an action potential, a period exists during which, no matter how strong the stimulus applied to the neuron is, it cannot generate another action potential. This period is called the absolute refractory period. Following the absolute refractory period, but before the membrane potential returns to the resting potential, a second stimulus that is larger than what is normally required to elicit an action potential can produce a new action potential. This period following the absolute refractory period is called the relative refractory period. The longer the time after the end of the absolute refractory period, the less the magnitude of stimulation required to elicit a new action potential. When a stimulus of the normal magnitude is sufficient to produce another action potential, the relative refractory period is over. What causes the absolute and relative refractory periods? A new action potential **absolutely** cannot be initiated until the voltage-gated sodium channels return to their original configuration of the activation gate closed and the inactivation gate open. The inactivation gates return to the open position as E_m nears the resting potential. No matter how great the stimulus, whether it is a large synaptic potential or receptor potential or an electric current run through the membrane artificially, a new action potential cannot be initiated until the inactivation gates return to their open position. The time between the initiation of the first action potential until the voltage-operated sodium channels return to a position available for flow of sodium determines the absolute refractory period. The relative refractory period exists during the time that the inactivation gates of sodium channels begin to return to the open position, but the voltage-operated potassium channels remain open. While potassium is flowing out of both voltage-operated and the nongated K^+ channels, the stimulus required to open voltage-operated sodium channels must be stronger to open sufficient sodium channels to produce an action potential. As voltage-operated K^+ channels begin to close during the down slope of the action potential, stimuli that open fewer sodium channels at once become sufficient to initiate the positive feedback cycle of the voltage-operated sodium channels. When the voltage-operated K^+ channels return to the closed position, a normal-sized stimulus again can initiate the action potential.

Refractory periods have two major roles: they prevent what is called "backfiring" of action potentials and they allow for the coding of sensory stimulus intensity. When a membrane develops an action potential, current travels in all directions along the membrane. The axon does not "know" which direction the action potential should travel. As the action potential propagates from its site of initiation, it drives current in all directions including backward. Because the cell membrane is refractory, the area of membrane just behind the site of action potential regeneration cannot be depolarized again until the action potential has moved too far along the axon. Otherwise, we would see a never-ending cycle of adjacent areas of membrane depolarizing each other. Sensory coding is provided by the frequency of action potentials from the sensory neuron to the central nervous system (CNS). Because of the nature of the relative refractory period, the greater the stimulus is, the earlier in the relative refractory period the next action potential occurs. A small stimulus will cause a series of action potentials near the end of the relative refractory period, whereas a large stimulus causes the action potentials to occur earlier in the refractory period and, therefore, more frequently.

SUMMARY

Neurons have four functions: input, integration, conduction, and output. Three types of membrane potentials are necessary for these functions. In addition, when the cell is not performing these functions, the membrane exists at a steady-state condition of polarity across the membrane, called the resting potential. Synaptic and receptor potentials are local and are graded to the size of the stimulus. Action potentials are stereotyped in size and duration and are regenerative, thereby allowing them to be conducted along the length of an axon. Membrane potentials are determined by the way in which charge is separated across the membrane. The energy to produce separation of charge comes from the separation of ions produced by the Na-K pump. Different types of membrane potentials are the result of physiological regulation of the membrane's permeability to different ions. The resting potential is the result of the membrane being selectively permeable to K^+ at rest, causing the membrane potential to be close to the equilibrium potential for potassium. During an action potential, the permeability of the membrane for sodium increases so much that the membrane potential approaches the equilibrium potential for sodium. The voltage-operated sodium channel has both activation and inactivation gates. The inactivation gate closes the sodium channel shortly after the activation gate opens to end the positive feedback cycle of inward current and opening of voltage-operated sodium channels. Voltage-operated potassium channels hasten the depolarization process by allowing an outward current to occur as the sodium channel closes. Absolute refractory period exists when the inactivation gates of the voltage-operated sodium channels are closed. Relative refractory period follows the absolute refractory period. Relative refractory period is the result of the open voltage-operated potassium channels allowing outward current, thereby obligating a larger inward current from a receptor or synaptic potential to initiate an action potential.

BIBLIOGRAPHY

Anderson OS, Koeppe RE II. Molecular determinants of channel function. *Physiological Reviews.* 1992;72:S89-S158.

Armstrong CM. Voltage dependent ion channels and their gating. *Physiological Reviews.* 1992;72:S5-S13.

Catteral WA. Cellular and molecular biology of voltage-gated sodium channels. *Physiological Reviews.* 1992;72:S15-S48.

Gardner D. A time integral of membrane currents. *Physiological Reviews.* 1992;72:S1-S3.

Pollato BS, Wagoner PK. Voltage-dependent potassium channels since Hodgkin and Huxley. *Physiological Reviews.* 1992;72:S49-S67.

Pongs O. Molecular biology of voltage dependent potassium channels. *Physiological Reviews.* 1992;72:S69-S88.

STUDY QUESTIONS

1. Describe the four functions of neurons. What roles do the receptor potential, synaptic potential, and action potential play in these functions?

2. What are the stimuli for the production of the three types of membrane potential (receptor, synaptic, and action potentials)?

3. Explain the concepts of graded potentials and local potentials. Are action potentials either graded or local?

4. Explain the need for ion channels. How can ion channels be specific for one type of ion? What driving forces exist to produce net flow across ion channels?

5. Explain the term "electric potential." What must the cell do to produce a membrane potential? How is a resting potential produced in a glial cell? Where is energy used?

6. Explain the three types of gating mechanisms responsible for the action potential. What roles do the activation gate, inactivation, and voltage-operated potassium channel play?

7. Explain how the permeability changes in the voltage-operated sodium and potassium channels are related to the shape of the action potential. Is it possible for the magnitude or duration of the action potential to change?

8. Explain the causes of the absolute and relative refractory periods. What benefits do these refractory periods have to the cell?

T E N

Synaptic Transmission

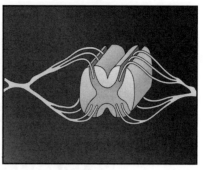

1. Describe the ionic mechanisms underlying the excitatory postsynaptic potential of central nervous system (CNS) neurons.

2. Compare the two types of summation and describe the need for summation.

3. Explain the ionic basis of two types of inhibitory postsynaptic potentials: hyperpolarizing and short-circuiting.

4. Explain the mechanisms by which acetylcholine is released from α motor neurons and the need for acetylcholinesterase.

5. Describe the structure of the motor end plate.

6. Explain the ionic basis of end plate potentials.

7. List the sympathetic and parasympathetic neurotransmitters.

8. Define the terms nicotinic and muscarinic receptors, and give their locations.

9. Contrast the different types of adrenergic receptors: the functions of α vs. β receptors and the pharmacologic significance of the two subtypes of β receptors.

10. List classifications of cutaneous nerves: Aα, Aβ, Aγ, Aδ, and C.

11. List classifications of muscular nerves: IA, IB, II, III, IV.

12. Describe the relationship between neuron diameter, presence of myelin, and conduction velocity for the two classification systems for neurons.

13. State the functions of different classes of sensory neurons:
    a. Aα—muscle mechanoreceptors
    b. Aβ—skin mechanoreceptors
    c. Aδ—temperature and sharp pain
    d. C—temperature, poorly localized pain, crude touch, tickle

14. Define longitudinal and axial conductance of a neuron.

15. Describe the effects of neuron cross-sectional area and length on longitudinal conductance.

16. Define capacitance, and list the factors determining capacitance of a neuron's membrane.

17. Describe the effects of myelin on axial conductance and capacitance.

18. List factors that determine nerve conduction velocity.

Most neurons communicate with each other by synaptic transmission. The synapse is a specialized region of contact between two cells. Neurons also communicate with effectors, including skeletal muscle, cardiac muscle, smooth muscle, and exocrine glands via synapses. Most synapses are chemical, although some electrical synapses exist in the nervous system.

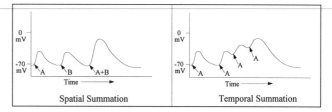

Figure 10-1. Summation of EPSPs on a postsynaptic membrane showing the effect of single EPSPs from neurons A and B, and spatial summation that occurs when both neurons A and B create EPSPs simultaneously on the left. In the right panel, temporal summation of EPSPs from neuron A alone is depicted.

CENTRAL NERVOUS SYSTEM TRANSMISSION

Both excitatory and inhibitory synapses exist on neurons within the central nervous system (CNS). Synaptic boutons or knobs occupy small patches of membrane on which specific excitatory and inhibitory ion channels are located. More than 20 substances have been identified as neurotransmitters within the CNS. Glutamate is the most widespread excitatory transmitter in the CNS. Several receptor subtypes have been described just for glutamate.

Other neurotransmitters include norepinephrine (NE), serotonin, dopamine (substantia nigra), and many peptides. Glycine is a common inhibitory transmitter in the spinal cord. Glycine produces inhibition by opening ligand-operated Cl^- channels, thereby stabilizing the membrane near E_{Cl} according to the Goldman equation.

When excitatory neurotransmitters in the spinal cord, such as glutamate or substance P, bind to their receptors, they cause nonspecific monovalent cation channels to open. Both Na^+ and K^+ are capable of flowing through these channels. However, because the driving force for Na^+ to flow into the cell is much greater than the driving force for K^+ to flow out of the cell, the immediate region of the receptor is depolarized to about –15 mV. Each presynaptic nerve terminal releases only a few vesicles so the synaptic potential of neurons, called the excitatory postsynaptic potential (EPSP), is much smaller than the end plate potential observed in skeletal muscle cells. In skeletal muscle, release of the neurotransmitter from the single lower motor neuron synapsing with the muscle cell is sufficient to produce an action potential in the skeletal muscle cell. Skeletal muscle cells receive stimulatory signals only; no mechanism exists at the level of the neuromuscular junction to inhibit the skeletal muscle cell's activity. Therefore, the most efficient way of signaling a skeletal muscle to contract is for the nerve to produce a sufficient signal with each action potential of a motor neuron.

In contrast to skeletal muscle cells, neurons receive messages from multiple neurons, which may be either excitatory or inhibitory (the phenomenon of conver-

gence). The "decision-making" process (integration) by the neuron is produced by adding up many small signals, rather than a single large signal. Depolarization of a neuron to create a signal to send elsewhere requires what is called summation in either the form of many neurons releasing excitatory neurotransmitter synchronously or in the form of fewer neurons releasing neurotransmitter at a high rate of repetition (Figure 10-1). For convenience, we can discuss summation as taking forms called temporal and spatial summation. More likely, for a given neuron, both occur simultaneously.

Temporal summation refers to the repetitive firing of single presynaptic neurons, meaning that the effects of one neuron are being summed over time. Spatial summation refers to the firing of many presynaptic neurons simultaneously. Spatial refers to the idea that many presynaptic neurons are summed over different spaces on the postsynaptic membrane. Should sufficient temporal and spatial summation occur to depolarize the axon hillock, an action potential is initiated at the axon hillock. Due to the presence of voltage-operated sodium channels as described in Chapter Nine, the action potential is propagated down the axon to the output region of the neuron.

An inhibitory signal received by the postsynaptic membrane is called an inhibitory postsynaptic potential (IPSP), whereas an excitatory signal is called an EPSP. Inhibitory neurotransmitters function either by producing IPSPs or by "short-circuiting" the membrane. An IPSP makes the cell membrane more negative (hyperpolarizes it) so that a greater inward current of positive charges is required to reach the threshold for generating an action potential. Hyperpolarization can be achieved through binding of inhibitory neurotransmitters to postsynaptic receptors that cause K^+ channels to open. Increased permeability to K^+, according to the Goldman equation, will drive E_m toward E_K. The other mechanism, short-circuiting the membrane, acts to stabilize the postsynaptic membrane near the resting potential.

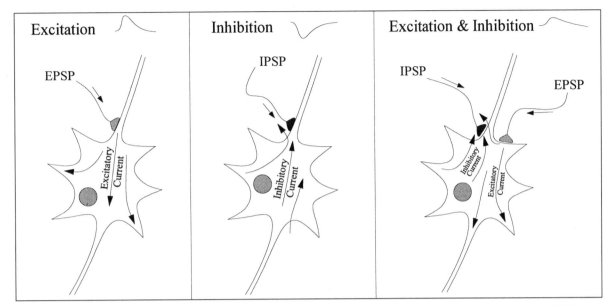

Figure 10-2. Ionic currents produced by an EPSP, an IPSP, and a simultaneous EPSP and IPSP. The IPSP produces a hyperpolarization due to an outward positive current or inward negative current. The third panel shows the process of "short circuiting" a membrane with an IPSP in which inward current is made ineffective by allowing the current to leak out of the cell before it reaches the axon hillock.

The membrane is stabilized by increasing the membrane's permeability to Cl⁻, which, according to the Goldman equation, reduces the effectiveness of the permeability of the membrane to other ions. Stabilization of neuron cell membranes can be achieved by inhibitory neurotransmitters that open Cl⁻ channels. Because the equilibrium potential for chloride ions, E_{Cl}, is approximately −88 mV, a greater number of ion channels are holding the membrane potential near its resting potential. In addition, the opening of chloride channels will slightly depolarize the membrane due to the movement of Cl⁻ into the cell. The effectiveness of an EPSP caused by increased permeability to Na⁺ is reduced by short circuiting because the inflow of positively charged sodium ions will be counteracted by inward movement of negatively charged chloride ions. This process of undermining the effectiveness of inward current is referred to as "short-circuiting" in analogy to an electric circuit that loses its effectiveness because the electric current is allowed to flow somewhere other than the desired direction. The flow of K⁺ out of the cell and Cl⁻ into the cell both cause the membrane to hyperpolarize. An EPSP increases the probability that a neuron will produce an action potential, and an IPSP decreases the probability of reaching threshold (Figure 10-2).

NEUROMUSCULAR SYNAPSES

Skeletal muscle is innervated by what are called α

motor neurons or lower motor neurons. The term α is derived from the size of the neuron (discussed later in this chapter). Lower motor neuron refers to a neuron with its cell body in the anterior horn of the spinal cord and an axon that extends to the skeletal muscle cells. This is distinguished from upper motor neurons that reside solely within the CNS, running from the "upper" area of the brain to the "lower" area in the spinal cord to synapse with a pool of lower motor neurons. Lower motor neurons also originate from the brain stem for muscles innervated by cranial nerves (eg, muscles of facial expression and mastication [chewing]). Both upper and lower motor neurons are required for skeletal muscle function. Damage to lower motor neurons results in flaccid (limp) paralysis. As we will see later in the unit on skeletal muscle reflexes, damage to upper motor neurons results in a condition called spasticity, characterized by an exaggerated response to the stretch reflex.

Two areas of synapse are responsible for neuromuscular function: the synapse between upper and lower motor neurons and the neuromuscular junction. The structure of the neuromuscular junction is shown in Figure 10-3. Dendrites and cell bodies of lower motor neurons receive synapses from a variety of sources. Some upper motor neurons release neurotransmitter that produces IPSPs; others produce EPSPs. Interneurons within the spinal cord relay sensory information that results in either inhibitory or excitatory neurotransmitter

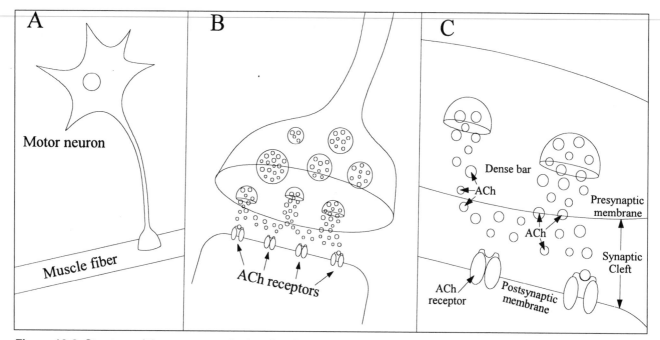

Figure 10-3. Structure of the neuromuscular junction. Dense bars with surrounding ACh vesicles awaiting an action potential to stimulate exocytosis are immediately across the junction from the synaptic clefts with their ACh receptors.

release. Some of these produce what we call reflexes because these responses are involuntary and occur before we have conscious perception of the stimulus.

The neuromuscular junction is a synaptic connection between a lower motor neuron and a muscle fiber. Because one lower motor neuron has synapses with many skeletal muscle fibers (range from 10 to thousands), the neuromuscular junction acts as a chemically mediated electric amplifier. This means that a small amount of current that generates an action potential in one lower motor neuron can produce action potentials in a large number of muscle fibers. Neuromuscular transmission involves four processes:

1. Release of the chemical transmitter acetylcholine (ACh) from the presynaptic nerve terminal
2. Diffusion of the transmitter to the postsynaptic membrane
3. Binding of ACh to the postsynaptic receptor to produce a conductance increase in the postsynaptic membrane to Na$^+$ and K$^+$
4. Inactivation of ACh by acetylcholinesterase to end the signaling mechanism and allow the muscle cell to repolarize

The neuromuscular junction is a highly specialized synapse that reduces the diffusion distance between the output of the motor neuron and the muscle cell membrane. Special areas called dense bars can be observed in the presynaptic membrane of the motor neuron terminal. Synaptic vesicles containing ACh collect around the dense bars. Directly across the synapse from the dense bars, troughs called postsynaptic folds are positioned on the postsynaptic membrane of the muscle cell. Within the troughs, the acetylcholine receptors are localized.

SYNTHESIS, STORAGE, AND RELEASE OF ACH

Acetylcholine is synthesized from acetyl CoA and choline by the enzyme choline acetyltransferase. Acetyl CoA is derived from the citric acid cycle; choline is derived from dietary phospholipids and is pumped into the nerve terminal by a sodium-dependent, secondary active transport system. Choline acetyltransferase, as well as other proteins synthesized in the cell body, is transported to the nerve terminal by axonal transport. ACh is stored in synaptic vesicles; each contains about 10,000 molecules of ACh. During the process of exocytosis, vesicles bind to release sites directly across from the acetylcholine receptors of the postsynaptic membrane of the muscle cells, fuse with the presynaptic membrane, and release ACh into the synaptic cleft. Depolarization of the nerve terminal by the action potential propagated from the spinal cord or brain stem stimulates exocytosis via voltage-operated calcium channels near the release site of ACh. When the motor neuron's terminal is depolarized by an action potential, calcium enters the cell and stimulates exocytosis. Under

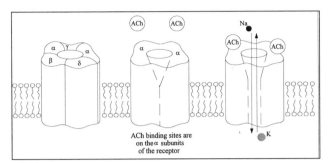

Figure 10-4. Structure of the nicotinic ACh receptor of skeletal muscle cells. Three views of the whole receptor within the membrane, the five proteins making up the channel, and a cross-section showing the closed configuration. The configuration of the protein complex changes shape when two ACh molecules bind to the sites on the α subunits of the receptor, allowing sodium and potassium ions to cross the membrane to produce the end plate potentials.

normal circumstances, approximately 300 vesicles release their contents in response to a single action potential. The transmitter diffuses across the synaptic cleft, binds to the postsynaptic receptor, and produces an action potential in the skeletal muscle cell. Subsequent action potentials will again result in release of ACh. This process can repeat itself more than 100 times per second (100 Hz), which is greater than that required for normal muscle function. The time between depolarization of the motor neuron and opening of nonselective monovalent cation channels in the muscle cell is termed synaptic delay. The delay is due primarily to the process of vesicle fusion and transmitter release (exocytosis), whereas the time for transmitter to diffuse across the 15 nm synaptic cleft is negligible.

POSTSYNAPTIC EFFECTS OF ACH

The postsynaptic receptor consists of a binding site for ACh and a receptor-operated ion channel (Figure 10-4). The channel allows both sodium and potassium to flow through it (nonselective monovalent cation channel). When ACh binds to the postsynaptic receptor, it causes nonspecific monovalent cation channels to open similar to those described for the EPSP. Na^+ flows down its concentration gradient into the cell. A lesser amount of K^+ flows down its concentration gradient out of the cell with the result of a graded, local depolarization, called the end plate potential. Because the channel is equally permeable to Na^+ and K^+, a localized area of the membrane depolarizes to a value intermediate between the K^+ equilibrium potential and the sodium equilibrium potential to about -15 mV. Because the entire membrane of the skeletal muscle cell is covered

with voltage-operated sodium channels, in contrast to the neuron in which these are located at the axon hillock and beyond, the number of nonspecific monovalent cation channels opened with a single presynaptic action potential is sufficient to depolarize the skeletal muscle fiber to threshold and produce an action potential.

Acetylcholine is inactivated by the enzyme acetylcholinesterase to end the signal from the motor neuron. The nonspecific monovalent cation channels must close to allow the skeletal muscle cell membrane to repolarize so subsequent action potentials can be developed on the skeletal muscle cell. Depending on the muscle and the individual, the membrane needs to depolarize at a rate as rapid as 50 per second or more to produce a normal muscle contraction. This principle is discussed fully in Chapter Sixteen.

Drugs and toxins can affect all of the processes involved in neuromuscular transmission. Black widow spider venom destroys synaptic vesicles. Thus, it produces a massive release of ACh followed by paralysis. Botulinum toxin causes paralysis by blocking the release of ACh from the nerve terminal. Neostigmine and related drugs block the action of acetylcholinesterase, prolonging the action of ACh at the end plate. Curare is a competitive blocker of ACh at the receptor binding site, producing paralysis. Drugs such as curare and related compounds are used therapeutically to produce skeletal muscle paralysis. ACh antibodies decrease the number and the effectiveness of ACh receptors in the disease myasthenia gravis. One treatment for myasthenia gravis is to give neostigmine or related drugs to allow the ACh released to open the available ion channels for a longer time.

AUTONOMIC NEUROTRANSMISSION

Acetylcholine and norepinephrine (NE) serve as the major neurotransmitters within the autonomic nervous system. ACh is used by the preganglionic fibers in both the parasympathetic and sympathetic divisions of the autonomic nervous system and by the postganglionic fibers of the parasympathetic division. Norepinephrine is used by most of the sympathetic postganglionic fibers (Figure 10-5). One notable exception is the release of ACh by postganglionic sympathetic neurons innervating sweat glands. The majority of autonomic nervous system synapses use nondirected synapses that do not make close contact with their postsynaptic cells. The terminal branches of axons form varicosities along their length from which the transmitter is released. The varicosities

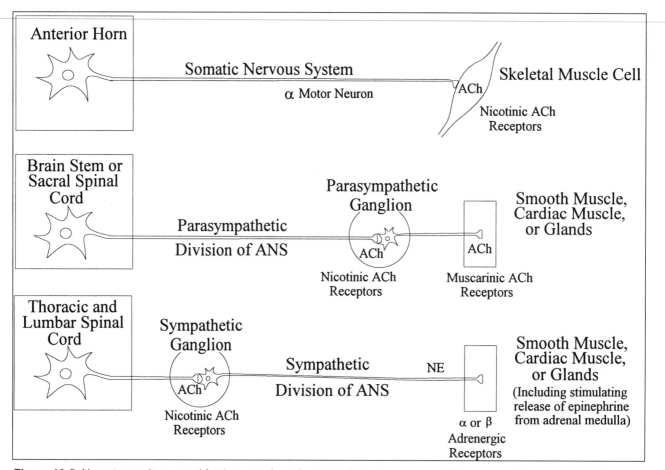

Figure 10-5. Neurotransmitters used for the somatic and autonomic motor systems. ACh is used at the neuromuscular junction, at both sympathetic and parasympathetic ganglia and by postganglionic parasympathetic neurons. Norepinephrine (NE) is used by postganglionic sympathetic neurons. Note the type of ACh receptors differ among the autonomic ganglia, neuromuscular junction, and target organs of the postganglionic parasympathetic neurons.

are 1 to 2 mm in diameter and occur at intervals of 3 to 5 mm. Inactivation of neurotransmitters of the autonomic nervous system is accomplished in several ways. ACh is hydrolyzed by acetylcholinesterase. NE is taken up by the presynaptic nerve terminal by an active transport process. The action of both transmitters may also be terminated by diffusion of the transmitter away from the synaptic area.

Although ACh receptors are found at the neuromuscular junction, autonomic ganglia and receptors for postganglionic parasympathetic neurons, these receptors have structural differences that can be exploited pharmacologically by designing drugs that bind more selectively to the different types of ACh receptors. ACh receptors on tissues innervated by postganglionic parasympathetic neurons are called muscarinic because they can be activated by a substance called muscarine. Because muscarinic receptors are competitively blocked by atropine and synthetic analogs, these drugs are used to block effects produced by the parasympathetic nerv-

ous system. Examples include preventing motion sickness, decreasing bronchial secretion, and increasing a slow heart rate. Many antihistamine drugs taken for symptomatic relief from colds and allergies also competitively block muscarinic receptors, resulting in a dry mouth and increased heart rate. ACh receptors in skeletal muscle end plates are called nicotinic because they will bind a substance called nicotine. Nicotinic receptors are competitively blocked by curare. Curare blocks neuromuscular transmission, resulting in paralysis of skeletal muscle, including muscles of respiration. The receptors within the ganglia of both the parasympathetic and sympathetic divisions of the autonomic nervous system are also nicotinic, but have somewhat different structures so that different competitive blocking drugs are more effective at the neuromuscular junction than at the autonomic ganglia. Curare is more effective at the neuromuscular junction, but hexamethonium is more effective at the autonomic ganglia and is the drug more commonly used to block autonomic ganglia.

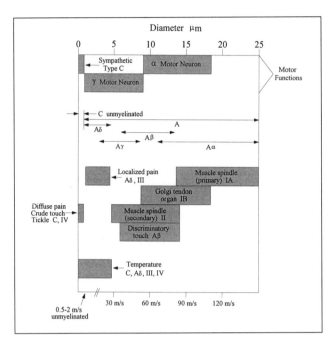

Figure 10-6. Classification schemes for sensory and motor neurons.

Muscarinic receptors used by postganglionic parasympathetic neurons produce a wide variety of postsynaptic effects. In the heart, binding of ACh to muscarinic receptors opens ligand-operated K^+ channels, causing hyperpolarization of heart muscle cells. In many smooth muscle cells, activation of muscarinic receptors by ACh causes the opening of nonselective cation channels, resulting in depolarization and contraction.

Adrenergic receptors are divided into two types, α and β, each of which has two subtypes: α_1 and α_2; and β_1 and β_2. The receptor types are distinguished pharmacologically by the particular class of drug that can activate or inhibit the receptor. NE binds better to α receptors than it does to β receptors. Epinephrine, the hormone secreted by the adrenal medulla, binds better to β receptors than it does to α receptors. The different receptor types produce their physiologic effects through different mechanisms. Activation of β adrenergic receptors causes the activation of adenylyl cyclase, which, in turn, produces cAMP from ATP. The cAMP then leads to a physiologic response. The two types of β receptors, β_1 and β_2, are found on different cells. For example β_1 receptors are found in cardiac muscle, and β_2 are found in bronchial smooth muscle. This difference in subtypes of β receptors can be exploited pharmacologically. A specific β_2 receptor agonist can be given to produce bronchodilation during an asthma attack with little effect on the heart. A specific β_1 antagonist can be given to decrease heart rate and force of contraction in a patient with hypertension without affecting the bronchial smooth muscle to any great extent.

Activation of an α_2 receptor causes the activation of a G protein that **inhibits** adenylate cyclase. Activation of α_1 receptors causes an increase in intracellular Ca^{++} concentration that, in turn, may cause muscle contraction or signal other events in the cell. More recent research has continued to find further subtypes of the subtypes of autonomic receptors that can be exploited by developing even more specific drugs.

CLASSIFICATION SYSTEMS OF NEURONS

In Chapter Eight, the organization of the nervous system was described. Within peripheral nerves, somatic sensory and motor neurons and autonomic nerves travel between the spinal cord and the periphery. Within peripheral nerves, a tremendous variation exists in the diameter of neurons. Early investigators discovered that clusters of nerve conduction velocity values of individual neurons existed within peripheral nerves and that this clustering differed from one peripheral nerve to another. Based on the different ranges of conduction velocity, researchers independently developed two classification schemes for classifying neurons. One system is based on neurons found in cutaneous nerves into A, B, and C fibers with subdivisions of $A\alpha$, $A\beta$, $A\gamma$, and $A\delta$. Researchers who studied nerves from muscles classified neurons into classes I, II, III, and IV with subclasses of IA and IB. For the most part, either classification scheme is sufficient to describe neurons, but some types of neurons are better described by one system than the other. For example, IA neurons carry information from one type of muscle receptor called the muscle spindle, which carries information concerning muscle length, and the IB neurons carry information concerning muscle tension from the Golgi tendon organs. On the other hand, chronic, poorly localized pain is carried by neurons described as either type IV or C, and acute, well-localized pain is carried by neurons described as either type III or $A\delta$ (Figure 10-6).

The basis for classification can be either diameter or conduction velocity. When a peripheral nerve carrying large numbers of several different types of neurons is electrically stimulated at one end, the resultant action potentials can be recorded at the other end after a period. Action potentials are not recorded simultaneously at the other end of each neuron in the peripheral nerve, but are recorded at different times in distinct populations. Two major factors determine conduction velocity: axon diameter and thickness of myelin surrounding the axon. The neurons with the greatest diameter conduct the action potential at the fastest rate. Myelin increases the velocity for two reasons. Myelin prevents the leakage of current out of the neuron so that action potentials regenerate only at the nodes of Ranvier, producing saltatory conduction. A second reason for increased action potential conduction velocity is that the presence of myelin causes less charge to build up along the cell membrane and fewer ions to leak out of the membrane, thereby allowing more of the ions to travel along the length of the axon. As a rule of thumb, conduction velocity in m/s equals neuron diameter in millimeters times six. A neuron 20 mm in diameter would have a conduction velocity of about 120 m/s; a neuron of 10 mm diameter would have a conduction velocity of 60 m/s, and so on. Type C or IV neurons do not have myelin sheaths and, therefore, conduct at a rate that is slower than that predicted by diameter alone, which is most likely caused by action potential regeneration at much shorter distances along the axon. Conduction velocity for unmyelinated fibers is 1 to 2 m/s for each millimeter of diameter. These neurons are associated with primitive, less precise functions, such as crude touch; tickle; chronic, poorly localized pain; temperature; and the sympathetic nervous system, whereas larger neurons are associated with more precise, well-developed functions including innervation of skeletal muscle and the receptors within muscles associated with reflexes. Preganglionic sympathetic neurons are the only type B neurons that have been described.

REVIEW OF ELECTRIC CIRCUITS

An understanding of the properties of electric circuits and of the classification of neurons is necessary to allow the clinician to recruit neurons of interest selectively with electric modalities, such as transcutaneous electrical nerve stimulation (TENS), neuromuscular electrical stimulation (NMES), and stimulation of denervated muscle by electrical muscle stimulation (EMS). The electrodiagnostic tests of chronaxie and nerve conduction velocity also require this knowledge. The measurement of chronaxie once was a common procedure to determine the integrity of a muscle's innervation. Today, the combination of electromyography and nerve conduction velocity has replaced chronaxie. The major concepts of electric circuits needed are those of charge, conductance (reciprocal of resistance), and capacitance.

Charge is the extensive property (quantity of electrical energy) of an electric system. Electrons have a negative charge; protons have a positive charge. In an electric circuit, charge is made to flow from an area of high

electrical potential (voltage) to an area of low electrical potential. If the difference in electrical potential can move 1 coulomb of charge a distance of 1 meter against a force of 1 Newton, the electrical force equals 1 joule/coulomb, which defines the volt. In living cells, electric current is carried by the net movement of ions. If the potential for positive ions to enter the cell exists, then the inside of the cell is negative with respect to the extracellular fluid. This is the normal situation for resting neurons. If positive ions enter a cell at one point, positively charged particles diffuse rapidly in all directions into the cell from the point of entry. This flow of positive ions constitutes an electric current. A bioelectric current behaves the same way as if a battery were connected to an electric circuit, except that the charge is carried by ions, not by electrons.

RESISTANCE

Resistance of an electric circuit refers to the difficulty in generating a current for a given difference in electric potential. The greater the resistance, the less current is produced for a given difference in electric potential. As discussed in Chapter Two, a better way of describing an electric system is by using the term conductance. Conductance and resistance are reciprocals. The greater the conductance (g), the greater the current generated for a given electric potential. Conductance is determined by a property of the conductor called conductivity and the geometry of the conductor. In an electric circuit, we consider wires to have negligible resistance or infinite conductance compared with resistors placed in the circuit. Metals, such as platinum, gold, silver, and copper, have high conductivity compared with other metals, such as aluminum. Therefore, aluminum wire generates more heat as current flows through it than does copper wire. Substances, such as air, rubber, plastic, and lipids, have very low conductivity and are considered insulators. Conductance increases with conductivity and cross-sectional area and decreases with length. The greater the cross-sectional area and the shorter the conductor, the greater its conductance. In neurons and muscle cells, current flows as the movement of ions from an area of like charge to that of the opposite charge. Resistance is not considered to be negligible. A neuron with a large diameter has a greater conductance or lower resistance to current flow than a small neuron. However, current does not flow only in the longitudinal direction, but also flows axially, from the center of a neuron through the membrane and into the extracellular space. The insulating properties of the cell membrane and myelin sheath determine the amount of axial flow. The greater the membrane resistance and the more of the cell covered by myelin, the greater is the axial resistance. The greater the axial resistance to current, the more current is available for longitudinal flow, and the faster the conduction velocity of the axon is. The analogy often used in this context is that of a garden hose with holes in it through which water can leak out axially. The leakage of water axially decreases the flow of water out of the other end of the hose. The greater the diameter of an axon is, the greater the cross-sectional area becomes relative to the surface area. Therefore, as diameter increases, longitudinal conductance increases, and axial conductance relative to longitudinal conductance decreases.

CAPACITANCE

Capacitance is a property of an electrical system describing the ability of a system to store charge and can be described as the slope of the relationship between electrical potential as the independent variable and charge stored as the dependent variable. As the voltage across a capacitor increases, the charge stored increases linearly according to the equation q (coulombs) = C (farads) ˇ E (volts). In an electric circuit, a capacitor consists of two conducting plates separated by an insulating layer. By analogy, the intracellular and extracellular fluids behave as the conducting plates, and the cell membrane behaves as the insulating layer of a capacitor. As the potential difference across a membrane increases, more charge builds up on the membrane, and the greater the capacitance of the cell membrane, the more charge is stored. If, during an action potential, charges are allowed to build up along the inner and outer surfaces, the flow of ions longitudinally along an axon is diminished. Therefore, the greater the capacitance of a membrane, the slower the action potential is propagated. In simple terms, membrane capacitance decreases conduction velocity.

Two geometric factors determine capacitance. First is the surface area. As surface area increases, more charge can be stored for any given potential across a capacitor. Secondly, capacitance decreases with distance between the plates of a capacitor. In practical terms, the greater the surface area and the thinner the insulator, the greater the capacitance. When current is allowed to flow across a cell membrane, some will flow along the axon longitudinally, causing the action potential to be propagated along the axon (longitudinal current), some will leak across the cell membrane in the axial direction (axial current), and some current (flow of ions) will go to build charge on the membrane (capacitive current). The charges drained off by capacitive and axial currents diminish the longitudinal current necessary to propagate the action potential. Moreover, the presence of charge stored on the membrane slows the reversal of charge on a membrane, which means that a neuron cannot produce action potentials as frequently if it has a high capacitance. In terms of electric circuits, capacitors act as low pass filters, allowing only low-frequency electrical changes to be transmitted. For axons to propagate action potentials at a high rate, capacitance must be minimized. Myelin decreases capacitance by increasing the thickness of insulator along the axon. A coating of myelin also improves longitudinal current by decreasing axial current. For practical purposes, the only places along an axon where current can leak out of the cell are at the nodes of Ranvier. For this reason, large axons with thick coats of myelin can produce more frequent action potentials than smaller diameter neurons or unmyelinated neurons. In demyelinating diseases, neurons may first lose the ability to produce rapid rates of firing before any pathology becomes evident.

The optimum situation for rapid longitudinal current flow and action potential velocity is one in which the diameter is large to reduce longitudinal resistance to current and myelin is thick to reduce axial current and decrease membrane capacitance. If axons conducted action potentials passively, the action potential would decrease with distance along an axon; some electric potential would be dissipated in overcoming longitudinal resistance, some current would be lost in an axial direction, and some current would be lost in charging the membrane (capacitive current). Thus, if current were initiated at one end of a neuron, it would eventually dissipate in a long axon. Active regeneration of the action potential occurs at each node of Ranvier between adjacent Schwann cells in peripheral nerves to prevent dissipation of the signal. The action potential appears to jump from node to node; thus, the name saltatory conduction ("jumping") has been used to describe conduction of action potentials along myelinated neurons.

CHRONAXIE

Each time an electric potential is placed across a membrane capacitance, current initially goes to charging the membrane. The amount of capacitive current depends on the capacitance of the membrane. For a membrane to be depolarized, a given amount of charge must cross the membrane. In theory, it would not matter whether a small current were applied for a long time or a strong current for a brief time. Charge (q) can be defined as current (charge/time) x duration (time). In reality, a minimum current that produces a net inward movement of positive charges into the cell must be applied to initiate an action potential because ions can leak across the membrane in both directions. To produce an action potential, charges must enter the cell at a rate sufficient to overcome leakage in the opposite direction. This minimum current is given the name rheobase. At current intensities greater than rheobase, progressively shorter durations of current need to be used to generate an action potential. A plot of the current needed at different durations of stimulation on a graph is called the strength-duration curve. The shape of the curve is hyperbolic; it fits the formula of X x Y = k. In other words, the product of X (duration) and Y (current) is a constant. This constant (k) is the minimum amount of charge that must be applied to produce a muscle contraction. For example, if the duration that produces a muscle contraction at a given intensity above rheobase is halved, intensity above rheobase must be doubled to produce a muscle contraction. If duration is reduced to one-third, intensity must be tripled and so on. This is the basis of a test that was once commonly used to determine if a muscle was normally innervated.

A normally innervated muscle can be made to contract if its α motor neuron is stimulated to produce an action potential. Branches of the neuron then cause each muscle cell to contract by causing an action potential in each muscle cell. Thus, the neuromuscular junction acts as an electric amplifier. If the peripheral nerve to a muscle is damaged so that it does not conduct an action potential, stimulating the motor nerve will not cause muscle to contract. However, muscle cells can be made to depolarize by producing an electric current through them directly. This situation requires a much greater amount of charge than that required to depolarize just the motor nerve. In this case, the equation I x t = q (X x Y = K) still applies, but the amount of charge (q) is much greater than in a normally innervated muscle. Not only must current be made to flow through individual muscle cells, but the capacitance of muscle cells is much greater than that of α motor neurons, which are not heavily coated with myelin. Therefore, at any given current intensity, a much longer duration is required in an denervated muscle than in an innervated muscle, or a much greater intensity is required for a given duration. This change in the required charge is quantified as chronaxie. Chronaxie is defined as the duration required to elicit a muscle contraction at an intensity twice that of rheobase, the minimum intensity that can elicit a contraction. In an innervated muscle, chronaxie is less than 1 ms. In a completely denervated muscle, it is greater than 15 ms. If a nerve is damaged, the value may be between 1 and 15 ms.

SUMMARY

Synaptic transmission is the sequence of events by which a chemical signal is sent by a neuron. Three types of synaptic transmission are described: synaptic transmission in the CNS, neuromuscular transmission, and autonomic synaptic transmission. In the CNS, synaptic transmission may be excitatory or inhibitory. Excitatory postsynaptic potentials (EPSPs) open nonspecific monovalent cation channels, resulting in a small, localized depolarization. Temporal or spatial summation of EPSPs is necessary to produce an action potential in the postsynaptic neuron. Inhibitory postsynaptic potentials (IPSPs) may be caused by opening K^+ channels to increase outward positive current, by opening Cl^- channels to increase inward negative current, or by short-circuiting the membrane by opening Cl^- channels. In neuromuscular synaptic transmission, a single action potential in the presynaptic neuron (the motor neuron) is sufficient to produce an action potential. The end plate potential is produced by the opening of channels similar to those described for the EPSP. In contrast to the EPSP, the end plate potential is sufficient to initiate the positive feedback cycle, resulting in an action potential on the surface of the skeletal muscle cell. The autonomic nervous system consists of pre- and postganglionic sympathetic and parasympathetic neurons. Preganglionic autonomic neurons release acetylcholine on nicotinic receptors on the postganglionic neurons, resulting in action potentials in the postganglionic neurons. The nicotinic receptors of the autonomic ganglia are blocked by different drugs than the nicotinic receptors of the neuromuscular junction. Postganglionic parasympathetic neurons release acetylcholine on muscarinic receptors. Muscarinic receptors perform different functions on different types of cells. Postganglionic sympathetic neurons usually release norepinephrine onto the postsynaptic membranes, although sweat glands receive acetylcholine. Adrenergic receptors include α and β types with two subtypes each. Stimulation of β receptors may be accomplished by sympathetic neurons or the hormone epinephrine, resulting in the production of cAMP. α receptors are commonly used to open Ca^{++} channels in smooth muscle cells. Neurons differ in properties related to the diameter of the neuron. Large neurons also have a coating of myelin, whereas the smallest neurons related to the most primitive functions of the nervous system do not.

The physical properties of neurons are related to the

electrical properties of conductance and capacitance. Longitudinal conductance increases with cross-sectional area of the neuron. Capacitance and axial conductance are reduced by coating axons with myelin. The largest diameter axons have the greatest conduction velocity because of low resistance to longitudinal flow, a high resistance to axial flow, and a low capacitance.

BIBLIOGRAPHY

Benfenati F, Valtorta F. Synapses and synaptic transmission. *News in Physiological Sciences.* 1993;8:18-23.

Berne RM, Levy MN. *Physiology.* St. Louis, Mo: Mosby-Year Book; 1998.

Ganong WF. *Review of Medical Physiology.* Norwalk, Conn: Appleton & Lange; 1995.

Guyton AC, Hall JE, Schmitt W. *Human Physiology and Mechanisms of Disease.* Philadelphia, Pa: WB Saunders; 1997.

STUDY QUESTIONS

1. Compare the excitatory and inhibitory postsynaptic potential in terms of ion flux.

2. Explain how the increased permeability to Cl^- can produce a stabilizing effect on membrane potential.

3. How are anticholinergic drugs, such as neostigmine, beneficial in myasthenia gravis?

4. Explain how the structure of the neuromuscular junction benefits the function of skeletal muscle.

5. Explain the need to develop β_2 specific drugs for treating airway disease.

6. Relate the properties of different classes of neurons with their functions.

7. Explain the relationship between axon diameter, cell body size, and conduction velocity.

8. Explain the benefits of myelination and the relationship between thickness of myelin and diameter.

LABORATORY EXERCISES

LABORATORY EXERCISE 10-1

NERVE CONDUCTION VELOCITY

Objective: Demonstrate the procedure of nerve conduction velocity (NCV) testing.

Materials:
EMG/NCV device
Electrode paste
Cable
Reference, ground, and active electrodes
Meter stick or metric tape measure

1. Turn equipment on and allow to warm up if necessary.

2. Attach the three electrodes to the cable. By convention the ground electrode is green, the active electrode is black, and the reference electrode is red.

3. Apply adhesive collars to all three electrodes. Place electrode paste in the cup of the electrode to just below the top.

4. Clean the back of the hand and the lateral aspect of one hand with isopropyl alcohol.

5. Apply ground electrode (green) to the back of the hand. Attach the active electrode (black) to the belly of abductor digiti minimi muscle and the reference electrode (red) over the distal tendon.

6. Set stimulator to deliver one impulse per second (PPS = 1). Set duration to 0.1 ms, stimulus intensity to 100 to 150 V. A higher intensity is usually required at the wrist than the elbow. Set gain to 2k mV/div. A sweep speed of 5 ms/div will provide a good tracing. Set filter to 2 10.

7. With the negative pole directed distally, apply the stimulator to the skin over the ulnar nerve near the wrist.

8. Move the stimulating electrode slightly if necessary to get the largest possible muscle action potential from the abductor digiti minimi. Measure time in tenths of ms between stimulus and rise of action potential. This time is called the distal latency. Decrease amplitude to zero. Remove the stimulation electrode and mark the position of the negative pole.

9. Place the stimulating electrode over the ulnar nerve on the posteromedial aspect of the elbow where the ulnar nerve passes under the medial epicondyle. Repeat step 8 at this location. Measure time between stimulus and rise of action potential to obtain the proximal latency.

10. Measure the distance between the distal and proximal locations with a meter stick or metric tape measure in millimeters.

LABORATORY EXERCISES

11. Compute nerve conduction velocity in meters/second. The time for the action potential to be propagated from the proximal point near the elbow and the distal point near the wrist is the difference between the proximal and distal latencies in milliseconds. Nerve conduction velocity equals distance between the points in millimeters divided by (proximal latency - distal latency). Convert units from millimeters per millisecond to meters per second. If distance is measured in millimeters and time in milliseconds, the milli- prefixes can simply be dropped; multiplying both numerator and denominator by 1000 does not change the number (1000/1000 = 1). If distance is measured in cm, then you would need to multiply by 10. Compare to the expected value of 63 ± 6 m/s.

LABORATORY EXERCISE 10-2

STRENGTH-DURATION CURVE

Objectives: Demonstrate the relationship between stimulus duration and intensity (strength of electrical stimulation). Find rheobase, chronaxie, and utilization time.

Materials:
Chronaxie meter
Electrode paste
Bipolar stimulation electrode

The purpose of chronaxie measurement is to determine if the α motor neurons are behaving as current amplifiers. By causing a peripheral nerve to depolarize with an external source of electricity, many muscle cells can be depolarized by chemical signaling from the α motor neuron to the muscle cells. Muscle cells can be stimulated directly to depolarize and cause a muscle contraction even in the absence of intact a motor neurons; however, a much larger current must be used because each muscle cell must be depolarized instead of causing motor neurons to be depolarized. The depolarization is actually caused by charge moving across the membrane of the excitable cell (muscle cell or neuron). Therefore, it is the combination of duration of the current and the magnitude of the current that drives charge across the membrane to depolarize these cells. The term *strength* in "strength duration" curve refers to the intensity in mA of the current required to generate a muscle response.

Electric current has units of charge per time and duration has units of time; the product of current and time (charge per time) x time equals charge. Because a threshold charge can cause a muscle contraction to occur, we can plot the magnitude of charge required to create muscle contraction for a given duration. Because this product is a constant, the plot will be that of a hyperbolic curve, which is describe mathematically as X x Y = k, or in this specific case, current x duration = a constant. However, a minimal current is required regardless of the duration that this current is applied. This current is called the rheobase. An index of the effectiveness of the motor neurons as current amplifiers is chronaxie. It is somewhat arbitrarily chosen as an index of the shape of the hyperbolic curve. Its computation is described below.

Turn on the TECA chronaxie meter (or equivalent device). Because this device operates with tubes, allow time for warm-up. Next, place electrodes over any superficial muscle and set controls as fol-

LABORATORY EXERCISES

lowing: duration vernier = 0, pulse duration = 1.0, duration multiplier = x 100, meter scale multiplier = x 1, interval between pulses = 1.0, selector = Chron, output switch = ON, intensity = 0.

Chronaxie is determined by plotting the intensity required to elicit a reproducible muscle contraction. Usually the minimal visible contraction is used for this purpose. Rheobase is determined as the minimum current that produces contraction at very long durations. The first few duration settings beginning with 100 ms should require the same intensity, which should be equal to rheobase. It is expected that these values will not be identical, so you will need to pick a value that seems to represent rheobase the most consistently. Slowly increase intensity from zero until muscle contraction occurs. Plot the intensity required for a duration of 100 ms. Turn intensity back to zero before removing the electrode to avoid shocking the patient.

Decrease pulse duration to 0.7 and repeat stimulation, recording intensity required for a duration of 70 ms (.7 times 100 ms). Continue at durations of 50, 30, 10, 7, 5, 3, 2, 1, 0.8, 0.6, 0.4, 0.3, 0.2, and 0.1 ms. If the required intensity is beyond 25 mA, stop the procedure.

Draw a smooth curve through the points on the graph. A hyperbolic curve should be generated. In the determination of chronaxie we should find that a combination of current and duration produces a muscle contraction. A current of twice the amplitude above rheobase should require one-half the duration and so on. Determine rheobase as the minimum current that can elicit a muscle contraction. Draw a horizontal line at a current that is twice that of rheobase. Chronaxie is the duration at which the horizontal line drawn at twice rheobase intersects the strength-duration curve.

What is the implication of the shape of the strength-duration curve? Was chronaxie within normal limits (WNL < 1.0 ms)?

ELEVEN

Sensation

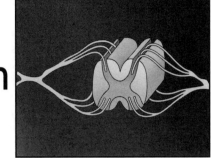

OBJECTIVES

1. List the five types of receptors and their functions.

2. Describe the two processes of stimulus transduction: production of a receptor potential and generation of action potentials.

3. Describe the relationship between stimulus intensity and receptor potential (Weber-Fechner or Steven's law) and the usefulness of these relationships.

4. Explain how relative refractory period and receptor potential interact to determine action potential frequency.

5. Define receptor adaption, fast adapting, and slow adapting receptors.

6. Explain how receptor adaptation provides the central nervous system with useful information.

7. Explain how the central nervous system can interpret the quality of a sensation from a series of action potentials.

8. List the five major types of skin mechanoreceptors, their locations, their adaption characteristics, and functions.

9. Compare and contrast the sensations of proprioception and kinesthesia.

10. Explain the relationships among proprioception, vision, and equilibrium.

11. Describe complex sensations of touch: stereognosis, two-point discrimination, barognosis, and graphesthesia.

12. Explain how temperature is encoded by cutaneous thermal receptive neurons.

13. Describe the functions of the semicircular canals, utricle and saccule, including their adequate stimuli and signal transduction.

For the nervous system to respond appropriately to stimuli from the environment and to events occurring within the body, we require mechanisms to gather information. This process is called sensation. Most movement is a result of sensation either directly, such as reflexes, or indirectly, as in walking to a thermostat to adjust temperature. It is common in rehabilitation to treat disorders that affect movement, such as stroke, by providing specific types of sensory experiences. Receptors ranging from very specialized structures to bare nerve endings respond to stimuli by producing receptor potentials. The receptor potentials, if sufficiently intense, lead to the production of action potentials. Action potentials, in turn, lead to the output response of the afferent nerve, which is usually release of neurotransmitter on one or more cells in the central nervous system. We must then interpret the signals produced by the afferent nerves to draw conclusions concerning the environment. The process of drawing conclusions based on sensation is what we call perception.

In this chapter, the mechanisms producing the sensations of touch, vibration, temperature, balance, body position, and body movement will be discussed. The processes to be discussed include the production of the receptor potential, conversion of the receptor potential into a series of action potentials, adaptation of the receptor, and pathways for afferent information into the central nervous system (CNS). Nociception, the sensation of pain, will be discussed separately in Chapter Twelve.

CLASSIFICATION OF RECEPTORS

Sensory endings (input mechanisms) include specialized receptors and well-differentiated nerve endings. These sensory endings are classified based on the type of stimulus to which they respond. Five types of receptors include 1) mechanoreceptors, 2) chemoreceptors, 3) photoreceptors, 4) thermoreceptors, and 5) nociceptors. Mechanoreceptors are responsible for the sensations we call touch on the skin, but have many more uses. Examples include the detection of arterial pressure and the fullness of the bladder. Many mechanoreceptors are involved in providing information that does not lead to conscious perception, such as arterial pressure. Mechanoreceptors are also involved in hearing, equilibrium, joint position, awareness of body movement, muscle tension, and muscle length. Chemoreceptors usually do not lead to conscious perception. The exceptions are the senses of smell and taste. Chemoreceptors are very important in our ability to maintain homeostasis. They provide information about concentrations of oxygen and carbon dioxide and about pH, osmolarity, glucose

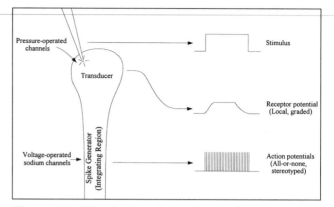

Figure 11-1. Stimulus transduction in a mechanoreceptor. A stimulus produces opening of pressure-operated channels, which produce a graded receptor potential. The receptor potential remains steady as long as the stimulus is applied, and the receptor potential causes action potentials to be generated in the integrating region of the sensory receptor.

concentration, and other chemicals. Information from photoreceptors is used by the visual system to interpret patterns of light and appear to be involved in other functions, including circadian and seasonal cycles and mood. Thermoreceptors are used to gather information concerning temperature and exist both on the skin and inside the body. Thermoreceptors provide information on thermal comfort and provide the information necessary to regulate body temperature. Temperature regulation has been discussed fully in Chapter Seven. Nociceptors are the receptors that produce the sensation of not only pain, but also "discomfort" as one might experience from sitting in the same position for a prolonged time. Lack of nociception is responsible in large part for development of ulcers on the diabetic foot and pressure sores. Nociception will be discussed separately in Chapter Twelve.

STIMULUS TRANSDUCTION

The process by which a stimulus is converted by an afferent neuron to a series of action potentials is called stimulus transduction. Transduction consists of two processes: a transducer producing a receptor potential graded to the size of the stimulus and a spike generating region converting the receptor potential into a proportional number of action potentials. The result of stimulus transduction is an action potential frequency proportional to the size of the stimulus (Figure 11-1).

The response to the stimulus, the receptor potential, is not linearly related to the size of the stimulus, but increases approximately with the log of the stimulus. Two different equations have been developed to quan-

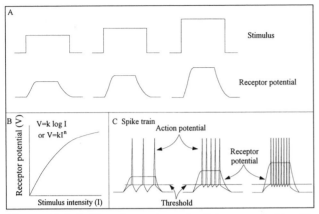

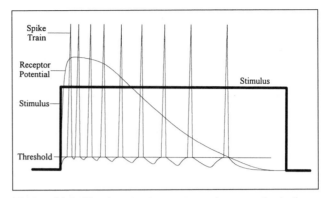

Figure 11-2. A: Size of receptor potentials generated by different levels of mechanical stimulus. B: The shape of the relationship between stimulus intensity and receptor potential is not linear, but receptor potential increases approximately with the log of the stimulus intensity, allowing a wider range of stimulus intensities to be encoded. C: The frequency of action potentials is proportional to the receptor potential. As long as the receptor potential remains above threshold, the spike-generating region of the cell continues to produce action potentials during the relative refractory period. The larger the stimulus, the earlier in the relative refractory period an action potential is produced.

Figure 11-3. Phasic receptor response to a constant stimulus in which receptor potential and action potential frequency decrease. Contrast to the tonic receptor's response to a constant stimulus in Figure 11-2.

tify this relationship. The Weber-Fechner relationship is stated V = k log I; the Steven's relationship is written V = k In, in which V is the receptor potential, k and n are constants for the type of receptor, and I is the stimulus intensity. As a result of how stimulus intensity is encoded, a wider range of stimulus intensity can be encoded than would be if the response were linear. As a consequence of this relationship, we can detect a constant relative, not a constant absolute difference in stimulus intensity. If, for example, we can differentiate between the mass of a 5-gram object and a 6-gram object, but we cannot differentiate between an object with a mass of 5000 g and one of 5001 g; we can, however, perceive the difference between 5 kg and 6 kg. The second part of signal transduction involves converting the receptor potential to a series of action potentials. In a sensory neuron that does not adapt (adaptation is discussed below), the receptor potential remains constant as long as the stimulus is present. If the receptor potential is great enough, the integrating portion of the cell produces an action potential. The action potential is transmitted centrally to the CNS. If the receptor potential persists beyond the neuron's absolute refractory period, another action potential may be produced. The maximum rate at which a neuron can produce action potentials is determined by the neuron's absolute refractory period. No matter how great the receptor potential is, another action potential cannot be developed until the

inactivation gates of the voltage-operated sodium channels return to their resting state. However, a new action potential can develop during the relative refractory period. The greater the receptor potential is, the earlier during the relative refractory period the next action potential is produced. This means that the frequency of action potentials developed by a sensory neuron increases with the size of the graded receptor potential. These events are summarized in Figure 11-2.

ADAPTATION OF RECEPTORS

In the previous discussion, it was stated that if the receptor did not adapt, the receptor potential remains constant as long as the stimulus remains constant. Adaptation refers to a decrease in receptor potential in the face of a constant stimulus. The adaptation characteristics of various receptors are different. Some adapt very slowly; these are called tonic receptors. Phasic receptors decrease the rate of action potentials for a given intensity of stimulus very rapidly (Figure 11-3). Some phasic receptors adapt so quickly that they only produce an action potential when the stimulus first appears and then again when the stimulation stops. The presence of tonic and phasic types of receptors allows the nervous system to interpret various types of information. Tonic receptors encode the magnitude of the stimulus by sending a frequency of action potential, whereas phasic receptors produce an action potential frequency proportional to the rate at which the stimulus changes. For example, the Pacinian corpuscle, a type of cutaneous receptor, adapts very quickly to a mechanical deformation and produces only one action potential when the corpuscle is deformed and again when the deformation is removed. Due to the adaptation characteristics of the Pacinian corpuscle, this receptor functions well for the detection of vibration in which the Pacinian corpuscle is rhythmically deformed and allowed to return to the resting shape. Most receptors show at least a small amount of adaptation in which the action potential frequency decreases for a short time, followed by a steady rate of firing. The higher initial rate can then be interpreted by the central nervous system as a change in the stimulus, and the slower rate that follows can be used to interpret the magnitude of the stimulus.

INTERPRETATION OF SENSORY INFORMATION

The CNS receives information from the periphery in the form of a series of action potentials from sensory neurons. The CNS must then somehow extract meaning from the series of action potentials. Through the process of learning, the CNS associates action potentials from certain neurons with specific stimuli. Because all sensory neurons use action potential frequency to communicate, no method exists for determining the quality of the sensation. That is, visual, auditory, tactile, and chemical receptors do not differ in the type of signals sent to the CNS. Instead, the CNS learns what type of information each sensory neuron conveys. This coding for different sensations is called a labeled line. The neuron does not do anything specific to tell the CNS what type of information it is conveying. The brain learns that if a certain neuron changes its action potential frequency, a certain type of sensation has changed. Each neuron carries only one type of sensation. The type of sensation **perceived** is determined by which neuron changes its action potential frequency, regardless of the actual sensation. For example, photoreceptors convey information to the brain concerning light. We have learned that if neurons receiving information from photoreceptors are stimulated, the stimulus must have been light. However, if pressure is placed on the eye, one does not perceive pressure, one perceives light (seeing stars). The labeled line also has an impact on sensation following recovery from a peripheral nerve injury. If axons regenerating within a peripheral nerve reinnervate different sensory endorgans than they did before the injury, one may experience confusion in sensation. The person who recovers from a peripheral nerve injury may require sensory reeducation to relearn what information each neuron conveys to the CNS.

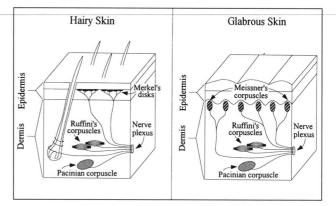

Figure 11-4. Touch receptors of the skin. Merkel's disks are located in the superficial dermis at the epidermal border and respond to steady skin indentation. Meissner's corpuscles are also superficial and respond to touch and low-frequency vibration. Meissner's corpuscles are not found in hairy skin, but are replaced by hair receptors with a similar function. The deep skin receptors, Pacinian corpuscles, and Ruffini corpuscles are located in both hairy and nonhairy skin. Pacinian corpuscles respond to high-frequency vibration. Ruffini corpuscles respond to stretching forces and are directionally sensitive.

TOUCH

Four major receptors are involved in producing the simple sensation of touch. These include Pacinian corpuscles, Meissner's corpuscles, Ruffini endings, and Merkel disks (Figure 11-4). Pacinian and Meissner corpuscles are rapidly adapting receptors with specialized endings. Pacinian receptors are found deep in the skin and respond to high frequency vibration within a range of 60 to 500 Hz. Meissner corpuscles respond to lower frequency vibration up to 80 Hz and may be used to detect movement of the skin. Meissner corpuscles are located in nonhairy skin, also called glabrous skin. On hairy skin, the Meissner corpuscle is replaced by hair receptors with similar properties to the Meissner corpuscle. Ruffini endings and Merkel disks are slowly adapting receptors. Merkel disks have small receptive fields, are superficial, and are useful for localizing continuous pressure. Ruffini receptors are found deep in the skin and respond to deep pressure and stretch. A useful feature of Ruffini receptors is their directional sensitivity. Ruffini endings are common joint receptors. Because Ruffini receptors are slowly adapting, directionally sensitive, and found in joints, information conveyed by Ruffini endings leads to the sensations of proprioception and kinesthesia.

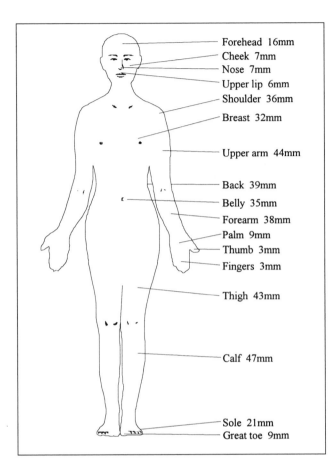

Figure 11-5. Mean threshold for two-point discrimination at different locations on the body.

PROPRIOCEPTION AND KINESTHESIA

Two types of sensation related in nature, kinesthesia and proprioception, provide information concerning joints. Proprioception is the sensation of static position of a joint that comes from receptors in joint capsules, ligaments, and skin surrounding the joints. Proprioception may be conscious or unconscious; "conscious proprioception" is received by the cortex and "unconscious proprioception" is directed to the cerebellum. Because damage to ligaments and joint capsules results in impaired proprioception, rehabilitation of joint injuries needs to include proprioceptive and kinesthetic training. Kinesthesia is the conscious awareness of direction and rate of movement of body parts. Kinesthesia is largely the result of stimulation of Ruffini endings around the joint and of Golgi tendon organs, which monitor muscle tension. Operation of Golgi tendon organs is described further in Chapter Eighteen.

Proprioception of different body parts is used in behaviors called righting reactions, in which one part of the body is aligned with other body parts. Examples include righting of the head on the body and the trunk with the lower body. Proprioception is also related to the ability to find and maintain a midline position. Head injury or cerebrovascular disease may result in the inability to perform righting reactions. Of particular importance is neck proprioception. Information concerning the orientation of the head with respect to the body is needed to integrate the information received from the visual and the vestibular systems. Because balance is the result of input from vision, the vestibular system, and proprioception, immobilization of the head for prolonged periods can result in impaired dynamic balance due to diminished neck proprioception. People with certain neurologic diseases watch their feet while walking. Lack of proprioception can also lead to joint destruction. In some neuropathies, the loss of pain and proprioception leads to joint damage called Charcot's joints or neurogenic arthropathy.

COMPLEX SENSATIONS OF TOUCH

Stereognosis is the ability to recognize objects by feeling them. A person with a CNS deficit may retain proprioception and thermal sensation, but have astereognosis. Small, culturally familiar objects, such as keys, coins, and safety pins, are used for testing this ability. Two-point discrimination is a measure of the smallest distance between two stimuli that can be identified as two distinct stimuli. The value for normal two-point discrimination varies substantially from one area of skin to another. It is very small on the fingers and very wide on areas such as the back (Figure 11-5). Barognosis is the ability to recognize weight (pressure). This is measured by comparing relative weights serially in the same hand or by comparing two weights simultaneously in different hands. Graphesthesia is the ability to recognize patterns, including letters or numbers, traced on the skin.

TEMPERATURE

Thermoreceptors are found both peripherally in the skin and within deep structures. Skin thermoreceptors provide information used to sense environmental temperature, to determine the level of thermal comfort, and to regulate body temperature. Cutaneous receptors serve as warnings to avoid damaging the skin and feed information forward concerning the environmental temperature so that the thermoregulatory system can prevent a fall in internal temperature. Both cold and

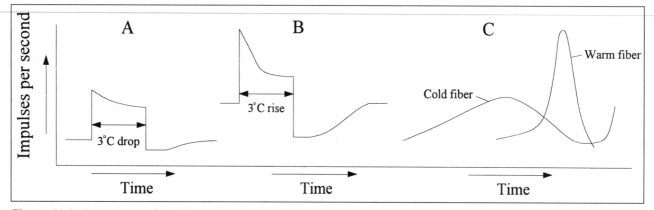

Figure 11-6. A: response of a cold receptor to a step change in temperature. An initial adaptation signals a change in temperature; the steady, increased firing rate signals the magnitude of the change to the CNS. B: response of a warmth receptor. C: the steady-state firing rates of cold and warm receptors at different temperatures. Note each type has a peak response at a particular temperature. Information from both types of receptors are necessary at extremes of temperature for successful interpretation of temperature.

warm sensations are derived from neurons without specialized end-organs. Temperature information is transmitted by slowly conducting C and Aδ neurons. Warmth and cold receptors are slowly adapting so they can convey both changes in temperature and develop a steady action potential frequency when temperature is held constant. Cold receptors respond within a range of approximately 5°C to 45°C with a peak action potential frequency of about 25°C. Warm fibers respond within a range of about 30°C to 45°C with a peak response at about 42°C. A combination of information from both types of receptors is necessary to detect temperature over a range of 5°C to 45°C. Very high or low temperatures stimulate pain receptors and, therefore, give the same sensation (Figure 11-6).

VESTIBULAR SYSTEM

Organs located in the "inner ear," or labyrinth, are associated by location and innervation with hearing. The organs of balance are immediately adjacent to the cochlea; all these organs are innervated by the vestibulocochlear nerve (cranial nerve VIII). An acoustic neuroma, a benign tumor of Schwann cells of the eighth nerve, can affect both hearing and equilibrium. Equilibrium is produced by sensations originating from three sets of organs. Semicircular canals detect angular acceleration of the head in all three planes. The utricle detects horizontal acceleration of the head, and the saccule is stimulated by vertical acceleration.

Three semicircular canals in each inner ear are arranged at right angles to each other, representing all three planes (Figure 11-7). Within a widened area of

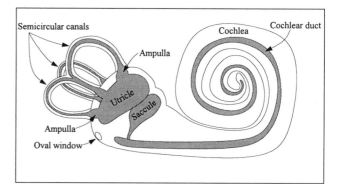

Figure 11-7. Location of the organs of the inner ear. Three semicircular canals exist at right angles to each other to represent all three dimensions. The actual sensory device is located in the widened area at the base of each canal, called the ampulla. At a constant velocity, all elements within the semicircular canal move at the same rate, and a steady action potential frequency is picked up from all six ampullae. Also, note the position of the saccule and utricle in the same region. The semicircular canals and other structures are surrounded by the temporal bone and are lined with a membranous structure.

each semicircular canal called the ampulla is a special sense organ called the cupula. The cupula is essentially a gelatinous mass in which hair cells, similar to those used by the cochlea for hearing, are located. The hair cells respond to bending and are directionally sensitive. Bending in one direction causes depolarization, whereas bending in the other causes hyperpolarization. The semicircular canals use the inertia of fluid within the canal and the cupula to sense angular acceleration. With acceleration of the head, everything attached to the labyrinth, including the cupula and hair cells, move with the head. However, the inertia of the fluid that is not

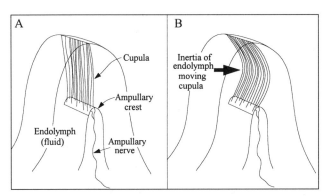

Figure 11-8. Structures within the ampulla that cause the receptor potential to be altered. The ampullary nerve carries the information obtained from bending of cilia within the cupula. A: Steady state exists with endolymph and cupula moving at the same rate. B: The head is accelerated moving the cupula into the still endolymph, resulting in bending of the cilia and either an increase or decrease in action potential frequency in the ampullary nerve. Deceleration will cause the endolymph to continue moving in the same direction as the cupula slows, bending the cilia in the opposite direction and causing the opposite action potential frequency response to occur. Information from all six semicircular canals is integrated with visual and proprioceptive stimuli to interpret the movement pattern.

attached to the bony skull initially causes the fluid to remain still as the cupula is accelerated with the head. This lag in movement of labyrinth fluid deforms the cupula, bending the hair cells (Figure 11-8). Once a constant angular velocity is obtained, the fluid within the canals reaches the same velocity as the cupula, the hair cells are no longer bent, and the firing rate of the hair cells returns to resting level. The mechanism works in a similar fashion during deceleration. When the head stops a rotary movement, or slows, fluid continues to move at the same velocity, whereas the cupula slows or stops. Hair cells are bent in the opposite direction from which they bent during acceleration. Again, when constant velocity of the head is reached, the hair cells are no longer bent, and action potential frequency returns to its resting level. The brain must interpret six signals related to angular acceleration of the head. Depending on the type of movement, the change in action potential frequency may be the opposite in the two ears or the same. When nodding "yes" (flexion and extension of the neck), the same information is received on both sides; however, when shaking the head "no" (rotation of the neck) and touching the ears to the shoulders (lateral flexion), opposite signals come from the two sides of the head.

The bilateral utricles and saccules provide information concerning linear acceleration in either the horizontal or vertical plane, such as what occurs when driving a car or riding an elevator, as opposed to rotary acceleration detected by the semicircular canals. The utricle and saccule also use directionally sensitive hair cells, but instead of using fluid and a cupula, they use an organ called a macula. The macula consists of a gelatinous material in which otoliths are embedded. Otoliths are calcium carbonate crystals that increase the mass and, therefore, the inertia of the macula. In the utricle, the macula lies in the horizontal plane. Horizontal acceleration and inertia of the otoliths produce similar effects on the hair cells as occurs during rotary acceleration in the semicircular canals. In the saccule, the macula is oriented vertically. Vertical acceleration in the face of inertia of the macula stimulates the hair cells to produce depolarization or hyperpolarization depending on the direction of vertical acceleration (Figure 11-9).

The signals received from the semicircular canals, utricle, and saccule must be learned and integrated with the senses of vision and proprioception. Motion sickness appears to be a consequence of incongruity between the visual and vestibular inputs. Visual information can be used to supplement or replace vestibular information. However, in general, two of the three systems produce sufficient information to maintain dynamic balance in everyday activities. To some degree, the lack of vestibular sensation or proprioception can be compensated by vision. When the person with a deficit in one system closes the eyes, balance is lost. Both vision and proprioception are sensitive enough to correct body position before enough acceleration of the body occurs to detect large swaying movements. The Romberg sign is used as a test of lower extremity proprioception based on this ability. An individual closes the eyes with the feet placed close together in standing. Vestibular input results from acceleration of the head. With a deficit in proprioception, the head is allowed to accelerate before posture is corrected, and a large increase in sway can be easily observed. With intact proprioception, little sway will be observed.

A temporary loss of input from the vestibular system results in the condition called vertigo, in which a person may become dizzy and nauseated. A permanent loss of input from the vestibular system causes the individual to relearn to interpret the signals from the vestibular system. Diminished input regarding a person's position in space may cause a person to become insecure and feel off-balance or even dizzy. This situation, in contrast to vertigo, is called dysequilibrium and may result from a situation as simple as a person not wearing prescribed eyeglasses or from a head cold. Presyncope is a type of dizziness that is not caused by the vestibular system, but by the cardiovascular system. Presyncope refers to the situation in which cerebral blood flow is sufficiently

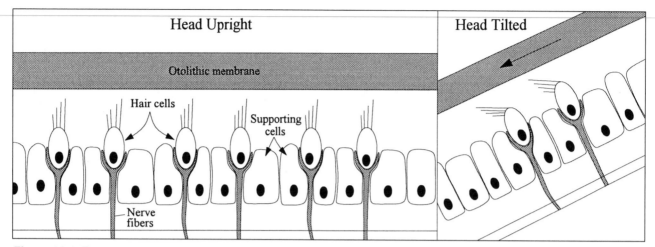

Figure 11-9. The otolithic membrane associated with the utricle. The saccule has a similar structure but is oriented vertically. Horizontal acceleration of the otolithic membrane across the hair cells changes action potential frequency in the utricle. The utricle will also respond to a tilting of the head by bending of cilia. The mechanism of the saccule is similar to the utricle.

diminished to disturb cognitive function briefly, resulting in dizziness for a short period. Orthostatic hypotension, due to loss of blood as may occur following surgery, often results in presyncope when a patient first begins to assume an upright posture. These individuals may need only to stand up gradually, may require tilt-table treatments, or may even require transfusion of blood.

SUMMARY

Sensory systems provide input to the CNS. Mechanoreceptors, chemoreceptors, photoreceptors, thermoreceptors, and nociceptors provide information, which is processed by the CNS to form perception. Stimulus transduction converts a stimulus to a series of action potentials. For a nonadapting receptor, the receptor potential is proportional to the log of the stimulus. The greater the receptor potential, the closer together in time the action potentials can be due to the refractory period of the neuron. Discrimination of sensation is proportional over a wide range of stimulus intensity. Adaptation of receptors allows perception of the rate of application of a stimulus and the steady-state magnitude of the stimulus. The type of stimulus to be perceived is learned from the specific neurons excited by certain types of stimuli. Simple touch is mediated by two slow-ly adapting receptors, one superficial and one deep and two rapidly adapting receptors. Kinesthesia and proprioception provide information concerning joint position and movement. Proprioception, vision, and vestibular systems are all used to maintain balance. The vestibular system consists of semicircular canals, the utricle, and the saccule. Semicircular canals detect rotary acceleration of the head in all three planes. The utricle detects horizontal acceleration and the saccule detects vertical acceleration.

BIBLIOGRAPHY

Berne RM, Levy MN. *Physiology*. St. Louis, Mo: Mosby-Year Book; 1998.

French AS, Torkkeli D. The basis of rapid adaptation in mechanoreceptors. *News in Physiological Sciences*. 1994;9:158-161.

Ganong WF. *Review of Medical Physiology*. Norwalk, Conn: Appleton & Lange; 1995.

Guyton AC, Hall JE, Schmitt W. *Human Physiology and Mechanisms of Disease*. Philadelphia, Pa: WB Saunders; 1997.

Hole JW Jr. *Essentials of Human Anatomy and Physiology*. 4th ed. Dubuque, Iowa: Wm. C. Brown Publishers; 1992.

Schauf C, Moffett D, Moffett S. *Human Physiology: Foundation and Frontiers*. St. Louis, Mo: Times Mirror/Mosby College Publishing; 1990.

Solomon EP, Davis PW. *Human Anatomy and Physiology*. Philadelphia, Pa: WB Saunders; 1983.

STUDY QUESTIONS

1. How are neurons able to code different sensory modalities if all the neurons use action potentials to signal a sensory event?

2. Describe how the refractory periods define the minimum and maximum frequencies of sensory neuron output.

3. Contrast the kinds of information that slowly adapting and rapidly adapting receptors provide.

4. Explain why neck proprioception is important for function of the vestibular system.

5. Why do people who have had their cervical spines immobilized display poor balance when the immobilization is discontinued?

6. Why do you think it is important to test for both simple sensory input, such as light touch, and complex sensations, such as graphesthesia?

7. Explain why a person buried in snow or a pilot flying through clouds cannot tell up from down. In these situations, what could you do to tell which direction is up?

8. Why do individuals going at a fixed speed lose sense of velocity?

9. Why does a person get a sense of weightlessness in a rapidly descending elevator?

TWELVE

Pain

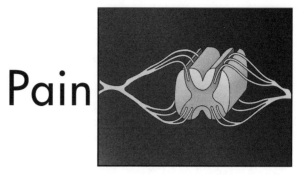

OBJECTIVES

1. Define and compare phase one, phase two, and phase three pain.

2. List stimuli capable of producing the sensation of pain.

3. Define hyperalgesia, and provide a plausible explanation of its presence.

4. Define referred pain, and discuss possible causes.

5. Describe the pathways of phase one and phase two pain information to the central nervous system (CNS).

6. Describe pain-associated reflexes: sharp cutaneous pain, visceral pain, and the pain-spasm positive feedback cycle.

7. Discuss phase-three pain and the causes of complex regional pain syndromes, phantom limb pain, and central pain, including the phenomenon of mechanical allodynia.

8. Describe the essential elements of the gate-control theory of pain: mechanoreceptors, gate cells, transmission cells, and C pain fibers.

9. Describe the descending analgesic pathways to the dorsal horn, including cells of the periaqueductal gray, serotonergic neurons, opiate receptors of the dorsal horn, enkephalin, endorphin, and the use of stimulation-produced analgesia.

Pain is often described as an important protective sensation; it is well known that the absence of pain can lead to extensive tissue damage. Important examples are joint destruction in neuropathies (Charcot's joints or neurogenic arthropathy), pressure ulcers following spinal cord injury, and neuropathic foot ulcers in diabetic patients' feet. Moreover, many people seek health care professionals due to pain. The difficulty in providing appropriate interventions for pain is that it is more than a sensation; it has a large emotional component, and quantifying it is difficult. Part of the problem lies in the perception of nociception as shaped by cultural and personal experience. The second problem is that pain is not a simple sensation and may be caused by many stimuli. To complicate the problem further, pain may persist after the stimulus is gone and change in quality over time.

To address this change over time, some investigators have developed a system of describing pain as occurring in three phases. The phases are sequential, but do not always progress to the next phase (ie, phase three must be preceded by phases one and two, phase two must be preceded by phase one; but phase one pain does not always progress to phase two, and phase two rarely progresses to phase three).

Phase one is a brief localized noxious stimulus, such as a pin prick. This type of pain is graded to the stimulus size, is well localized, and is brief. Phase two is a chronic, lower intensity pain with psychologic consequences caused not by some immediate stimulus, but by tissue damage or inflammation. Phase three is the most perplexing type of pain and is sometimes called neuropathic pain. It can usually be traced to damage to peripheral nerves or to parts of the central nervous system related to pain. This third category includes phenomena such as central pain syndromes, trigeminal neuralgia, phantom limb pain, and complex regional pain syndrome. In phase-three pain, the degree of pain perceived by the individual is reported to be much greater than the history would suggest. Unusual painful sensations also occur with neuropathic disease, such as advanced diabetes mellitus, and is characterized by a burning sensation from the areas of lost sensation, usually the feet.

STIMULI

Pain-receptive neurons are called nociceptors. Their cell bodies are found in the same locations as other sensory neurons in the dorsal root ganglia and the trigeminal ganglia. However, they do not have specialized end organs, such as those of highly specialized mechanoreceptors described in Chapter Eleven, but appear to have chemical receptors. Phase-one pain information is carried by small, myelinated Aδ fibers. Typical stimuli for the Aδ neurons include strong mechanical events, such as pin prick or heavy pressure, and thermal stimulation above 45°C or below 15°C. The stimulus that produces phase-one pain lasts as long as the stimulus persists and is easily localized.

Chemical stimuli and tissue damage, including inflammation, stimulate nociceptors with C fibers. Stimulation of C fibers gives rise to phase-two pain. Phase two lasts longer than the stimulus is present and

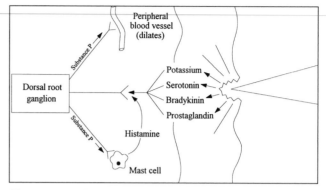

Figure 12-1. Chemical mediators of pain released with tissue damage.

is not as well-localized as phase-one pain. Because extracts of damaged tissue have been shown to produce intense pain when injected into skin, one might conclude that chemicals released by damaged tissue mediate phase-two pain. Recently, capsaicin, the active ingredient in chili peppers, has been demonstrated to be a mediator of this type of pain. Specific capsaicin receptors have been isolated and cloned and are being used in pain research. Other chemicals known to contribute to phase two pain include substance P, potassium, serotonin, bradykinin, histamine, and prostaglandins (Figure 12-1). Nociceptors are also stimulated by ischemia caused by pressure over bony prominences. This nociception causes us to shift our weight unconsciously when sitting and may be the cause of distress commonly seen in the classroom when individuals are asked to sit for hours on end. Both debilitation and loss of sensation can lead to development of pressure ulcers.

HYPERALGESIA

Hyperalgesia refers to decreased threshold and spread of pain to neighboring, noninjured areas. In particular, pain caused by tissue damage can produce hyperalgesia (Figure 12-2). Following injury, nerve growth factor increases the activity of capsaicin. Moreover, potassium and prostaglandins released by tissue damage stimulate C fibers to release substance P, which sets up a positive feedback mechanism. The release of substance P causes release of other chemical mediators of pain and inflammation including serotonin from platelets and histamine from mast cells, which contribute to spread of edema and pain from the area of injury. Substance P release by nociceptors is blocked by morphine. In addition, bradykinin, a potent chemical pain producer, is converted from plasma kininogen following tissue damage. Bradykinin activates both Aδ and C pain fibers and

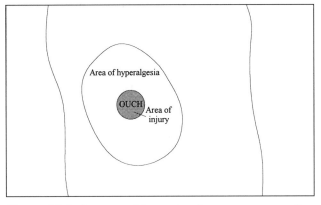

Figure 12-2. An area of hyperalgesia occurs surrounding the actual area of tissue injury, which may be caused by diffusion of chemical mediators of pain from the site of tissue injury.

increases prostaglandin synthesis and release from damaged cells. Prostaglandins play an important role in maintaining phase-two pain, apparently by sensitization of nociceptors. Aspirin and other drugs that inhibit prostaglandin synthesis reduce inflammatory pain. Topical application of capsaicin is now being used for pain relief. Capsaicin receptors appear to be down-regulated by overexposure to capsaicin.

REFERRED PAIN

The perception of pain on familiar cutaneous areas in response to painful stimuli applied to unfamiliar viscera is called referred pain. Individuals may seek pain relief and be referred to a rehabilitation professional for pain that originates from viscera. The classical example of referred pain is the distribution of angina. Coronary insufficiency produces a crushing sensation felt over the chest and radiating down the left upper extremity, up to the jaw, and through to the back. However, in some individuals, the pain may be localized to a more specific musculoskeletal area, such as the shoulder (Figure 12-3). A good history and physical exam is needed to rule out referred pain. For example, shoulder pain that occurs during walking, but not during resisted shoulder movement, should raise the suspicion of angina. Pain over the right shoulder may be due to gall bladder pain, and flank pain that is actually caused by infection of the kidney (pyelonephritis) may be mistaken for "low back pain." Any systemic signs of infection, such as fever, loss of appetite, and sleepiness, should alert the clinician to the possibility of pain being referred from internal structures.

The area to which pain is referred is always a structure innervated at the same spinal cord level. During

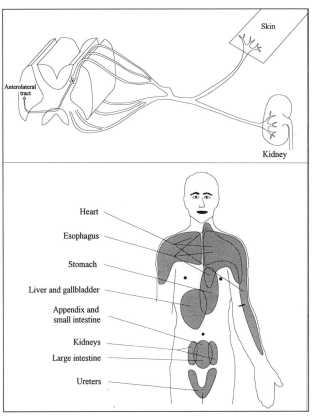

Figure 12-3. Well-described areas of referred pain. The skin perceived to be the origin of the pain is innervated by sensory neurons originating at the same spinal cord level as the actual site of pain.

development, many structures innervated at a given spinal cord level migrate. For example, the heart and shoulder are both innervated at the same level and exist at similar locations in the body, whereas the kidneys at one point in development are pelvic organs that migrate superiorly. One explanation for referred pain involves convergence of nociceptors for viscera and skin on the same ascending neurons. Sensation is mapped on the cerebral cortex in the familiar homonucleus. Skin, muscle, and joints (somatic regions) are stimulated frequently, and the cortex "knows" which of these body parts are receiving stimulation. Cortical cells receiving information from internal organs do not receive this learning process. Lack of stimulation of these cells likely results in few synapses with ascending sensory neurons, which allows branches from the nearby somatic regions of the sensory cortex to synapse with the cortical cells receiving signals from the viscera. We then learn that when cortical cells that are "wired" to viscera are stimulated, a familiar somatic area is being stimulated. However, when pain information is actually received from these viscera, we cannot distinguish whether the

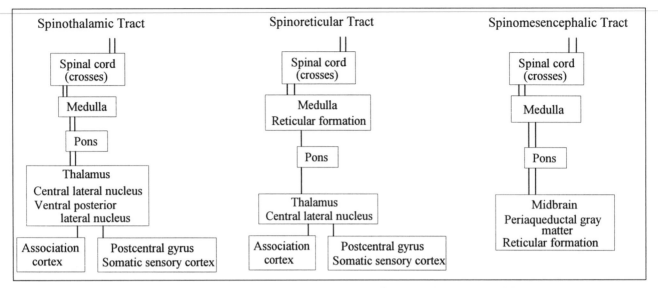

Figure 12-4. Three major ascending pathways transmitting nociception from the dorsal horn to higher centers.

information came from the viscera or the "adopted" branches from somatic structures. Our familiarity with skin sensation leads to the conclusion that pain originates in the skin area. Just as infants learn by integrating different senses and experiences with the area of skin stimulated, we learn through other senses which viscera are being stimulated. Because of the lack of information to learn visceral pain, the brain may interpret the pain as coming from areas of the skin that their cortex maps in proximity to those of the affected viscera.

PAIN PATHWAYS

Pain information is carried by neurons to the area of the spinal cord called the substantia gelatinosa where the nociceptive neurons synapse with a large number of other neurons. A second neuron carries the pain information from the spinal cord in a bundle of neurons called the spinothalamic tract. Phase-one and phase-two pain have slightly different pathways. Within the spinothalamic tract, phase-one pain carried originally by the Aδ fibers is transmitted by the second order neuron directly to the thalamus via the phylogenetically newer neospinothalamic tract (lateral spinothalamic tract). A third neuron in the chain from the periphery to the cerebral cortex carries phase-one pain to the cortex to provide conscious perception of sharp, well-localized pain. The paleospinothalamic tract (medial spinothalamic tract) carries information via second-order neurons from the peripheral C fibers into a primitive network of neurons called the reticular formation, which, at some point, is relayed to the cortex and is perceived as dull,

poorly localized pain. Pathways are illustrated in Figure 12-4.

PAIN-ASSOCIATED REFLEXES

Pain stimuli result in several reflexes, depending on whether it is phase one, two, or three. Phase-one pain produces the withdrawal reflex in which a stimulated limb is withdrawn from the source of pain. This reflex is graded in response to intensity. A greater pain stimulus causes more of the body to be involved in the withdrawal response. Pain involving the skin, joint, or muscle is accompanied by an increase in blood pressure. Pain involving the viscera causes a decrease in blood pressure. Phase-two and -three pain are associated with increased skeletal muscle tone and vasoconstriction. Skeletal muscle contractions and vasoconstriction cause ischemia, leading to increased pain. The increased pain can lead to more contraction of muscle and increased vasoconstriction, setting up a positive feedback cycle between pain and muscle spasm (Figure 12-5). Therapy in this case can be aimed at breaking the cycle of pain and spasm from either or both directions. Treatments, such as massage, heat, ice, neuromuscular electrical stimulation, transcutaneous electrical nerve stimulation, stretching, and others, are used to decrease either pain or muscle spasm.

PHASE-THREE PAIN

Perception of pain that greatly exceeds the stimulus

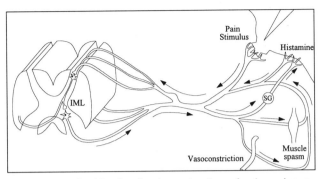

Figure 12-5. Positive feedback mechanism of pain and muscle spasm and vasoconstriction. Pain stimulates sympathetic preganglionic neurons in the intermediolateral column and anterior horn (motor neuron) cells, producing muscle spasm. Muscle spasm then produces increased pain. S = stimulus, IML = intermediolateral column (preganglionic sympathetic cell bodies), H = histamine, and SG = sympathetic ganglion.

or is produced by stimuli not considered painful is classified as phase-three pain. Phase-three pain can be caused by either peripheral nerve damage or damage to the central nervous system (CNS) itself from cerebrovascular disease or spinal cord injury. Phase-one and phase-two pain are easily traced to peripheral injury; phase three is a symptom of neurological abnormality. However, not all injuries to peripheral nerves result in phase-three pain, nor is all phase-three pain linked to injury of the nervous system. Amputation results in severing nerves, and many people who have limbs amputated experience phantom pain. In this condition, pain is felt in the amputated part or in an area not amputated, but denervated due to the amputation. A group of disorders, called complex regional pain syndromes (CRPS), can also be classified as phase-three pain. CRPS type II (formerly known as causalgia) occurs in some individuals who have traumatic injury to a major nerve trunk. CRPS type I follows injuries such as fractures or soft tissue injury that cannot be traced directly to nerve injury. Not all individuals who experience these injuries are afflicted with CRPS. These syndromes occur with much higher frequency in emotional, sympathetic responders and in people with dependent personalities. The link between personality and susceptibility to CRPS is not understood at this time. These syndromes have in common chronic pain, hypersensitivity, and sympathetic dysfunction, including swelling, loss of hair, nail changes, and skin texture changes indicating poor nutrition of the involved extremity. Certain infectious and metabolic diseases have also been linked to phase-three pain, including herpes zoster (shingles) and diabetes mellitus.

Phase-three pain appears to be caused by both central and peripheral changes to the nervous system. A

reorganization of central nervous system pain mapping occurs, and the CNS receives a large amount of abnormal input. In many individuals, blocking sympathetic nerves by anesthesia of sympathetic ganglia is sufficient to stop the process after a series of injections. In other individuals, sympathetic blockade does not help. Compression through the affected limb or distraction by carrying weights helps many others. In the evolution of the syndrome, stimulation of Aβ fibers, which normally carry touch and pressure sensations, causes a type of pain called mechanical allodynia. This can be shown by selectively blocking Aβ fibers. Ischemic blockade stops mechanical allodynia when Aβ fibers no longer conduct, but Aδ and C fibers still conduct.

The central component of complex regional pain syndromes, central pain syndromes, and phantom pain is likely due to remapping of pain in the cortex. When a nerve is injured, the axon dies back, and synapses with other neurons are lost. Other neurons, especially those innervating neighboring neurons, develop branches to produce synapses where the innervation was lost. Neurons of the cerebral cortex mapped to a missing body part will be adopted by healthy neurons bringing sensory information from intact body parts. Stimulation of the intact body part will produce signals sent to both the intact body part's sensory cortex and to the sensory cortex of the missing part. This phenomenon can be demonstrated by mapping sensory perception with touching of intact surfaces. For example, a person with an arm amputation may be touched on various areas on the face and perceive the touching as coming from amputated fingers.

Changes also occur in the periphery. Following damage to a neuron, sodium ion channels specific to pain receptors accumulate at the site of injury. Release of nerve growth factor (NGF) following injury may be responsible. Down-regulation of capsaicin receptors is one approach being pursued by investigators, as well as drugs to block the sodium ion channels specific to pain neurons. Other researchers have discovered one particular type of phosphokinase C (PKC) responsible for transmission of nonphase-one pain. Mice lacking PKC gamma respond to phase-one pain, but do not develop phase-three pain. Central pain can be caused by damage to any part of the somatosensory system. Central pain does not require any peripheral input and does not respond to any procedures that would prevent the input of nociception, including peripheral nerve block, spinal anesthesia, dorsal rhizotomy (surgical section of the dorsal root), or cordotomy. Causes of central pain include traumatic injury to the spinal cord, especially above L1, and strokes or head injury producing damage to nociceptive pathways, and some surgical procedures

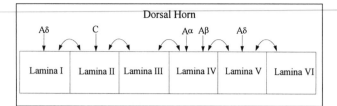

Figure 12-6. Convergence and divergence of nociceptive information in the dorsal horn. Interneurons in lamina I receive information from Aδ nociceptors directly and indirectly from C nociceptors via lamina II interneurons. Aδ neurons also synapse with lamina V cells with which skin and muscle mechanoreceptors also synapse. Lamina I cells directly project sharp pain information to the thalamus, whereas lamina V cells project information that may be modulated by stimulation of mechanoreceptors and phase I pain receptors.

designed to alleviate pain can cause central pain due to damage produced in the pain pathways.

TRANSCUTANEOUS ELECTRICAL NERVE STIMULATION

The central branches of nociceptors terminate in the superficial layer of the dorsal horn of the spinal cord at which integration of nociceptive signals begins. The interneurons of the dorsal horn that receive nociceptive input also have input from descending pathways and from other spinal interneurons, including those from skin mechanoreceptors (Figure 12-6). Pain stimuli can, therefore, be modulated at the level of the spinal cord.

The gate control theory of pain developed by Melczak and Wall in 1965 was an important contribution to the knowledge of pain and led directly to development of transcutaneous electrical nerve stimulation (TENS) as a method to control pain. The gate control theory relies on the presence of an inhibitory interneuron or a "gate cell" (Figure 12-7). The gate control will be explained in its most simple details to make sense of how TENS functions to relieve pain. More extensive descriptions of the gate control theory of pain can be found in the references. According to the theory, the smaller C fiber synapses with a "transmission cell" that conveys the nociceptive information to the brain. The transmission cell also receives input from the inhibitory gate cell. Mechanoreceptors stimulate the gate cell to inhibit the transmission cell. A painful stimulus excites the transmission cell to convey pain to the CNS via C fibers, and, if sufficient stimulation of the transmission cell is received, information is forwarded to the brain, and pain is perceived. If, however, the Aα and Aβ mechanoreceptive fibers entering the spinal cord at the

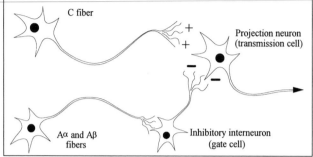

Figure 12-7. A simplified adaptation of the gate control theory of Melczak and Wall. Diffuse nociceptive information received via C fibers is routed to an interneuron (projection neuron) in the substantia gelatinosa. Stimulation of the inhibitory interneuron (gate cell) inhibits the transmission of pain from C fibers to the projection cell and to higher centers (closing the gate to pain). Stimulation of C fibers both stimulates the transmission cell and inhibits the gate cell, but stimulation of mechanoreceptors of the skin and muscle (Aα and Aβ fibers) stimulate the gate cell, thereby diminishing transmission of pain to higher centers.

same dorsal root are stimulated, pain is reduced by excitation of the gate cell, which inhibits the transmission cell. The gate control theory explains phenomena such as the rubbing of a painful area or "running off the pain." Based on predictions of the pain control theory, TENS devices were developed. TENS, as originally conceived, electrically stimulates mechanoreceptive neurons preferentially, which causes excitation of gate cells, inhibition of transmission cells, and decreased perception of the pain caused by tissue injury. Based on these assumptions, conventional TENS should work best on phase-two pain, but not phase one or phase three. TENS used to excite only mechanoreceptive neurons is called conventional TENS. Other uses of TENS have been developed in an effort to control phase-one and phase-three pain. The brief intense mode of TENS works very well on phase-one pain, producing nearly complete anesthesia and may be used during painful procedures, such as debriding a wound, reducing a dislocation, extracting a tooth, mobilizing a painful joint, and other applications. Low-frequency TENS is used on some types of phase-three pain and does not work by the gate control theory of pain. Low-frequency TENS operates on the idea that strong stimulation of nociceptive input can excite descending analgesic pathways and cause release of endogenous opiates (see next section below). It is also possible that low-frequency TENS causes capsaicin release. In common usage, low-frequency TENS is used for pain that has lasted longer than 72 hours, and conventional TENS is used for pain that has lasted less than 72 hours.

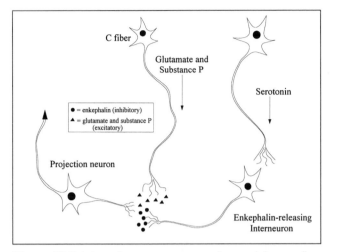

Figure 12-8. Interactions among ascending and descending analgesic pathways. Descending analgesic pathways releasing serotonin stimulate enkephalin-releasing interneurons to produce both pre- and postsynaptic inhibition of pain information carrying afferent neurons. The C fiber releases fewer vesicles of excitatory neurotransmitter on the projection neuron, and the projection neuron becomes less sensitive to the excitatory neurotransmitter released by the C fiber.

MECHANISMS OF ANALGESIA

In the mid 1970s, endogenous opiate-like substances were isolated from several species, including humans. Morphine, a derivative of opium, had already been used for pain control for many years, but it is very addictive. Receptors for opiates, such as morphine, exist both in the brain and in the spinal cord. In the spinal cord, receptors for opiates can be found on both sides of synapses between nociceptive neurons and dorsal horn interneurons (pre- and postsynaptic membranes) (Figure 12-8). Opiates decrease the amount of neurotransmitter released by nociceptors onto dorsal horn cells and directly inhibit dorsal horn cells by hyperpolarizing them. Enkephalin is an endogenous opiate with a short half-life that functions as a neurotransmitter. Enkephalin is released by interneurons within the dorsal horn to inhibit pain. Enkephalin-releasing interneurons may represent the gate cells proposed in the gate control theory of pain.

Pain can also be modulated by descending pathways from the brain. Descending pain control neurons release serotonin presumably onto the dorsal horn interneurons that release enkephalin to inhibit the transmission of pain from the periphery to the brain (Figure 12-9). Electrical stimulation of neurons found in the periaqueductal gray matter that synapse with cells in the rostro-

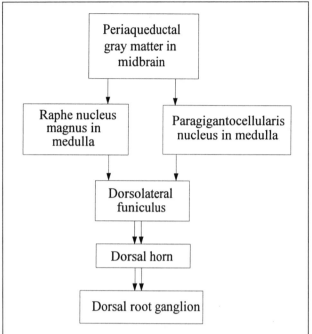

Figure 12-9. Descending nociceptive pathways. In the spinal cord, these pathways inhibit nociceptive projection neurons both directly and through stimulation of enkephalin-releasing interneurons.

ventral medulla produces analgesia. The neurons in the rostroventral medulla appear to be the neurons that release serotonin and excite the dorsal horn interneurons that, in turn, inhibit the transmission of pain to the brain. Stimulation of the rostroventral medulla also produces analgesia. These descending pathways have been exploited for pain control. Electric stimulators are implanted in some individuals for stimulation-produced analgesia (SPA) as a treatment for chronic pain. Binding of opiates to receptors in the brain produces a similar effect to stimulation-produced analgesia (Figure 12-10). Production of opiates, such as endorphins, by the brain in response to pain appears to act by stimulating the descending serotonergic pathway, which in turn causes release of enkephalin onto dorsal horn cells. β endorphin is found in neurons of the hypothalamus that send projections to the periaqueductal gray. Endorphins, which have a much longer half-life than enkephalin, may have a hormonal type of effect and bind to opiate receptors in the dorsal horn directly as well as stimulating descending pathways of analgesia. The production of endogenous opiates appears to be responsible for the analgesia observed in situations, such as battlefield injuries, and may be the mechanism by which low-frequency TENS produces analgesia.

SUMMARY

Three phases of pain are described. Phase one corresponds to graded, localized pain. Phase two is due to tissue injury, lasts longer, and is poorly localized. Phase three represents a derangement of the nociceptive and mechanoreceptive systems following injury to a peripheral nerve or to the CNS. Hyperalgesia is the spread of pain to areas adjacent to an area of tissue injury due to the release of substances from damaged tissues. Phase-one pain is conveyed to the thalamus via the neospinothalamic tract and from the thalamus to the cortex. Phase-two pain, carried by the older paleospinothalamic tract, is routed through several structures, including those that give a psychologic aspect to chronic pain. Pain produces withdrawal of the stimulated body part, increases blood pressure if pain is somatic, and decreases pain if it is visceral. Pain can set up a positive feedback cycle between pain and muscle spasm. The gate control theory of pain explains how stimulation of mechanoreceptors of the skin inhibits pain. TENS devices were developed as a result of the gate control theory of pain. Pain can be modulated by descending analgesic pathways. Endogenous opiates secreted by the brain stimulate neurons in the periaqueductal gray matter, which, in turn, stimulate serotonergic rostroventral medulla neurons. Serotonergic neurons stimulate dorsal horn interneurons that release enkephalin that acts to inhibit transmission of pain from the dorsal horn to the brain.

BIBLIOGRAPHY

Berne RM, Levy MN. *Physiology.* St. Louis, Mo: Mosby-Year Book; 1998.

Carsten SE. Neural mechanism of hyperalgesia: peripheral and central sensitization. *News in Physiological Sciences.* 1995;10:260-265.

Cervero F. Sensory innervation of the viscera: peripheral basis of visceral pain. *Physiological Reviews.* 1994;74:95-138.

Ganong WF. *Review of Medical Physiology.* Norwalk, Conn: Appleton & Lange; 1995.

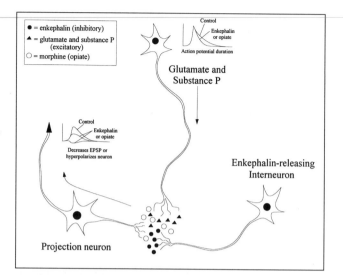

Figure 12-10. Effects of enkephalin and opiates on nociceptive information in the spinal cord. Enkephalin-releasing cells produce both presynaptic and postsynaptic inhibition by decreasing the size of the EPSP produced by the nociceptive neuron and by hyperpolarizing the transmission cell. Circulating opiates produce the same effects as enkephalin, are longer acting, and reduce the effectiveness of the action potential generated in the axon of the nociceptive fiber, thereby diminishing the EPSP generated by the nociceptive cell.

Guyton AC, Hall JE, Schmitt W. *Human Physiology and Mechanisms of Disease.* Philadelphia, Pa: WB Saunders; 1997.

Handwerker HO, Kobal G. Psychophysiology of experimentally induced pain. *Physiological Reviews.* 1993;73:639-671.

Hole JW Jr. *Essentials of Human Anatomy and Physiology.* 4th ed. Dubuque, Iowa: Wm. C. Brown Publishers; 1992.

Hopkins K. Getting at the molecular roots of pain. *The Scientist.* 1999; Jan:12-13.

Schauf C, Moffett D, Moffett S. *Human Physiology: Foundation and Frontiers.* St. Louis, Mo: Times Mirror/Mosby College Publishing; 1990.

Solomon EP, Davis PW. *Human Anatomy and Physiology.* Philadelphia, Pa: WB Saunders; 1983.

Treed R, Magerl W. Modern concepts of pain and hyperalgesia: beyond the polymodal C-nociception. *News in Physiological Sciences.* 1995;10:216-228.

STUDY QUESTIONS

1. Provide examples in which an individual will develop only phase-one pain, will develop phase one and phase two, and will develop phases one, two, and three pain.

2. Why is distinguishing referred pain important? If a person complains of left shoulder pain only during walking and not during lifting, what might you conclude?

3. A person with a history of urinary tract infections is referred to you for low back pain. No specific movement pattern exists that elicits pain, and the person complains of fever and feeling ill in general. What else could be the problem?

4. What do complex regional pain syndrome, phantom limb pain, and central pain have in common? Based on the proposed mechanism from these, should using the involved extremity be expected to improve or worsen the condition?

5. Contrast the effects of enkephalins and endorphins in terms of onset of action, localization, and length of action. If conventional TENS works by producing enkephalins and low-frequency TENS works by releasing endorphins, describe how you expect the onset and duration of pain relief to differ between these two types of TENS.

LABORATORY EXERCISE 12-1

TRANSCUTANEOUS ELECTRICAL NERVE STIMULATION (TENS)

TENS was developed directly as a result of the gate control theory of pain, which proposes that stimulation of large mechanoreceptive neurons stimulates a "gate cell" that inhibits the transmission cell. The nociceptive C fiber synapses on the transmission cell, but the inhibition of the transmission cell due to stimulation of mechanoreceptors of the skin decreases the effectiveness of nociception.

Acute pain is sharp, localized, and its intensity and duration are accurately identified. Acute pain (phase-one pain) is transmitted by Aδ fibers to the lateral spinothalamic (neospinothalamic) tract.

Chronic pain is dull, deep, diffuse, and difficult to judge in terms of its intensity and duration. Chronic pain is transmitted by C fibers to the medial spinothalamic (paleospinothalamic) tract.

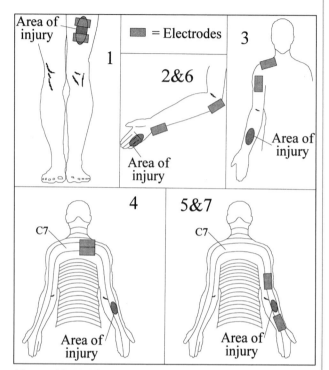

Figure 12-11. The basis of electrode placement in TENS.

The original mode developed to exploit the gate control theory of pain is called conventional TENS. This type of stimulation is effective on phase-two pain due to tissue injury. Two other modes have since been developed to control other types of pain. These include the low frequency mode and brief intense mode. Manufacturers have also added "modulating modes" in the belief that the nervous system "accommodates" to the rhythmic transcutaneous current and by altering one or more of the stimulation parameters, accommodation can be prevented. Preventing accommodation is thought to make TENS effective for a longer time.

Modes:
1.   Conventional (high frequency)
     Rate: 50 to 100 Hz
     Duration: 40 to 75 ms
     Amplitude: sensory
     Activates: Aα and Aβ sensory fibers
     Designed to work via gate control theory of pain, release of enkephalins.
     Works within 1 to 20 minutes, lasts up to 2 hours.
     Used for 30 to 60 minutes whenever necessary (PRN) for pain that has occurred within 72 hours.

LABORATORY EXERCISE

2. Low frequency
    Rate: 1 to 4 Hz
    Duration: 150 to 250 ms
    Amplitude: Strong motor to noxious to patient's tolerance for 45 to 60 minutes
    Activates: Aδ and C pain fibers
    Designed to work via release of endorphins to stimulate descending pain control pathways and inhibit nociception at the spinal cord level.
    Works within 20 to 60 minutes, lasts 2 to 6 hours.
    Used for 45 to 60 minutes PRN for pain that has lasted more than 72 hours.

    The 72-hour cut-off between conventional and low-frequency TENS is arbitrary and has no known physiologic basis at this time.

3. Brief intense
    Rate: 100 to 150 Hz
    Duration: 150 to 250 ms
    Amplitude: Highest tolerated, can be gradually increased as tolerated
    Activates: Everything
    Designed to produce a rapid onset of deep anesthesia. Used for temporary use during painful procedures. Switch to either high or low frequency mode to continue pain relief after procedure.
    Works almost immediately, lasts until turned off.
    Used for maximum of 15 minutes.

4. Modulating modes. Constantly change amplitude, duration, frequency, or a combination. SD (strength-duration) mode alters both amplitude and duration to maintain constant amount of charge per pulse according to SD curve. The product of amplitude (mA) and duration (ms) equals charge.

Electrode placement:

For TENS to be effective in relief of pain, electrodes must be placed on the skin so that the current passes through the axons of Aα or Aβ fibers that enter the same dorsal root ganglion as the nociceptive neurons transmitting the pain. Passing the current either through the actual site of pain or through peripheral nerves serving the painful areas will be the most effective. Below, seven ways to place electrodes are given. You may mix different ways using one or two leads (two or four electrodes) to get the best effect. Unless the area is large, one lead is usually sufficient.

1. Directly over the site of injury or pathology, providing the skin is intact.

2. Over the trunk of the peripheral nerve innervating the area of injury or pathology. The nerve must be superficial (eg, peroneal or ulnar nerve).

3. Over the nerve plexus from which the nerve innervating the area of pain originates. In particular the brachial plexus can be very useful for pain anywhere in the upper extremity. An electrode is placed over Erb's point (the area between the clavicle and trapezius where the brachial plexus is the most superficial).

4. Over the sensory nerve roots innervating the site of pain (using a dermatome chart).

LABORATORY EXERCISE

5.   Within the same dermatome as the site of pain (assuming affected nociceptors are entering the same dorsal root as the stimulated mechanoreceptive neurons).

6.   Over the motor point of an injured or painful muscle. The motor point is the location at which one obtains a muscle contraction with the lowest current. Presumably this location is directly over the nerve of the muscle, which also contains sensory neurons of the muscle ($A\alpha$ fibers).

7.   Arranged so that the current will run between two electrodes through the area of pain.

Some people advocate use of acupuncture points for TENS. One point of particular interest is bladder 60 (B 60), located on the lateral heel between the lateral malleolus and Achilles' tendon.

TENS problems:

1.   Use two channels for chronic shoulder pain.

2.   Use one channel for a sprained ankle.

3.   Use either one or two channels for debridement of foot ulcers.

4.   Use one channel for a painful tibialis anterior.

5.   Use one channel for pain during reduction of a dislocated finger.

T H I R T E E N

Sleep and States of Consciousness

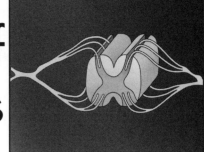

OBJECTIVES

1. Describe the types of brainwaves and when they are appropriate.

2. Describe the EEG, EOG, and EMG characteristics of the different phases of sleep.

3. Describe how sleep patterns change with age.

4. Define syncope, lethargy, stupor, and coma.

5. Describe the basic characteristics of the Glasgow coma scale and Rancho Los Amigos level of consciousness.

6. Define brain death.

7. Describe the characteristics of fibromyalgia and how they relate to sleep disorders.

At present, higher nervous system function cannot be explained at the cellular level. Recordings of gross activity of the brain are, however, correlated to various types of brain activity and level of consciousness. Electrical activity of the brain is recorded in a standard way through electroencephalography (EEG). Additional information about state of consciousness is also gained from monitoring eye movement (EOG—electrooculography) and skeletal muscle activity (EMG—electromyography).

Four basic rhythms of brain electrical activity have been described. Additional waveforms picked up by the EEG will not be considered here. Alpha (α) waves have a frequency of 8 to 13 per second. They are recorded in normal individuals who are awake and relaxed. α waves are lost during sleep and intense mental activity. β waves have a frequency greater than 14 per second and may be as high as 25 to 50 per second. β waves may be recorded during intense mental activity. Θ waves are slower than α waves and have a frequency of 4 to 7 per second. They are recorded over the parietal and temporal lobes in children or during emotional stress in adults. δ waves have the lowest frequency, less than 3.5 per second to less than 1 per second. δ waves may be recorded during deep sleep in a normal individual in infancy or may be a sign of cerebral dysfunction in adults. These waves are depicted in Figure 13-1.

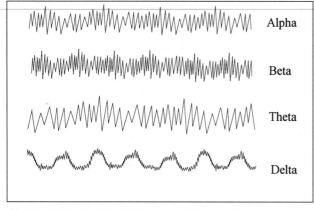

Figure 13-1. Normal electroencephalographic waves.

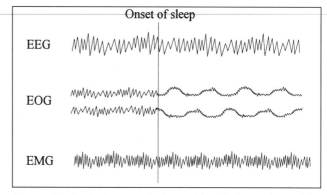

Figure 13-2. Electroencephalographic, electrooculographic, and electromyographic changes with the onset of sleep.

SLEEP

Sleep may be defined as a state of unconsciousness from which one can be aroused. Sleep is usually divided into two types: slow wave (or nonREM) sleep and rapid eye movement (REM) sleep. Slow-wave sleep is further divided into four stages of progressively slower brain activity. During slow-wave sleep, as the name implies, the EEG shows Θ and δ waves. The eyes, as demonstrated by EOG, have a slower rate of movement or may be still. During slow-wave sleep, tone is sufficient to provide for some postures, but is too low for standing or unsupported sitting. During slow-wave sleep, major postural adjustments, such as turning over in bed, occur about every 20 minutes. Cardiac and pulmonary rhythms are slow but regular during slow-wave sleep, with a generalized increased parasympathetic activity, which includes increased gastrointestinal activity.

During REM sleep, the EOG shows a high level of activity, thus the name rapid eye movement sleep, but postural tone virtually disappears. Irregularities in cardiac and pulmonary rhythms occur, which are associated with increased sympathetic activity; heart rate and blood pressure increase, and gastrointestinal activity decreases. One parasympathetic activity, erection, occurs during virtually every REM cycle in the male. Nocturnal penile tumescence is often used to investigate the cause of erectile dysfunction. During REM sleep, dreaming occurs. If a person awakes during REM sleep, dream recall is good (75% to 95%). However, if a person is awakened from slow wave sleep, dream recall is only 0 to 51%. Characteristics of different sleep states are depicted in Figure 13-2.

During a normal sleep cycle (Figures 13-3 and 13-4), a regular alternation between slow wave and REM sleep occurs. Sleep normally begins with slow-wave sleep, progressing from stage 1 (transitional sleep) to stage 4 (deep sleep) and then to stage 2 (moderate sleep). It is progressively more difficult to arouse an individual from stage 1 to stage 4 sleep. After approximately 1.5 to 2 hours, stage 2 sleep is followed by REM sleep. REM sleep periods last 15 to 20 minutes, then return to stage 2. During a typical night, one's sleep consists 20% to 25% REM sleep, 50% stage 2 sleep, and 15% of stage 3 or 4 (δ wave sleep). As sleep progresses toward morning, almost all of the sleep consists of alternation between stage 2 and REM sleep, and the duration of each REM sleep cycle increases. It may be more difficult to arouse a person from REM sleep than from stage 2 sleep, but one is more likely to awaken spontaneously from REM sleep than from slow-wave sleep.

With age, the duration of sleep and amount of time spent in REM compared with slow-wave sleep changes. Even before birth, a pattern of decreased time sleeping occurs. The time sleeping decreases rapidly until adulthood, but still slowly decreases. A greater rate of change occurs in REM sleep with age. Eighty percent of sleep in premature infants is REM sleep. The percentage decreases rapidly to about 20% in adults, but tends to remain steady as the total time spent sleeping decreases with age until a second decline in percentage of sleep as REM sleep occurs after the age of 80.

Brain centers responsible for sleep have yet to be clearly identified. Several theories of sleep have been proposed involving various centers, including release of serotonin. Recently, rhythmic changes in production of two related prostaglandins correlated with sleep have been reported. Prostaglandins E2 and D2 are synthesized in two different parts of the hypothalamus. PGE2 is produced in the posterior hypothalamus in the awake state, and PGD2 is produced in the preoptic area during sleep. Because changes in prostaglandin metabolism

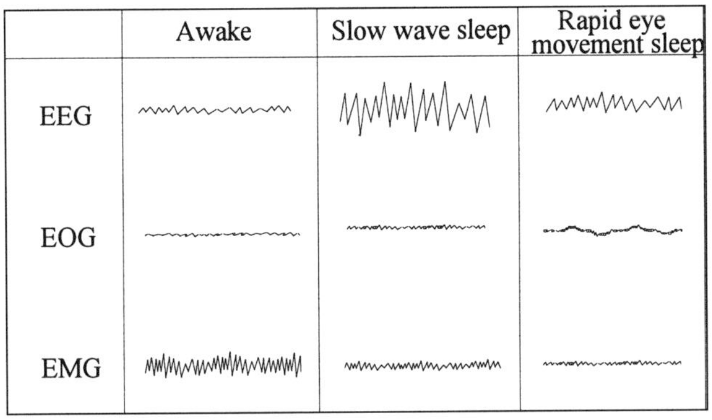

	Awake	Slow wave sleep	Rapid eye movement sleep
EEG			
EOG			
EMG			

Figure 13-3. Stages of sleep.

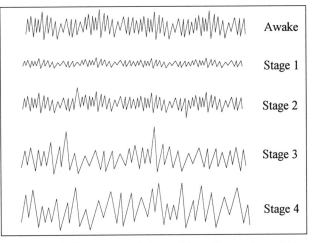

Figure 13-4. Electroencephalographic patterns characteristic of the stages of sleep.

have been observed in some sleep disorders, therapy may be aimed at altering levels of specific prostaglandins in the future.

Although the physiologic role of sleep is unknown, it does appear that a specific need for slow-wave and REM sleep exist. Sleep deprivation leads to deterioration of mental and motor performance in the awake state. The amount of stage 4 sleep is correlated with prior wakefulness, indicating a "catching up" early in sleep. A person who is deprived of REM sleep does not only exhibit the physical symptoms of sleep loss, but does recover lost REM sleep when allowed. Sleep patterns are interrupted frequently in hospitals, which may decrease a patient's motor performance. The combination of sleep interruption and loss of day/night cycles in inten-

sive care units has been linked to inappropriate perceptions and behavior termed "ICU psychosis."

CLINICAL LEVELS OF UNCONSCIOUSNESS

Syncope, lethargy, stupor, and coma are specifically defined clinical levels of unconsciousness. Syncope is a transient loss of consciousness usually due to hypoperfusion of the brain from which a person can be readily

Glasgow Coma Scale

	EYE OPENING	VERBAL RESPONSE	MOTOR RESPONSE
6			Obeys command to move
5		Response indicates orientation	Moves limbs to remove stimuli
4	Spontaneous eye opening	Response indicates confusion	Flexes upper extremity to pain
3	Opens eyes to sound	Produces speech	Flexion associated with decorticate rigidity
2	Opens eyes to pain	Unintelligible sounds	Abnormal extensor posturing
1	Never opens eyes	No verbal responses	No motor response

In 1974, a method of assessing individuals with head injury was developed and named the Glasgow Coma Scale. Points are given based on eye opening, verbal response, and motor response. A coma is diagnosed if a person scores 7 or lower, and a score of 9 or greater rules out coma. A person scores 4 points for spontaneous eye opening, 3 points for opening eyes to sound, 2 points for opening eyes to pain, and 1 point if eyes are never opened. Scoring for verbal response includes 5 points for a response that indicates orientation, 4 points for a response that indicates confusion, 3 points for producing speech but not able to carry on a conversation, 2 points for unintelligible sounds such as moans, and 1 point for no verbal responses. Motor responses are scored as 6 points for obeying a command to move, 5 points for moving a limb to remove a stimulus, 4 points for flexing the upper extremity in response to a painful stimulus, 3 points for producing the flexion associated with decorticate rigidity in response to pain, 2 points for abnormal extension posturing, and 1 point for no motor response.

aroused. Lethargy is indifference to common stimuli, such as talking, shouting, shaking, or noxious stimuli, whereas a person in a stupor is responsive only to shaking, shouting, or noxious stimuli. A person in a coma is totally unresponsive to any type of stimulus.

Loss of consciousness is usually due to either a widespread depression of the cerebral hemispheres or depression or destruction of critical brain stem areas. This depression or destruction is usually the result of one of three types of problems:

1. Masses or destructive lesions in and around the brain stem, such as tumors or hemorrhage.
2. Masses in and around the cerebrum that compress the diencephalon (thalamus and hypothalamus), including tumors and subdural hematoma.
3. Metabolic disorders, including anoxia (lack of oxygen), ischemia (lack of blood flow), concussion, infection (encephalitis or meningitis), toxins, and enzyme deficiencies.

Coma usually carries a poor prognosis. In one study of 2650 patients with coma, apnea, and isoelectric (flat) EEG in the absence of drug intoxication or hypothermia, a 0% survival was reported. Patients with coma due to drug intoxication or in the presence of hypothermia have a much better prognosis.

BRAIN DEATH

Because the brain is so vulnerable to hypoxia or other metabolic disorders, many times, brain death may occur in the presence of otherwise normally functioning organs. One set of criteria for brain death was set forth by the National Institute of Neurological and Communicative Diseases and Stroke of the National Institutes of Health in 1977. They include coma with cerebral unresponsiveness, apnea, dilated pupils, absent cephalic reflexes, and electrocerebral silence. Cerebral unresponsiveness refers to the absence of purposeful response to externally applied stimuli as listed above for the definition of a coma. Apnea is the absence of spontaneous ventilation, which requires mechanical ventilation to support life. Cephalic reflexes include pupillary and other reflexes involving the cranial nerves, and electrocerebral silence refers to an EEG that fails to reach a threshold level of electrical activity considered to exist in a living brain. What is done following determination of brain death has become an issue of medical ethics as well as one of the courts and has produced several widely publicized stories.

NARCOLEPSY

Narcolepsy is a condition in which a person has irresistible attacks of sleep that may last 5 to 30 minutes. It occurs in 0.04% to 0.09% of the population, but does not appear until the teenage or adult years. Unfortunately, attacks may occur at inopportune times such as during driving. A person with narcolepsy incorporates parts of REM sleep and the transition between sleep and wakefulness during waking activity. In contrast to normal sleep, a person with narcolepsy may directly enter REM sleep. Another symptom of narcolepsy, besides sleep attacks and sleep-onset REM, is the phe-

Rancho Los Amigos Levels of Cognitive Functioning

Another scale used in classifying responses to individuals who have sustained injury to the brain is the Rancho Los Amigos Level of Cognitive Functioning. This scale has eight levels denoted with Roman numerals. Level I ("no response") is a lack of response to any stimulus. Level II is called a "generalized response," which is a nonpurposeful response to all stimuli in the same way and may include any one of a number of responses including movement, vocalization, or changes in vital signs. "Localized response" is level III in which a person reacts in a way specific to the stimulus or may follow simple commands, but otherwise is in a low level of consciousness. In level IV ("confused-agitated"), a person shows a higher level of consciousness, but has decreased ability to process information and behaves in a bizarre and even hostile manner and is unable to participate in therapy. "Confused-inappropriate" is level V, and the person can respond to simple commands, but not complex tasks and is easily distracted. Verbalization is inappropriate, and the person may wander off if physically able. Level VI is called "confused-appropriate," and a person can perform goal-directed activity but requires cues. The person may be able to perform old tasks, but not new tasks. In level VII, "automatic-appropriate," the person is appropriate and oriented, but lacks insight, judgment, and problem-solving skills. Level VIII is called "purposeful-appropriate." This person is capable of independence but may operate at diminished social, emotional, and intellectual abilities. Knowledge of level of consciousness is helpful in treatment planning, determining how much assistance is needed during therapy, and, most importantly, for discharge planning and community reentry.

nomenon of cataplexy in which a person suddenly loses muscle tone. Cataplexy typically occurs during increased emotion including laughter and anger. In addition, two phenomena occurring in the transition between sleep and wakefulness are associated with narcolepsy in a minority of people. Sleep paralysis is the inhibition of muscle activity, and hypnagogic phenomena are auditory or visual hallucinations that occur at the onset of sleep. It has been shown that sleep patterns are abnormal in narcolepsy, especially a fragmentation of REM sleep. However, the problems of narcolepsy appear to be more complex than deprivation of REM sleep.

SUMMARY

Sleep consists of two major types—slow-wave sleep and REM sleep. Slow-wave sleep is divided into progressively deeper and slower brainwave frequencies from stage 1 to stage 4. Deep slow-wave sleep is accomplished early on, whereas, later on, sleep consists primarily of alternating periods of stage 2 and REM sleep. REM sleep is characterized by eye movements and loss of muscle tone. Both deep slow-wave sleep and REM sleep appear to be necessary, although it is not clear why. Loss of deep sleep is made up by increasing the percentage of

Fibromyalgia

Fibromyalgia is a condition associated with sleep disturbance and musculoskeletal pain. It is frequently missed on diagnosis and misdiagnosed as another musculoskeletal disease. Similar to forms of arthritis, pain worsens with rest and improves with activity, and many people display decreased active range of motion of the neck, shoulder, low back, and hips. The individual with fibromyalgia complains of tender points of muscles, which improve with superficial heat and worsen with cold. Fibromyalgia is also associated with deranged sleep, characterized by frequent waking and loss of stage 4 deep sleep. Individuals awake exhausted, as if they received no sleep. Interestingly, fibromyalgia-like symptoms can be produced in other individuals by disrupting stage 4 sleep. An estimated 3 to 6 million individuals in the United States are affected by fibromyalgia. Of these, approximately 80% are women, with an average onset in the fourth decade of life, but it may occur in childhood or in senescence. Most individuals with fibromyalgia display a decreased aerobic fitness, but it is not clear if the decreased aerobic fitness is part of the disease, or decreased activity due to stiffness causes the decreased fitness. Many people believe that aerobic activity may, to some degree, restore normal sleep patterns and decrease symptoms of the disease. It has been noted that people with high aerobic fitness are not susceptible to the fibromyalgia-like symptoms caused by disruption of stage 4 sleep.

Diagnosis of fibromyalgia is difficult and relies on identifying 11 of 18 particular tender points. These include nine bilateral locations: the occiput, cervical spine, trapezius, supraspinatus, second costochondral junction, lateral epicondyle of the elbow, gluteal muscles, greater trochanter, and medial fat pad of the knee. A person should have chronic, widespread pain for longer than 3 months, involving all four quadrants, absence of other systemic disease, and pain with 4 kg/cm pressure at 11 of the 18 tender points. Treatment of fibromyalgia consists of patient education, tricyclic antidepressant drugs, and physical therapy. Physical therapy treatment includes symptomatic pain relief, postural improvement, aerobic activities, and relaxation techniques. Symptomatic intervention is useful to increase participation in other interventions, but it must be made clear that the person should not become dependent on symptomatic treatment but should be limited to flare-ups that often accompany physical or emotional stress. These symptomatic treatments include superficial heat, massage, mobilization, spray and stretch, and electrical modalities, such as neuromuscular electrical stimulation, high-volt pulsed current, interferential current, and transcutaneous electrical nerve stimulation. A worksite and home ergonomic evaluation and exercises for correcting the "pain posture" of forward head, protracted shoulders, and posterior pelvic tilt are needed for long-term relief. In addition, improved aerobic fitness has been shown in some preliminary studies to help relieve symptoms. These individuals need to start at a low level and increase activity gradually and involve low-impact, low-load activities, such as exercise in water, to avoid increased soreness that may cause them to drop out of the exercise program. Relaxation may consist of biofeedback, Jacobsen's exercises, relaxation tapes, and some forms of manual therapy. Increased participation in an exercise program also relies on identifying barriers to exercise, including depression and anxiety and education concerning the downward spiral of pain and fatigue causing inactivity, inactivity causing deconditioning, and deconditioning causing more pain and fatigue.

stage 3 and 4 sleep after prolonged wakefulness. Both total time sleeping and percentage of sleep that is REM sleep decrease with age. Different levels of consciousness described included syncope, lethargy, stupor, and coma. Coma carries a poor prognosis. Coma combined with apnea, loss of pupillary reflexes, and a flat EEG is virtually diagnostic of brain death. Narcolepsy is a state is which normal inhibition of REM during wakefulness leads to attacks of sleep with rapid onset of REM sleep and is associated with the phenomena of cataplexy, sleep paralysis, and hypnagogic phenomena.

BIBLIOGRAPHY

Berger RJ, Phillips NH. Sleep and energy conservation. *News in Physiological Sciences.* 1993;8:276-281.

Berne RM, Levy MN. *Physiology.* St. Louis, Mo: Mosby-Year Book; 1998.

Franzini C, Zoccoli G, Cianci T, Lenzi P. Sleep-dependent changes in regional circulations. *News in Physiological Sciences.* 1996;11:274-280.

Ganong WF. *Review of Medical Physiology.* Norwalk, Conn: Appleton & Lange; 1995.

Guyton AC, Hall JE, Schmitt W. *Human Physiology and Mechanisms of Disease.* Philadelphia, Pa: WB Saunders; 1997.

Krueger JM, Fang J, Hansen MK, Zhang J, Obl F Jr. Humoral regulation of sleep. *News in Physiological Sciences.* 1998;13:189-194.

Kubin L, Davies RO, Pack AI. Control of upper airway motor neurons during REM sleep. *News in Physiological Sciences.* 1998;13:91-97.

STUDY QUESTIONS

1. How can you distinguish among lethargy, stupor, and coma? Is it possible for a person in a coma to participate in rehabilitation?

2. Explain the relationships among sleep, aerobic fitness, and fibromyalgia.

3. Explain why people engage in "head-bobbing" during boring lectures.

4. In what ways do the Glasgow Coma Scale and Rancho Los Amigos level of consciousness give similar information? How do they differ?

5. Why do you think a person in a coma needs to be seen by a rehabilitation professional?

Integumentary System

The integumentary system has critical passive and active roles. Passively, it acts as a barrier to prevent damage from the external environment and loss of body fluid to the external environment. Actively, it is part of the thermoregulatory system as blood flow through superficial veins and activation of sweat glands are regulated through local reflexes and central control. The skin also maintains itself through the presence of immune cells, melanocytes to regulate the amount of light penetrating the skin, sebaceous glands to maintain the suppleness of skin, and sensory neurons to protect the skin from injury. Malnutrition, incontinence, and lack of mobility present tremendous challenges to maintaining the health of the skin. For this reason, the gastrointestinal system and micturition have been described in other chapters. The next unit focuses on the musculoskeletal system, which is also necessary to maintain healthy skin.

FOURTEEN

Skin

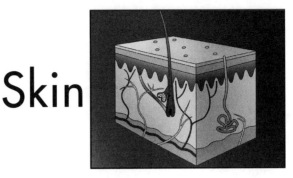

Skin is the largest and perhaps least appreciated organ system of the body. The failure to appreciate the contributions of the skin to homeostasis fully until the last 15 to 20 years is the major reason that people who burned more than 50% of their skin commonly died, but today, many individuals can survive burn injuries destroying up to 90% of the skin's surface area.

FUNCTIONS OF SKIN

The skin not only serves as a mechanical barrier between the external environment and the underlying tissues but is intricately involved in a defense role and several other important functions. The skin impedes passage into the body of most materials that come into contact with the body surface, including most bacteria and toxic chemicals. Skin contains some immune cells and antibodies that can initially control the proliferation of

bacteria until the immune system can mount a more specific response. In addition, the skin contains enzymes that can modify some compounds, such as carcinogens.

A second, and largely unappreciated until recent years, barrier function is that of retaining moisture. Among other layers, skin maintains a keratinized layer that is airtight and fairly waterproof, thus impervious to most substances. Therefore, it serves to minimize loss of water and other vital components from the body. This protective layer's function in holding in body fluids becomes obvious when considering severe burns. Large quantities of body fluids and plasma proteins can be lost from the exposed burned surface. The resulting circulatory disturbances can be life-threatening.

A third function of skin is maintenance of body temperature. From a thermoregulatory point of view, the body is often considered to have a central core surrounded by an outer shell. The inner core consists of the abdominal and thoracic organs, the central nervous system, and the skeletal muscle, which maintain a constant temperature in spite of variations in the environmental temperature. However, temperature of the skin and subcutaneous fat tissue, both constituting the outer shell, can vary significantly. Alteration of the skin temperature maintains the core's thermal constancy, especially in the face of the widely varying temperature of the external environment. This thermoregulatory function of the shell can be altered by varying blood flow through the skin. Blood heated by the central core is pumped to the skin from the heart, bringing a variable amount of heat to the skin. Thermoregulation allows skin blood flow to vary tremendously, from 400 ml/min up to 2500 ml/min. The skin's blood vessels, by allowing heat to be carried to the surface, decrease the effectiveness of skin as an insulator by allowing heat to be lost by radiation, conduction, and convection. In a cold environment, the skin acts as an insulator for heat. Vasoconstriction reduces blood flow through the skin, thereby decreasing the amount of heat carried to the skin, which has the effect of increasing the insulating property of the skin. Reduced heat loss through the skin keeps more heat within the core environment where it is insulated from the external environment. Conversely, in a warm environment, vasodilation of the skin vessels permits increased flow blood to the skin, which promotes heat loss.

To augment the dissipation of heat by the skin, sweat is secreted through specialized appendages of the skin, known as sweat glands. This active, evaporative heat loss process is under sympathetic nervous system control. Sweat is a dilute salt solution extruded onto the skin's surface via sweat glands. The heat of the skin is transferred to the sweat, which adds energy to the solution, causing it to achieve sufficient energy to leave the liquid phase and enter the gaseous phase, that is, to evaporate. However, sweat must be evaporated from the skin for heat loss to occur. If sweat drips off the skin or is simply wiped off, no heat loss is accomplished. This mechanism of energy transfer from skin to liquid sweat to water vapor is capable of transferring enough heat to allow a person to maintain body temperature at environmental temperatures in excess of 100°C. Because evaporation of sweat is required for this mechanism of heat loss, the movement of water vapor from skin to air must be unimpeded. The most important factor determining the extent of evaporation of sweat is the relative humidity of the surrounding air. Relative humidity refers to the percentage of water vapor present in the air compared to the greatest amount that the air can hold at that temperature. A very high relative humidity impedes sweat evaporation, thus heat loss from the skin, because the air is almost fully saturated and has little ability to take up additional moisture from the skin. Therefore, maintaining body temperature at a comfortable level when humidity is high is more difficult. We can, however, hasten the movement of water vapor from the skin to the air by using the process of convection. By moving air, as with a fan, greater rates of evaporation of sweat from the skin can be achieved, resulting in greater loss of heat from the skin. Some individuals, especially wrestlers, exploit this effect of humidity on sweat evaporation by wearing water impermeable garments while in a hot environment or while exercising to increase body temperature, thereby increasing sweat rate and loss of body mass. This imprudent practice results in the dangerous combination of elevated body temperature and dehydration.

A final function of the skin is its role as an endocrine gland producing the important hormone cholecalciferol, or vitamin D. Upon exposure to sunlight, vitamin D is produced by the skin from a precursor related to cholesterol. This chemical messenger is subsequently released into the blood to act at the distant target site, the intestine. There, it plays an essential role in calcium absorption. Because skin exposure to sunlight is limited much of the time, other sources of vitamin D, such as dietary, are required to meet the demand. Regardless of its source, vitamin D is biologically inactive upon first entering the blood stream. Two steps involving the liver and the kidneys are involved in the activation process. Once activated, vitamin D is then capable of performing its most important function—to increase calcium absorption in the intestine. Lack of vitamin D causes osteomalacia, or a softening of the bones, which are inadequately mineralized. In children, a lack of this important vitamin is known as rickets and causes bones to become too soft to support the child's weight, resulting in bowing of long bones of the lower extremities.

STRUCTURE OF SKIN

Skin consists of more or less distinct layers with specific roles in the homeostatic mechanisms of their respective organs. Skin is typically divided into three layers: the epidermis, the dermis, and subcutaneous fat (Figure 14-1). Epidermis is not vascularized, and its cells are sacrificed to produce an outer waterproof layer. The dermis consists of vascularized tissues, surrounding the accessory organs (sweat glands, sebaceous glands, hair follicles) and nerves. The subcutaneous fat consists of insulation between the skin and the underlying tissue, such as muscle, bone, tendon, or ligament. The epidermis and dermis are connected along ridges that serve to increase the surface area and adhesion between the two

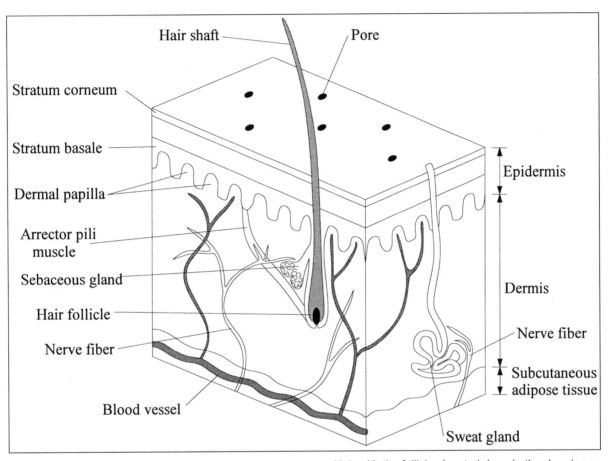

Figure 14-1. Structure of skin, including accessory structures. Hair with the follicles located deep in the dermis are shown with the associated arrector pili muscles that cause the hairs to become erect and form "goose flesh" in the cold. Sweat glands with their coiled portion deep in the dermis and openings onto the surface of the skin are also depicted. Sebaceous glands are associated with hair follicles and secrete their oily sebum onto the skin to help retain moisture. Also note the relative thickness of the dermis, which is about 10 times thicker than the epidermis, the presence of sensory receptors in the dermis, and blood vessels in the dermis.

layers. On the palms of the hands, which we subject to large shearing forces, the ridges of dermis covered with epidermis are large enough to observe as fingerprints.

Although epidermis is only about the thickness of a sheet of paper, it contains four or, in some areas, five distinct layers. The stratum basale (basal layer) is the deepest layer, next to the dermis. This is the reproductive layer in which mitosis constantly produces new cells and moves the old cells upward. The migration of cells to the surface takes about 14 days to occur. Once in the outer layer, cells remain for approximately another 2 weeks before being lost. The next layer is the stratum spinosum, so named because of the prominent desmosomes seen under the microscope. The next layer is flatter and has produced large quantities of keratin granules; this layer is called the stratum granulosum. The next layer, the stratum lucidum, can only be seen in the soles and palms. In the outermost layer of skin, cells are no longer

living; the nucleus and other organelles have been destroyed, and the cells are almost filled with keratin granules to form the horn-like stratum corneum layer, which serves to waterproof the skin. Waterproofing provides a barrier to both infection and loss of moisture to the external environment. The dermis does not have distinct layers, but consists largely of collagen fiber bundles, blood vessels, nerves, and the origins of the accessory structures. Blood supply to the skin is usually greatly in excess of that needed for nutrition to the skin, but the high rate of blood flow is necessary for temperature regulation.

The subcutaneous fat layer is loosely connected to itself but adheres to the dermis and the underlying fascia. This allows skin to dissipate both pressure and shearing forces. In areas where bony prominences such as the heel and greater trochanter are immediately adjacent to the subcutaneous fat layer without much muscle mass, the ability of the skin to dissipate pressure is compromised. The disproportionate pressure placed on these areas mechanically occludes blood flow to these areas, causing tissue death. These areas of dead tissue are called pressure sores or pressure ulcers. The obsolete term decubitus ulcer is often still used to describe these areas. In many cases, subcutaneous tissue may be necrotic or severely compromised before the epidermis shows signs of pressure damage.

The subcutaneous fat layer provides thermal as well as mechanical insulation. Arctic animals are capable of survival in extremely cold environments largely due to a thick layer of subcutaneous fat. Fat also acts as an energy store. By volume, fat stores approximately 20 times as much energy as the storage form of carbohydrate in animals, called glycogen.

CELLS OF THE SKIN

The skin consists of several basic types of cells, in addition to blood vessels, nerves, and sensory receptors for pain, touch, and temperature. These cells include Langerhans cells, melanocytes, keratinocytes, fibroblasts, and mast cells (Figure 14-2). Langerhans cells are the resident macrophages of the skin, representing approximately 3% of the epidermal cells. They present antigen to helper T cells, thereby increasing their responsiveness to the skin associated antigen. As such, these cells often respond to noninjurious molecules, resulting in conditions called contact dermatitis. A second type of cell, also representing 3% of the epidermal cells, is the melanocyte. Melanocytes produce the brown pigment melanin, the amount of which is responsible for the different shades of skin color. In addition to the hereditary component of melanin production, the amount of this pigment can be temporarily increased in response to exposure to ultraviolet sun rays. This additional melanin production, by absorbing harmful ultraviolet rays, produces what we know as a "tan." The most abundant epidermal cells are the keratinocytes, representing 94% of the cells of the epidermis. As the name implies, keratinocytes are specialized to produce keratin. The cells form the outer protective layer that is both airtight and fairly waterproof. In addition to this protective function, they are responsible for generating hair and nails as well as performing an immunologic function. That is, they secrete interleukin-1, which influences the maturation of T cells localized to the skin.

Mast cells are resident skin cells similar to the basophil, a white blood cell. Mast cells produce and release the compound histamine under mechanical stress

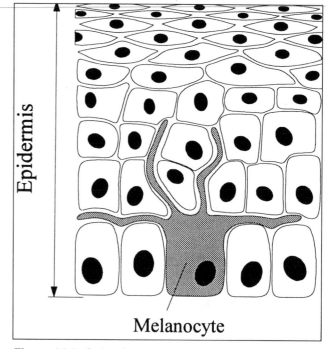

Figure 14-2. Cells of the epidermis. A melanocyte with its dendrites distributing melanin to surrounding keratinocytes is depicted. No Langerhans cells are shown.

or when signaled by inflammatory cells. Histamine increases the permeability of small blood vessels (chiefly venules), which allows fluid and proteins to escape from blood vessels. Histamine also increases blood flow in the area in which it is released. Scratching of the skin is often sufficient stimulus for release of histamine, which results in red streaks where the skin was scratched that can last for several minutes.

The cells within the dermis are not in direct contact with each other. Rather, they are held together and surrounded by the extracellular matrix, a meshwork consisting of fibrous proteins embedded within a watery, gel-like substance. There are three major types of protein fibers within this organic matrix. Collagen, by forming cable-like fibers or sheets, promotes the tensile strength of skin. Elastin is a rubberlike protein fiber, found most abundantly within tissues that are subject to much stretch and recoil. Finally, fibronectin promotes cell adhesion, thus helping to hold cells in position. Fibroblasts secrete both the proteins that produce the fibers and the molecules making up the gel, called the extracellular matrix. Fibroblasts are also important in wound healing. Following inflammation, fibroblasts undergo rapid cell division to replace lost cells and secrete the proteins of the fibers and molecules of the extracellular matrix to bring about repair.

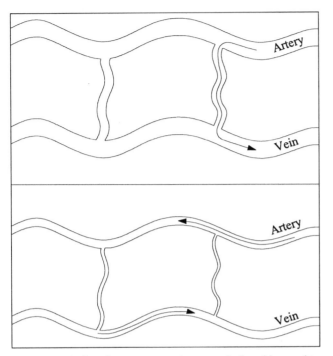

Figure 14-3. Arteriovenous anastomoses in the skin used to dissipate heat. In a warm environment (top), the sympathetic nerves decrease their signaling to the vessels, allowing flow to enter the AV anastomosis and the venous plexus, which behaves as a radiator to dissipate heat in the skin. In a cold environment (bottom), the sympathetic nerves constrict the arteriolar vessels and decrease blood flow through the venous plexus, thereby allowing more heat to be retained.

APPENDAGES OF SKIN

The appendages of the skin include the sweat glands, sebaceous glands, hair follicles, and nails. Although sebaceous glands and hair follicles are located in the dermis, they are lined with epidermal cells, which can be a source of new cells to repair wounds. Sweat glands are coiled structures located deep in the dermis that behave somewhat like renal tubules but are under control of the sympathetic nervous system. Stimulation of the sympathetic nerves stimulates the glands to secrete a fluid similar in composition to the renal tubular fluid. Just as aldosterone causes reabsorption of sodium and, passively, chloride ions in the renal tubules, reabsorption also occurs in the sweat glands, rendering sweat hypotonic. Sebaceous glands secrete sebum, an oily substance that helps to waterproof and lubricate the skin to prevent drying out and cracking. Sex hormones increase the production of sebum during puberty and may increase it to the point of clogging the ostium of the gland, which allows the gland to be infected by Propionibacterium acnes. This infection produces the condition known as acne. Hair follicles occur in association with sebaceous glands. The base of the hair follicle is located deep in the dermis. One can exploit this information to help determine the depth of a burn injury. If a hair pulls out easily, the injury has extended the full thickness (third degree or full thickness burn) of the skin. If resistance is felt, the injury is a deep partial thickness burn injury. The formation of scar tissue following wounding of the skin leads to avascular, lightly pigmented, and dry skin due to the lack of accessory structures in scar tissue.

BLOOD SUPPLY OF SKIN

Skin in areas, such as fingertips, palms of the hands, toes, soles of the feet, ears, nose, and lips, has specialized structures to aid in temperature regulation. In addition to the normal small arterial vessels called arterioles, large networks of venous vessels called venous plexuses exist. Without innervation, blood flow largely bypasses the capillary network and allows blood to be directed into these venous vessels that behave as the pipes on a radiator to lose heat from the blood to the skin (Figure 14-3). Under comfortable thermal conditions, the sympathetic nerves prevent flow into the venous plexus to prevent excess heat loss. When the surrounding air is cold, blood flow is significantly decreased throughout the skin to prevent heat loss from the blood. However, in a warm environment, the smooth muscle of the arterioles and pathways into the venous plexus relaxes as the sympathetic nerves are inhibited by central temperature-controlling mechanisms. In addition, local reflexes involving temperature receptors of the skin promote relaxation of these blood vessels. Therefore, local heating of skin can produce increased blood flow to an area of skin, and increased body temperature increases blood flow throughout the entire skin surface.

The epidermis is not supplied with blood vessels; therefore, superficial thickness (sunburn-type) burns do not cause blistering of the skin. When the outer part of the dermis with its blood vessels is injured in a second-degree burn (superficial partial thickness burn), large quantities of fluid escape from damaged blood vessels producing the blisters associated with this type of burn.

INJURY TO THE SKIN

Practice patterns for the integumentary system include primary prevention of integumentary damage, superficial injury, partial thickness, full thickness, subcutaneous tissue loss, and lymphedema. For burns and pressure ulcers, we have specialized terminology to report the severity of the wound. A first-degree burn injures only the epidermis, this is also known as a superficial burn. A second-degree burn results in inflammation of the dermis as well as injury to the epidermis. Fluid leaking from the inflamed dermis collects between the dermis and epidermis to produce the blisters associated with superficial partial thickness/second-degree burns. Second-degree burns are also very painful, because pain-transmitting neurons survive the injury. Deep partial thickness burns allow some blood flow to remain at the lower level of the dermis. When one pushes on this area, blanching occurs indicative of the presence of blood flow in the deepest dermis. No equivalent to deep partial thickness exists in the first, second, third degree system. A third-degree or full thickness burn has damaged the appendages to the skin as well as the blood vessels. Healing proceeds from the edges of the wound, and, once a wound becomes full thickness and larger than an area the size of the back of the hand, grafting of skin from one part of the body to the burned area may be necessary. Pressure ulcers are classified as stage I if reddening of the skin persists after pressure is removed, stage II if damage extends into, but not through, the dermis, stage III if damage extends through the dermis and into subcutaneous fat, but not beyond the underlying fascia. A stage IV pressure ulcer extends beyond the fascia into underlying muscle, bone, ligament, or tendon. When staging a pressure ulcer, a common mistake is to "reverse stage" a wound as it fills in. Once a wound is assigned a stage when the wound bed can be visualized, the wound should always be graded as such. The scar tissue that fills the wound does not specifically replace the tissue that was originally present. Therefore, if a pressure ulcer originally extended to the bone, it should always be staged as a stage IV pressure ulcer.

Several etiologies of skin injury exist, which may be placed in the following categories: mechanical injury or trauma, thermal injury, vascular insufficiency, radiation injury, chemical injury, and toxic injury. Mechanical injury includes open (compound) fractures, degloving, in which skin is torn and peeled off the body, lacerations, abrasions, incisions (including knife injuries), and gunshot wounds. Any acute traumatic injury carries the risk of infection due to the presence of foreign material and necrotic tissue. Thermal injury includes elevated temperature caused by contact with a hot object, flash burn (contact with hot gas, i.e., fireball), scald (liquid, steam), and decreased temperature (frostbite). Both the very young and elderly are at greater risk due to either decreased mobility or lack of knowledge of the consequences of exposure to heat. Toddlers in particular are

at great risk of scalding in either the kitchen or bathroom. Vascular insufficiency may take the form of arterial insufficiency in which tissue necrosis occurs due to ischemia of the extremities, often in the form we call gangrene. Venous insufficiency causes malnutrition of the skin and skin necrosis due to the leakage of protein from elevated venous and capillary pressure that results from compromised calf muscle pumping. Venous insufficiency is caused by one of three problems: obstruction of venous vessels by thrombi, clots, tumors, obesity, or pregnancy; insufficient venous valves that allow backflow of venous blood; or loss of voluntary muscle movement in an extremity. Excessive pressure over a bony prominence causes insufficiency of capillary blood flow, resulting in what are called pressure ulcers, formerly known as decubitus ulcers. Radiation injury is usually caused by radiation therapy to treat cancer. Chemical burns are usually the result of industrial accidents in which caustic agents contact the skin. Toxic injuries include poisons, such as brown recluse spider toxin. Although an antitoxin is now available, brown recluse toxin can cause rapid necrosis through fatty tissue in a short time. Some bacteria cause necrotizing fasciitis and have been termed "flesh-eating" bacteria.

Management of wounds includes debridement (removal of necrotic tissue), cleansing wounds, and dressing changes as well as prevention of new wounds and preventing functional limitations and disabilities caused by wounds. Debridement can be done in four basic ways: nonselective mechanical debridement, sharp debridement, chemical debridement, and autolytic debridement. Mechanical means include the use of whirlpools, irrigation, or more specific devices that produce pulsatile lavage with concurrent suction (basic concept of carpet cleaners in which a jet of water is used for cleaning and is vacuumed from the carpet concurrently). One common type of nonselective mechanical debridement is the wet-to-dry dressing. Gauze is moistened, placed in the wound, and then allowed to dry into necrotic tissue. The dry gauze is then pulled out with necrotic tissue to debride necrotic tissue rapidly. Chemical debridement uses chemicals that selectively break down substances in the wound including protein and collagen. Dried necrotic tissue (eschar) can be scored with a scalpel prior to administering a chemical debrider to increase the surface area over which the agent works. Sharp debridement includes the use of instruments, such as forceps, scissors, and scalpels, to remove necrotic tissue selectively. Sharp debridement is considered an advanced skill, requiring specialized training beyond entry-level education. Autolytic (self-destruction) debridement is performed by enzymes produced by cells within the wound. This type is slower, but painless, and requires the use of occlusive dressings that retain wound exudate.

Wound healing consists of four basic phases: inflammation, proliferation, epithelialization, and remodeling. After the injury, inflammation allows the destruction of foreign material and microbes. Neutrophils are usually the first cells to the site of injury and function to destroy microbes. Macrophages come later and aid in wound healing by removing debris and attracting and promoting proliferation of fibroblasts. Fibroblasts secrete the molecules that form the ground substance and fibers of the scar tissue that fills the tissue loss. The tissue that is generated forms in small piles, resembling the pebbled surface of a basketball, and because of the formation of leaky, new blood vessels, it is beefy red and shiny. This tissue is called granulation tissue. Within the developing scar tissue, fibers are generated in random directions and provide little of the tensile strength of normal skin. During the proliferation phase, myofibroblasts in the wound pull the wound edges toward the middle, producing wound contraction. Concurrent with and continuing after the wound has completed granulation, is the process of epithelialization. As granulation tissue fills in from the sides of the wound, new epithelial cells are regenerated to cover the scar tissue below. Although mature scar tissue has many of the same components of dermis, it lacks the accessory structures and blood vessels of natural dermis. The remodeling phase consists of reinforcement of collagen in the direction of stress and removal of collagen bundles that are unstressed so that a mature scar has approximately 80% of the strength of normal skin.

If necrotic tissue is allowed to dry, an eschar is formed. A scab is a type of eschar composed of a large number of red blood cells that give a scab its color. In the presence of eschar, the migration of cells to fill the wound and re-epithelialize it is greatly slowed. One could say that we must make the "eschar go" or the wound will heal at a snail's pace. For this reason, the emphasis in modern wound healing is the model of moist wound healing in which the microenvironment of a wound is managed to maintain temperature near 37°C and to retain moisture and molecules produced by cells in the wound by trapping them under a wound dressing. Many wound dressings are available to promote moist wound healing. Moreover, the more frequently a wound is handled, the more we promote inflammation and slow healing. Ideally, we strive to handle the clean, granulating wound as little as possible, such as every 5 days or less frequently.

A few general rules guide wound management. One states that we debride black wounds (eschar), clean yellow wounds (moist necrotic tissue or pus), and protect red wounds (granulating). Another important rule pertains to occluding wounds. Occlusion refers to retention of exudate within the wound to promote moist wound healing. Several dressings are available to do this. Because occlusion promotes growth, we want to occlude wounds that are not infected but do not want to occlude infected wounds. On infected wounds, we generally use gauze soaked in antibiotic solution for several days. After the infection is cleared, we can safely begin the use of occlusive dressings. In general, once a wound is debrided, it is unlikely to become infected. Necrotic tissue is a tremendous breeding ground for bacteria, and its removal is a major factor is preventing infection.

Dressing decisions are based on four judgment branch points. The first point is whether a wound is infected. If a wound is infected, we first treat the infection. Using antimicrobial agents and nonocclusive dressings slows growth but assists in removing the infection. Once a wound is no longer infected, we move to the next decision point, which is the need for debridement. If a wound has a large quantity of necrotic tissue, or the presence of necrotic tissue is determining the length of a hospital stay, wet-to-dry dressings and other forms of nonspecific mechanical debridement are used to remove necrotic tissue as rapidly as possible, usually in an acute-care facility. In a situation in which length of stay is not an issue, such as home health or outpatient, the use of occlusive dressings and promotion of autolytic debridement is prudent. The third decision branching point is whether subcutaneous tissue loss is present and filling the wound is necessary to ensure that the wound heals from the inside toward the surface. If a wound is clean and granulating, a biocompatible substance is placed in the wound to prevent the wound from healing over a void in the skin. If large amounts of necrotic tissue remain in the wound, a wet-to-dry dressing is usually employed to fill the cavity. If the wound heals over, the resultant cavity is very likely to become infected and form an abscess. If a wound is partial or full-thickness, but without subcutaneous tissue loss, simple, flat dressings can be placed over the wound for several days at a time until healing is complete. The final branch point is that of managing exudate. To allow a dressing to remain in place for several days, one must select a dressing that can maintain a proper level of exudate by one of three processes: allowing evaporation through the dressing, absorbing the exudate, or trapping exudate below the dressing surface without allowing fluid to wet the skin around the wound and damage it. Wound management is a very rewarding aspect of clinical practice and relies heavily on understanding and promoting the physiology of wound healing.

skin by increasing blood flow, and loss of heat to a cold environment is minimized by a decrease in blood flow to the skin.

SUMMARY

Skin functions to protect the internal environment from loss of moisture, parasites, and excessive changes in body temperature. Skin also synthesizes the inactive form of vitamin D, which is converted to the active form by the kidney. Vitamin D is required to absorb calcium from the diet. Cells of the skin described were the Langerhans cell, melanocytes, keratinocytes, mast cells, and fibroblasts. Langerhans cells are immune cells of the skin. Melanocytes synthesize and distribute melanin to pigment the keratinocytes, which are 94% of the epidermal cells. Keratinocytes migrate through four or five layers of skin to the surface, where they perform a waterproofing role. Fibroblasts secrete the proteins that make up the organic matrix of skin, including the fibers that provide tensile strength and elasticity. Blood vessels are important in the skin in the role of thermoregulation. To rid the body of heat, blood carries more heat to the

BIBLIOGRAPHY

Bergstrom N, Allman RM, Alvarez OM, et al. *Clinical Practice Guideline: Pressure Ulcers in Adults: Prediction and Prevention*. 3rd ed. Rockville, Md: AHCPR Publishing; 1992.

Bergstrom N, Allman RM, Alvarez OM, et al. *Clinical Practice Guideline: Treatment of Pressure Ulcers*. 15th ed. Rockville, Md: AHCPR Publishing; 1994.

Gogia PP. *Clinical Wound Management*. Thorofare, NJ: SLACK Incorporated; 1995.

Guyton AC. *Human Physiology and Mechanism of Disease*. 5th ed. Philadelphia, Pa: WB Saunders Co; 1992.

Hess CT. *Nurse's Clinical Guide: Wound Care*. Springhouse, Pa: Springhouse Corporation; 1993.

McCulloch JM, Kloth LC, Feedar JA. *Wound Healing: Alternatives in Management*. 2nd ed. Philadelphia, Pa: FA Davis Company; 1995.

Scott-Burden T. Extracellular matrix: the cellular environment. *News in Physiological Sciences*. 1994;9:110-115.

Sussman C, Bates-Jensen BM. *Wound Care: A Collaborative Practice Manual for Physical Therapists and Nurses*. Gaithersburg, Md: Aspen Publishers Inc; 1998.

STUDY QUESTIONS

1. Based upon the functions of skin, why is a person with full-thickness burns at high risk for infection and hypovolemic shock?

2. With a full-thickness injury, what happens to the coloration, ability to sweat, sensation, moisture, and hair growth in the scar?

3. Discuss why blisters only form with an injury to the skin that inflames the dermis.

4. What functions are served by the high blood flow to the papillary layer of the dermis?

Musculoskeletal System

The musculoskeletal system is comprised of "passive" elements (bone, tendon, and ligaments) and an active element (skeletal muscle). The variations in the stiffness of these structures at appropriate times allow for posture and movement. Muscles contract, increasing the tension on tendons, bones, and ligaments. The partial contraction of muscle produces a level of muscle tone that, balanced with that from other muscles, may balance the skeletal structures in such a way that gravity is opposed, producing what we call posture. Muscle may also produce enough tension through itself and the passive elements to overcome gravity. Muscle may produce a tension that allows control over how rapidly gravity or another force moves the body (ie, lowering an object with control). The musculoskeletal system provides the active element of the ventilatory pump (muscles of ventilation) and the bony attachments of the chest wall. It also controls micturition by opening the neck of the bladder and, when failing to do so, leads to stress urinary incontinence. Loss of muscle activity of the lower extremities leads to venous disease in the lower extremities with the risk of blood clots and the potential for death due to pulmonary embolism and lesser problems, such as swelling of the legs, varicose veins, and ulcers of the legs. This unit explores first the passive elements of the musculoskeletal system and their adaptations to stress and lack of stress, followed by the structure of skeletal muscle, how strength is controlled, and how skeletal muscle functions as the interface of the neuromuscular and musculoskeletal systems to provide appropriate and controlled posture and movement.

FIFTEEN

Bone and Dense Connective Tissue

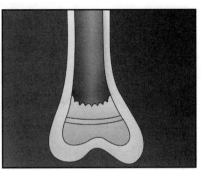

Glenn Irion, PhD, PT, CWS and Sarah N. Jerome, PhD, RRT

OBJECTIVES

1. List the major functions of bone: physical support and protection, movement, production of blood and other immune cells, and calcium metabolism.

2. Describe the cellular and noncellular components of bone and dense connective tissue.

3. Describe the vascular anatomy of bone.

4. Describe the layers of bone.

5. Describe the development and growth of bone.

6. Contrast the structure of different dense connective tissues.

7. Describe the responses of bone and dense connective tissue to stress and lack of stress.

Bone and dense connective tissue are the "passive" elements of the musculoskeletal system as opposed to the active element, skeletal muscle. Bone also has a protective role for the central nervous system and the thoracic and abdominal viscera. The dense connective tissues (tendon, cartilage, and ligament) have supportive roles in the musculoskeletal system, allowing movement and posture. In this chapter, however, it will be shown that bone and dense connective tissue are far from being passive.

FUNCTIONS OF BONES AND DENSE CONNECTIVE TISSUE

In addition to the roles of bone in movement and posture, bone contains marrow, which produces the cellular elements of the blood and other immune cells that will be discussed in a later chapter. Bone also represents a large store for serum calcium, which must be maintained carefully at a concentration of approximately 2.5 mM. Excess calcium and phosphate can be deposited in bone or excreted by the kidney. When blood concentration of calcium falls, parathyroid hormone causes calcium to be released by bone to be used by the rest of the body.

DENSE CONNECTIVE TISSUE

Musculoskeletal structures, in addition to bone and muscle, include tendons, ligaments, and cartilage. These tissues consist of **dense connective tissue**. These tissues are characterized by the large proportion of the tissue consisting of fibers, especially collagen. The orientation of fibers within these tissues corresponds to the function of these tissues. Tendons, which transmit large forces from muscles to bones, have densely packed parallel fibers. The addition of stress, such as resistance training, increases the thickness of the collagen fiber bundles, whereas immobilization results in decreased diameters of individual fascicles as well as diameter of the tendon. Ligament and joint capsules have a less regular fiber orientation that allows some movement of the joints. Stress placed on ligaments and capsules also increases the thickness of these tissues and their resistance to tearing. Immobilization weakens all of these dense connective tissues and increases the risk of tearing and injury.

COMPONENTS OF DENSE CONNECTIVE TISSUE

Fibers

The major fiber in dense connective tissue is collagen. Collagen is secreted as procollagen from fibroblasts. Following secretion of procollagen, the units are transformed into tropocollagen and are linked into a strand of collagen. The collagen fibers are arranged in a triple helix (Figure 15-1) similar to a hair braid with cross-links between the strands to increase the strength of the fibers. The most common form of collagen found in skin, tendon, bones, and ligaments is called type I collagen. Other types of collagen are produced in the human body but are found in other tissues or occur early in maturation. Tropocollagen molecules aggregate into microfibrils. Several microfibrils are bound together to make up a subfibril, and several subfibrils make up a fibril. Each fascicle of a tendon consists of many fibrils, and several fascicles make up a tendon. The organization of tropocollagen molecules produces a regular pattern of light and dark striations along the length of collagen fibers with crimps along the fibers.

Different forms of collagen are given Roman numerals to distinguish them. Type I collagen, the predominant form in dermis and bone, is characterized by

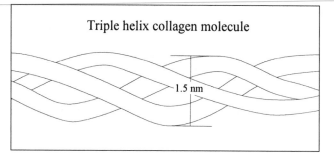

Figure 15-1. Triple helix structure of collagen fibers. Chains of collagen molecules are reinforced by the braiding and cross-links between the three strands.

closely packed fibers and is produced by fibroblasts, osteoblasts, odontoblasts, and chondroblasts. It performs well in resisting tension. Type II collagen is the predominant form in hyaline and elastic cartilage. It does not produce distinct cable-like fibers, but exists in a loose collagenous mass with fibrils embedded in ground substance. This type is produced by chondroblasts and interacts intimately with the molecules of the ground substance to produce a tissue that resists compressive forces. Type III collagen is found in smooth muscle, endoneurium (connective tissue of peripheral nerves), arteries, the uterus, and other organs. It is characterized by loosely packed, thin fibrils that resist tension in extensible organs and vessels. Type IV collagen is found in endothelial and epithelial tissues. The final type, type V, is found only in the placenta.

Cells

Among the collagen fibers are the cells that produce collagen. Fibroblasts are found in the dermis of the skin, tendons, joint capsules, and ligaments. In bone, osteoblasts create the organic matrix, consisting primarily of collagen fibers, whereas the cells of cartilage are termed chrondroblasts.

Ground Substance

The ground substance is the amorphous tissue between bundles of collagen, which, similar to dermis, consists of a gel-like material. Certain molecules of the ground substance are able to hold approximately 1000 times their weight in water. Only 1% of the dry weight of a tendon is ground substance in contrast to the looser connective tissue of the dermis. Glycosaminoglycans, proteoglycans, and glycoproteins are the primary molecules of the ground substance. Glycosaminoglycans bind water in the ground substance to prevent free water movement. Proteoglycans provide the lubricant function necessary to allow fibers to move across one another and allow tissue extensibility. Glycoproteins, especially laminin and fibronectin, attach cells to the fibers.

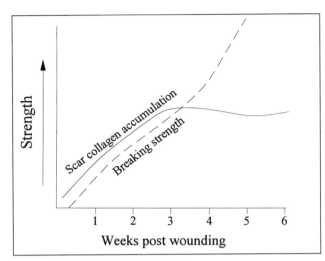

Figure 15-2. Relationship between collagen accumulation and breaking strength in a tendon. Note that breaking strength and collagen accumulation are initially directly related, but breaking strength continues to increase after collagen accumulation reaches a plateau. The further increase in breaking strength appears to be caused by organization of the collagen fibers and interaction with the ground substance.

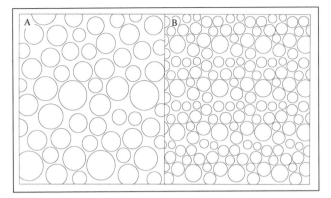

Figure 15-3. Effect of removal of stress on collagen bundles of a tendon. Note the atrophy of collagen bundles when a limb is immobilized.

With age, collagen fibers increase in strength. As lab animals increase in age, a greater force is required to produce a given increase in tendon length. During healing from an injury, a progressive increase in strength of tendons is observed (Figure 15-2). This change is thought to be the result of three factors: increased diameter of the individual fibers, improved alignment of fibers along lines of stress, and increased strength of bonding within the fibers. To a large degree, the increase in strength results directly from increased diameter of the fibers. However, strength continues to increase after fibers reach their maximum length. The increase in strength is postulated to be caused by interaction with elements of the ground substance binding to the collagen molecule.

A major factor determining strength of tendons and other dense connective tissues is stress. Increased stress increases collagen fiber thickness in tissues including tendons and ligaments, whereas decreased stress, as in immobilization in a cast, causes not only decreased diameter of individual collagen fibers, but also further weakens dense connective tissue by creating a disorganization of collagen fibers (Figure 15-3).

STRESS-STRAIN RELATIONSHIP OF DENSE CONNECTIVE TISSUE

Stress-strain refers to the applied force necessary to produce a given increase in tissue length. Shown graph-

ically (Figure 15-4), the force transmitted along a tendon (stress) for a given increase in tendon length (strain) consists of five regions. The toe region demonstrates little increase in tension (stress) in a tendon as it is lengthened (increase in strain). The appearance of the toe region is speculated to be due to straightening of the crimps of collagen fibers. The next region, termed the linear region, demonstrates a consistent stiffness (slope of the stress/strain relationship) and is thought to be due to physical stretch of collagen fibers up to their physiologic limit. Further increase in length produces a diminished slope in the region termed either yield region 1 or progressive failure region. In this region of the stress/strain relationship, a greater increase in length is required to produce an increase in tension (ie, the fibers are beginning to fail, yield to the stress, or, stated another way, are yielding to the stress on them by beginning to fail). In the yield region 2, or major failure region, collagen fibers weaken to the point that a tendon begins to thin and fray. The final region is called the complete rupture region. This region represents the maximum strength of a tendon and the stress at which a tendon ruptures.

In general, the toe region consists of the first 1% to 2% increase in length/strain, the linear range exists between 2% and 6%, yield occurs between the linear range and up to 8%, whereas rupture occurs when a tendon is stretched by about 10%. The actual load leading to rupture is about 6 kg/mm^2 of tendon cross-section. The amount of force required to straighten the crimps in collagen fibers (ie, move through the toe region), has been estimated to be equal to the force produced by a maximum voluntary contraction of the muscle. The force necessary to place a tendon into the linear region with risk of injury to the tendon requires an external force to be placed on the tendon greater than the weight that a person can hold isometrically. Tendon injuries may result from excessively forceful stretching, an effort to lower an excessive weight (eccentric contraction), or a sudden load being placed on a musculoskeletal unit.

The stress-strain relationship is usually described under static conditions. When tendon is stretched cyclically or is placed under a constant load that does not immediately damage the tendon, the tendon stretches. The term used to describe the phenomenon by which tissue lengthens under prolonged stretch is termed creep. Creep also occurs in smooth muscle, such as that making up the walls of organs such as the bladder and uterus. In experimental models, prolonged 1% strain for 1 hour was observed to cause damage to tendons, and 3% strain causes damage in a shorter time. Warming a tendon increases the lengthening with stress, but also increases the chance for a tendon to rupture at very high temperatures and strain. Applying heat (ultrasound or diathermy) to dense connective tissue followed by forceful stretching, greater than 2% strain, may result in permanent damage to the tissue.

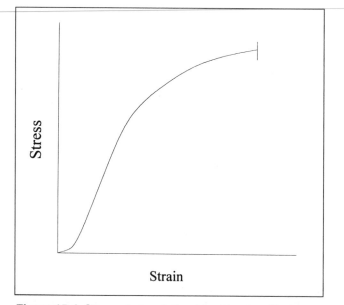

Figure 15-4. Stress-strain relationship of tendon. Strain represents increased tendon length. The tension required to lengthen the tendon is plotted as stress in units of kg/mm². Five areas described are the toe region, linear region, yield 1 region (progressive failure), yield 2 region (major failure), and complete rupture region.

CARTILAGE

Cartilage gives structure to the outer ear, much of the bridge of the nose, the nasal septum, and connects the lower ribs to the sternum. Cartilage also directly supports the function of bone in joints. Cartilage lines the borders of bones that must glide across each other to produce movement. A specialized cartilage, fibrocartilage, acts as a cushion in joints including between the two pubis bones, in the knee, and in the joints between adjacent vertebral bodies. Cartilage is a more rigid type of tissue than skin because of the large quantity of collagen fibers, but it lacks the mineralization that gives bone its ability to withstand compression. Cartilage cells are called chondrocytes, and they, much like osteocytes, occupy small spaces called lacunae in the cartilage. Just as bone is surrounded by periosteum, cartilage is sur-

rounded by perichondrium. Unlike bone, which has a blood supply, cartilage has no blood vessels, except for those in the perichondrium. Damage to cartilage is very slow to be repaired because of the lack of direct blood flow.

LIGAMENTS AND CAPSULE

In contrast to the active fiber-producing cells of dermis and tendon, ligaments and capsules have a smaller density of cells, which are mainly the mature form, called a fibrocyte. Fibrocytes have a lower activity of fiber component production. Moreover, ligaments and

---

Case Study

A 42-year-old man is playing tennis when he feels a sudden pain above the back of his right heel. He is unable to plantarflex his ankle (point the toes). Immediately before the injury, he stepped backward forcefully onto his right foot. He describes himself as a weekend athlete, engaging mainly in game-type activities, but not training on a regular basis.

What was the cause of his pain and loss of plantarflexion?

What action caused the injury to occur?

How might regular weight training have prevented this injury?

capsules, in general, have a lower vessel density than other connective tissues.

Ligaments are generally grouped into two types: those that connect viscera to each other or to the body wall, and those that connect one bone to another. The latter, or skeletal ligaments, consist of distinct bands of connective tissue that bind two bones or bony parts. Often, at joint sites that have cavities, these ligaments will blend with the capsular wall of the joint cavity. Therefore, in these cases, they can be considered as specialized thickenings of the fibrous capsule.

Because skeletal ligaments must withstand significant pull at the joints they cross, most of their fibers run in the same direction. Most of these ligaments consist of closely packed collagen fibers that allow for little stretch. These fibers are generally white in color. Some ligaments, however, are yellow in color, due to the presence of elastic fibers. This allows for stretch with movement in one direction and shortening with movement in the opposite direction. Thus, they tend to remain taut rather than lax. If a joint capsule with its associated ligaments is torn or stretched excessively, joint movement can be impaired, resulting in pain and damage to the joint. If an injury creates enough discomfort for a person to avoid moving a joint, the well-organized collagen bundles of the joint capsule will be slowly replaced by random collagen bundles. This condition of hypomobility itself may become painful and reinforce the lack of movement until the person has very little movement available in a joint. Mobilization techniques used by therapists or, if severe enough, manipulation under anesthesia by a physician may be required to regain movement.

TENDONS

Tendons are defined as structures that connect skeletal muscle to another structure, usually bone. Therefore, while one end of the tendon is always attached to muscle, the fibers of the other end of the tendon blend with the periosteum of the bone. Some tendons of muscles not associated with bones, such as muscles of facial expression, blend with the dense connective tissue that forms below the dermis of the skin.

The composition of tendons, like that of most ligaments, is one of very dense collagenous tissue in which collagen bundles run in one direction to withstand great pull. Because the densely packed parallel bundles of fibers are held together by very few cross fibers, tendons are subject to easy tearing. Due to limited vascularity and regeneration, a torn tendon or ligament heals through scar tissue formation. The predominance of collagen fibers gives a tendon its white, shiny appearance. Thus, tendons and ligaments often tend to blend with each other when they are close together. Indeed, ligaments may be reinforced by a tendon that blends with it.

Compared to the parallel fiber arrangement in tendons, ligaments and capsules have a dense weave of collagen fibers that must slide across one another to confer extensibility. Mobility in capsules and ligaments can be lost by injury that produces remodeling of collagen fibers, loss of water, and proteoglycans.

Case Study

A 31-year-old man working as a chef slipped and fell at work on a greasy floor. He was initially diagnosed with a low back muscle strain and was unable to return to work for 3 weeks. He was not referred for any therapy by his physician and spent the bulk of the next 3 weeks in bed. Upon return to work, he complained of constant, moderate back pain and could not work an entire shift. He was referred to a pain center where he received a series of trigger-point injections with local anesthetic in hopes of returning him to work. He failed to improve and was referred for therapy. Examination revealed a hypomobile segment of the thoracic spine. Areas above and below the midthoracic spine allowed movement of the vertebra with mobilization by the therapist. The area between T4 and T7 could not be mobilized by the therapist manually. The mobility was restored by a high-velocity technique, and the chef was able to return to work, eventually resuming full-time duties.

What was the cause of this person's hypomobile thoracic spine segment?

Did the 3 weeks of bed rest help or hinder his return to work?

Why was a high-velocity technique necessary to restore thoracic spine mobility?

ATROPHY AND CONTRACTURE OF DENSE CONNECTIVE TISSUE

Immobilization, denervation, or any condition that diminishes the stress on dense connective tissue results in loss of tensile strength. Decreased strength is caused by both decreased collagen fiber diameter and loss of organization. Tensile strength can be restored by restoring normal stress on the tissue. A second phenomenon is contracture, in which remodeling results in a shortening of dense connective tissue and decreased joint range of motion. Remodeling of unstressed dense connective tissue produces shorter tissue. Research indicates that contracture takes much longer to occur than does fiber atrophy. After approximately 4 weeks of immobilization, significant losses of tensile strength and range of motion occur, which are reversible in about 3 weeks, whereas immobilization for 7 weeks or longer will require specialized therapy to restore range of motion to affected joints. These include joint mobilization and prolonged, low-load stretch, such as dynamic splinting. Physical agents, such as ultrasound and diathermy, can produce sufficient alteration in chemical bonds of collagen to allow lengthening. However, heat increases the risk of rupture of dense connective tissue when combined with high stretching force. Ultrasound used at a nonthermal intensity disrupts bonds within collagen fibers and may be combined with stretch to lengthen shortened dense connective tissue. In some cases, rupture of inappropriate dense connective tissue is desired, and heat and high forces may be effective for that purpose.

CELLS OF BONE

The cells within bone, known as osteoblasts, produce an organic matrix similar to that produced by fibroblasts within skin and dense connective tissue. This matrix is composed primarily of collagen fibers in a semisolid gel. This matrix is responsible for giving bone its tensile strength, that is, its resiliency to breakage when tension is applied. An inorganic component, a network made of calcium phosphate salt called hydroxyapatite, is deposited in the organic matrix of bone. Whereas the organic matrix gives bone its tensile strength, the inorganic component, or calcium phosphate crystal precipitate within the matrix, gives bone its compressive strength. This characteristic allows bone to hold its shape when squeezed or compressed. Osteocytes are mature, entrapped osteoblasts that have become entombed by the inorganic matrix that it has deposited around itself. Small canals, which supply nutrients, are

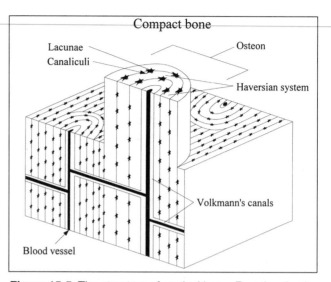

Figure 15-5. The structure of cortical bone. Functional units called osteons are built around Haversian canals. Lacunae containing osteocytes form rings around each canal within an osteon. Canaliculi between lacunae allow the processes of the osteocytes to communicate with surrounding osteocytes and allow movement of extracellular fluid through the osteon. Volkmann's canals provide pathways between Haversian canals for transmission of blood vessels. Osteons are cemented together to form the cortical bone.

formed by the osteocyte within the calcified matrix, thus allowing them to remain alive. Osteocytes are localized in small islands, to be described later, in which the osteocytes are capable of communicating with each other (Figure 15-5).

Osteocytes respond to electric stimuli by increasing bone mass. This function of osteocytes can be exploited by using electrical stimulators to increase the rate of fracture healing in cases in which healing is slow or nonexistent (delayed union or nonunion of a fracture). Osteocytes also respond to the electric current caused by the compression of its crystal structure. This principle is called the piezoelectric effect and is used in the phonograph in which a needle resting on the surface of a record compresses a crystal, producing a current that is amplified and routed to audio speakers. Mechanical stresses applied to bone cause bone mass to increase along the lines of stress applied to the bone. Conversely, the lack of mechanical stress on bone results in the loss of bone mass, which is termed osteoporosis. Osteopenia is a general term for lack of bone mass and includes the conditions known as osteoporosis and osteomalacia. Osteoporosis is characterized by normally mineralized, thin bone; osteomalacia represents bone that is soft secondary to the lack of inorganic salts to strengthen the organic matrix. The inorganic salts of bone can be selectively dissolved experimentally to leave only the organic

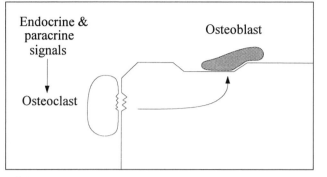

Figure 15-6. Remodeling process of bone. Endocrine and paracrine signals activate osteoclasts to reabsorb bone. Osteoclasts originate from cells related to the macrophage. Macrophages help finish the clean-up operation. After removal of bone occurs, osteoblasts are attracted to the area to form new areas of bone by first producing the organic matrix. The osteoblasts later mature into osteocytes and direct mineralization of the new matrix.

matrix (you may perform this at home using vinegar). When this process is performed, a rubbery bone results that has no compressive strength, can be easily bent and twisted, but cannot be pulled apart. The inorganic matrix functions much as a brick, which can withstand tremendous compression but breaks easily with tensile stress or twisting.

While bone is constantly being deposited by osteoblasts, it is continually being absorbed by osteoclasts (Figure 15-6). Osteoclasts are large, multinucleated cells derived from monocytes formed in the bone

marrow. Normal functioning bone has a balance of osteoclastic and osteoblastic activity, which maintains the strength of bone. Areas of bone with little mechanical stress are taken up by osteoclasts, as new areas of organic matrix are produced by osteoblasts and calcified by osteocytes. Up to approximately 20 to 30 years of age, bone mass increases then stabilizes around the age of 35 to 40. Without sufficient mechanical stresses, bone mass progressively diminishes with age. In women, bone mass decreases rapidly after menopause, resulting in postmenopausal osteoporosis. By the age of 80, men have similar degrees of bone mass loss as women. The loss of bone mass with age is called senile osteoporosis. In addition to the effects of mechanical stress, age, and menopause, several other factors can increase osteoporosis. The loss of calcium during pregnancy as the developing fetus extracts calcium from maternal blood and breastfeeding increases the risk of developing osteoporosis. In addition, short, white women of northern European descent and those who smoke are at risk for osteoporosis.

STRUCTURE OF BONE

Bone is considered to have four layers: the periosteum, cortical (or compact bone), cancellous (or trabecular bone), and in long bones, which have hollow centers, the endosteum. The periosteum is the outermost layer of any type of bone. It is not hardened by calcifi-

---

Case Study

A 36-year-old man fractured his tibia when his left leg was trapped between his truck and a mounted tire for earth-moving equipment when the tire fell over at a work site. Due to slow healing, including smoking, his left lower extremity was immobilized for 8 weeks. Following immobilization to allow fracture healing, the man regained very little range of motion of his left knee. Attempts to regain range of motion by stretching at home, moist heat, and ultrasound failed to improve his range of motion significantly. He underwent surgical manipulation of the knee under general anesthesia, but he failed to perform his home program following surgical manipulation and, again, lost his knee range of motion. Mobilization of his knee joint and patella restored much of his knee flexion, but failed to improve his knee extension. A dynamic splint was applied to provide low-load stretch to supplement his therapy. He regained sufficient range of motion to return to work in 8 weeks.

How did the prolonged immobilization of the knee contribute to his loss of range of motion?

Why did stretching, heating, and ultrasound fail to restore range of motion in this individual?

What is the purpose of surgical manipulation in this case?

Why did the surgical manipulation fail?

Why did the dynamic splint succeed where the manipulation and previous therapy failed?

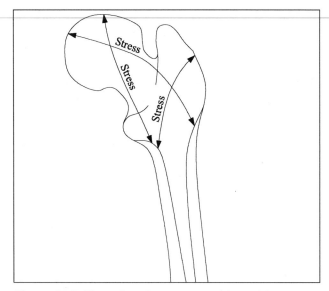

Figure 15-7. The trabecular structure of the epiphyses and metaphyses of long bones showing the transferring of stress to the cortical bone.

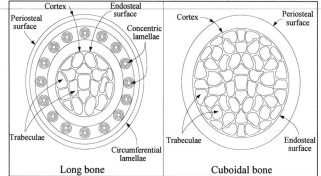

Figure 15-8. Basic structure of long bones (left) and cuboidal bones (right) in cross-section to demonstrate the relative contributions of cortical and cancellous bone.

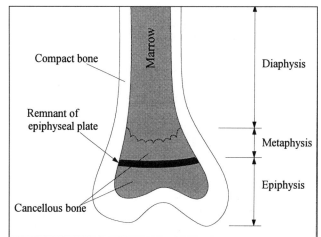

Figure 15-9. The parts of a long bone: the diaphysis, consisting of cortical bone; the metaphysis, consisting of outer cortical and inner cancellous bone; the epiphyseal plate; and the epiphysis, located at the ends of long bones with inner cancellous bone and outer cortical bone.

cation and is highly vascular and innervated. Excessive heating of the periosteum with ultrasound or diathermy will produce an exquisite periosteal pain. The periosteum often is involved in the initial healing phase of bone, forming what is called external callus to help the bone repair itself following a fracture. Cortical bone is densely packed and calcified to give a bone strength against forces of compression. Cortical bone represents 80% of bone mass, and cancellous bone, although it represents 80% of bone volume, only represents 20% of bone mass. The entire surface of bone is covered with cortical bone. Cancellous bone is found throughout bones other than long bones. It has spaces and a bony, spongelike network that serves to distribute forces to the cortical bone in a fashion that can be likened to struts or buttresses (Figure 15-7). Cancellous bone is also found in the ends of long bones, and its presence serves as the boundary between the shaft and ends of the long bone. Within the cavity of the long bone, a layer called endosteum is found. It, like the periosteum, is a connective tissue that is not ossified. The endosteum is also involved in fracture healing by producing internal callus to provide some strength until the fracture is healed. The medullary cavity of long bones is filled with bone marrow. It can be exploited to aid fracture healing by driving what is called an intramedullary rod or bone nail into it to keep fragments of long bones, such as the femur, tibia, radius, and ulna, in place during healing and allow earlier weightbearing and ambulation.

Bone is divided into three basic types: flat, cuboidal, and long bones. Flat and cuboidal bones consist of cor-

tical bone with cancellous bone throughout the inside (Figure 15-8). Cuboidal and flat bones exist primarily within the axial skeleton and the proximal bones attaching directly or indirectly to the vertebral column. Cuboidal bones include the vertebra and several bones of the wrist and ankle. The bones of the skull, ribs, scapulae, and pelvis are flat bones. In adults, the marrow of the flat bones, vertebra, and the cancellous ends of long bones are the sources of blood cells (red marrow). Long bones are generally found in the extremities.

Long bones have three parts called the diaphysis (or the shaft), the metaphysis, and the epiphysis (Figure 15-9). The bone parts are named for the area of bone that provides for increased length of long bones during growth. The physis, or growth plate, is located between the epiphysis, at each end of the bone, and the metaphysis, which is located between the growth plate and dia-physis. A typical long bone will consist, from one end to the other, of an epiphysis, metaphysis, diaphysis, meta-physis, and epiphysis along the long axis of the bone. Both the epiphysis and metaphysis are filled with cancel-lous bone. Although the length of a long bone may not increase in an adult, mechanical stresses placed on the bone cause the metabolic rate and blood flow to this area of bone to be quite high. Therefore, this area of bone is the most likely to develop cancer because of the constant growth and to become infected by bacteria car-ried in the blood.

The organic matrix produced by osteoblasts forms concentric layers called lamella around tubelike struc-tures called Haversian canals (see Figure 15-5). The osteoblasts mature and are called osteocytes. Whereas the osteoblasts are responsible for creating the organic matrix, the osteocytes direct the deposition of the calci-um salt onto the matrix. Approximately 10 days are required to form a new matrix and completely calcify the new bone. Both osteoblastic activity (deposition of matrix and mineralization) and osteoclastic activity (demineralization and destruction of matrix) occur at the surfaces of bone. Each osteocyte resides in an open-ing surrounding the Haversian canal, called a lacuna. Thus, several rings similar to rings of a tree can be seen with several lacunae within each ring. Openings in the matrix that connect lacunae are called canaliculi. Canaliculi allow the dendrites of osteocytes to physical-ly touch each other in a three-dimensional structure. The series of rings around each Haversian canal form the functional and structural unit of bone called an osteon. The cementing of osteons together forms cortical bone. Chemical signals from osteocytes recruit osteoclasts to produce reabsorption of bone; osteoblasts recruited to the same area fill in the area along the lines of stress detected by the osteocytes. Several hormones influence bone production, including growth hormone, insulin, both estrogens and androgens (male hormones), vita-min D, and several growth factors. Bone formation is inhibited by parathyroid hormone and cortisol. Resorption of bone is stimulated by parathyroid hor-mone, vitamin D, cortisol, thyroid hormone, and some mediators of inflammation. Estrogens and androgens both inhibit resorption of bone.

The ends of long bones are covered with a layer of articular cartilage, which does not appear in an x-ray. A normal joint will appear on the x-ray to have a signifi-cant gap between the two bones. This gap largely repre-sents the articular cartilage in addition to any specialized fibrocartilage, such as that of the knee. In osteoarthritis, the articular cartilage may be worn down to the actual

bone, and the gap that we expect to see will be absent, showing bone rubbing on bone.

BLOOD SUPPLY OF BONE

Bone receives a supply of blood from vessels in the periosteum, but also requires a flow of blood into the bone. Nutrient arteries enter the bone in nonarticular areas (ie, where the bone does not form a joint with an adjacent bone). In most bones, especially long bones, this is easily accomplished through nutrient foramina, which can be seen grossly. In small bones that articulate with several bones, such as the scaphoid of the wrist and navicular of the foot, the blood supply is relatively small. Fractures of these bones are often slow to heal because of this relative lack of blood flow, which can be com-pounded by damage to the nutrient arteries during the fracture. In addition to the nutrient arteries, long bones generally also have blood vessels that enter the meta-physes and epiphyses. Certain arteries, such as that entering the head of the femur, can be irreparably dam-aged during a fracture or dislocation, resulting in death of the head of the femur and causing the need to replace the hip or other joint. These areas are also often dam-aged by sickle cell disease and administration of corti-costeroids for diseases such as lupus.

DEVELOPMENT OF BONES

Flat bones of the skull develop in a different manner than long or cuboidal bones. Long bones, cuboidal bones, and flat bones outside the skull develop by a mechanism called enchondral ossification, whereas flat bones of the skull develop by a process termed mem-branous ossification. A long bone (and others) begins as a mass of cartilage in the basic shape and location of the bone. The cartilage mass is invaded by blood vessels, and the cartilage cells are destroyed and replaced with bone cells over a period of months to years. Many bones, especially the navicular of the foot, show up par-tially or not at all on x-rays at birth. One area not replaced in long bones is the epiphyseal plate. The area of cartilage called the growth plate provides the new cells that add length to long bones during development. At the age when bone length no longer increases (usu-ally late teens), the epiphyseal plates close off, and adult height is achieved.

Membranous ossification is the process by which flat bones of the head and face are created. Relatively flat membranes develop one or more centers of ossification from which spicules of bone are developed and spread to the borders of the bone. Several diseases exist in which this process occurs prematurely. The skull becomes rigid and interferes with continued brain growth. The fontanels of the skull are indicators of the progression of ossification of the skull. Premature closure of the fontanels is a red flag for one of these developmental diseases. Membranous ossification is also used to increase the thickness of all three types of bone. Long bones increase in length by enchondral ossification, but increase in thickness by membranous ossification. While bones increase in their size by membranous ossification, the bone is remodeled to remove cortical bone from the inside, thus preventing the bone from becoming too thick and heavy. In the disease osteopetrosis (condition of stonelike bone), the failure to reabsorb bone leads to thick, brittle bones without space for the bloodforming marrow.

SUMMARY

Functions of bone include physical support and protection; moving in conjunction with muscles, tendons, ligaments, and cartilage; producing blood and other immune cells; and acting as a store for calcium. Dense connective tissue consists of cells, fibers, and ground substance. Dense connective tissue responds to stresses by increasing thickness of fibers, and lack of stress leads to atrophy and disorganization of fibers. Heating and stretching of dense connective tissue can be used for remodeling or may result in injury. Bone cells described include the osteoblast, osteocyte, and osteoclast. Osteoblasts secrete the organic matrix of bone, which surrounds these cells. The osteoblasts mature into osteocytes that direct deposition of the salts that give bone its strength against compression. Osteoclasts are cells related to macrophages that remove areas of bone to allow remodeling of bone as a tissue. Bone develops and grows by the processes of membranous ossification and enchondral ossification. Bones of the face and skull develop by membranous ossification, and others develop by enchondral ossification. Long bones increase in length by enchondral ossification at the growth plate. Long bones increase in width via membranous ossification on the outer surface while osteoclasts remove bone from the inside. Other bones increase in dimensions via membranous ossification as well.

BIBLIOGRAPHY

Berne RM, Levy MN. *Physiology.* St. Louis, Mo: Mosby-Year Book; 1998.

Ganong WF. *Review of Medical Physiology.* Norwalk, Conn: Appleton & Lange; 1995.

Guyton AC, Hall JE, Schmitt W. *Human Physiology and Mechanisms of Disease.* Philadelphia, Pa: WB Saunders; 1997.

Hole JW Jr. *Essentials of Human Anatomy and Physiology.* 4th ed. Dubuque, Iowa: Wm. C. Brown Publishers; 1992.

Schauf C, Moffett D, Moffett S. *Human Physiology: Foundation and Frontiers.* St. Louis, Mo: Times Mirror/Mosby College Publishing; 1990.

Scott-Burden T. Extracellular matrix: the cellular environment. *News in Physiological Sciences.* 1994;9:110-115.

Solomon EP, Davis PW. *Human Anatomy and Physiology.* Philadelphia, Pa: WB Saunders; 1983.

Stein GS, Lian JB, Stein JL, VanWijnen AJ, Montecino M. Transcriptional control of osteoblast growth and differentiation. *Physiological Reviews.* 1996;76:593-629.

STUDY QUESTIONS

1. Why is a gap between the femur and tibia normally seen on an x-ray? What is the interpretation of an x-ray without a gap?

2. Why is it possible to rupture an Achilles' tendon when one forcefully dorsiflexes during physical activities?

3. How is it possible for an avulsion fracture (tearing of the bone at a tendinous junction) to occur?

4. Why might forceful stretching of an extremity following deep heating be imprudent?

5. What do you suspect happens to bone and dense connective tissue during prolonged periods of weightlessness?

6. How can osteoporosis be prevented?

SIXTEEN

Skeletal Muscle Structure and Function

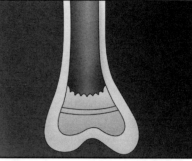

OBJECTIVES

1. Describe the relationship between muscle cell size, energy efficiency, capacity for oxidative metabolism, and speed of contraction.

2. Describe the locations of the connective tissue of the muscle: endomysium, perimysium, and epimysium.

3. Define the terms fascicle, sarcomere, and myofibril.

4. Describe the functional importance and origins of Z line, M line, H zone, A band, and I band, and describe how the different zones change during sarcomere shortening.

5. Describe the elements of the thick and thin filaments.

6. Describe the structure and function of the transverse tubules and sarcoplasmic reticulum.

7. Describe the need for the transverse tubules.

8. Describe how the sarcoplasmic reticulum alters intracellular calcium ion concentration.

9. Explain the roles of troponin and tropomyosin in excitation-contraction coupling.

10. Describe the four stages and steps of cross-bridge cycling: association, power stroke, dissociation, and return stroke.

11. Describe the functions of ATP and calcium in the cross-bridge cycle.

12. Discuss the importance of asynchronous cross-bridge cycling and the attachments of thick and thin filaments in three dimensions.

13. Explain how the sarcoplasmic reticulum produces relaxation.

14. Explain why a single twitch cannot develop much force.

OVERVIEW

Muscle acts as a transducer to convert chemical energy into mechanical energy, producing the force necessary to provide movement, support, and other mechanical functions. The function of muscle can be summarized by the equation describing force, $F = ma$. Shortening of a muscle produces a force to accelerate a mass. Muscle can be used to apply a force against another force called a load. Depending on the force produced by the muscle through its connections and the load on the muscle, shortening results in one of three processes: 1) net movement in the opposite direction of acceleration of the load, 2) a deceleration or slowing of the load in its original direction, or 3) zero acceleration if the force (or tension) of the muscle equals the force produced by the load. The third possibility is known as an isometric contraction. The three different results of muscle contraction will be addressed in Chapter Seventeen, along with the factors that determine muscle strength. Briefly, the ability of muscle to produce force depends on factors intrinsic to the muscle: its size, measured in cross-sectional area, and contractility (or contractile strength), which is measured in Newtons/cm^2 or more commonly in kg/cm^2 times the acceleration of gravity. In addition, three other factors determine muscle performance. Preload is the force placed on a muscle to stretch it before it contracts. Afterload is the load against which the muscle contracts. The third factor is the way in which muscle is attached to other structures, usually the bony lever system to which skeletal muscle is attached via tendons. These factors are also discussed in Chapter Eighteen. The steps involved between the signal from the central nervous system to contract (excitation) and contraction are known collectively as excitation-contraction coupling (E-C coupling). Most of these steps are well known at this time for skeletal muscle. E-C coupling is described in this chapter.

A factor that influences performance in a muscle that has been active is fatigue. Fatigue and the relationship between fatigue and the classification system of skeletal muscle fiber types is discussed in Chapter Eighteen. Once the function of individual muscle cells is described, the function of skeletal muscles as they act on bony lever systems is detailed in Chapter Eighteen. Chapter Eighteen also deals with sensory structures located within skeletal muscle and the reflexes with which the muscle receptors are involved. In this chapter, the focus is on the structure of muscle and the three basic classes of vertebrate muscle.

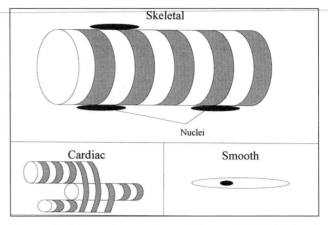

Figure 16-1. Three types of muscle fibers. Both skeletal and cardiac muscle are striated, but skeletal muscle cells are much larger in diameter and length. Skeletal muscle cells are spindle-shaped, whereas cardiac muscle cells have a stair-step appearance. Smooth muscle cells lack striations due to their different internal architecture and are much smaller than skeletal or cardiac muscle cells.

TYPES OF MUSCLE

Muscle tissue is typically categorized into three classes: skeletal muscle, cardiac muscle, and smooth muscle (Figure 16-1). All three types can then be divided into subcategories. Skeletal muscle and cardiac muscle possess internal structures that give these tissues their stereotyped striated appearance. Smooth muscle, in contrast, has an internal architecture that is not arranged linearly and is, therefore, not striated. Skeletal muscle is the type of muscle that one typically thinks of as muscle. It develops force between two bones, allowing movement of body parts. In addition, skeletal muscle may act on tissues other than bones to produce movements, such as facial expression. One property that all skeletal muscle has in common is its innervation. Each skeletal muscle cell receives a branch from a nerve cell called an α motor neuron, which is part of the somatic nervous system. Action potentials propagated along the α motor neuron signal skeletal muscle to contract. In contrast, cardiac muscle and smooth muscle are innervated by the autonomic nervous system, and muscle contraction is not determined directly by a single message from the nerve.

The three types of muscle also vary in two other basic areas: cell size and speed of contraction. The different classes of muscle and their subtypes fall systematically along a continuum of size and speed. Moreover, these two properties are related. In general, the largest cells contract the most rapidly, and the smallest cells are

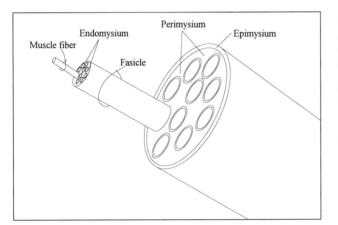

Figure 16-2. Functional units of skeletal muscle. The muscle is surrounded by a layer of connective tissue called epimysium. Within the muscle, units called fascicles are separated by connective tissue called perimysium. Individual muscle cells within each fascicle are separated by connective tissue called endomysium.

the slowest. The slower (and smaller) cells tend to be the most energy efficient. Skeletal muscle cells are the largest and contract the fastest, whereas smooth muscle cells are the smallest and slowest. Cardiac muscle cells are intermediate in size and speed as well as in some other properties that will be discussed later, such as mechanisms of E-C coupling and muscle mechanics.

SUBTYPES OF MUSCLES

Skeletal muscle cells are classified according to 1) speed of contraction into fast- and slow-twitch muscle; 2) the dominant form of metabolism for regenerating ATP into oxidative and glycolytic fibers; and 3) resistance to fatigue into fatigable and fatigue-resistance cells. Classification schemes are varied but generally identify the same subtype populations. The fatigue classification tends to be redundant when compared with the type of metabolism. Currently, the most popular type of classification of skeletal muscle is into the categories of **fast-glycolytic** muscle fibers, **fast-oxidative** muscle fibers, and **slow-oxidative** muscle fibers. The older classification terminology into type I and type IIa and IIb conveys no useful meaning and should be discarded. These subtypes are described further in Chapter Eighteen.

The heart (Chapter Nineteen) consists of cardiac muscle cells, an inside lining of endothelial cells (endocardium), a fibrous outside lining (pericardium), and fibrous tissue to separate the upper chambers (atria) from the lower chambers (ventricles). Other than the valves, inside and outside linings, and the tissue separating the upper and lower chambers, the heart is composed of cardiac muscle cells and their connective tissue

through which blood vessels and nerves travel. Cardiac muscle is subdivided into cells that are specialized for three basic functions: contraction, which accounts for 99% of the cells; pacemaking; and conduction of action potentials from cell to cell at a faster rate than cells specialized for contraction. This other 1% comprises the tissues known as the sinoatrial node, atrioventricular node, bundle of His, bundle branches, and Purkinje fibers. The last three make up what is termed the ventricular conduction system, through which action potentials are conducted in a systematic, predictable pattern.

Smooth muscle (Chapter Twenty-Eight) makes up contractile tissues other than the heart that are not usually under voluntary control. These tissues are generally associated with controlling the diameter of hollow organs, such as the digestive system, the respiratory system, the urogenital system, and blood vessels. These muscle cells are influenced by either sympathetic or parasympathetic nerves and in some cases by both, as well as circulating hormones and complex mechanisms that are beyond the scope of this book. Especially notable in the alimentary canal is a complex nervous system that controls reflexes, contains numerous neurotransmitters and hormones, and is only influenced, not controlled, by the autonomic nervous system. Smooth muscle is arbitrarily divided into single-unit and multi-unit types. Single-unit types are characterized by large groups of cells that act as a group, receive sparse autonomic innervation, but communicate extensively (usually by gap junctions) so that innervation of only a few cells alters activity of many cells. Multi-unit cells are innervated separately and do not tend to have gap junctions. Single units are found commonly in tissues such as the gastrointestinal system and small blood vessels. Multi-unit cells are found in the intrinsic eye muscles, large blood vessels, and upper airways. Smooth muscle is described more in Chapter Twenty-Eight. The remainder of this chapter will deal with skeletal muscle.

COMPONENTS OF SKELETAL MUSCLE

A typical arrangement of a skeletal muscle is shown in Figure 16-2. Muscles are divided macroscopically by dense fibrous connective tissue called perimysium into units termed fascicles. In cross-section, fascicles are obvious to the unaided eye. In turn, each fascicle is composed of several hundred to thousands of subunits separated by connective tissue called endomysium. Each subunit is an individual muscle cell or myocyte or muscle fiber. In cross-section, one can microscopically identify small fibers called myofibrils within each muscle cell. Longitudinally along muscle fibers, divisions called sarcomeres can be observed. The sarcomere is the basic functional unit of skeletal muscle cells.

MYOFIBRILS

Two types of filaments are found within skeletal muscle cells. These are termed thick and thin filaments. The filaments are arranged in a regular pattern with a well-described structure and consist of several proteins. Within each myocyte, these filaments are packaged into highly regular bundles called myofibrils. The space between these bundles allows room for structures and supplies to maintain myofibril function, including tubular structures (described below), mitochondria, glycogen, and fat droplets. Looking at the cross-section of a myocyte microscopically, one can see that each thick filament is surrounded by six thin filaments, and each thin filament is surrounded by three thick filaments. It is the sum of the small forces produced by the interaction of the millions to billions of thick and thin filaments that results in the force transmitted from the muscle to the skeleton that translates into movement.

SARCOMERES

Looking at the skeletal muscle cells longitudinally, instead of in cross-section, the characteristic banding pattern from which the term striated muscle originated becomes obvious. Note that both skeletal and cardiac muscles are striated. They are both striated because they share the same basic organization of myofibrils into sarcomeres. Although smooth muscle shares many of the same functional contractile elements, it does not appear striated because of a different intracellular organization of the myofibrils. Along the striated muscle fiber, a regular pattern of dark and light areas appears (Figure 16-3). At the center of each dark band, a short, lighter area can be observed with a line in its center. At the center of each light band, a dark line is apparent.

Striations are produced by presence of what are termed A and I bands and H zones. The regular pattern of light and dark areas are the result of the regular organization of the thick and thin filaments, in a longitudinal manner. In addition to being the functional unit of the skeletal muscle fiber, the sarcomere is a repeating unit 2 to 3 μm long that runs the length of a skeletal (or cardiac) muscle cell.

The sarcomere is defined as that area within the cell membrane between two Z lines. Z lines are the dark lines observed in the middle of the light bands. The light bands are termed I bands for isotropic in contrast to the darker A bands or anisotropic bands. Because Z lines serve as the boundary for a sarcomere and because Z lines are found in the center of the I band (light band), I bands extend from a point about halfway to the center of one sarcomere in a resting cell to about halfway toward the center of the next sarcomere. A bands are darker, not only because thick filaments are found in the A bands, but also because thin filaments extend from the Z line and overlap in this region of the sarcomere. A lighter area within the A band, called the H zone, exists because, in a resting muscle, thin filaments do not extend to the center of the sarcomere. Between the ends of the thin filaments extending from one Z line and those from the other Z line, no overlap of thick and thin filaments occurs; therefore, the lighter H zone can be detected.

The Z lines have a function beyond marking the ends of the sarcomeres. This dense area serves to anchor the thin filaments together and maintain the spatial relationship among the thin filaments. A similar function is performed by the M line in the A band. Thick filaments are anchored in the center of the sarcomere. The size of the A band is determined by the area occupied by the thick filaments; therefore, the size of the A band remains constant. However, two areas may exist in which only one filament is found (ie, no overlap of thick and thin filaments). The lighter area in the center of the A band, known as the H zone, consists of only thick filaments without the overlapping thin filaments; the I band consists of thin filaments only. When a muscle contracts, thin filaments are pulled across thick filaments, resulting in an increased overlap of thick and thin filaments. When this occurs, the distance between the end of the thick filaments and the Z line decreases, and the distance between thin filaments originating from either end of the sarcomere decreases. In other words, although the A band does not change in size during muscle contraction, the I band and H zone decrease in length as the thick filaments pull thin filaments toward the center of each sarcomere. As this process occurs, Z lines are pulled closer to each other, and the entire muscle shortens. The details of this process are discussed in the following chapter.

CONNECTIVE TISSUE ELEMENTS

Connective tissue serves to couple the force generated by sarcomere shortening into force applied to the bony lever system of the skeleton. Between each muscle cell, or fiber, a network of connective tissue called endomysium serves to transmit force developed by one cell to the neighboring cells. A large group of cells, termed a fascicle, is enclosed by connective tissue that transmits force among fascicles. This tissue is given the

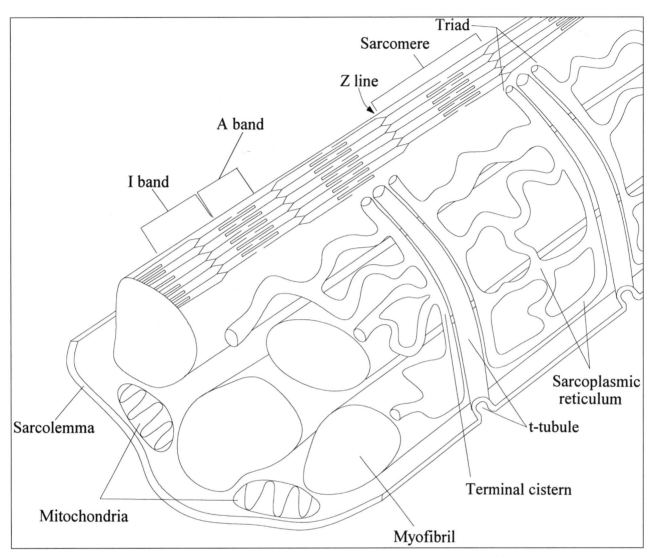

Figure 16-3. The internal structure of a skeletal muscle cell. The striations (light and dark bands) are produced by a regular pattern of overlapping filaments within the muscle fibers. Also diagramed are the components of the tubular system, the t-tubules, and sarcoplasmic reticulum, which act together to cause contraction and relaxation of the muscle cells.

name perimysium. A third level of connective tissue serves to bind the entire muscle and to transmit force developed by the muscle to the tendons, which in turn transmit force to bones. This tissue is given the name epimysium.

These tissues are important for two primary reasons. First, they hold the cells together in an organized manner to allow the shortening of sarcomeres to pull on an elastic tissue that eventually pulls on bones. Secondly, this connective tissue provides space for blood vessels and nerves to tunnel through to individual muscle fibers. The role of the connective tissue in transmitting force from sarcomere to bone will be discussed in Chapter Seventeen.

ARCHITECTURE OF THE SARCOMERE

Although actin and myosin are the primary components of the thick and thin filaments, these filaments consist of several proteins. The proteins responsible for the shortening of sarcomeres are myosin in the thick filaments and actin in the thin filaments. Actin is a very common structural protein, found in many places besides muscle cells. The **thin filament** is approximately 1 μm long and consists of three proteins that regulate muscle function, which will be discussed below. **Thick filaments** are somewhat long, about 1.5 μm, and consist primarily of the protein myosin. **Myosin** has a shape

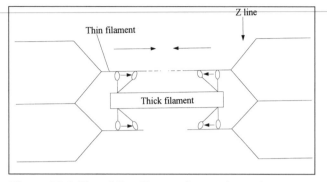

Figure 16-4. The sliding filament theory of muscle contraction. Attachment of thick filaments to the thin filaments causes a change in the shape of the myosin molecule that results in the thin filament being pulled toward the center of the thick filament and the movement of Z lines closer to each other.

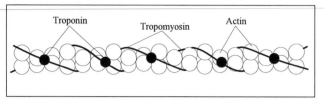

Figure 16-5. The components of the thin filament. A double helix of actin molecules has a thread of tropomyosin running through the groove in the helix and preventing myosin heads from attaching to binding sites on the actin molecules. Troponin molecules are located at regular intervals along the thread of tropomyosin.

that is often likened to that of a golf club. Myosin molecules aggregate with the handles, forming the rod-like thick filament, with globular heads protruding from the thick filament and oriented toward either Z line with a "bald-spot" in the center of the A band at which no globular heads are located. Also found on the globular head of the myosin molecule is the enzyme myosin ATPase. This enzyme is responsible for degrading ATP to ADP to provide the energy necessary for the chemical reactions that culminate sarcomere shortening. In Chapter Eighteen, differences in the properties of myosin ATPase in different types of muscle fibers will be discussed.

Anchoring of thick and thin filaments occurs at the M line and Z line, respectively. The presence of the M and Z lines is critical to muscle function. The pulling of thin filaments across thick filaments results in shortening of sarcomeres and production of force by skeletal muscle. If thick and thin filaments were free to move about within muscle cells, no net force could be generated. Muscle cells are designed to pull two adjacent Z lines closer to each other (Figure 16-4). This pulling is accomplished indirectly by pulling thin filaments toward the center of the sarcomere. Thin filaments serve as handles for the thick filaments to pull Z lines toward the center of sarcomeres from both ends, resulting in a shorter, thicker sarcomere. At the same time, thin filaments on the other side of the same Z lines are pulled in the opposite direction.

The result of thousands of Z lines being pulled in opposite directions is that all Z lines are pulled toward whatever end of the muscle is fixed and away from that end of the muscle that is free to move. If both ends of a muscle are fixed (isometric contraction), then both ends of the muscle move toward the center of the entire mus-

cle. The M line of the A band serves a similar function for thick filaments. It binds thick filaments together in the center of the sarcomere. Therefore, Z lines are pulled toward M lines. M lines must withstand the force developed by actin and myosin interaction to allow sarcomere shortening, just as a pulley bolted to an overhead beam must support the force that moves the load attached to the pulley.

ELEMENTS OF THE THIN FILAMENT

The structure of the thin filament is more complex than that of the thick filament (Figure 16-5). Thin filaments are composed of globular proteins called g-actin. G-actin then aggregates into a double helix filament called f-actin. The thin filament, about 1 µm long, runs from near the center of one sarcomere, through the Z line, and toward the center of the adjacent sarcomere. A second protein, tropomyosin, is found in the cleft formed by the double helix arrangement of the actin molecules. Under resting conditions, tropomyosin covers a site to which myosin can bind, thereby preventing muscle contraction. At regular intervals along the tropomyosin molecule is a third protein of the thin filament termed troponin. Troponin has three parts, one of which is a binding site for Ca^{++}. The other two parts of troponin interact with the Ca^{++} binding site to displace tropomyosin from the actin-binding site when Ca^{++} is bound to troponin. Ca^{++} is the signal for muscle contraction; troponin is the regulatory protein for muscle contraction; and tropomyosin is the molecule that is responsible for preventing muscle contraction from occurring until sufficient Ca^{++} is present within the muscle fiber cytoplasm (sarcoplasm). The steps are depicted in Figure 16-6.

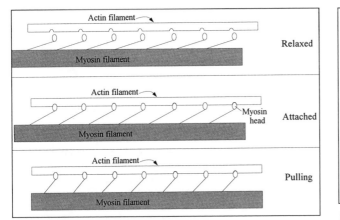

Figure 16-6. The events of Figure 16-4 are shown in sequence.

THE SARCOPLASMIC RETICULUM AND T TUBULES

The cytoplasm or intracellular fluid space of a skeletal muscle cell is also called the sarcoplasm. Within this space, a network of tubules called the sarcoplasmic reticulum is located beneath the cell membrane and surrounding the myofibrils. The sarcoplasmic reticulum uses ATP to remove Ca^{++} from the sarcoplasm actively, but also can be stimulated to release Ca^{++}, thereby permitting muscle contraction. Therefore, the sarcoplasmic reticulum (SR) functions actively to take up, store, and, when signaled, release Ca^{++}.

The SR is composed of a series of sac-like structures that store Ca^{++}. These sac-like areas are in close proximity to another structure of the muscle cell, the t-tubule. T-tubules are continuous with the cell membrane and, when viewed from directly above, appear as tunnels into the cell. T-tubules, being continuous with the cell membrane, also depolarize when an action potential is propagated along the membrane. It is thought that t-tubules function to carry the electric signal for muscle contraction through the relatively thick skeletal muscle fiber to the sarcoplasmic reticulum.

EXCITATION-CONTRACTION COUPLING

The signal for skeletal muscle cells to contract was discussed in Chapter Ten. Briefly, an action potential of the α motor neuron innervating a skeletal muscle cell causes release of acetylcholine onto the motor end plate, which, in turn, causes an action potential to be propagated along the muscle cell membrane. The series of events that occur, beginning with depolarization of the myocyte membrane and leading to sarcomere shortening, is termed **excitation-contraction coupling** (E-C coupling). E-C coupling can be divided into five stages: 1) propagation of an action potential along the muscle

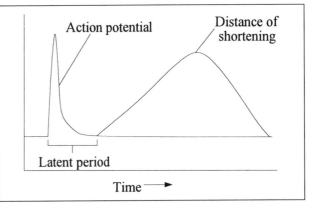

Figure 16-7. The signal for muscle contraction (the action potential) and the mechanical event (contraction) are plotted on the same graph to show the temporal relationship. The time between generation of the action potential on the membrane of the muscle cell and the actual shortening of muscle cells is called the latent period. Factors influencing the latent period are discussed later in the text.

cell membrane and t-tubules; 2) release of Ca^{++} from the sarcoplasmic reticulum (SR); 3) cross-bridge cycling, the series of steps during which sarcomere shortening occurs (it is called cross-bridge cycling because myosin forms a **cross-bridge** with actin); 4) reuptake of Ca^{++} by the SR; and 5) relaxation. Cardiac muscle E-C coupling shares most of the same steps as skeletal muscle and will be described in Chapter Twenty. Smooth muscle E-C coupling is varied and complex and is described separately in Chapter Twenty-Eight.

Depolarization of the cell membrane and t-tubules may be termed excitation. Membrane depolarization is the signal to allow actin and myosin to interact. Binding of acetylcholine to specific receptors located at the motor end plate culminates in interaction between actin and myosin molecules, which then produces muscle shortening, or contraction (Figure 16-7). An action potential is propagated in all directions from the motor endplate along the muscle cell membrane. The t-tubule, which appears as an invagination in the surface of the membrane, is continuous with the membrane and conducts the wave of depolarization toward the interior of the muscle cell. Depolarization of the t-tubule has been found to be the critical step in the entire process of E-C coupling in skeletal muscle.

Using a fine glass micropipet that can carry a depolarizing current, one can demonstrate that depolarization of the t-tubule is necessary and sufficient for sarcomere shortening. In mammalian resting skeletal muscle cells, t-tubules are located at the junction of the A and I bands (the farthest point toward the end of the sarcomere that the thick filament extends). Only when the glass pipet is located at the A-I junction does contraction occur. A strong contraction is produced in the half-sarcomere beneath the membrane, and a weak contraction occurs in the other half. We may conclude from this type of experiment that depolarization of the t-tubule is the event that directly leads to the next step of E-C coupling.

RELEASE OF CA⁺⁺ FROM THE SARCOPLASMIC RETICULUM

The t-tubule makes specialized contact with the sarcoplasmic reticulum. On either side of the t-tubule, lateral sacs of two networks of SR are found. This arrangement is commonly referred to as a triad. The SR actively transports Ca^{++} from the cytoplasm, sequestering it so that in a resting muscle cell, cytoplasmic Ca^{++} concentration is approximately 1/10,000 of the extracellular Ca^{++} concentration (less than 10^{-7} M). The portion of the SR making intimate contact with the t-tubule is called the lateral sac or terminal cisterna of the SR. This appears to be the site of Ca^{++} storage within the SR when the cell membrane is at its resting potential. When t-tubules are depolarized, calcium ions enter the cell through surface channels. These calcium ions activate receptors within the SR called Ryanodine receptors. Ryanodine receptors are similar to IP3 receptors described in Chapter Five, but cause much more rapid opening of calcium ion channels than IP3, which is critical to skeletal muscle functions. Calcium ions then rapidly enter the sarcoplasmic space to signal actin-myosin interaction. In skeletal muscle, sufficient Ca^{++} is released with every action potential so that virtually all troponin molecules bind Ca^{++}, allowing all myosin molecules to bind to actin. In contrast, in cardiac muscle, not all myosin heads are normally able to bind to actin following membrane depolarization. Instead, intracellular Ca^{++} concentration of cardiac muscle cells can be regulated to vary force developed by the heart. The binding of Ca^{++} released by the SR to troponin begins the process termed cross-bridge cycling. These processes by which calcium ions signal release of Ca^{++} from the SR (calcium-induced calcium release) has been known for many years in cardiac muscle cells and is described more fully in Chapter Twenty.

Cross-bridge cycling, as the name implies, is a series of steps repeated sequentially with no beginning or end. Cross-bridge cycling, once started, will continue under two conditions: 1) sufficient cytoplasmic Ca^{++} to bind to troponin and 2) ATP remains available. The release of Ca^{++} from the SR allows cross-bridge cycling to begin. Removal of Ca^{++} by active transport back into the SR

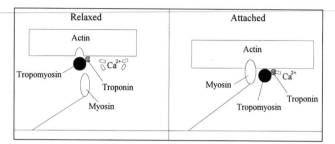

Figure 16-8. The permissive role of intracellular calcium ions in muscle contraction. As Ca^{++} concentration rises, the probability of binding of Ca^{++} to troponin increases to the point that near saturation of troponin occurs. Binding of Ca^{++} to troponin changes the shape of tropomyosin and allows the myosin heads to have access to binding sites on actin, thereby initiating muscle contraction.

stops cross-bridge cycling. Actin, located on the thin filament, has a specific site to which myosin, located in the thick filament, can bind. At rest, the protein tropomyosin, also located on the thin filament, interferes with binding of myosin molecules of the thick filament with actin of the thin filament. A third protein of the thin filament, troponin, changes its shape when Ca^{++} binds to it. The shape change of troponin then, in turn, moves tropomyosin away from the actin binding site, thereby allowing cross-bridge cycling to occur.

At rest, with a Ca^{++} concentration less than 10^{-7} M, the probability of a Ca^{++} ion binding with troponin is so small that, at any given time, very few cross-bridges can cycle, and no meaningful force is generated by the muscle cell. However, when a muscle cell is depolarized and the SR releases large quantities of Ca^{++}, Ca^{++} concentration increases to greater than 10^{-5} M. At this concentration, the probability of a Ca^{++} ion not being located on every troponin molecule is very low. When Ca^{++} is at a saturating level, every time a Ca^{++} ion comes off troponin, another Ca^{++} ion binds to troponin almost immediately. While troponin is saturated, all actin-binding sites on the thin filaments are available to be bound by myosin heads to generate force. As Ca^{++} is taken up by the SR and sarcoplasmic Ca^{++} concentration falls, the probability of troponin having a calcium ion on it diminishes toward zero (Figure 16-8).

CROSS-BRIDGE CYCLING

During the time that troponin molecules are saturated by Ca^{++}, the four events of cross-bridge cycling are repeated (the events are depicted in Figure 16-9):

1. Myosin heads attach to actin molecules to form a cross bridge.

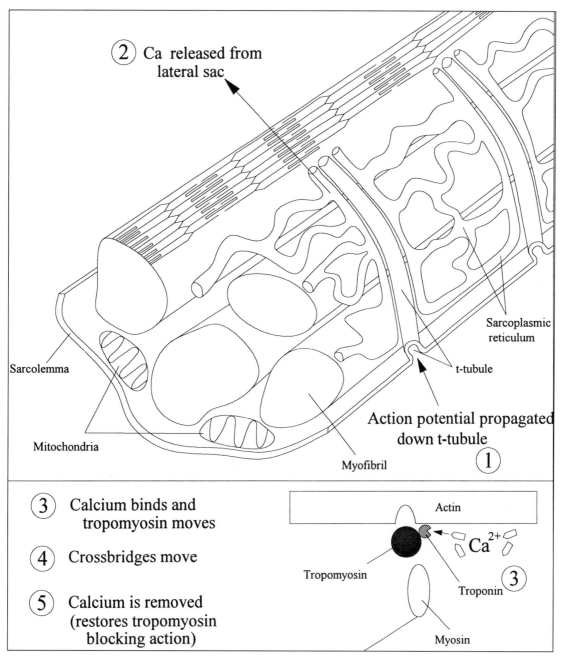

(2) Ca released from
lateral sac

Sarcoplasmic
reticulum

Sarcolemma

t-tubule

Action potential propagated
down t-tubule

Mitochondria

(1)

Myofibril

(3) Calcium binds and
tropomyosin moves

Actin

(4) Crossbridges move

Ca^{2+}

Tropomyosin

Troponin (3)

(5) Calcium is removed
(restores tropomyosin
blocking action)

Myosin

Figure 16-9. The sequence of events of the cross-bridge cycle.

2. Myosin changes its shape to pull actin molecules and, therefore, thin filaments toward the center of the sarcomere, producing the power stroke of the cycle.
3. Cross-bridges with actin are broken.
4. ATP is broken down into ADP + P_i to return myosin to the activated shape it had prior to its interaction with actin, producing the return stroke of the cycle.

After using ATP, each active cross-bridge can attach to and pull a thin filament at a new location closer to the Z line. With each cross-bridge cycle, the Z lines of each end of each sarcomere are pulled closer together.

Myosin molecules are not synchronized with each other, but operate independently of each other in an asynchronous manner. Synchronization cannot occur because of the requirement of binding of Ca++ to troponin. Ca++ does not remain permanently attached to troponin. Instead, these ions constantly bind and detach and other ions bind to the same sites. This movement of Ca^{++} ions prevents all actin-binding sites from becoming available to myosin cross-bridges at the same time. Therefore, different myosin molecules exist at different stages of the cross-bridge cycle at any given time. This asynchronous nature of cross-bridge cycling prevents the slippage of thin filaments between power strokes. As some myosin molecules pull a given thin filament, other myosin molecules are either detaching, performing a return stroke, or attaching to a more distant site on the same thin filament. This can be accomplished because each thick filament is surrounded by six thin filaments and each thin filament is surrounded by three thick filaments. Therefore, each thin filament is simultaneously pulled by three different thick filaments, and each thick filament pulls on six different thin filaments at the same time. This asynchronous movement can be likened to a tug-of-war. If all the members of one team were to release the rope to change their grips to new locations on the rope, the rope would rapidly slip away. The asynchronous nature of cross-bridge cycling also requires spring-like properties to exist within the cross bridge formed between myosin and actin molecules.

BREAKING CROSS-BRIDGES

The role of ATP in cross-bridge cycling is often misunderstood. Intuitively, one might suspect that energy is used in the step of cross-bridge cycling during which sarcomere shortening occurs and that the source of this energy is ATP. Energy is used indirectly from ATP to produce the pulling action of thick filaments on the thin filaments; ATP is actually used in the step prior to shortening. As discussed in Chapter Three, ATP is used to alter the structure of proteins by placing a strongly negative group onto a protein. In the case of cross-bridge cycling, ATP is used to alter the shape of myosin to perform the return stroke of the cross-bridge. The binding of myosin to actin then unleashes the chemical force stored in the myosin molecule by the use of ATP to perform the "power stroke" of cross-bridge cycling. The hydrolysis of ATP to ADP + P_i can be thought of as "energizing" the myosin molecule, giving it the potential energy to pull actin toward the center of the sarcomere as soon as actin and myosin bind. Binding of a fresh ATP molecule to myosin is required for myosin to detach from actin so that the cycle can continue.

If ATP levels fall low enough, the cycle stops before cross-bridges are broken following the power stroke. Completion of the power stroke in which actin is bound to myosin in the shortened position produces what is called a rigor complex. When muscle cells die, they release Ca^{++}, allowing the cross-bridge cycle to begin. Myosin binds to actin, thin filaments are pulled toward the center of the sarcomere, but there is no ATP to bind to myosin ATPase to allow detachment of cross-bridges from the thin filaments. This causes the muscle stiffness observed some time after death. When this condition occurs, it is termed rigor mortis.

UPTAKE OF Ca^{++} BY THE SARCOPLASMIC RETICULUM

In addition to the roles of the SR in Ca^{++} storage and release, the SR actively removes Ca^{++} from the cytoplasm for storage in the terminal cisternae. This Ca^{++} is technically within the cell membrane, but is sequestered outside the sarcoplasmic space, so it cannot interact with the myofilaments. Active transport of Ca^{++} into the SR also requires ATP. Shortly after the release of Ca^{++} that follows membrane depolarization, the SR begins to take Ca^{++} back up, thereby reducing cytoplasmic Ca^{++} concentration back to its resting level. As the SR takes up Ca^{++}, the probability of Ca^{++} being bound to each troponin molecule decreases. As fewer troponin molecules have Ca^{++} bound to them, fewer cross-bridges can be formed between actin on the thin filament, and fewer cross-bridge cycles can occur. As reaccumulation of Ca^{++} occurs, less force is developed by sarcomeres until the cell is returned to its resting state. The process by which the number of active cross-bridges decreases with time after an action potential is called relaxation. For the same reason, force builds steadily as Ca^{++} is released and more cross-bridges become active.

RELAXATION

Relaxation occurs due to the reaccumulation of Ca^{++} by the SR. A single action potential produces an event called a twitch, or clonic contraction. Although the action potential may last only 1 to 2 ms on the surface of the muscle cell, the events that produce a twitch may last from 50 to 250 ms, depending on the type of muscle cell (see Figure 16-7). Fast twitch muscle cells may go through the steps of excitation-contraction coupling back to relaxation within 50 ms, whereas cardiac muscle cells may require 250 ms. The length of the twitch is determined primarily by the rate at which Ca^{++} is taken up by the SR, whereas the rate at which the cross-bridge cycle occurs is determined by the enzyme myosin ATPase, which breaks down ATP to ADP and inorganic phosphate. Both the rate of cross-bridge cycling and the duration of the twitch are related to muscle cell size. Cross-bridge cycling in fast twitch muscle is faster than it is in slow twitch or cardiac muscle, and a twitch is completed faster as well.

Relaxation is not part of the cross-bridge cycle, but results from the gradual decrease in the number of myosin molecules involved in cross-bridge cycling. Ca^{++} ions release and bind to troponin constantly, without regard for any specific steps involved in E-C coupling or cross-bridge cycling. What changes is the concentration of Ca^{++} in the cytoplasm. As Ca^{++} concentration increases, the probability of Ca^{++} being bound to troponin increases, more cross-bridges can cycle, and force produced by the muscle increases. As the SR reaccumulates Ca^{++}, the probability that Ca^{++} will be bound to troponin decreases, the number of cross-bridges cycling decreases, and the force produced by a muscle decreases.

FORCE DEVELOPED BY A TWITCH

When thick filaments begin pulling thin filaments toward the center of the sarcomere, force is not instantaneously developed throughout the muscle's connective tissue and transmitted to the bony levers. Force increases with time as the muscle cells shorten and elastic components of the muscle tissue are stretched, much as a rubber band attached to a weight is stretched before the weight is lifted. In human muscle stimulated to produce a single action potential and thereby producing a twitch, relaxation occurs before maximum force can be developed. For this reason, a muscle cannot transmit all of the force that it is capable of generating during a single twitch, developing only about one-third of the force of a physiologic contraction. This concept is discussed in more detail in Chapter Seventeen.

SUMMARY

Muscle tissue acts as a transducer to convert chemical energy into useful force. Factors that determine muscle performance are called preload, afterload, and contractile state. The way that skeletal muscles are attached to the skeleton also determines muscle performance. Muscle may be divided into skeletal muscle, cardiac muscle, and smooth muscle. Each type may then be divided further into subtypes. Skeletal muscle is the largest, fastest, and least energy-efficient. As a general rule within all types and subtypes of muscle, the larger the cell, the faster the contraction speed, and the less energy-efficient it is. Skeletal muscle is classified into three categories according to speed of contraction and

the predominant form of metabolism: slow-oxidative, fast-oxidative, and fast-glycolytic fibers.

Skeletal muscle is given its characteristic striated appearance because of the physical arrangement of the myofibrils, which are made of the proteins actin and myosin. Skeletal muscle and cardiac muscle cells consist of functional units called sarcomeres. A sarcomere extends from one Z line to another. The striations are produced by the presence of A and I bands and H zones that are the result of how the thick and thin filaments overlap. When muscle contracts, the overlap of thick and thin filaments increases, and Z lines are brought closer to each other.

Connective tissue elements between the muscle cells transmit force to the skeleton to perform useful muscle activity. The sarcoplasmic reticulum and t-tubules are responsible for the process called excitation-contraction coupling. The sarcoplasmic reticulum stores Ca^{++}, releases it when the t-tubules are depolarized, and takes Ca^{++} back up to produce relaxation. Excitation-contraction coupling is the series of steps that occur between depolarization of the muscle cell membrane and the generation of force. E-C coupling consists of five steps: membrane depolarization, release of Ca^{++} by the SR, cross-bridge cycling, reuptake of Ca^{++} by the SR, and relaxation. Depolarization of the cell membrane is carried deep into the cell via the t-tubule. Depolarization of the t-tubule produces release of Ca^{++} by the SR. Binding of Ca^{++} to troponin on the thin filament allows energy stored in myosin molecules by the hydrolysis of ATP to be used once myosin contacts actin. At rest, actin cannot bind to myosin because of the presence of tropomyosin blocking the actin-binding site. Binding of Ca^{++} to troponin physically moves tropomyosin out of the way and allows myosin to bind to actin. Binding of myosin to actin, then results in shortening of the muscle cell. Shortly after the SR releases Ca^{++}, it immediately begins to take up Ca^{++}. As Ca^{++} is taken up by the SR, fewer interactions between actin and myosin can take place, and the muscle begins to relax.

BIBLIOGRAPHY

Booth FW, Tseng BS. Olympic goal: molecular and cellular approaches to understanding muscle adaptation. *News in Physiological Sciences.* 1993;8:165-169.

Cecchi G, Bagni MA. Myofilament lattice spacing affects tension in striated muscle. *News in Physiological Sciences.* 1994;9:3-7.

Cooke R. Actomyosin interaction in striated muscle. *Physiological Reviews.* 1997;77:671-697.

Cope TC, Pinter MJ. The size principle: still working after all these years. *News in Physiological Sciences.* 1995;10:280-286.

Fitts RH. Cellular mechanism of muscle fatigue. *Physiological Reviews*. 1994;74:49-94.

Franzini-Armstrong C, Protasi F. Ryanodine receptors of striated muscle: a complex channel capable of multiple interactions. *Physiological Reviews*. 1997;77:699-729.

Fuchs F. Mechanical modulation of the calcium regulatory protein complex in cardiac muscle. *News in Physiological Sciences*. 1995;10:6-12.

Grinnell AD. Dynamics of nerve-muscle interaction in developing and mature neuromuscular junctions. *Physiological Reviews*. 1995;75:789-834.

Marder E, Calabrese RL. Principles of rhythmic motor pattern generation. *Physiological Reviews*. 1996;76:687-717.

Millman BM. The filament lattice of striated muscle. *Physiological Reviews*. 1998;78:359-391.

Proske U. The mammalian muscle spindle. *News in Physiological Sciences*. 1997;12:37-42.

Rette D, Staron RS. The molecular diversity of mammalian muscle fibers. *News in Physiological Sciences*. 1993;8:153-157.

Shulman GI, Landau BR. Pathways of glycogen repletion. *Physiological Reviews*. 1992;72:1019-1035.

Weiss P, Jeannerod M. Getting a grasp on coordination. *News in Physiological Sciences*. 1998;13:70-75.

STUDY QUESTIONS

1. Describe the relationship between muscle cell size and
   a. Speed of contraction
   b. Capillary blood supply
   c. Energy efficiency
   d. Fatiguability

2. Identify components of muscle and associated functions:
   a. Whole muscle, tendon, and epimysium
   b. Fascicle, neurovascular structures, and perimysium
   c. Myocyte, capillaries, and endomysium

3. Identify components of sarcomeres and their functions:
   a. Thin filament
   b. Z line
   c. Thick filament
   d. M line

4. Explain the origin of the A, I, and H bands.

5. When muscle contracts, what happens to the size of the A, I, and H bands?

6. Identify the components of the thin filament (actin, tropomyosin, troponin). What functions do they perform?

7. Identify the components of the tubular system (transverse tubules and sarcoplasmic reticulum). Describe their functions.

LABORATORY EXERCISE

LABORATORY EXERCISE 16-1

NEUROMUSCULAR ELECTRICAL STIMULATION (NMES)

NMES is electrical stimulation of skeletal muscle via intact motor neurons in contrast to electrical muscle stimulation (EMS) performed on denervated muscle.

Normal voluntary muscle contractions are intermittent tetanic contractions with asynchronous recruitment of different motor units. A motor unit is a motor neuron and all of the muscle cells innervated by that motor neuron. NMES produces synchronous recruitment of motor units. Which neurons are recruited by the NMES devices (or any other transcutaneous devices including TENS) depends on the size of the neuron and the distance from the skin. Recruitment of fibers with transcutaneous current depends on the electrical properties of different classes of neurons. The amount of current that enters different neurons is directly related to the surface area of their axons within the peripheral nerves. Neurons with large diameter axons are recruited first; small unmyelinated neurons, such as pain and temperature sensory neurons, and sympathetic neurons are last to be recruited.

This principle is directly opposite of the size principle of recruiting motor neurons, in which a small neuron with a low conductance will be recruited before a large neuron with a high conductance for the same amount of synaptic input. As amplitude is increased, the large cutaneous sensory fibers are recruited first. This level of amplitude is called the sensory level. With increasing amplitude, more distant and smaller neurons are recruited. Because the electrodes are placed on the skin, the first neurons to be depolarized by the current produced by the stimulator will be the mechanoreceptors of the skin, even though these fibers are somewhat smaller than the farther motor neurons. The first motor neurons to be recruited will be the largest, most fatigable neurons. This level of amplitude is called a low motor level of stimulation. The last motor neurons recruited by NMES are those recruited first voluntarily and are the most fatigue-resistant. Recruitment of all of the motor neurons deep below the skin may require sufficient current to recruit nociceptive fibers near the skin's surface. Therefore, the intensity required to recruit maximum strength of contraction is usually at a noxious level of stimulation.

To avoid recruitment of unwanted neurons, try to find a place over the muscle of interest at which the least amount of current is required. This area is called the motor point. This point is usually the location at which the nerve enters the muscle. Strength of contraction can be increased by increasing amplitude (current), duration, or frequency. Other ways include moving the electrodes farther apart to force the current deeper into the muscle and using smaller electrodes to increase the current density (current per surface area of the electrode).

Preparation:
1. Self-adhesive electrodes ("stick-ons") are reusable for some time. They must be moistened and stored in an airtight bag when finished. Skin must be prepared with alcohol. Stick-ons are very convenient. No straps or tape are needed. They can be cut to fit different areas. These electrodes will wear out with time and become uncomfortable.

2. Sponge electrodes need to be moistened before use and wrung out and allowed to dry following use to prevent mildew. Plastic covers of two electrodes may touch each other. The skin does not have to be prepared with alcohol. Sponges need to be snug to have good contact,

but do not cut off blood flow. Sponge electrodes can be awkward to apply. Sponges also present a hygiene problem. Some facilities that use sponge electrodes store them in warm antibiotic solution.

3. Carbonized rubber electrodes require electrode gel, but can be moved around over the skin surface to find optimum location. They need to be taped in place once the proper location is found.

4. Do not apply on skin that has been recently shaved. Nicked skin will conduct a current better than intact skin.

5. Be sure the amplitude is set to zero before starting and before changing parameters to any extent.

Amplitude:
1. Sensory—patient can only feel stimulus.

2. Motor—higher intensity, patient can feel and muscle movement can be seen or felt.

3. Noxious—unpleasant feeling at higher intensity, produces strong motor response.

Frequency (rate):
- 1 to 10 Hz produces a series of muscle twitches (clonic contractions).
- 10 to 25 Hz produces an unfused tetanic contraction (treppe), which is a shuddering type of movement. Treppe continues until the stimulator is turned off.
- >25 Hz produces one sustained tetanic contraction until the stimulator is turned off or severe fatigue occurs.

These numbers may vary depending on the muscle used and the individual patient and serve only as a guideline for where to start. Rate should be set to evoke the desired response (type of contraction), and not to some arbitrary frequency. As a general rule, small muscles, such as those of the hand and forearm tend to fuse into tetanic contractions at low rates and large muscles such as the quadriceps may require a frequency as great as 50 Hz to produce a tetanic contraction.

Ramp/surge modulation: Current is stopped and started.

NMES devices can be set to stimulate for a time (on time) and allow a rest period (off time).

Surge: A number of pulses determined by the frequency and on time (eg, frequency = 25 Hz, on time = 2 s; surge consists of 50 pulses).

Ramp: To increase comfort, pulse amplitude or duration is gradually increased (ramp up) at the beginning of a surge and gradually decreased at the end of a surge (ramp down). Different devices allow differing amounts of control over the ramp up and ramp down. Technically, the on time is only the time during which current amplitude and duration are constant. However, on many NMES devices the on time set actually includes on time, ramp up, and ramp down.

LABORATORY EXERCISE

Use of on time : off time ratio

- 1:5 does not fatigue muscle
- 1:4 produces some fatigue
- 1:3 is commonly used in the clinic; patient should be able to maintain for 30 to 60 minutes
- 1:1 will cause rapid fatigue

Electrode placement:
Electrode placement can be performed in various ways depending on the muscle and response desired.
1. Two equally sized electrodes over the muscle of interest.

2. One electrode over each of a pair of synergistic muscles (eg, deltoid and supraspinatus)

3. Smaller, active electrode over muscle of interest, larger inactive (or dispersive) electrode over a nonmuscular area on same side of body.

4. The closer and smaller the electrodes, the more superficial the current.

5. The larger and farther apart the electrodes, the deeper the current.

Generic instructions:
1. Plug in or check batteries.

2. Turn amplitude to zero or off.

3. Find appropriate electrodes.

4. Prepare appropriate site.

5. Plug leads into electrodes and NMES device.

6. Some devices have a "constant" button. Hold in to set amplitude, frequency, and duration if applicable without waiting for device to cycle back to on time.

7. Set rate (frequency), amplitude (intensity or current), duration (pulse width) to appropriate values. Not all devices allow duration to be adjusted.

8. Set ramp up and ramp down if applicable.

9. Set surge frequency if using intermittent tetanic stimulation.

10. Do not change amplitude during off time.

Clinical uses of NMES:
1. Increase blood flow to an area. One may use individual twitches (clonic contractions), unfused tetanic contractions (treppe), or intermittent tetanic contractions. Unfused tetanic contractions may be the most effective.

2. Decrease muscle spasm by using any of the three types of contraction in #1. Constant tetanic contraction will produce fatigue the most rapidly, but unfused tetanic contractions may be the most effective.

LABORATORY EXERCISE

3. Intermittent tetanic contractions are used for:
    a. Facilitating a normal but denervated muscle
    b. Muscle reeducation
    c. Muscle strengthening
    d. Maintaining or increasing range of motion

Synchronous vs. reciprocal:
Synchronous refers to using same parameters on two leads simultaneously. This may be used on large muscles, muscle groups, or on synergists. Reciprocal refers to switching between leads so that the on time of one channel is the off time of the other. A few NMES devices are designed so that a rest period during which neither channel is active can be obtained. Most devices simply switch in such a way that when one channel is on, the other is off, which gives a 1:1 ratio of on time to off time. This ratio is very fatiguing.
The VMS II, Myocare, and Respond Select can be set for a rest period between contractions. The reciprocal mode is useful for range of motion and muscle reeducation of antagonists. VMS II: set on time for both channels and off time between each channel. Myocare: set on time for each channel and off time between each channel. Respond Select: set on time, off time, and delay between channels to obtain either synchronous or reciprocal.

Contraindications for NMES:
*   Transthoracically

*   On a patient with a pacemaker

*   Over carotid baroreceptors

*   Transcerebrally

*   Over uterus of a pregnant person

*   Over or near cancer

*   Over superficial bone producing periosteal pain

*   Over broken or irritated skin

*   On a patient who reacts negatively

Exercises:
*   Reciprocally for wrist flexion and extension
*   One channel for supraspinatus and deltoid
*   Reciprocal for inversion and eversion of the foot
*   Strengthening of weak dorsiflexors
*   Reeducation of quadriceps post-knee arthroplasty
*   Two channels for lumbar muscle spasms
*   Two channels for neck muscle spasms

SEVENTEEN

Regulation of Muscle Strength

1. Define the four factors determining muscle strength: size, contractility, preload, and afterload. Indicate which are intrinsic and which are extrinsic.

2. Describe the mechanical differences between placing sarcomeres in parallel and in series and different orientations of cells within a muscle.

3. Explain the length-tension relationship: the increase, plateau, and decrease of tension at different lengths.

4. Explain the need for preload on a muscle as it relates to the length-tension relationship.

5. Compare an isometric with an isotonic set up, including what is measured and the latency between stimulation and the appearance of an index of muscle performance.

6. Describe the force-frequency relationship, including the three types of contraction, where in the range of stimulation frequency force increases, and the role of the sarcoplasmic reticulum.

7. Explain the role of the series elastic component in the force-frequency relationship.

8. Explain how concentric, isometric, and eccentric contractions are produced by a muscle.

9. Describe the force-velocity relationship, including the importance of the force at which velocity is zero and the velocity when load is zero.

10. Explain how latency changes as a consequence of the load in an isotonic contraction.

11. Explain how displacement of a load changes as a consequence of the load in an isotonic contraction.

In Chapter Sixteen, structure and excitation-contraction coupling of skeletal muscle were examined. In this chapter, factors that determine how much force a muscle can generate will be analyzed systematically. The principles described in this chapter are derived from experiments using muscles removed, at least in part, from their nervous and bony connections. Chapter Eighteen will examine how an innervated muscle attached at both ends to bones behaves. This chapter focuses on four properties of isolated muscle. Two factors are **intrinsic** to the muscle: size (cross-sectional area) and contractility (kg/cm^2 or N/cm^2). Two **extrinsic** factors can be considered coupling factors between muscle performance and the load placed on a muscle. These factors are called **preload** and **afterload**. Another coupling factor, the attachment of muscle to bony levers, is considered in Chapter Eighteen.

INTRINSIC PROPERTIES OF STRIATED MUSCLE

Beginning with the most obvious point, the bigger a muscle, the stronger the muscle. But which dimension of muscle size determines strength? One might intuitively choose mass or volume, but it has been demonstrated clearly that the critical dimension is **cross-sectional area**. If one measures the tension developed by a muscle and then shortens the muscle by cutting its ends, its measured strength does not change. However, if the muscle is split longitudinally, its strength decreases in proportion to the remaining cross-sectional area. The key to muscle strength is the number of sarcomeres pulling in parallel. The number of sarcomeres pulling in series is not relevant to strength. In other words, the number of sarcomeres pulling independently on the ends of the muscle (side-by-side) determines strength; sarcomeres pulling on each other do not affect strength. If we look at sarcomeres operating in series, we can see that a single sarcomere produces force by pulling Z lines from either end toward the center of the sarcomere. At the same time, the sarcomeres on either end of the first sarcomere are pulling equally hard on the same Z lines. Therefore, a second sarcomere pulling on one end of the middle (first) sarcomere negates the force produced at the other end by the third sarcomere pulling the middle sarcomere in the opposite direction. The net force produced by three or any number of sarcomeres in series is, therefore, the same as that produced by a single sarcomere. Although adding sarcomeres in series does not increase force, it does increase the amount of shortening that a muscle can undergo. Adding sarcomeres in parallel, on the other hand, increases strength.

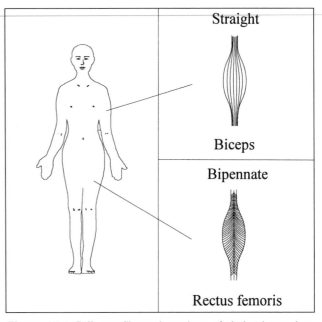

Figure 17-1. Different fiber orientations of skeletal muscles. A straight fiber orientation produces greater sarcomere shortening of the muscle, whereas a bipennate orientation yields greater force due to increased numbers of cross-bridges in parallel per cross-sectional area, but produces less shortening of the muscle.

The contractile state or **contractility** of a muscle can be determined by measuring its maximum force of contraction and dividing by its cross-sectional area. Contractility is the force that a fresh muscle can generate independent of change in its length. A change in muscle performance secondary to a change in its length, a change in the load placed on the muscle, or a change due to previous contractile activity is not a change in contractility. Most muscles can develop a force of approximately 3 kg/cm^2 or 29 N/cm^2 of cross-sectional area. This number varies little between individuals or even species. One factor that complicates determination of a muscle's contractility is the orientation of fibers within a skeletal muscle (Figure 17-1). If a muscle's fibers run parallel to the axis defined by its tendons, one can simply divide a muscle's volume (cm^3) by its length to obtain its cross-sectional area. However, many muscles have fiber arrangements that deviate markedly from parallel. Arrangements, such as that found in the bipennate gastrocnemius, are examples of strategies to increase muscle strength per volume. A bipennate structure of the same volume as a parallel arrangement can produce twice the strength per volume due to the increased number of sarcomeres that can operate in parallel. However, the bipennate muscle cannot shorten as much as a muscle arranged parallel to its axis because the bipennate muscle has fewer sarcomeres in series.

In skeletal muscle, sufficient Ca^{++} is released with each action potential to allow each actin-binding site to be available to a myosin head. The nervous system can choose the appropriate number of skeletal muscle cells (we will see how in Chapter Eighteen) to produce the appropriate amount of force. In contrast, cardiac muscle cells do not, under normal conditions, release sufficient Ca^{++} to allow all myosin molecules to bind to actin. Cardiac muscle strength can be regulated by alterations in its contractility. In the heart, every cardiac muscle cell is active every heartbeat. By physiologically altering the contractility of cardiac muscle cells, the force produced by the heart can be varied as needed. In skeletal muscle, force is, for the most part, regulated by recruiting more or fewer cells to contract. In the heart, force is regulated by using all the cells, but varying the contractility by varying intracellular Ca^{++}.

EXTRINSIC PROPERTIES OF MUSCLE

The extrinsic properties consist of those that serve to couple muscle function with a load placed upon the muscle. These properties include preload and afterload.

PRELOAD

A load may be considered a force acting in a direction opposite to the force produced by shortening of sarcomeres. Therefore, preload may be considered as the force placed on a muscle before the muscle contracts. Preload serves to stretch sarcomeres, thereby producing a passive tension across a muscle. Preload may be defined in terms of either sarcomere length prior to contraction or the force necessary to produce a given sarcomere length (Figure 17-2). This force may be expressed in Newtons or kg x gravity. In the heart, preload can also be expressed in terms of chamber volume or pressure immediately prior to contraction. What is the value in altering sarcomere length prior to contraction? The answer lies in the concept of the length-tension relationship. According to the length-tension relationship, an optimum length at which maximum active tension can be developed exists. At lengths longer or shorter than optimum length, force is less (Figure 17-3).

The length-tension relationship refers to how changes in sarcomere length affect the force that a muscle can generate. This principle is different from that discussed previously regarding muscle cross-sectional area and strength. In that discussion, it is stated that muscle length does not affect muscle strength. That is, the number of sarcomeres arranged end-to-end is irrelevant in muscle strength; only the number of sarcomeres arranged side-by-side determines strength. Often, the length-tension relationship is discussed in the context of changing muscle length. When a muscle is stretched, it becomes longer because each sarcomere is stretched, not because the number of sarcomeres in series changes. When the length-tension relationship is discussed, one should speak in terms of sarcomere length rather than muscle length to avoid this confusion. When a muscle is stretched by an external load prior to contraction (a preload is placed on a muscle), muscle length, including sarcomere length, is increased.

If one begins with a muscle that is completely slack, no preload is present, and little force is developed when the muscle is stimulated to contract. Muscle can then be stretched so that some tension exists, and when stimulated, the muscle responds with more force. Within a certain range of length and passive tension, the muscle produces the most force when stimulated. This length is called the muscle's optimum length and occurs when sarcomere length is 2.0 to 2.5 µm. At lengths greater than this, force produced by a muscle progressively decreases with increasing length. Most of the length-tension relationship can be explained simply by the spatial relationship between thick and thin filaments as sarcomere length changes (Figure 17-4). The length-tension relationship is a different means of altering muscle strength that should not be confused with contractility. To avoid any confusion, contractility is best defined as a change in muscle strength independent of muscle length.

The thick filament consists of approximately 250 myosin molecules oriented toward two Z lines from the M line. Within the center of the thick filament, extending a short distance from the M line, there is a small area at which no myosin heads exist. From this point to both ends of the thick filament, myosin heads can bind to actin, form cross-bridges between the thick and thin filaments, and pull thin filaments toward the center of the sarcomere. The more cross-bridges pulling on each thin filament, the more tension is developed by the muscle. Therefore, the most force is produced when sarcomeres are stretched to a configuration in which each myosin head has access to a thin filament. That length is 2.0 to 2.5 µm. As sarcomeres are stretched longer than this, heads of myosin molecules nearest the M line no longer have a thin filament accessible, and, as length increases, fewer myosin molecules have potential binding sites. The plateau in the length-tension relationship is explainable due to the "bald" spot in the center of the thick filament where the "handles" of the myosin molecules are found, but no heads are present.

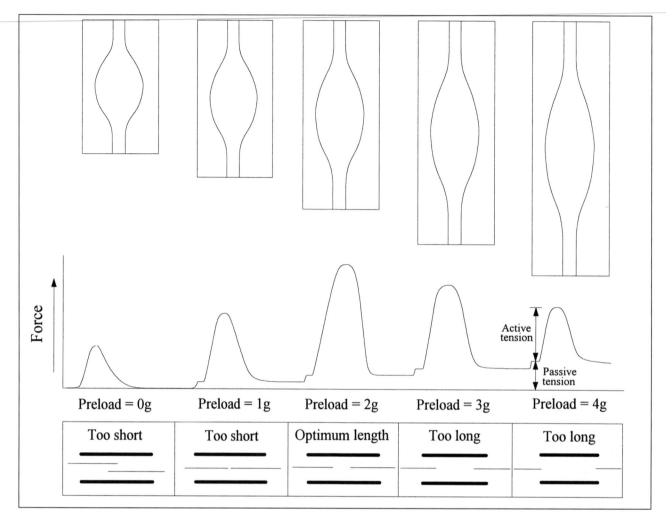

Figure 17-2. In isometric setup, preload can be given in terms of muscle length before contraction or in terms of the force necessary to obtain that length. The effect of preload on the spatial relationship of the thick and thin filaments is depicted in the lower panel.

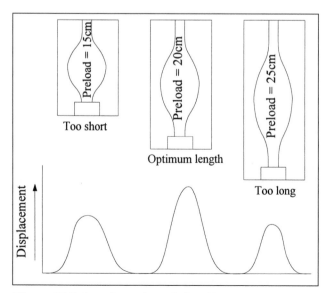

Figure 17-3. Length-tension relationship.

Figure 17-4. The tension developed by a contracting muscle at different lengths can be explained partially by the degree of overlap of thick and thin filament.

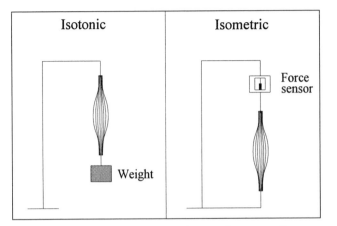

Figure 17-5. Isotonic and isometric muscle preparations.

Why active tension decreases with lengths shorter than that which produces maximum overlap of thick and thin filaments is more complex. Some of the decrease may be explained based on overlap of thin filaments from opposite ends of the sarcomere, interfering with pulling of thin filaments toward the center of the sarcomere. Moreover, as cells become shorter, volume does not change; cells become proportionally thicker. As muscle cells become thicker, the distance between thick and thin filaments and between the sarcoplasmic reticulum and the center of the cell increases. This change in cell proportions means that the power stroke of the cross-bridge cycle cannot displace the thin filament as much and that Ca^{++} must diffuse a greater distance to allow cross-bridge cycling to occur throughout the cell.

AFTERLOAD

Just as preload may be defined as a force acting in a direction opposite to that developed by muscle prior to contraction, afterload is a force acting opposite to that produced by muscle contraction that exists **after** a muscle is stimulated to contract. In other words, it is a force that a muscle must overcome before an observable shortening of muscle can occur. To understand the relationships between muscle size, contractility, preload, and afterload, it is necessary to first describe the differences between isometric and isotonic experimental preparations.

ISOMETRIC CONTRACTION

In an isometric setup, a muscle is placed in a rigid frame to which both ends of a muscle are attached. At one end of the frame, a tendon is attached to a force transducer to record the tension across the muscle. The other end of the muscle is attached to an adjustable post to change muscle length. When the muscle is activated, an increased tension can be recorded but no change in muscle length can occur. In the isometric setup, one can alter preload by increasing or decreasing stretch on the muscle. Preload can be recorded either as muscle length or the passive tension on the muscle before stimulation. Afterload in this setup, for all purposes, may be considered infinite. The rigid frame produces a force equal and opposite to that developed by the muscle, preventing any shortening of the muscle. Because muscle length cannot change, the contraction is isometric.

A muscle is allowed to change length in an isotonic setup. One end is attached to a rigid frame. The other end, instead of attaching to a transducer, is attached to a weight. Muscle length is varied by adjusting a platform that supports the weight before stimulating the muscle to contract. The weight supported by the platform is the afterload. The tension across the muscle due to partial support of the weight is the preload. Muscle performance in an isotonic setup is determined by how far the attached weight is moved by the activated muscle.

The length-tension relationship is demonstrated best using an isometric preparation. One can measure tension easily across a muscle before contraction, then stimulate the muscle to contract. During muscle contraction, tension increases. The increase in tension above preload is the active tension developed by contraction of the muscle. By subtracting passive tension (preload) from total tension, active tension can be calculated. One can then plot a curve relating preload (passive tension) to active tension. This relationship is the length-tension relationship. See Figure 17-5 for a comparison of the two set-ups.

FORCE-FREQUENCY RELATIONSHIP

A second relationship displayed best using an isometric preparation is the force-frequency relationship. Stated briefly, the tension developed by a muscle is dependent on the frequency of action potentials occurring on the muscle cell membrane. A single action potential produces a mechanical response termed a twitch. A single action potential lasts 1 to 2 ms, whereas a twitch may take 50 to 200 ms to complete (Figure 17-6 [A]). Therefore, one may introduce a second action potential during a twitch. The resulting increase in force is known as summation. As stimuli are delivered more rapidly to muscle cells, the force generated increases until, at a rapid enough rate of stimulation, one prolonged contraction with a maximum strength

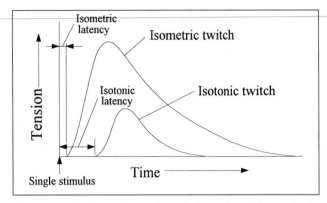

Figure 17-6. A: an isometric twitch produced by a single stimulus. The recorded mechanical event begins almost immediately and is recorded as an increase in tension, as the ends of the muscle are fixed. B: an isotonic twitch produced by a single stimulus. The recorded mechanical event has a detectable latency before the load attached to the muscle is moved.

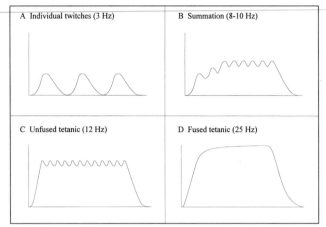

Figure 17-7. Force-frequency relationship. A: individual twitches. B: summation with greater frequency. C: unfused tetanic contractions (treppe). D: fused tetanic contraction.

three to five times that of a single twitch is observed. This result is termed a tetanic contraction. In human muscle, this typically occurs between 12 and 20 action potentials per second or at a stimulation rate of 12 to 20 Hz. At lower rates of stimulation, one observes unfused tetanic contractions, also known as treppe. Ripples in the force output correspond to individual stimuli used to generate action potentials. The process of summation, treppe, and tetanic contractions can be explained based on muscle structure and the sliding filament theory. During a single muscle twitch, Ca^{++} is released, allowing contraction to occur. The force is then used to pull the surrounding elastic tissues of the endomysium, perimysium, and epimysium, resulting in stretching of the tendons on either end of the muscle. The stretch placed on the tendons increases the tension within them, just as stretching a spring or rubber band. The tendon pulls on a force transducer, and force is measured. However, before cross-bridge cycling can take up all the slack in the surrounding elastic tissues, the sarcoplasmic reticulum takes up Ca^{++}, resulting in relaxation before maximum force can develop.

If a second action potential occurs before relaxation occurs, Ca^{++} is released anew, and cross-bridge cycling can continue for a longer period than a single twitch allows. Because some slack in the elastic tissues has already been taken up, cross-bridge cycling following a second stimulus results in greater force. If the muscle is stimulated frequently enough that the sarcoplasmic reticulum cannot take up Ca^{++} fast enough to cause any relaxation, the muscle continues to contract, resulting in a tetanic contraction. The muscle has sufficient time to develop its maximum force during a tetanic contraction, which is three to five times greater in force than a single

twitch. During tetanic contractions, Ca^{++} levels remain above that required to saturate troponin. Treppe is produced by a frequency of action potentials that allows a short period of relaxation. As a result, the Ca^{++} level within the cells drops slightly below saturation level for troponin for a short time between each action potential, and evidence of the beginning of relaxation between stimuli can be observed (Figure 17-7). Treppe at the muscle level looks like shaking and can be used therapeutically to help tense muscle relax.

The second part of the explanation for summation and tetanic contraction lies in a construct termed the series elastic component. The muscle can be thought to consist of a contractile element, which consists of the thick and thin filaments; a parallel elastic component, consisting of the elasticity within the actin-myosin crossbridges that provides resistance to stretching; and the series elastic component, making up the tendons. During an isometric twitch, **total** muscle length cannot change. The contractile component of the muscle shortens, pulling on the series elastic component, and the series elastic component is stretched by the same distance that the contractile element shortens. Stretching the series elastic component increases the tension across it, which is, in turn, transmitted to the force transducer and recorded. If a muscle is allowed to relax between each action potential, the series elastic component must be restretched with every action potential. With a stimulation frequency of 12 to 20 Hz or greater, the series elastic component can be stretched until its tension equals the maximum force that cross-bridge cycling can generate. One can show this effect by palpating the biceps tendon in the cubital fossa when the muscle is relaxed and while the muscle undergoes an isometric

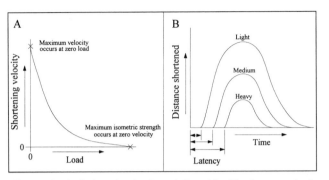

Figure 17-8. A: Load-velocity relationship. Maximum velocity occurs at zero load. Maximum isometric strength is determined isotonically as the load that produces a zero velocity. B: Effect of load on latency and degree of shortening. A heavy load requires more cross-bridge cycling to move the load, resulting in a longer latency and less shortening available for the load to move.

contraction. At rest, the tendon is slack and can be moved easily about the fossa. When the muscle contracts isometrically, the tendon becomes very stiff and cannot be moved within the fossa.

RELATIONSHIPS DEMONSTRATED BY ISOTONIC RECORDING

In isometric contractions, no shortening of muscle occurs, and no movement of a mass occurs; therefore, no work is done in the sense of the definition of work in physics. Isotonic contraction results in movement of a load. If the force generated by the muscle in an isotonic setup equals the load, no movement occurs; the contraction is isometric. If the force developed by the muscle **exceeds** the load, the load will be moved according to the definition of force, F = m x a (force equals mass times acceleration). For example, if a muscle produces a force of 10 N greater than the load produced by a 20-kg weight, the weight will be accelerated 0.5 m/s². If instead, the muscle produces less force than the load placed on it, the mass will be accelerated in a negative direction (eg, toward gravity). This type of contraction is used to control the descent of a load as occurs when an object is set down or when one changes from a standing to a sitting posture. When a muscle contraction produces a positive acceleration of an object, the contraction is termed **concentric** or a shortening contraction. If acceleration equals zero, the contraction is isometric, and when acceleration is negative, the term **eccentric**, or lengthening contraction, is used because the muscle is stretched to a greater length in spite of the activity of the muscle.

The situations described above relate to what is called the load-velocity relationship. More specifically, the load-velocity relationship is displayed in an isotonic muscle preparation in which the muscle is stimulated to produce its maximum force. One places different loads on the muscle, stimulates the muscle to contract, and measures the change in length per time or the velocity of contraction (Figure 17-8). Two important points exist on the load-velocity curve. By extrapolating the curve to a load of zero, we can estimate the maximum velocity of muscle contraction, which is determined by the rate of cross-bridge cycling. Cross-bridge cycling rate is determined largely by the isozyme of myosin ATPase present in the muscle. The second important point on the curve is where velocity equals zero. The point of zero velocity can be used as an index of strength. At this point of zero velocity, we know precisely how much force the muscle is producing. At any other point on the curve, muscle performance is complicated by energy expended in acceleration of the load. The force at zero velocity is termed maximum isometric tension and is equal to what one would record during an isometric setup.

Two related phenomena demonstrated by isotonic recording are the results of a load on the **amount** of shortening and the **latency** of shortening. In an isometric setup, no shortening occurs, and tension produced by the muscle is immediately recorded upon the initiation of cross-bridge cycling. In an isotonic setup, one records how far a load is moved, which is equivalent to how much the muscle shortens. A light load is moved sooner and farther than a heavier load; the latency is less, and the muscle shortens more. As load increases, latency increases, and shortening decreases. Compare latency of these in Figure 17-6 (A and B).

If we attach a force transducer to the isotonic setup, we can also see that, as load increases, force produced by the muscle continues to increase until load equals maximum isometric tension. If the afterload is greater than maximum isometric tension, active tension does not increase further; instead, the muscle lengthens (eccentric contraction). When the muscle is stimulated, shortening of the contractile element does not initially shorten the muscle, but must first stretch the series elastic component. Stretching the series elastic component has the same effect as Hooke described for a spring. As the series elastic component is stretched, tension (restoring force) increases in proportion to the stretch. The load will not move until force across the tendon exceeds the load. When this occurs, contractile element shortening results in shortening of the muscle and movement of the load. Therefore, the first part of the sarcomere shortening caused by cross-bridge cycling goes into stretching the SEC before any movement of an external object can occur and is, therefore, isometric.

Whatever available sarcomere shortening that can be accomplished following stretch of the SEC results in movement of the load. The distance that the load is moved is equal to the amount of sarcomere shortening that occurs after the SEC is stretched. If a load equals maximum isometric tension, the load will not move; the distance that the contractile element shortens will be equal to the distance that the SEC lengthens. If the load is less than maximum isometric tension, some contractile element shortening results in movement of the load. The lighter the load, the more, the sooner, and the faster the load is moved. Conversely, as load increases, the load moves less, the latency is longer, and the load moves more slowly. At maximum isometric tension, the distance the load moves is zero, the latency is infinite, and the velocity is zero (see Figure 17-8). At loads greater than maximum isometric tension (producing an eccentric contraction), the distance moved and velocity are less than zero (negative). No latency can be measured in an eccentric contraction; movement occurs in the negative direction as soon as the support for the load is removed.

We can voluntarily produce any of these contractions (concentric, isometric, or eccentric) for a load less than maximum isometric contraction. At a certain level of muscle activity, we can hold a load in one position, producing an isometric contraction. By producing more effort, we can accelerate the load in the positive direction, against gravity. The greater the effort, the faster the load is accelerated. By putting forth less effort than that needed for isometric contraction, we can lower a weight. The less effort we place against a load, the faster the load moves in the negative direction. We use eccentric contraction as often as we use concentric contractions. Whenever we lift something, we use concentric contraction. To put something down, including our own bodies, we control the object's descent by using eccentric contraction rather than just dropping an object.

The types of contractions and relationships between muscle tension and length, frequency of stimulation, velocity, shortening, and latency are similar in skeletal and cardiac muscle and will be briefly reviewed in the chapter of mechanical properties of the heart. Smooth muscle mechanics will be discussed separately in Chapter Twenty-Eight.

SUMMARY

Four factors influence the performance of skeletal muscle: the intrinsic property of contractility, muscle cross-sectional area, and the extrinsic properties of preload and afterload. Muscle strength is proportional to cross-sectional area, not mass or volume. Mass and volume are determined by both cross-sectional area and length of a muscle. Muscle strength is increased as cross-sectional area is increased. Increasing the length of a muscle increases the amount that the muscle can be shortened during contraction. Some muscles are arranged in configurations such as bipennate to optimize the cross-sectional area available in a volume of muscle, but sacrifice the amount of shortening available. Preload is a force that stretches a muscle prior to contraction. If a preload stretches a muscle to its optimum length, the muscle produces its maximum force. Stretching a muscle beyond optimum length or allowing a muscle to be slack reduces the force available. The intrinsic property of contractility refers to the strength of muscle independent of differences in sarcomere length. Afterload is the load against which a muscle must contract to make the load move. Increasing the afterload decreases velocity of contraction, increases latency, and decreases the distance a load can be moved. Concentric muscle contraction refers to a contraction in which the bony levers connected to a muscle are approximated or an object is accelerated against gravity. An isometric contraction refers to a contraction in which the force generated through the bony lever is equal to the load against which the muscle is contracting. An eccentric contraction refers to a contraction in which the muscle produces less force than the load and the muscle lengthens during contraction. At light loads, we can produce any of the three; at heavier loads, we have less choice in the amount of acceleration of an object. The force-frequency relationship refers to the increased force of contraction that occurs as depolarizing stimuli are presented more frequently to the muscle. A single twitch does not allow enough time for a muscle to develop its maximum force. At a frequency of approximately 20 Hz, Ca^{++} levels are not allowed to fall low enough between stimuli to produce any relaxation. At intermediate frequencies (about 10 Hz), a slight relaxation between stimuli results, a phenomenon called unfused tetanic contraction, or treppe.

BIBLIOGRAPHY

Booth FW, Tseng BS. Olympic goal: molecular and cellular approaches to understanding muscle adaptation. *News in Physiological Sciences.* 1993;8:165-169.

Cope TC, Pinter MJ. The size principle: still working after all these years. *News in Physiological Sciences.* 1995;10:280-286.

Fitts RH. Cellular mechanism of muscle fatigue. *Physiological Reviews.* 1994;74:49-94.

Grinnell AD. Dynamics of nerve-muscle interaction in developing and mature neuromuscular junctions. *Physiological Reviews*. 1995;75:789-834.

Jami L. Golgi tendon organ in mammalian skeleton muscle: functional properties and central actions. *Physiological Reviews*. 1992;72:623-666.

Marder E, Calabrese RL. Principles of rhythmic motor pattern generation. *Physiological Reviews*. 1996;76:687-717.

Proske U. The mammalian muscle spindle. *News in Physiological Sciences*. 1997;12:37-42.

Rette D, Staron RS. The molecular diversity of mammalian muscle fibers. *News in Physiological Sciences*. 1993;8:153-157.

Shulman GI, Landau BR. Pathways of glycogen repletion. *Physiological Reviews*. 1992;72:1019-1035.

Weiss P, Jeannerod M. Getting a grasp on coordination. *News in Physiological Sciences*. 1998;13:70-75.

STUDY QUESTIONS

1. What does the equation for force ($F = m\,a$) mean in terms of muscle function? What is a load? What happens if force produced by a muscle is 1) greater than the load; 2) less than the load; 3) equal to the load?

2. Explain why latency occurs in isotonic contractions, but not in isometric contractions.

3. Explain the difference between treppe and fused muscle contractions. Why would treppe produce a more relaxing therapy than a fused tetanic contraction?

4. What is the functional importance of eccentric contractions? Isometric contractions?

5. Explain the functional significance of zero velocity in the load-velocity relationship. What do you think happens to this point as a result of strength training?

LABORATORY EXERCISES

LABORATORY EXERCISE 17-1

MUSCLE MECHANICS

Objectives:
1. Demonstrate frequency-tension relationship including summation and tetanization.

2. Demonstrate relationship between muscle fatigue and frequency of contraction.

Materials:
Neuromuscular electric stimulator
Force transducer with platform for hand
Self-adhesive electrodes

1. Turn on recorder and stimulator.

2. Place small self-adhesive electrode over the abductor pollicis brevis and the large electrode on the back of the hand.

3. Place the hand on platform so that contraction of the abductor pollicis brevis pulls on the force transducer. Do not apply more than 2 kg (5 lb) of force on the transducer.

4. Produce a single twitch of the abductor pollicis brevis by gradually increasing the intensity until a maximal twitch occurs.

5. While recording, gradually increase the frequency until tetanization is observed. Mark frequency on the tracing as frequency is increased. Turn stimulator off.

6. Set the stimulator to an on time of 1 second and an off time of 5 seconds. Record tetanic contractions at a slow chart speed until fatigue appears. Rest for 1 minute. Repeat procedure at an off time of 4 seconds. Rest, then repeat at decreasing off times until a 1:1 ratio of on time to off time is reached.

7. How is summation produced?

8. Why are there oscillations in force at the intermediate frequencies? Why do the oscillations disappear with higher frequencies?

9. How much greater was force during tetanization than during a single twitch?

10. What role does the series elastic component play in the greater force attained during tetany than a single twitch?

11. At which ratio of on time to off time did fatigue occur most rapidly? Why?

LABORATORY EXERCISES

LABORATORY EXERCISE 17-2

LENGTH-TENSION RELATIONSHIP

Objective: Investigate the relationship between muscle length and tension.

Materials:
Graph paper
Handgrip dynamometer

1. Set stirrup on handgrip dynamometer to a width of 3.0 cm.

2. Determine maximum force at that setting.

3. Increase width to 3.5 cm and measure handgrip strength.

4. Continue to increase width of dynamometer in 0.5 cm increments.

5. Take greatest of at least two determinations at each dynamometer width.

6. Plot handgrip strength vs width of dynamometer.

7. At what dynamometer setting was handgrip greatest? Why?

8. Did this vary from person to person? Why?

LABORATORY EXERCISE 17-3

MUSCLE LENGTH AND VOLUME

Objective: Describe the function of the series elastic component.

Materials:
Tape measure
Assorted weights
Graph paper
Spring

1. Rest the arm on a tabletop keeping the elbow at 90°. Measure the circumference of the arm at its largest point. Maximally contract the biceps muscle without changing the joint angle. Measure circumference again. If biceps length does not change, why does circumference increase?

2. Lift different weights with an attached spring. Plot length of spring (dependent variable) against weight as the independent variable. Why does spring length change? How is this related to the function of the series elastic component?

EIGHTEEN

Whole Muscle Function

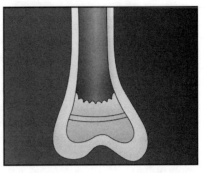

1. Discuss the three major mechanisms for regenerating ATP, including their limitations, their timing, and their efficiency during aerobic and anaerobic activities.

2. Define fatigue, and list possible causes of fatigue during short, intense, and long duration activities.

3. Define a motor unit; explain why it is the functional unit of a muscle from the perspective of the central nervous system.

4. Describe the development of motor units and the distribution of motor unit sizes.

5. Discuss the benefits derived from having many small motor units and small numbers of large motor units.

6. Describe the basis for classification of motor units by speed of contraction, oxidative vs. glycolytic metabolism, color, and fatigability, and order of recruitment during voluntary activity vs. neuromuscular electrical stimulation.

7. Describe how preload is altered during voluntary muscle activity.

8. Describe the three classes of lever systems and the advantages and disadvantages of a third class lever.

9. Compare the processes of co-contraction and reciprocal innervation; describe how these are used in skilled vs. novel movements.

10. Define active and passive insufficiency of a muscle. Provide examples of muscle groups and actions.

11. Describe the structures and locations of Golgi tendon organs and muscle spindles.

12. Discuss the negative feedback loops of which the Golgi tendon organs and muscle spindles act as sensors.

13. Describe the stretch reflex, including the actions of synergists and antagonists.

14. Describe the functions of gamma motor neurons, including their role in increasing muscle tone during muscle activity.

15. Describe how the effectiveness of the stretch reflex is altered in upper and lower motor neuron diseases.

16. Describe the phenomenon of spasticity and interventions used to control it.

Skeletal muscle may be called upon to provide a range of activities, such as the continuous muscle tone necessary to maintain posture to intermittent bursts of high-power output needed for lifting heavy weights or sprinting. Between, we may classify activities as low-intensity aerobic activities, such as walking, to high-intensity activities that can be sustained aerobically for only about 3.5 minutes, such as running 1500 meters. Aerobic activities are those that can be sustained by using oxygen to regenerate the needed adenosine triphosphate (ATP); anaerobic activities can use ATP at a rate faster than what can be regenerated by consumption of oxygen alone. During muscle activity, ATP is required to maintain cross-bridge cycling. ATP binds to myosin to allow myosin to dissociate from actin to continue the cross-bridge cycle. Calcium uptake by the sarcoplasmic reticulum (SR) and active transport by the Na-K pump also require ATP.

MECHANISMS FOR REGENERATING ATP

Three major mechanisms exist to regenerate ATP from adenosine diphosphate (ADP). They are oxidative phosphorylation, substrate phosphorylation (glycolysis), and creatine phosphate. Creatine phosphate (CP) is used as a reservoir for phosphate. Sufficient creatine phosphate concentration is available at rest to perform the reaction ADP + CP → ATP + creatine via the enzyme creatine kinase for about 10 seconds. When ATP is in abundant supply, ATP is used in the reverse direction to regenerate CP. When ATP is used faster than it is regenerated by oxidative or substrate phosphorylation causing ATP concentration to fall, the creatine kinase reaction maintains ATP at the expense of CP for a short time. Although CP can only support ATP concentration for a short time, this 10 seconds or so is long enough to allow the rate of ATP production via oxidative and substrate phosphorylation to catch up with use of ATP. Therefore, extremely high levels of ATP use can occur for enough time to run a 100-meter dash or to lift a heavy weight for a few seconds.

Some well-trained athletes can sustain near maximal running speed for more than 43 seconds. This means that other rapid means of regenerating ATP must be available. Substrate phosphorylation is a process in which a substrate, glucose, is used to donate a phosphate group to ADP. Substrate phosphorylation is very inefficient, producing only a net of two ATP molecules per glucose molecule. The advantage of substrate phos-

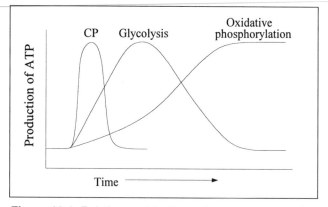

Figure 18-1. Relative contributions of energy sources during moderate exercise. Initially, ATP is rephosphorylated by breakdown of creatine phosphate as glycolysis begins to increase. Oxidative phosphorylation is slower to increase, but becomes the dominant source of energy as exercise proceeds.

phorylation is how quickly substrate phosphorylation can augment ATP concentration compared with oxidative phosphorylation. A disadvantage is the production of NADH and pyruvic acid as products. Under aerobic conditions, pyruvate generated by substrate phosphorylation from glucose would enter the Krebs cycle to produce an additional 34 ATP molecules per glucose molecule. Because NAD is needed to continue substrate phosphorylation, NADH must be converted to NAD by converting pyruvic acid into lactic acid, thereby rendering the muscle tissue acidic. High rates of metabolism can be supported by substrate phosphorylation, but at the cost of a heavy acid production. The success of an individual in running 400 meters is, to a large degree, dependent on the ability of the person to buffer the acid generated by running nearly full speed for more than 40 seconds.

Oxidative phosphorylation can maintain ATP concentration indefinitely. The maximum metabolic rate that can be sustained for a minimum of 3 minutes is determined by the maximum rate at which oxygen can be used (maximum oxygen consumption or VO_2 max). Each molecule of fuel that enters the Krebs cycle produces 17 molecules of ATP, but only a small amount of ATP is generated in the Krebs cycle itself. Most of the ATP is gained by oxidizing the proton acceptors used in the Krebs cycle, NADH and $FADH_2$. Each NADH yields three ATP molecules, and each $FADH_2$ yields two ATP molecules. Activities, such as running 1500 to 5000 meters, that last for 3 minutes or longer are mainly dependent on how much oxygen can be used to regenerate ATP from ADP by oxidative phosphorylation.

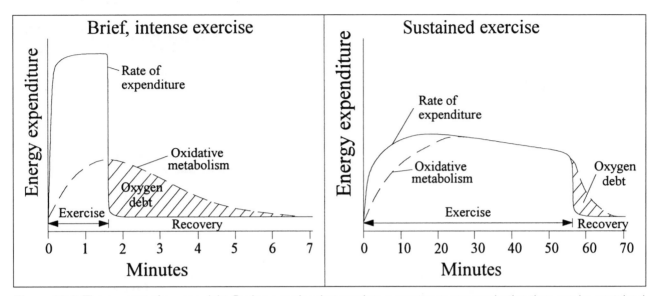

Figure 18-2. The concept of oxygen debt. During exercise that requires a greater energy production than can be sustained by oxidative phosphorylation, energy is produced anaerobically. The difference between energy use and production of energy by aerobic metabolism is called the oxygen debt. Following exercise, oxygen consumption remains elevated. On the right, an example of very high intensity activity with a large oxygen debt is depicted. Note the area labeled oxygen debt is approximately equal to the deficit depicted as the difference in rate of expenditure and oxidative metabolism. On the left, an example typical of moderate exercise that can be sustained aerobically is depicted.

OXYGEN DEBT

Because of the slow response of oxidative phosphorylation to increased demand for ATP, initial demands for ATP are met first by creatine phosphate, followed by anaerobic glycolysis until a steady state in which oxidative phosphorylation can produce ATP at the same rate that it is being used can be attained (Figure 18-1). The oxygen that would be required to generate the amount of ATP produced by breakdown of CP and anaerobic glycolysis at the beginning of exercise is termed oxygen debt. The actual physiologic mechanisms involved in oxygen debt and its payback are still not known. What is known is that, at the end of exercise, oxygen consumption remains elevated beyond that required by the person who just completed exercise. The excess oxygen consumption following exercise is nearly equal to the oxygen debt incurred at the beginning of exercise (Figure 18-2).

FATIGUE

Fatigue may be defined in many ways. A simple definition that seems to work for most cases is that fatigue is a decrease in force produced by a muscle secondary to contractile activity. Fatigue is often assumed to be a failure of the contractile mechanisms to keep up with the demands placed upon them. Instead, we should consider the possibility that fatigue is a regulated phenomenon that serves to prevent the consequences of ATP depletion. In ischemia, ATP depletion leads first to reversible cell injury and swelling of cells due to decreased Na-K pump activity, followed by irreversible cell damage. Fatigue prevents ATP concentration from being driven down to dangerous levels by decreasing ATP use. In the laboratory, it can be shown that increasing the rate of blood flow to a contracting muscle will decrease fatigue (Figure 18-3). If a muscle is stimulated to contract tetanically at a high rate, the force produced by the muscle quickly decreases to about 35% of the maximum force generated by a single contraction. Elevating muscle blood flow by raising arterial blood pressure produces a proportional increase in the force generated, a partial reversal of fatigue.

SHORT-DURATION ACTIVITY

Fatigue during short-term, intense activity is generally explained based on the acidosis produced by high levels of substrate phosphorylation with the production of lactic acid. Acidosis appears to depress contractile activity by one or a combination of three factors:

1. Decreased Ca^{++} release by the sarcoplasmic reticulum.
2. A change in the shape of troponin, rendering Ca^{++} release less effective.
3. A direct effect on the myofibrils.

Caffeine, which activates ryanodine receptors, can temporarily reduce muscle fatigue, perhaps by increasing Ca⁺⁺ release from the SR of fatigued muscles.

LONG-DURATION ACTIVITY

Lower-intensity, longer-duration activities such as races of 10,000 meters or longer appear to be related to depletion of substrates needed for oxidative phosphorylation. A sudden decrease in muscle activity during intense, aerobic activity has been termed "hitting the wall." As discussed in Chapter Seven, glucose is provided to the entire body through glycogen stored in the liver and the process of gluconeogenesis in which substances other than glycogen are converted to glucose. Muscle cells store their own supply of glucose as glycogen also, but muscle cells cannot release their glucose back into the circulation for other cells to use. When the liver is depleted of glycogen, the entire body suffers a lack of substrate for oxidative phosphorylation, which results in fatigue.

THE MOTOR UNIT

The sarcomere has been described as the functional unit of muscle from the perspective of muscle mechanics. However, from the perspective of the central nervous system, the functional unit is the motor unit. A motor unit is defined as a motor neuron with its cell body in the anterior horn of the spinal cord (brain stem for muscles of the head and neck) and the individual muscle cells innervated by that motor neuron. When a motor neuron is depolarized to threshold, it releases acetylcholine on all of the muscle cells that receive a branch from that neuron. Therefore, the nervous system produces increments in force equal to the force generated by a motor unit; it cannot increase force by a fraction of a motor unit. Our ability to grade force in an isolated muscle is limited by the incremental nature of recruiting additional motor units. With attachment of muscles to bones, other ways are available for grading force. One way is the co-contraction of muscles on opposite sides of a joint, in which one muscle, for example the biceps, is opposed by the triceps muscle. A second means of grading force is to alter the preload (muscle length) by the positioning of body parts.

NUMBER AND SIZE OF MOTOR UNITS

A group of cell bodies of motor neurons innervating a given muscle is found in close proximity in the anterior horn of the spinal cord. Both excitatory and inhibitory neurons synapse with these neurons. During

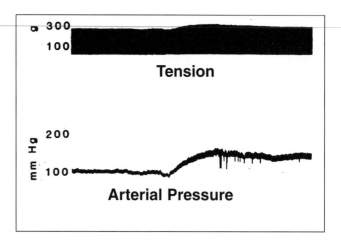

Figure 18-3. The effect of skeletal muscle blood flow on muscular fatigue. With a steady arterial pressure and skeletal muscle blood flow, the tension produced by intermittent tetanic contractions is constant. Experimentally increasing skeletal muscle blood flow by increasing arterial pressure produces a proportional increase in the tension developed by the muscle, indicative of the protective nature of muscle fatigue.

development, many motor neurons send axons to the muscles of the limbs and trunk running along peripheral nerves that branch to muscles. The branches of motor neurons compete with each other for muscle cells in an apparently random fashion. It is uncommon to find muscle cells of the same motor unit next to each other. When one stains a muscle biopsy sample for different biochemical markers indicative of certain properties, one finds a mosaic-like microscopic appearance because muscle cells of the same motor unit have the same biochemical features.

α motor neurons that innervate only a few muscle cells develop small cell bodies and small diameter axons, whereas motor neurons innervating many skeletal muscle cells develop large cell bodies and large axons. The distribution of motor unit sizes (number of muscle cells or diameter of axon) does not follow a normal or Gaussian distribution in which most of the motor units would be medium-sized with few small or large motor units. Instead, the distribution resembles that of a Poisson distribution in which a large number of small motor units are found with a decreasing number of large motor units. A Poisson distribution describes phenomena with a frequency distribution skewed in one direction. For example, the distribution of the number of children in a pregnancy has a vast majority of pregnancies with one child, many fewer with two, and so on. This Poisson distribution of motor units with a large number of small motor units and a small number of large motor units has the benefit of allowing small gradations in force by recruiting small motor units initially when small increments in force are needed at low to intermediate levels of required muscle force. When high levels of muscle force are required, large increments of force can be added by recruiting the large motor units later. The way motor units are recruited will be described later in this chapter.

CLASSIFICATION OF MOTOR UNITS INTO MUSCLE FIBER TYPES

Because all of the muscle cells in a motor unit are recruited simultaneously, the muscle cells within a motor unit receive the same stimuli responsible for the development of the characteristics that determine a fiber type and, therefore, have the same biochemical and mechanical properties. Motor units are divided into three major categories based on speed of contraction (mechanical property) and either type of metabolism or fatigue characteristics (biochemical property). The most commonly used classification scheme is based on the speed of cross-bridge cycling (speed of contraction) and whether the muscle cells have high levels of oxidative or glycolytic enzymes. Using this classification, we have three types:

1. Slow oxidative
2. Fast oxidative
3. Fast glycolytic

No slow glycolytic type exists. Slow speed of contraction and glycolytic metabolism are not compatible in the same cell. Knowledge of different muscle fiber types comes largely from studies performed on rodents. One reason for this is that rodent skeletal muscle does not have a mosaic pattern like human muscle, but motor units of the same type tend to be layered with slow oxidative closest to the bone (deepest), fast glycolytic the most superficial, and fast oxidative at an intermediate depth within a given muscle. In human muscle, few fast oxidative motor units are found. For the most part, we have either slow oxidative motor units or fast glycolytic motor units.

A second type of classification is based on the color of the muscle. The presence of cytochromes used in oxidative phosphorylation and myoglobin, an oxygen-binding protein similar to hemoglobin, gives oxidative muscle cells a red color. Glycolytic muscle tends to have a pale color. These color differences in muscle tissue are readily apparent in chicken muscles. The dark meat of a chicken consists of oxidative muscle of the thigh and leg, whereas white meat is observed in the breast of this non-flying bird. Using the color scheme, slow oxidative motor units are called slow twitch red, fast oxidative are called fast twitch red, and fast glycolytic are called fast

twitch white. One may also base classification on the fatigability of the motor units, although this classification, too, is redundant. Oxidative motor units do not fatigue as much as glycolytic motor units. Slow oxidative are slow fatigue-resistant, fast oxidative are fast fatigue resistant, and fast glycolytic are fast fatigable. One last classification scheme must be mentioned because it is still used by some. This classification is based on the order of recruitment during voluntary muscle activity. Slow oxidative motor units are called type I, and fast glycolytic are called type II. However, during neuromuscular electrical stimulation, it should be noted that the order of recruitment is opposite of what occurs during voluntary muscle contraction.

Slow oxidative motor units are recruited first during muscle activity. These motor units contract slowly compared with the larger, fast glycolytic motor units and use ATP at a slower rate. For a given amount of force generated, slow oxidative motor units use less ATP. Muscle cells of slow oxidative motor units are smaller in diameter and receive a greater blood flow per cell volume during activity. In addition, slow oxidative motor units have much greater concentrations of oxidative enzymes and lower concentrations of glycolytic enzymes than fast glycolytic motor units (Figure 18-4). The greater efficiency and greater capacity for oxidative metabolism and blood flow during exercise give slow oxidative motor units a greater resistance to fatigue. These characteristics of the different motor units are related to the type of activity performed by the different motor units. The smallest motor units, which are recruited first, are the most fatigue resistant. As larger motor units are recruited to add to the force generated by the motor units that are already active, the characteristics tend to change from slow, oxidative, and fatigue-resistant to fast, glycolytic, and fatigable. Because the smallest motor units are active more often than the largest motor units, the development of fatigue-resistant characteristics aids in their function. Experiments in which neurons of slow motor units were surgically crossed with those of fast motor units resulted in changes in the muscle cells consistent with the idea that the pattern of innervation is responsible for the characteristics of the muscle cells. With time, the previously fast motor units now innervated by small motor neurons took on the characteristics of slow contraction and oxidative metabolism, and the muscle cells that were once slow oxidative cells became fast and glycolytic. Electrical stimulation studies have shown that when fast glycolytic motor units are stimulated in the same manner as slow oxidative motor units are recruited in vivo, the motor units take on the same characteristics as slow oxidative motor units.

RECRUITMENT OF MOTOR UNITS (SIZE PRINCIPLE)

The size principle was elaborated by Dr. Elwood Henneman, based on studies of individual motor units of cat muscle. Motor neurons with small diameter axons and low conduction velocity were recruited first, followed by increasingly larger, faster conducting motor neurons with increased synaptic input to the motor neurons of a given muscle. Subsequently, it was determined that the diameter of the motor neuron is proportional to both the number of muscle cells innervated by an motor neuron and the size of the neuron's cell body in the anterior horn of the spinal cord. The smallest motor neurons are selected by the central nervous system (CNS) because of their high resistance to ion flow. To reach threshold to produce an action potential, sufficient excitatory synaptic input must be present to cause the axon hillock of the a motor neuron to depolarize to threshold. To produce this change in membrane potential, an increased number of excitatory postsynaptic potentials are produced by descending neurons to overcome the inhibitory postsynaptic potentials produced by descending neurons and local interneurons. The high-resistance, small-diameter motor neurons have a greater change in membrane potential for a given amount of current allowed to enter due to EPSPs. The recruitment pattern based on size of the motor neuron was termed the size principle. The size principle simplifies the decision-making process of the CNS. The CNS determines how much force the muscle needs to generate to produce the desired effect of muscle contraction. Rather than choosing a specific number of motor neurons, all the CNS needs to do is to increase or decrease the synaptic input to the pool of motor neurons innervating a particular muscle.

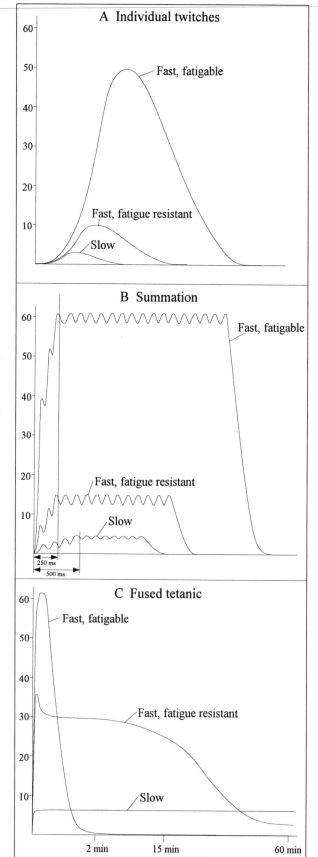

Figure 18-4. Differences in motor units of varying proportions of muscle fiber types. A: Twitch tension; the greatest twitch tension is generated by fast glycolytic motor units and the least by slow oxidative motor units. B: Tension with summation; again, fast glycotic motor units produce the greatest tension and slow oxidative, the least. C: Sustained tetanic contractions; fast glycolytic motor units produce the greatest tension but fatigue rapidly. Slow oxidative motor units produce much less tension but are able to sustain this tension. Fast oxidative glycolytic produce a greater tension than slow oxidative, but fatigue.

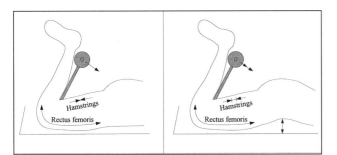

Figure 18-5. Passive and active insufficiency. With the combination of knee flexion and hip extension, the hamstring muscles experience a loss of strength due to short sarcomere length (active insufficiency); hip flexion improves hamstring strength by increasing sarcomere length. The rectus femoris loses strength under the same conditions due to excessive sarcomere length as the muscle is stretched across both the knee and hip joints to produce passive insufficiency.

FORCE-FREQUENCY RELATIONSHIP

The first motor units recruited have slowly contracting and relaxing muscle cells. In addition, the motor neurons innervating these cells can only produce action potentials at a slow rate because of the properties of small-diameter neurons. Because the muscle cells innervated by small motor neurons have slow contraction and relaxation rates, they do not require a high action potential frequency to maintain intracellular Ca^{++} levels at a concentration sufficient to produce tetanization. As greater amounts of neurotransmitter are released on the motor neuron pool, neurons capable of producing end plate potentials at a higher rate are recruited. These motor neurons innervate muscle cells with sarcoplasmic reticulum that takes up Ca^{++} faster and, therefore, requires a higher action potential frequency to tetanize. In either case, sufficient stimulus to the motor neuron pool will result in a contraction approaching a tetanic contraction initially in the recruited motor units, progressing to a fused tetanic contraction as synaptic input to the motor neuron pool increases. The small motor neurons will be depolarized frequently enough to produce action potentials frequently enough in the muscle cells to produce a tetanic contraction. Greater release of neurotransmitter results in recruitment of motor neurons capable of generating a higher rate of action potentials that produce tetanic contraction of the larger, faster motor neurons. Through years of practice, we learn how much synaptic input to place on which motor neuron pools to achieve the desired result.

PRELOAD (LENGTH-TENSION RELATIONSHIP)

Each muscle has connections to bones that we call the origin and insertion in a somewhat arbitrary manner. When muscle contracts, it pulls equally on both attachments. However, muscles do not operate in an independent manner; other muscles can also produce force on the same bones. We can position a muscle at different lengths by placing an external force on a muscle before it contracts (preload), or we may stretch a muscle using other muscles to alter the distance between a given muscle's attachments. Through experience, we learn how much force our muscles generate at different lengths. Unconsciously, we adjust muscle length before initiating a movement to develop the force we want. A more difficult task is to select the appropriate synaptic input to a motor neuron pool if the muscle length is not under voluntary control, such as a novel position or rapid adjustment to an unforeseen circumstance. For example, it is much easier to make a free throw in basketball than it is to make a shot from the same distance while moving around a defender.

ACTIVE AND PASSIVE INSUFFICIENCY

Muscles may be classified based on the number of joints over which they cross. Three of the quadriceps muscles, for example, cross only the knee joint, whereas the rectus femoris crosses both the hip and knee joints. Two-joint muscles, therefore, can be stretched over a greater range than one-joint muscles. This range allows a two-joint muscle, such as the rectus femoris, to become too short to develop significant tension during combined hip flexion and knee extension or to become too long during combined hip extension and knee flexion to develop much force. When a two-joint muscle is contracting and becomes too short, the process is called **active insufficiency. Passive insufficiency** occurs when a muscle is passively stretched to a sarcomere length that is too long. Both active and passive insufficiency can occur at the same time in a pair of antagonists (Figure 18-5). A good example is the combined movement of hip extension and knee flexion. This movement produces active insufficiency of the hamstrings and passive insufficiency of the rectus femoris. One may observe an individual performing hamstring curls often flexes at the hip at the end of knee flexion to complete the lift.

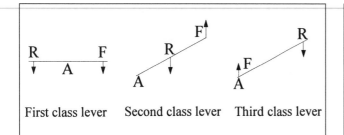

First class lever   Second class lever   Third class lever

Figure 18-6. Three classes of lever systems. The mnemonic ARF can be used to distinguish them. In a first-class lever system, the axis is between the resistance and force. The third-class lever system is characteristic of many musculoskeletal units of the body in which the tendon (the force transmitting structure) is proximal and the load is distal along the bony lever.

LEVER SYSTEMS

Previous discussion of muscle performance has been limited to measurement from muscles attached directly to a force transducer or to a load directly through a tendon. However, our muscles operate through bony lever systems to produce force against a load. In physics, three-lever systems are described. These systems are called first-, second-, and third-class levers. A simple way to remember the types of levers is "ARF" (Figure 18-6). The three components of a lever are the axis, resistance (load), and force. ARF refers to the component in the middle of the lever system. A first-class lever, such as a seesaw, has the axis in the center and the resistance and force on either end. A second-class lever, a wheelbarrow for example, has the resistance in the middle, the axis on one end, and the force on the other. Most musculoskeletal levers are third-class levers. The force is in the middle, and the resistance and axis are at the ends. In a first-class lever system, equilibrium is achieved by placing a force and resistance on opposite sides of the axis with the same direction, usually downward. In a third-class lever, in contrast, the force and resistance are on the same side of the axis, the resistance is farther from the axis, and the force and resistance have opposite directions (Figure 18-7). The distance of the axis from the resistance is called the resistance arm. Likewise, the distance from the axis to the force is called the force arm. Torque is the product of distance and force. For a lever system to be in equilibrium, the torque produced by the resistance (load) is equal to load times resistance arm, and the torque produced by the force is force times force arm. In a first-class lever in which the force arm is equal to the resistance arm, equilibrium exists if the force equals the resistance. When the resistance and force arms are of unequal length, the force and resist-

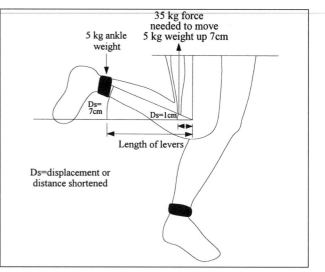

Figure 18-7. A typical third-class lever musculoskeletal unit. A muscle must develop a much greater tension than the resistance (in this case an ankle weight) to balance the lever system. In this case, a tension equal to seven times the load is required. This mechanism is costly in terms of tension generated, but multiplies the distance that the muscle displaces the bony lever.

ance must be inversely proportional to the difference in force and resistance arm. For example, if the resistance arm is 35 cm long and the force arm is 5 cm long, and if the resistance is equivalent to 10 kg, the force must be 10 x (35/5) = 70 kg (times the acceleration of gravity) for equilibrium to exist. The effects of differences in the length of the resistance and force arms are the same in a third-class lever system. For example, if the biceps tendon is inserted 5 cm from the elbow and a load of 10 kg is held in the hand 35 cm from the elbow, the biceps must generate a force equal to 10 x (35/5) kg = 70 kg to hold the weight still.

This third-class lever system produces a mechanical disadvantage in that the muscles attached in this way must produce a much greater force than the load. However, a mechanical advantage exists in terms of how much a muscle must shorten to move a load. In our biceps example above in which the biceps tendon is inserted 5 cm from the elbow and the load is held 35 cm from the elbow, the biceps needs to shorten only 1 cm to move the load 7 cm upward.

A second consideration of the lever system is how the length of the resistance arm changes with joint angle. The length of the resistance arm is not the distance along the bone between the axis and the load, but is an imaginary line perpendicular to the direction of the acceleration of the load (usually downward with gravity) from the axis to the load. Therefore, the resistance arm is greatest when the joint angle is perpendicular to the acceleration of the load (eg, a 90° angle of the elbow if the individual is upright). As the joint angle deviates from perpendicular, the resistance arm decreases in length with the sine of the joint angle. For example, if the elbow is held at an angle of either 30° or 120°, the resistance arm is halved from its value at an angle of 90°. Neglecting other forces, such as effects on sarcomere length and rotary components of force, less effort needs to be generated as the joint angle deviates from 90°. These effects need to be examined, at least on a qualitative basis, when prescribing exercises for patients/clients.

CO-CONTRACTION AND RECIPROCAL INNERVATION (INHIBITION)

Co-contraction refers to the simultaneous recruitment of motor units from agonists and antagonists (muscles on opposite sides of joints that oppose each other's force). Co-contraction stabilizes joints by compressing a joint and resisting any unexpected changes in force. However, movements that include co-contraction are produced by a muscle that must overcome both an external load and the opposition of the antagonistic muscle. Therefore, a movement using co-contraction is less smooth and cannot accelerate a load as well as one in which a muscle is unopposed. Reciprocal innervation refers to a concept that antagonistic muscles are innervated so that recruitment of motor units from one muscle automatically inhibits the muscle's antagonist. Most movements tend to use some co-contraction. Novel or unpracticed movements tend to use a large co-contraction component. In a highly skilled movement, especially one that requires high velocity, a reciprocal innervation type situation is found. Through practice, one learns how many motor units to recruit to initiate a movement and how many motor units of the antagonist to recruit to stop the movement and the timing of recruitment of the agonists and antagonists. Learning the necessary motor unit recruitment patterns produces smooth, high-velocity movements needed for many types of athletic events, such as tennis or golf strokes.

SKELETAL MUSCLE SENSORY RECEPTORS

Two types of sensory receptors found in skeletal muscle are used to provide information needed for feedback. Muscle spindles detect changes in muscle length, and Golgi tendon organs detect changes in musculotendinous tension. Muscle spindles are found among the skeletal muscle fibers within the belly of a muscle and are arranged in **parallel** with the muscle fibers, whereas Golgi tendon organs are located in tendons near the junction with muscle cells and are arranged in **series** with the muscle (Figure 18-8). Muscle spindles have both afferent and efferent neurons. Within the spindle, stretch receptors in **series** with special muscle fibers called intrafusal fibers are found. The muscle fiber within the spindle is called an intrafusal fiber to distinguish it from the skeletal muscle cells described previously called extrafusal (outside the spindle) fibers. The intrafusal fiber is innervated by a motor neuron of smaller diameter called a γ (gamma) motor neuron, in contrast to the larger motor neurons innervating extrafusal fibers called α motor neurons. Activation of the motor neurons stretches the muscle spindle. Muscle spindles have two afferent neurons, one called a primary afferent and the other called a secondary afferent. We will not try to distinguish between the two in this discussion. The Golgi tendon organ (GTO) has only a single afferent neuron. Both of the muscle sensory receptors have neurons that can be classified as A neurons.

Both types of receptors are stimulated by stretch. By virtue of muscle attachment to bones at both ends of the muscle, some stretch is always present on muscles. Changes in stretch change the frequency of action potentials generated by these receptors. The muscle spindle is deformed when the length of extrafusal fibers increases relative to the spindle and responds by increasing the frequency of action potentials carried by its afferent neurons. The spindle decreases its action potential frequency if the extrafusal fibers decrease in length relative to the muscle spindle (Figure 18-9). If a muscle is stretched, the muscle spindle increases its action potential frequency. If the extrafusal muscle fibers contract, the action potential frequency generated by the muscle spindle decreases (Figure 18-10). The GTO increases its action potential frequency when deformed by stretching of the musculotendinous junction, which occurs when a muscle is passively stretched or when the extrafusal fibers contract (Figure 18-11).

Both types of receptors are involved in negative feedback mechanisms. The muscle spindle acts to keep muscle length at a value determined by the central nervous system (CNS). An unexpected load that causes a deviation in muscle length from the expected causes a change in the direction to restore length to the desired value. The GTO is involved in a reflex to prevent excessive tension in a muscle. Deformation of either type of receptor by passive stretch of a muscle increases action potential frequency, whereas muscle contraction produces opposite effects on the two types of receptors. Contraction shortens muscle, decreasing stretch on the muscle spindle, but contraction stretches tendons and the GTO. Without the activation of γ motor neurons, muscle contraction would lead to decreased action potential frequency from the muscle spindle and increased action potential frequency from the GTO. However, during a voluntary muscle contraction, both the α and γ motor neurons are recruited, causing short-

ening of both the extra- and intrafusal muscle fibers. Shortening of extrafusal fibers in parallel with the spindle puts the spindle on slack, but shortening of the intrafusal fiber in series with the receptive region of the spindle pulls up the slack in the receptor, preventing a decrease in action potential frequency from occurring in the muscle spindle (see Figure 18-9 b and c).

The muscle spindle is involved in two important reflexes: the stretch reflex and the load reflex. The load

Spasticity

Thousands of neurons synapse with motor neurons in the anterior horn of the spinal cord. These include neurons that originate from the brain and are carried in the bundle called the corticospinal tract. These neurons, called upper motor neurons, carry both excitatory and inhibitory messages to the motor neurons. The term upper motor neuron is used to distinguish them from the motor neurons that directly innervate skeletal muscle and are called lower motor neurons. Other neurons synapsing with the motor neuron are the sensory fibers of the muscle spindle and interneurons relaying information from other sensory structures, such as Golgi tendon organs, touch, and pain receptors. This information produces an amount of activity in the muscle called tone. We can think of tone as the resistance to passive movement. Tone is low during sleep and very low during REM sleep. Tone increases greatly when we are startled. The muscle spindle is largely responsible for producing tone by generating a steady action potential frequency at rest, which helps us to overcome gravity and maintain posture. This tone is increased when the muscle is stretched, for example, if your arm slips off the arm of a chair.

Damage to the lower motor neurons results in paralysis with flaccidity (no postural tone due to the lack of innervation of muscle cells) and a loss of the deep tendon (stretch) reflex. Damage to the upper motor neurons, on the other hand, often leads to the development of very high tone and hyperreflexia. The muscle spindle represents an excitatory input to the motor neuron opposed at rest by inhibitory messages from upper motor neurons and other sensory structures. Following an event such as a stroke or spinal cord injury, synapses from upper motor neurons are lost, and the space that they free up on the motor neuron becomes available for other neurons to send "sprouts" to create new synapses. Many of these new synapses come from muscle spindles, creating a condition of too much excitatory input and muscle tone that we call spasticity. The increased input of muscle spindles not only increases tone, but it also makes the stretch reflex very sensitive. Spasticity can create so much tone that a tremendous effort is required to move the extremity passively. Slow stretch activates Golgi tendon organs and can cause tone to diminish. If a person receives sensory input to the affected extremity, the development of spasticity can be decreased. This is often done through simple means, such as placing the extremity in a position of weightbearing. One may speculate that weightbearing promotes sprouting of neurons other than muscle spindle afferents to affected lower motor neurons. Spasticity appears to involve other factors that are not understood well at this time. Spasticity seems to develop in certain muscles preferentially. When a stroke affects an entire side of the body, spasticity occurs in specific patterns involving mainly flexor muscles of the upper extremities and extensors of the lower extremities.

Modified Ashworth Scale for Grading Spasticity

Grade	Description
0	No increase in muscle tone.
1	Slight increase in muscle tone manifested by a catch and release or by minimal resistance at the end of the range of motion when the affected part(s) is moved in flexion or extension.
1+	Slight increase in muscle tone manifested by a catch, followed by minimal resistance throughout the remainder (less than half) of the range of motion.
2	More marked increase in muscle tone through most of the range of motion, but affected part(s) easily moved.
3	Considerable increase in muscle tone, passive movement difficult.
4	Affected part(s) rigid in flexion or extension.

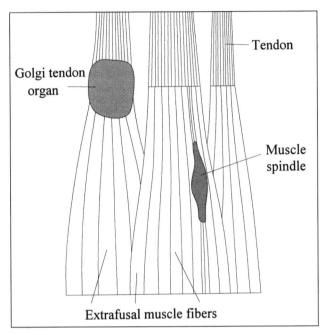

Figure 18-8. Location of muscle sensory receptors. Note that the Golgi tendon organ is located in series with the extrafusal muscle fibers, whereas the muscle spindle is located parallel to extrafusal muscle fibers.

reflex refers to the condition in which an unexpected load is placed on a muscle. Stretching of the muscle by the unexpected load causes a stretching of the muscle spindle. The muscle spindle's neuron synapses with the α motor neurons of the same muscle, increasing the synaptic input on the motor neuron pool proportionally to the stretch on the muscle spindle caused by the unexpected load. The increased synaptic input increases the force generated by the muscle to correct for the unexpected load (Figure 18-12). The stretch reflex is what one tries to elicit when testing deep tendon reflexes. Although one taps on the tendon, it is the muscle spindle that produces the reflex. Rapid stretch of a muscle by tapping the tendon stretches the muscle spindle, which in turn facilitates the α motor neuron pool of the same muscle and the muscle's synergists, and simultaneously inhibits the muscle's antagonists, producing an observable muscle contraction.

During certain activities that require increased stability, such as balance activities or other activities in which the muscle length may change rapidly or unpredictably, γ motor neurons are activated to increase the sensitivity of the muscle spindle (Figure 18-13). This process is called gamma bias and serves to increase the muscle tone for any given level of stretch of the muscle spindle. Novel activities elicit gamma bias and co-contractions of muscle. Learning of a novel activity requires a decrease in gamma bias to allow a reciprocal inhibition

to allow muscles to work more efficiently instead of "fighting" their antagonists.

The GTO is involved in a reflex called the tendon reflex that may prevent muscle injury due to excessive tension on a muscle. Stretch of the GTO inhibits the same muscle and its synergists and simultaneously facilitates the muscle's antagonists. The tendon reflex may be used to decrease muscle spasm or spasticity by slow stretch of the muscle or pressure on the tendon. The tendon reflex is also useful for maintaining tension of a muscle in the face of fatigue. When muscle tension decreases due to fatigue, the GTO is less active, resulting in decreased inhibition on the motor neuron pool of the same muscle. The decreased inhibition allows more motor units to be recruited to compensate for fatigue.

SUMMARY

ATP is used during muscle activity for cross-bridge cycling, uptake of Ca^{++}, and maintaining the concentrations of sodium and potassium. Mechanisms available for regenerating ATP from ADP include breakdown of creatine phosphate, substrate phosphorylation, and oxidative phosphorylation. Breakdown of creatine phosphate is the most rapid means of regenerating ATP but is useful for only a short time. Glycolysis (substrate phosphorylation) can rapidly, but inefficiently, produce ATP. Oxidative phosphorylation can produce ATP indefinitely, but requires a longer time to catch up to the rate of ATP use. Metabolic activity in excess of the rate of oxidative metabolism is called oxygen debt. At the end of exercise, an excess of oxygen consumption approximately equal to the oxygen debt occurs. Fatigue is the decline in force production by muscle following a period of muscle activity. During intense activity, acidosis appears to be responsible for fatigue. During prolonged, less intense activity, substrate depletion may cause fatigue. A motor unit is an motor neuron and all the muscle cells innervated by the motor neuron. Motor units may be classified as slow oxidative, fast oxidative, or fast glycolytic. Slow oxidative are the most efficient, oxidative, and fatigue resistant. The slowest oxidative motor units are active more than other motor units. The order of recruitment of motor units from small to large appears to be responsible for the biochemical and mechanical characteristics of the different motor units. The size principle describes the manner in which motor units are sequentially recruited as more force is demanded by the CNS. Small, slowly conducting motor neurons innervating small numbers of small skeletal muscle cells are recruited first followed by progressively larger, faster

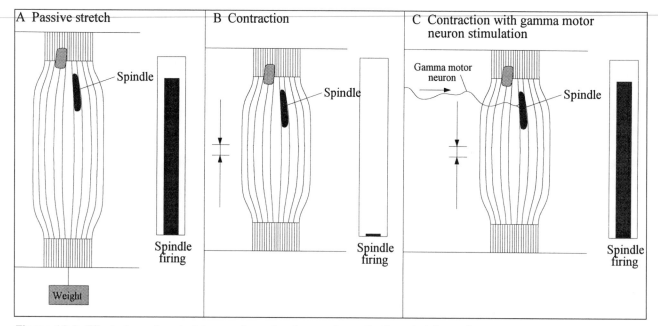

Figure 18-9. Effect of passive stretch, muscle contraction, and coactivation of alpha and gamma motor neurons. Note that muscle spindles are located parallel to extrafusal muscle cells and respond to passive stretch with increased firing and muscle contraction with decreased firing. With coactivation of alpha and gamma motor neurons, tension remains on the muscle spindle, thereby maintaining the spindle's firing rate.

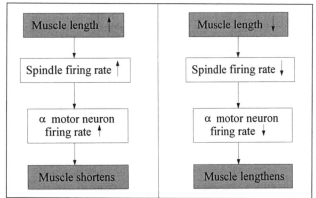

Figure 18-10. Responses of the muscle spindle to alterations in muscle length.

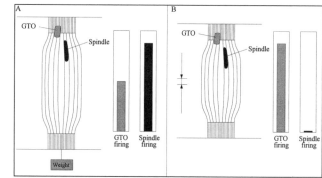

Figure 18-11. Comparison of the effects of passive stretch and muscle contraction on muscle spindles and Golgi tendon organs.

conducting motor neurons innervating large numbers of large skeletal muscle cells. The frequency of action potentials required to tetanize the motor units increases with the size of the motor unit. Small motor units tetanize at a relatively low action potential frequency, whereas the large muscle cells innervated by the largest motor neurons have a faster sarcoplasmic reticulum and require a greater action potential frequency to be tetanized. Through learning, we can place our muscles at the optimum length prior to contraction by preloading a muscle with both the load and antagonistic muscles. A two-joint muscle experiences passive insufficien-

cy when it is stretched too much across two joints and active insufficiency when it shortens too much. Many of our muscles are used to produce force on third-class bony lever systems. In this arrangement, the muscle must generate a much greater force than the load to move the load, but the muscle needs only to shorten a fraction of the distance that the load is moved. Co-contraction refers to the simultaneous recruitment of antagonistic muscles to provide stability. Reciprocal innervation refers to the inhibition of a muscle's antagonist to perform highly skilled, high-velocity movements.

Two types of sensory receptors are located in skele-

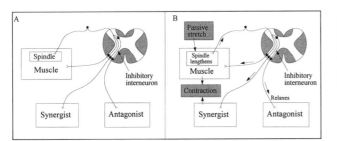

Figure 18-12. The components of the load reflex. Unexpected loading of skeletal muscle stretches muscle spindles, resulting in facilitation of the stretched muscle and its synergists while inhibiting the stretched muscles' antagonists.

Behavioral state	Cat resting	Cat sitting	Cat walking	Cat beam walking
Gamma activity	0	0	+	+++

Figure 18-13. Activation of gamma motor neurons during different activities. Novel activities or those requiring stability result in greater activity of gamma motor neurons, which, in turn, increases the sensitivity of muscle spindles.

tal muscle. The muscle spindle monitors muscle length; the GTO monitors tension in the musculotendinous junction. Both receptors respond to stretch with increased action potential frequency. During voluntary contraction, the muscle spindle's intrafusal fiber and the surrounding skeletal muscle fibers both shorten with no net change in stretch on the muscle spindle. An unexpected load (load reflex) or a rapid stretch of the muscle by tapping the tendon (stretch reflex) causes an increased action potential frequency leading to greater synaptic input on the motor neuron pools of the stretched muscle and its synergists as well as inhibition of its antagonists. During certain activities, the sensitivity of the muscle spindle is increased by activation of gamma motor neurons in anticipation of the activity (gamma bias). Golgi tendon organs are stretched during muscle contraction or passive stretch. Increased action potential frequency from the GTO causes inhibition of the same muscle and its synergists and a facilitation of the muscle's antagonists.

EMG Biofeedback
B. Nathaniel Grubbs, MS, PT

The use of biofeedback to optimize rehabilitation outcomes is a common practice in physical therapy. Biofeedback modalities, as utilized in physical therapy, reveal to patients information concerning physiological events, most commonly in the form of a visual, an auditory, or a combination of both signals. The aim of biofeedback training is to teach patients to manipulate these otherwise involuntary or unfelt physiological events by manipulating the displayed signals. The most common form of biofeedback used in physical therapy is electromyographic biofeedback (EMGBF). The physiological event monitored in EMGBF is propagation of action potentials along muscle cell membranes following depolarization of motor neurons in the monitored muscle. Surface sensors (electrodes) placed over a target muscle detect membrane depolarization (excitation) as the muscle is recruited. Most EMGBF units used in physical therapy require two active sensors and a single ground (reference) sensor. Myoelectric activity detected in the two active sensors is compared to activity detected in the ground sensor by a differential amplifier.

Following detection and amplification, the signal is processed in such a way that allows for the electromyographic activity to be displayed to the patient in a variety of ways. Visual representation of the EMG signal may take the form of a line traveling across a monitor, needle deflection, a bank of lights, or even as a component of a video game (contingent upon computer interfacing). Auditory tones, beeps, or clicks may also provide the client with feedback. During EMGBF training, the patient attempts to alter the visual or auditory display as directed by the physical therapist, thereby resulting in an alteration of the measured physiological activity (motor unit recruitment).

The most basic goals for the physical therapy patient undergoing EMGBF training are to either increase (facilitate) or decrease (inhibit) myoelectric activity. Following proper skin preparation, the active sensors are placed along the long axis of the target muscle(s), and a baseline EMG activity level is established. Thereafter, the patient is instructed by the physical therapist to alter the visual or auditory signal appropriately. Clinical examples of the use of EMGBF include facilitation of vastus medialis function in the treatment of patellofemoral dysfunction, improved control of pelvic floor musculature in the treatment of urinary incontinence, facilitation of dorsiflexion in neurologically involved patients with "foot-drop," relaxation therapy for hypertonic muscles, and muscle re-education in patients following tendon transplant procedures.

STUDY QUESTIONS

1. Consider the following track events: the 100-meter dash, the 1-mile run, and the 10,000-meter run. What do you think are the primary limiting factors of performance as related to fatigue?

2. The world record for the 400-meter run has declined tremendously over the past 40 years. What factor related to fatigue do you think determines the time? What adaptations at the cellular level of skeletal myocytes are necessary to allow today's athletes to overcome this limitation?

3. Why does a person who has been bed-bound become fatigued so quickly when walking?

4. What benefit does having small motor units in the muscles of the hand have? What sort of characteristics do these muscles have?

5. What benefit is there to having large motor units in the quadriceps? What characteristics do you suppose these muscles have?

6. How do you suspect the characteristics of motor units in a person running long distances compare with those in a person who sprints, jumps, or lifts weights?

7. Explain the benefit of recruitment of small motor units progressing to large motor units as demands for muscle force increase.

8. During most athletic events, note that a component of the event usually involves a quick stretch of muscles before they contract forcefully. How does a quick stretch of muscle improve its performance?

9. Give examples of how gamma bias can improve or diminish performance of motor function.

10. Explain how the stretch reflex can prevent someone from falling and how the load reflex can prevent a person from dropping an object.

11. Based on the idea of sprouting, why do you think that weightbearing and other types of sensory input reduce the hyperreflexia that occurs after a stroke?

LABORATORY EXERCISES

LABORATORY EXERCISE 18-1

ESTIMATION OF MUSCLE STRENGTH BASED ON MUSCLE SIZE

Objective: Demonstrate the relationships between muscle size and lever systems in determining the load that a muscle can move.

Materials:
Isokinetic knee extension device
Tape measure

Estimate strength of quadriceps based on cross-sectional area and contractility of 3 kg/cm^2. Assume quadriceps cross-section is an ellipse. Measure width at mid-thigh in centimeters. Subtract a double layer of skin and subcutaneous fat. Measure distance from top of thigh to estimated top of femur. Subtract a single thickness of skin and subcutaneous fat. Estimate cross-sectional area as π [(width + height)/4]^2. Multiply by 3 kg/cm^2 to estimate what maximum force should be (Fmax). Next, measure distance from tibial plateau to the tibial tuberosity. Measure the distance from the tibial plateau to where the pad of a knee extension machine makes contact with the shin. You should be able to move a weight equal to Fmax x distance to the tibial tuberosity/distance to the pad of the knee extension machine. What factors could introduce error between estimated and measured quadriceps strength?

LABORATORY EXERCISE 18-2

ELECTROMYOGRAPHY

Objectives:
1.   Record an electromyogram (EMG).
2.   Describe the differences between concentric, isometric, and eccentric contractions.
3.   Explain the difference between maximal and submaximal isometric contractions.
4.   Describe how external load changes with joint angle.
5.   Explain the relationship between EMG activity and motor unit recruitment.
6.   Demonstrate how different muscles become active during different parts of a movement.
7.   Demonstrate the relationship between fatigue and recruitment.

The EMG is a recording of the difference in electrical potential between two electrodes placed into muscle (needle electrodes) or on the skin over a muscle (surface electrodes). Potentials recorded this way are biphasic in nature. The EMG is a recording of electrical activity originating from skeletal muscle related to muscle contraction. The asynchronous discharge of different motor units superimposed on biphasic waves produces a complex waveform called an interference pattern. The waveform of the EMG will vary in amplitude and frequency in a predictable fashion with changes in muscle activity, which makes the EMG a useful clinical and research tool.

Clinically, the EMG is usually displayed on an oscilloscope and the signal is also sent to a speaker so that variations in amplitude and frequency can also be heard. This was done previously during

LABORATORY EXERCISES

the nerve conduction velocity procedure. Permanent records will be made on paper during these exercises. Records can also be stored on tape or computer discs for later analysis. The EMG can be quantified by rectification and integration of the signal (making all deflections go in one direction and averaging the signal over time). This process is done electronically by a module within the recording apparatus. The integrated EMG can also usually be displayed on the stored record for a more quantifiable determination of muscle activity.

During relaxation, a normally innervated muscle should be relatively quiet. However, changes in muscle activity will be reflected in changes in the EMG. As more muscle force is required, more motor units will be recruited and the frequency of muscle action potentials will increase. This results in increases in both the frequency and amplitude of the EMG.

For this laboratory exercise, we will use surface electrodes and an ink and pen recorder without a speaker, although sounds can be heard with headphones attached to the output jack of the recorder. Clinical EMGs will usually be recorded with needle electrodes to distinguish between neuropathies (nerve disease) and myopathies (muscle diseases) for differential diagnosis of neuromuscular disease.

Materials:
Two sets of EMG leads with surface (disc) electrodes
Electrode paste, alcohol, and gauze pads
Weights
Handgrip dynamometer
Physiologic recorder with high gain coupler and EMG integrator coupler

When recording an EMG from only one muscle, place the EMG cable into the high gain coupler to record the raw EMG. Place a cable in the output jack of the high gain coupler and connect the other end to the input of the EMG integrator coupler to record a signal that can be quantified. Place the switch on the EMG coupler to integrate. When recording two EMGs simultaneously plug a cable into the input of both modules and switch the EMG integrator module to "direct."

Methods:
EMG and isotonic, isometric, and eccentric contractions:
1. Find the motor point for the middle deltoid.
2. Prepare the skin over the middle deltoid, deltoid tuberosity, and seventh cervical vertebra with isopropyl alcohol.
3. Apply adhesive collars to the EMG electrodes and fill to near top with electrode paste. Attach electrodes to the skin over the seventh cervical vertebra, deltoid tuberosity, and motor point of the middle deltoid.
4. Record the EMG produced by the middle deltoid under resting conditions. This can be verified by the minimal waveform on the recorder. If there is excessive noise, ask for help.

A. Isometric contraction
Submaximal isometric contraction: with the subject standing, place the shoulder at 90° abduction. Adjust the gain on the channels used to ensure that maximal effort can be recorded without the pen deflecting beyond its range while the subject exerts maximal effort against an infinite load. While recording, add weight in 5 lb. increments, recording at each load up to the subject's ability to maintain the shoulder at 90° of abduction. Note if the load does not move, the contractions are isometric. How does the EMG compare at different loads? How may we define an isometric contraction in terms of force produced by the muscle and the load on the muscle?

LABORATORY EXERCISES

Maximal isometric contraction. Next, attempt to abduct the shoulder against an infinite load, such as a wall. Exert maximum effort at several joint angles while recording the EMG. Does the EMG change at different joint angles? Why should or should not the EMG change?

B. Isotonic contraction
With the subject in the standing position and the arm at the side, lift a moderately heavy weight (5 to 15 lbs.) through the entire range of motion (ROM) over a 3 to 4 second period. Note how the EMG changes through the ROM. Where in the ROM are the amplitude and frequency the greatest and the least? Stop momentarily at full abduction and 0° of abduction. Mark top (180°), bottom (0°), and 90° on the tracing.

C. Eccentric contraction
Compare the size of the EMG when raising the weight in B above (concentric contraction) to lowering the weight (eccentric contraction). How did the size of the EMG during concentric and eccentric contraction compare with maximal isometric contraction (A)?

D. Effect of joint angle
Record the EMG while holding the heaviest weight at five different joint angles. Hand the weight to the subject, record the EMG, and remove the weight. Assume a different joint angle and repeat. Allow the subject a minute to rest between each trial. Use 90°, two positions above 90°, and two positions below 90°. Where is EMG largest? How do the effects of length of the resistance arm, sarcomere length, and the horizontal component of a rotary movement affect the motor unit recruitment required at each joint angle?

E. Demonstration of EMG of synergistic muscles
Each group should perform at least one the three following exercises and ensure that each of the three exercises is performed by at least one group.

1. Supraspinatus and deltoid. Attach two sets of electrodes: one for the deltoid and another set for the supraspinatus. Observe the timing of EMG bursts during shoulder abduction with a moderate weight. Record EMG while lowering the weight (adduction). Where in the ROM are the two different muscles most active?

2. Pectoralis major and triceps. Attach one set of electrodes over the pectoralis major and another over the triceps of the same arm. Have the subject perform push-ups with the hands directly below the shoulder. Repeat with the hands together and again with the hands wider than the shoulders. Note which muscles are more active in the different positions.

3. Biceps and brachioradialis. Attach one set of electrodes over the biceps brachii and another over the brachioradialis of the same forearm. Record the EMGs while flexing the elbow. Record while lifting a moderate weight with the hand supinated and record again with the hand in the neutral position.

G. EMG and muscle fatigue
1. Place electrodes over the motor point of the flexor digitorum superficialis in the center of the forearm, over the distal part of the muscle and over the seventh cervical vertebra.

2. Determine maximum handgrip strength while recording the EMG and adjust the gain of the recorder if necessary.

LABORATORY EXERCISES

3. Compute what 75% and 50% of maximum handgrip strength are.

4. Maintain 75% of maximum handgrip while recording the EMG. Continue recording until force falls below 50% of maximum despite maximum effort. Give the subject verbal encouragement to aid performance. What happens to EMG with time? How does the subject compensate for fatigue?

H. Questions

1. Define:
    Recruitment
    Motor unit
    Isometric contraction
    Isotonic contraction
    Concentric contraction
    Eccentric contraction
    Fatigue

2. What factors determine whether a contraction is isometric, concentric, or eccentric? What factors limit our ability to perform these types of contraction?

3. What factors determine how much we can accelerate an external object?

4. Explain the factors that complicate rotary movements that are imposed by our joint structure.

5. During an isometric contraction, do we know how much force the muscle is producing? What other information do we need to know?

6. During an eccentric or concentric contraction, do we know how much force the muscle is producing? What other information do we need to know?

UNIT V

Cardiopulmonary System

The cardiovascular and respiratory systems act in concert to deliver nutrients and eliminate wastes, particularly oxygen and carbon dioxide. Both systems require energy to create the bulk flow within their respective systems. The cardiac pump consists of two one-way circuits in series, such that blood pumped by the right side of the heart pumps blood through the lungs to oxygenate blood and into the left side of the heart, which, in turn, pumps blood to the rest of the body and then to the right side of the heart. The cardiac pump consists of a muscular chamber for each circulation and valves to ensure unidirectional flow from veins to arteries. Cardiac pump dysfunction can result from weakness or disorganized contraction, valvular disease, or obstruction of the vessels. The ventilatory pump is a two-way circuit in which energy is used to allow the atmosphere to drive bulk flow of air into the lungs, and elastic recoil of the lungs drives bulk flow back out. The ventilatory pump consists of muscles of inspiration that pull the chest wall out, abdominal muscles necessary for the diaphragm to function optimally, ribs, and various muscles that stabilize and mobilize the ribs as appropriate. Ventilatory pump dysfunction can result from weakness of the muscles of ventilation, the abdominal muscles, or injury to the chest wall or pleura. This unit presents chapters that describe the basic principles of the cardiovascular system, function of the cardiac pump, principles governing the flow of blood, how the cardiovascular system is controlled, basic properties of the ventilatory pump, how the ventilatory pump is controlled, how the cardiac and ventilatory pumps work together to transport gases to and from the environment and cells, how the ventilatory pump and pH are controlled, and, finally, how the cardiovascular and respiratory systems respond to exercise stress.

NINETEEN

Introduction to the Cardiovascular System

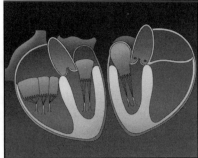

1. Describe the basic circuit of the cardiovascular system: left atrium, left ventricle, systemic arteries, arterioles, capillaries, veins, right atrium, right ventricle, pulmonary arteries, capillaries, and veins.

2. Describe the structure and roles of the four chambers of the heart.

3. Describe the structure and roles of the four cardiac valves.

4. Describe the structure of the cardiac myocyte: presence of striations, intercalated disc, gap junctions.

5. Compare the features that determine the oxidative capacity of skeletal muscle to cardiac muscle.

6. Describe phase 0, 1, 2, 3, and 4 of the ventricular cell action potential; compare with the action potential of skeletal muscle or neurons.

7. State the mechanisms responsible for each phase of the ventricular cell action potential.

8. Compare the fast response action potential of atrial and ventricular cells to the slow response action potential of SA node and AV node cells.

9. Define automaticity. List cells that display automaticity and their relative rate of depolarization.

10. Trace the normal sequence of cardiac excitation.

Put in simplest terms, the heart has a single function. That function is to pump blood from veins into arteries. The pumping of blood into arteries increases arterial pressure. The removal of blood from veins decreases venous pressure, and the difference in pressure between arteries and veins created by the heart drives the bulk flow of blood through the circulation. Circulation of blood provides the convection required to exchange substances between the internal and external environment and among tissues. Effectiveness of the heart as a pump depends on the ability of the heart muscle to produce rhythmic, coordinated contractions and healthy valves to ensure flow in only one direction with minimal resistance to forward flow.

The volume of blood pumped out of the heart into the arteries per time equals the volume pumped out of the veins and also equals the volume transported by bulk flow due to the difference in pressure from arteries to veins, thus completing a circuit. The cardiovascular system in a healthy individual produces a steady state in which the blood flow through the circulation is equal to the blood pumped into and from the heart. In other words, cardiac output equals venous return, and both equal the sum of peripheral blood flows. Using the equation for bulk flow, $Q = g\Delta P$ with Q equal to cardiac output (CO), using mean arterial blood pressure (MAP) through the cardiac cycle as ΔP, and the conductance of the peripheral blood vessels, we can summarize as CO = MAP x total conductance. Traditionally, the units to describe the conductance of the entire vascular system have been the reciprocal of conductance, total peripheral resistance (TPR). This is stated mathematically in analogy with Ohm's law as MAP = CO x TPR. Some examples of how this equation can be useful follow. In hypertension, a high total peripheral resistance requires a greater mean arterial pressure to drive a given cardiac output through the circulation. A low total peripheral resistance, which occurs during exercise due to vasodilation in working muscle, requires a greater cardiac output to maintain a given mean arterial pressure. In decompensated heart failure, mean arterial pressure falls due to the inability of the heart to create a sufficient cardiac output to match the total peripheral resistance. In hemorrhagic shock, the heart is stimulated in an attempt to increase cardiac output, and blood vessels are constricted in an attempt to maintain mean arterial pressure, resulting in a weak, thready pulse and injury to organs, such as the kidneys, that do not receive sufficient blood flow. Throughout discussions involving the circulatory system, we can refer to this equation and components of each part with the realization that what is pumped out of the heart, what is removed from the veins, and what circulates is equal over a short period. Thinking in sim-

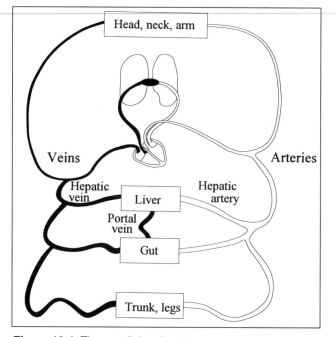

Figure 19-1. The parallel and series elements of circulation. The systemic and pulmonary circuits operate in series. Flow through one must equal the other, and obstruction of one diminishes flow through the other. Within the systemic circulation, blood flows to the different organs are in parallel.

ple terms of the heart as a pump also allows us to analyze cardiovascular disease in terms of effectiveness of cardiac pumping: valve function, rhythmic, coordinated contraction, resistance to outflow, or inadequate inflow to the heart.

The cardiovascular system consists of two circulatory systems in series (Figure 19-1). The systemic circulation, which is served by the left side of the heart, produces convective transport to all tissues of the body with a small contribution to the lungs called the bronchial circulation. The pulmonary circulation provides blood flow to the alveoli of the lungs where the exchange of gases with the atmosphere occurs. The pulmonary circulation rids the body of carbon dioxide and, in the process, picks up oxygen.

Different types of vessels are necessary to perform the various roles required of the circulatory system. Arteries distribute blood under high pressure to the different organs and have a smaller diameter than the veins that return blood from the tissues under low pressure. Large arteries convert the pulsatile pumping of the heart to a near steady flow at the tissue level. Smaller arteries and arterioles distribute blood to tissues according to the needs of the tissues. Most of the exchange of substances between blood and tissues occurs across capillaries, which branch from the smallest arterioles. The cap-

TABLE 19-1

Roles of the Components of the Cardiovascular System

COMPONENT	ROLE
Left ventricle	Pumps blood returning from lungs through systemic circulation under high pressure
Right ventricle	Pumps blood returning from the systemic circulation through the lungs under low pressure
Systemic circulation	Carries blood from the left ventricle to tissue other than lungs under high pressure, then back to the right atrium
Pulmonary circulation	Carries blood from the right ventricle through the lungs under low pressure, then back to the left atrium
Arteries	Deliver blood to different organs and areas within organs
Large arteries	Convert pulsatile pumping of ventricles into near-steady flow into organs
Small arteries	Divide flow among tissues according to tissue needs under local control
Capillaries	Allow exchange of substances between the blood and interstitial fluid around cells
Veins	Return blood to the atria under low pressure and low velocity, and have a much greater cross-sectional area than arteries

illaries then drain into small venous vessels called venules that converge into larger veins and finally into the superior and inferior vena cava of the systemic circulation, which empty into the right atrium or the four pulmonary veins of the pulmonary circulation (two from each lung), which empty into the left atrium.

BLOOD VESSEL STRUCTURE

Blood vessels and the heart are lined with endothelial cells that prevent blood cells from interacting directly with the substances within the vessel wall and, thus, prevent activation of the coagulation process (see Chapter Twenty-One for details). Smooth muscle cells within the wall respond to a large number of influences including neural (sympathetic division), hormonal (especially angiotensin II and epinephrine), and a multitude of paracrine regulators. Fibrous tissue on the outside of the vessel, including collagen and elastin, gives the vessel walls tensile and elastic strength. The relative contribution of these components to the vessel wall varies with the function of the blood vessel. Large vessels have thick layers of elastic and fibrous tissue giving them the compliance and strength needed for converting pulsatile flow into steady flow under high pressure. Smaller arteries and arterioles have a relatively thick layer of smooth muscle to regulate vessel diameter, thereby giving them the capability to regulate blood flow local-

ly. Capillaries have a single layer of endothelial cells, which minimizes diffusion distance. Veins are much more compliant than arteries so that their volume can be changed substantially without affecting pressure greatly, and larger veins have a substantial layer of smooth muscle so that their compliance can be regulated physiologically. The functions of each component are summarized in Table 19-1.

CHARACTERISTICS OF BLOOD VESSELS

Blood pressure decreases as blood moves from the large to the small arteries and into capillaries and finally through the veins. The loss of pressure is the direct result of energy lost as flowing blood interacts with the blood vessel walls. Because circumference does not increase as much as cross-sectional area with diameter of a blood vessel, the larger the diameter of the vessel, the fewer the interactions with the wall per volume of blood, and blood pressure falls less. As a consequence, blood pressure decreases negligibly from the aorta into arteries that serve organs and decreases little within the veins. Blood pressure measured from the brachial artery with a sphygmomanometer, therefore, gives an accurate estimate of pressure within the largest arteries. Veins are much larger than their accompanying arteries, several veins may drain the same tissue that an artery supplies, and the compliance of veins is much greater than that of arteries. For these reasons, much more blood volume exists on the venous side, compared with the arterial side of the circulation. Physiologic regulation of venous compliance can alter the relative volumes of the arterial and venous circulation. Changes in venous compliance, which will be discussed in Chapter Twenty-Two, allow preload on the heart and arterial blood pressure to be regulated simultaneously so that cardiac output, venous return, and peripheral blood flow can remain equal despite various challenges to the circulatory system. The different characteristics of arteries and veins also cause the pressure and velocity of the flowing blood to be greater in arteries than in veins, which can be observed when an artery bleeds contrasted with a bleeding vein. The slow flow of blood in veins can promote the chemical reaction involved in clotting under certain circumstances. A very large mass of clotted blood displaced from a vein may travel through the inferior vena cava, the right side of the heart, and lodge in the circulation of the lung (pulmonary embolus). In severe cases, death may result before anything can be done. Pulmonary embolism is the most likely cause of sudden death in rehabilitation patients.

STRUCTURE OF THE CARDIAC MYOCYTE

Cardiac myocytes, like skeletal myocytes, are striated cells. They possess the same structures that produce the striations and are organized into sarcomeres with A bands, I bands, H zones, M lines, and Z lines (Figure 19-2). As in skeletal muscle, contraction results from approximation of the Z lines. However, instead of pulling two tendons closer to each other, the shortening of cardiac myocytes increases pressure on the volume of the blood within the heart chambers.

Cardiac myocytes have properties that follow the continuum of myocyte properties previously described from fast glycolytic to slow oxidative skeletal muscle fibers to cardiac muscle. Cardiac myocytes are much smaller, have a slower contraction time, have a slower relaxation time than slow oxidative skeletal muscle, are extremely fatigue resistant, and have a tremendous capacity for oxidative metabolism. The small diameter of the cardiac myocyte both decreases the distance that oxygen needs to diffuse from capillaries into the myocyte and causes more capillaries to exist per cross-sectional area of muscle tissue than what is observed in skeletal muscle. These cells also have numerous mito-

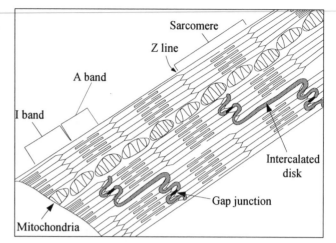

Figure 19-2. Diagram of the internal structure of a cardiac myocyte. Shown are the intercalated discs between cells, gap junctions, and numerous mitochondria.

chondria, and, because of their slow myosin ATPase, they are more energy efficient.

Ventricular cells have a stair-step appearance in contrast to the spindle shape of skeletal muscle and smooth muscle cells. This shape allows adjacent cells to attach to each other through membrane junctions known as intercalated discs. Along the intercalated discs, numerous gap junctions allow for cell communication. In contrast to skeletal muscle, which has a motor nerve to each cell, cardiac myocytes are not innervated to produce contraction. Innervation by the autonomic nervous system produces changes in the frequency and force of contraction, but does not cause contraction. Current from adjacent cells, through gap junctions, causes a wave of depolarization to signal myocyte contraction. Sarcoplasmic reticulum functions in the cardiac myocyte similar to smooth muscle, in that the sarcoplasmic reticulum does not contain sufficient calcium to produce a maximum contraction. The t-tubule observed in skeletal muscle is also found in cardiac muscle and functions in a way similar to that of skeletal muscle to signal the increased concentration of calcium within the cells. This process is more complex than that of skeletal muscle, and excitation-contraction coupling of cardiac muscle is described more fully in the next chapter.

CARDIAC CHAMBERS

The heart consists of four chambers: two upper chambers called atria and two ventricles (Figure 19-3). The right and left atria receive blood from the vena cava and pulmonary veins, respectively. Because no valves exist between the atria and great veins, the atria fill with

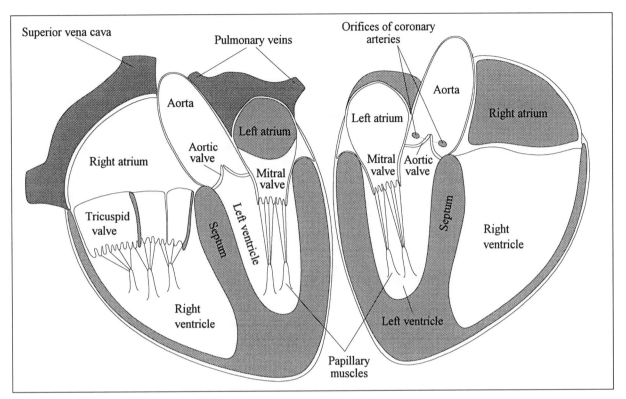

Figure 19-3. Schematic of the heart's internal structure including the four chambers and four valves.

blood throughout the cardiac cycle. The atria are thin-walled, but their contraction prior to the ventricular contraction is important to finish preloading the ventricles. Synchronous contraction of the atria is necessary to prevent stagnation of blood within the atria. The condition of atrial fibrillation, commonly caused by the hyperthyroid state of Graves' disease, is associated with increased risk of stroke due to the clotting of stagnant blood within the fibrillating atria. Because the veins and atria are not separated by valves, a small pulse can be observed in the jugular veins with atrial contraction as blood is pumped forward into the ventricles and backward into the veins. The ventricles and atria are separated by the atrioventricular valves and fibrous tissue. The left ventricle creates four to five times as much arterial pressure as the right ventricle, and the walls of the left ventricle are proportionally thicker. The left ventricle and the interventricular septum form a powerful cone-like mass of muscle, and the free right ventricle wall forms a pocket-like chamber on the right side of the septum. The left ventricle develops sufficient pressure to open the aortic valve to eject blood into the aorta, which then circulates through the systemic circulation to the vena cava and then to the right atrium. The right ventricle develops 20% to 25% of the pressure of the left ventricle to open the pulmonic valve to eject blood into

the pulmonary artery, which then circulates through the lungs and returns to the left atrium having unloaded large quantities of carbon dioxide while picking up oxygen.

HEART VALVES

Four heart valves exist in the plane of the heart between the atria and ventricles (Figure 19-4). The valves have two basic functions: to allow forward movement of blood with negligible resistance to flow and to prevent backflow, which is also known as regurgitation or insufficiency. The valves must be able to withstand ventricular pressure in the case of the atrioventricular valves, or both ventricular and arterial pressure in the cases of the aortic and pulmonic valves. The aortic and pulmonic valves are collectively known as the semilunar valves because each of their three cusps resembles half-moons. The atrioventricular valves include the mitral valve in the left heart and the tricuspid valve of the right heart. The atrioventricular valves are much larger than the aortic and pulmonic valves, and the valve leaflets are anchored to the ventricular apices by chordae tendineae and papillary muscles. They allow filling of the ventricles from the veins through the atria to the ventricles at a low pressure. Because atrial pressure is so low, a large

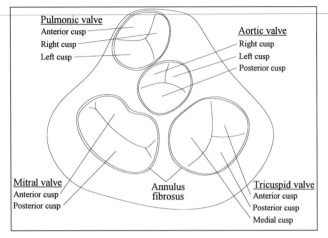

Figure 19-4. The four valves of the heart as viewed from the base. Note that the valves exist in a plane, and note the differences in diameter between the atrioventricular valves and semilunar aortic and pulmonic valves.

surface area is needed to produce sufficient flow across the valves. However, the large surface area means that the total force on the valves during ventricular contraction (pressure times area) could invert the valves if they were untethered. In addition, shortening of the ventricles from the apex toward the base (toward the atria) would allow the chordae tendineae, which tether the atrioventricular valves, to become slack and allow leaflet inversion. This is prevented by contraction of the papillary muscles to which the chordae tendineae are attached. Rupture of the chordae tendineae or papillary muscles can produce acute heart failure, in which ventricular contraction causes blood to be pumped both forward and backward, not allowing for sufficient arterial pressure to drive blood flow through the systemic or pulmonary circulation.

The semilunar valves permit ejection from the ventricles under high pressure and prevent backflow. The valves have three pocket-like cusps that catch a small backflow toward the heart, thus closing the semilunar valves. The backflow in the aorta is detectable on a recorded peripheral pulse as the incisura. When analyzing a tracing of peripheral blood pressure (discussed in Chapter Twenty Cardiac Laboratory Exercise 1), the incisura is used to mark the end of the ejection phase of the cardiac cycle. The incisura shows a rapid decrease in pressure as blood flows backward to fill the cusps of the aortic valve and a sharp increase in aortic pressure as the valves close and blood flow changes direction again, followed by a gradual decrease in aortic pressure as blood empties from the aorta by elastic recoil.

ELECTRIC ACTIVITY OF THE HEART

Different types of cells within the heart have different patterns of electrical activity. Ventricular cells have a resting potential similar to that of skeletal muscle. Atrial cells are less polarized, and the pacemaker cells of the sinoatrial node and the tissue that conducts atrial current into the ventricles, called the atrioventricular node, have electrical activity that more closely resembles that of smooth muscle. In addition to sodium and potassium ions, which were so important to explain membrane potentials in skeletal muscle and neurons, the membrane potentials of cardiac cells are also influenced by calcium due to the presence of voltage-operated calcium channels. Calcium has the potential for rapid movement into a cell in the presence of an open calcium channel. In resting ventricular cell membranes, permeability to potassium ions is much greater than it is to sodium or calcium ions. For this reason, the membrane potential (E_m) is near the K^+ equilibrium potential (E_K) of approximately -90 mV. However, certain types of cardiac myocytes are less polarized and do not display a steady resting potential. Some of these cell types depolarize spontaneously and can set the pace of contraction of the heart.

THE VENTRICULAR ACTION POTENTIAL

Five phases of the ventricular action potential can be described. They are numbered from phase 0 to phase 4. These membrane potential changes can be explained on the basis of membrane conductance changes, just as they were for the neuron. The major difference between a neuron's action potential and that of a cardiac cell is the effect of voltage-operated calcium channels. Phase 0 is the upstroke of the action potential. This phase is identical to the upstroke of the neuron's action potential and is caused by the opening of voltage-operated sodium channels. The Na channels activate at approximately -75 mV, and shortly after opening, the Na channels inactivate in the same way as they do in the neuron. Because activation is more rapid than inactivation, a brief inward sodium current results. Phase 1 is produced by the inactivation gate of the voltage-operated sodium channels, but stops before repolarization occurs. Phase 2 is triggered by depolarization and is the plateau phase of the action potential. Phase 2 occurs due to opening of slow Ca channels and closure of resting K channels. Voltage-

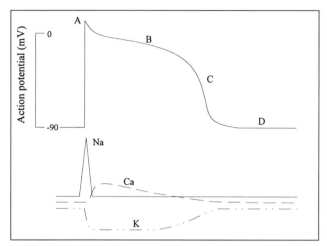

Figure 19-5. The ventricular cell action potential (top) and the ionic fluxes responsible for its generation (below).

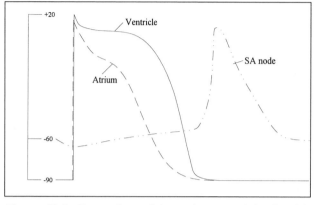

Figure 19-6. Comparison of the action potentials of atrial, ventricular, and SA nodal cells.

operated Ca channels are activated and then inactivated within a voltage range of –40 to +20 mV. The number of calcium channels open during a ventricular cell action potential is controlled by cAMP. The binding of norepinephrine or hormones to β adrenergic receptors increases the number of open calcium channels. Regulation of the number of calcium channels determines the strength of contraction of the ventricular cells. Cardiac muscle behaves similarly to smooth muscle in that its sarcoplasmic reticulum does not contain sufficient calcium to produce maximum contractility. Alterations in intracellular calcium concentration are used to regulate strength of contraction of the cardiac myocyte. Therefore, phase 2 is needed to allow extracellular calcium to enter the cells. Calcium is removed from the cell by both primary active transport and secondary active transport using a Na/Ca exchanger before the next depolarization. Phase 3 is the final repolarization phase of the action potential. It is produced by both inactivation of slow Ca currents and activation of a second population of K channels. The entire process may take up to 300 ms to complete as opposed to 1 to 2 ms in neurons and skeletal muscle cells. Phase 4 is the steady resting potential of the ventricular cell. Some cardiac myocytes do not demonstrate a steady phase 4, but depolarize spontaneously instead. The events at the level of the ion channels are shown in Figure 19-5.

ACTION POTENTIALS OF SPECIFIC CARDIAC CELLS

Ventricular muscle cells display a prominent plateau phase, which allows more Ca current to provide for muscle contraction compared with atrial muscle cells. Phase 4 depolarization, also called **automaticity**, is observed in specialized cardiac cells, including the sinoatrial node (SA node), atrioventricular node (AV node), and the large cells of the ventricular conduction system with their many gap junctions. These cells can initiate an action potential via spontaneous depolarization during phase 4. The SA node has a spontaneous rate of depolarization during phase 4 that would produce 100 action potentials per minute without influence of the autonomic nervous system or circulating epinephrine, whereas the AV node would do this about 60 times per second and the ventricular conduction cells would do this 30 to 40 times per minute. Therefore, the SA node is the pacemaker of the heart due to its faster inherent rate of depolarization. It reaches threshold and initiates an action potential before any other cells with automaticity. The action potential of the SA node is characterized by its phase 4 depolarization. The remainder of the action potential is Ca channel dependent. The AV node is similar to the SA node with a slow, Ca channel-dependent action potential, but displays slower phase 4 depolarization. AV node cells are very small and conduct the action potential slowly. The ventricular conduction system has the longest AP duration, and even slower phase 4 depolarization. These specialized cardiac myocytes are large cells with many gap junctions that conduct action potentials rapidly from one cell to the next. These action potentials are depicted in Figure 19-6.

IONIC BASIS OF AUTOMATICITY

At least three ion channels are responsible for the automaticity of SA node cells. They include potassium channels that open to produce repolarization and two types of calcium ion channels that contribute to the initial depolarization and cause the more rapid, sustained depolarization. As SA node cells reach the peak of depolarization, potassium channels open to cause repolarization. Upon repolarization, these channels close, and movement of potassium out of the cell declines, resulting in a slow depolarization. The depolarization opens one type of calcium channel (transient), continuing the slow phase 4 depolarization to about –50 mV. At this potential, the other set of calcium channels (long-lasting) begin to open and depolarize the cells at a greater rate as can be seen by the change in slope of depolarization at approximately –50 mV. To complete the cycle, potassium ion channels open to return membrane potential to its maximum value of phase 4.

CARDIAC CONDUCTION

The heart consists of fibrous tissue separating the upper and lower chambers and myocytes specialized for initiating and conducting action potentials or for developing force. The SA node, AV node, bundle of His, bundle branches and Purkinje fibers consist of specialized myocytes that are capable of spontaneous depolarization. Conduction cells of the ventricles can conduct action potentials and distribute the signal to contract at much faster rates than the other 99% of the myocytes specialized for contraction, thereby ensuring a smooth contraction of the heart from its apex to its base. The rate of action potential conduction is slow compared with that of myelinated axons (60 m/s or faster). In the ventricular conducting system, the action potential is propagated at 4 m/s, compared with 1 m/s in other ventricular cells. This difference in conduction can be observed in EKG patterns in which conduction occurs through ventricular muscle rather than the normal bundle of His, bundle branch, Purkinje cell sequence. Conduction is much slower in the SA node and AV node (0.05 m/s). Conduction of the action potential is increased by sympathetic stimulation and is decreased by parasympathetic stimulation.

Because many cells are capable of spontaneous depolarization, any of these cells are potential pacemakers for the heart. Cells with this property are said to have automaticity. Once a cell is depolarized and repolarizes, it begins phase 4 depolarization anew. Therefore, whichever cell has the fastest slope to its spontaneous depolarization will reach threshold first and will signal all of the other cells to contract. This cell becomes the pacemaker for the heart and is usually located in the SA node. Sympathetic stimulation increases the slope of

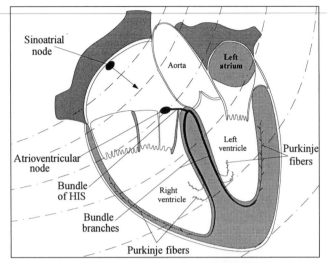

Figure 19-7. The conduction system of the heart. The action potential generated by the SA node is propagated to the AV node through atrial muscle then through the specialized conducting cells of the bundle of His, bundle branches, and Purkinje cells.

depolarization and, therefore, increases heart rate. Parasympathetic stimulation, on the other hand, decreases the slope of phase 4 depolarization and further polarizes cells with automaticity, which decreases heart rate. If the SA node is diseased, cells in the AV node can take over pacemaking duties but at a slower rate (about 60/min). The only pathway between the upper and lower chambers of the normal heart is through the AV node into the bundle of His. The locations of these tissues are shown in Figure 19-7. Conduction block of this pathway causes the ventricles and atria to have separate rates of depolarization as the specialized conducting cells of the ventricle are capable of initiating a ventricular beat but at a much slower rate (30 to 40 bpm). The speed and direction of propagation of the cardiac action potential determine the sequence of contraction of the cardiac chambers, and the electrical activity pattern that can be recorded from the skin is known as the electrocardiogram. Recording the electrical activity of the heart (electrocardiography) can give us clues about the way the heart is initiating and conducting action potentials. Certain conditions are detectable on the electrocardiogram as abnormal automaticity or abnormal conduction. Moreover, the rate can show problems, including an abnormal pacemaker of ventricular activity. For example, if the action potential originating in the SA node is blocked in the AV node, a ventricular rate of 30 to 40 beats per minute will result from a pacemaker in the ventricular conduction system.

The action potential begins in the SA node and propagates from cell to cell via gap junctions throughout the atria at a rate of 1 m/s with a mean direction of propagation from right to left because the SA node is found in the right atrium. Before the most-distant areas of the left atrium are depolarized, the wave of depolarization reaches the AV node. The AV node has the slowest conduction velocity of all cardiac tissues. The delay caused by the conduction through the small cells of the AV node allows the atria to complete their contraction before the ventricles contract. The His-Purkinje system is composed of myocytes that are specialized for rapid conduction of the action potential to signal ventricular muscle cells to contract. In the ventricular muscle cells, activation proceeds from endocardium to epicardium while repolarization proceeds from epicardium to endocardium. The direction of depolarization is influenced by the greater mass of the left ventricle, so that normal sequence of the average electrical signal produced during a heartbeat is downward and to the left. The sequence, the inherent rates of phase 4 depolarization, and rate of conduction are taken into account when an electrocardiogram is interpreted systematically. Some of these principles are discussed in Laboratory Exercise 20-1 on electrocardiography and the cardiac cycle.

SUMMARY

The heart acts as a pump to create sufficient pressure to drive flow through the systemic and pulmonary circulation to meet the transport needs of the tissues. The left heart pumps blood returning from the lungs to the rest of the body. Blood returning from the systemic circulation is received by the right heart and is pumped through the pulmonary circulation. The structure of the blood vessels differs with the function of the vessel type. Large arteries convert pulsatile flow into steady flow due to their elasticity. Smooth muscle of the arterioles is used to regulate the flow to different tissues according to needs. The capillary consists of a single layer of endothelium to maximize transport into the interstitial fluid. Veins have a high compliance, and this compliance is regulated to control preload on the heart and the relative volume of blood on the arterial and venous sides of the circulation. The left ventricle pumps against four to five times the pressure than the right ventricle does and has a proportionally thicker wall. The atria have thin walls, receive blood from the great veins, and contract prior to ventricular contraction to increase the preload on the ventricles. Cardiac myocytes are smaller, slower, more fatigue resistant, and capable of higher levels of oxidative metabolism than slow oxidative skeletal muscle fibers. Their small diameter allows a greater number of capillaries per volume to exist in the heart than in skeletal muscle. Large atrioventricular valves tethered by chordae tendineae and papillary muscles separate the atria from the ventricles. Papillary muscles contract when the rest of the ventricle contracts to maintain the tension on the chordae tendineae as the ventricle shortens in the apex to base dimension during contraction. Large valves are required between the atria and ventricles due to the low pressure in the atria. The semilunar valves between the ventricles and great arteries must withstand a greater pressure but can be smaller in diameter. The action potential of ventricular cells is much longer than in skeletal muscle but is similarly polarized to near E_K. It has five phases created by opening and closing of sodium, calcium, and potassium ion channels. Phase 0 is rapid depolarization due to opening of sodium channels. Phase 1 is a rapid, but incomplete, repolarization due to closing of the sodium channels. Phase 2 is a plateau due to opening of calcium channels that allow needed calcium to enter the cell for muscle contraction. Phase 3 is the final repolarization due to opening of potassium channels. Phase 4 is steady in ventricular cells but demonstrates spontaneous depolarization in SA node, AV node, and ventricular conduction myocytes. The automaticity of these cells is produced by calcium and potassium ion channels that are different from those producing the ventricular cell action potential. The pathway of cardiac conduction of the action potential begins in the SA node, is conducted cell-to-cell through the atria, and enters the AV node, which is the only pathway between the atria and the ventricles in the normal heart. The AV node slows conduction enough to allow the atria to finish contracting before the ventricles contract.

BIBLIOGRAPHY

Berne RM, Levy MN. *Cardiovascular Physiology*. 6th ed. St. Louis, Mo: Mosby; 1992.

Berne RM, Levy MN. *Physiology*. St. Louis, Mo: Mosby-Year Book; 1998.

Brobeck JR, ed. *Best & Taylor's Physiological Basis of Medical Practice*. 10th ed. Baltimore, Md: Williams & Wilkins; 1979.

Ellsworth ML, Ellis CG, Popel AS, Pittman RN. Role of microvessels in oxygen supply to tissue. *News in Physiological Sciences*. 1994;9:119-123.

Ganong WF. *Review of Medical Physiology*. Norwalk, Conn: Appleton & Lange; 1995.

Guyton AC, Hall JE, Schmitt W. *Human Physiology and Mechanisms of Disease*. Philadelphia, Pa: WB Saunders; 1997.

Guyton AC. *Human Physiology and Mechanism of Disease*. 5th ed. Philadelphia, Pa: WB Saunders; 1992.

Hole JW Jr. *Essentials of Human Anatomy and Physiology*. 4th ed. Dubuque, Iowa: Wm. C. Brown Publishers; 1992.

Schauf C, Moffett D, Moffett S. *Human Physiology: Foundation and Frontiers*. St. Louis, Mo: Times Mirror/Mosby College Publishing; 1990.

Solomon EP, Davis PW. *Human Anatomy and Physiology*. Philadelphia, Pa: WB Saunders; 1983.

STUDY QUESTIONS

1. If the heart ceases to pump, what happens to arterial pressure? What happens to venous pressure? What does it mean if arterial pressure and venous pressure are equal?

2. How does the structure of the arterial wall relate to its function? How does Hooke's law apply to the role of the aorta in the circulation? Use Hooke's law to explain how the aorta converts pulsatile pumping into steady blood flow in the periphery.

3. If cardiac output equals the sum of peripheral blood flow, what must happen if blood flow increases to one organ and cardiac output does not change? What must happen to cardiac output if blood flow increases to one organ, but blood flow to other organs does not change?

4. Using the equation CO = MAP x TPR, what happens to MAP if TPR decreases and CO stays the same? What must happen to CO during exercise if TPR falls to one-half its resting value and MAP does not fall?

5. If venous pressure acts as the preload on the heart, what happens to preload if veins contract and increase venous pressure? What happens to preload on the heart if the heart pumps out so much blood that venous pressure falls? Why is venoconstriction necessary when cardiac output is high?

6. Compare the flow of blood through the aorta and pulmonary artery in terms of volume, velocity, and pressure. Compare the flow of blood through the aorta and vena cava in the same terms.

7. Why are gap junctions important in cardiac myocytes?

8. Compare the roles of skeletal muscle and cardiac muscle in the framework of the following questions. Why must cardiac myocytes be so small? Why must they be so slow? Why must they have so many capillaries and mitochondria?

9. Why do we have jugular pulses?

10. If preload produced by atrial contraction is important for ventricular function, why is the conduction delay in the AV node, which allows the atria to complete contraction before the ventricles contract, important?

11. How does the structure of the left ventricle, compared with the right ventricle, relate to its function?

12. Why must the atrioventricular valves have a larger surface area than the semilunar valves? What would happen if the papillary muscles suddenly ruptured?

13. If the SA node becomes diseased, cells in what area become the pacemaker? What would the rate be? What does ventricular rate become if the AV node becomes blocked?

14. What occurs during the plateau phase of the ventricular cell that determines its contractility? Why do ventricular cells need such a long plateau phase compared with other cardiac myocytes?

TWENTY

The Cardiac Cycle

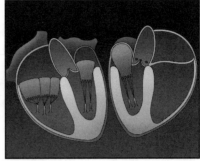

OBJECTIVES

1. Compare excitation-contraction coupling of cardiac muscle with that of skeletal muscle.

2. Explain the role of extracellular Ca^{++} in both excitation-contraction coupling and the regulation of cardiac myocyte contractility, the need for Ca^{++} channels, and the active transport of Ca^{++}.

3. Explain how preload is altered in the heart and the Frank-Starling mechanism.

4. Explain how afterload on cardiac muscle is varied.

5. Describe the effects of the autonomic nervous system on heart rate, contractility, and conduction. Describe how the following alter contractility: heart rate, digitalis, sympathetic stimulation, β agonists including hormones.

6. Define the normal range of heart rate, bradycardia, and tachycardia, and the effect of training on resting heart rate.

7. Describe the four phases of the cardiac cycle (isovolumic contraction, ejection, isovolumic relaxation, filling) in terms of ventricular and aortic pressure, aortic blood flow, ventricular volume, heart sounds, and electrocardiogram.

8. Explain the normal heart sounds and systolic and diastolic murmurs.

9. Describe the effects of valvular stenosis and insufficiency on preload and afterload.

10. Use a pressure-volume loop to describe the cardiac cycle.

11. Use ejection fraction as a means to quantify cardiac performance.

12. Describe how changes in afterload and contractility influence stroke volume.

13. Describe the effects of valvular stenosis and insufficiency on preload and afterload.

14. Use the law of LaPlace, wall stress (τ) = P x r/thickness, to describe oxygen demand by the heart under different conditions qualitatively.

15. Describe the major energy-consuming processes in the heart.

16. Describe how changes in preload, afterload, and contractile state affect the energy consumption of the heart.

EXCITATION-CONTRACTION COUPLING

Excitation-contraction coupling in the ventricular cells is largely the same process as that of skeletal muscle cells. The same components of the sarcomere, its thick and thin filaments, tropomyosin, and troponin, exist in cardiac muscle. Two major differences exist: the signal for contraction and contractility. In skeletal muscle, each myocyte is innervated so that an end plate potential can be developed to signal contraction. In cardiac muscle, the depolarization from one cell to its neighbors signals the contractile mechanism. In skeletal muscle, each action potential causes sufficient calcium to be released from the sarcoplasmic reticulum to saturate troponin, but a series of action potentials is necessary for the cells to develop maximum force. In cardiac muscle, an action potential usually does not cause enough calcium to be released to produce saturation of troponin. Instead, the strength of the ventricular contraction is regulated by changes in the concentration of calcium in the ventricular myocyte, thereby altering contractility. The importance of changes in contractility in the heart is related to the first difference noted between skeletal and cardiac muscle. In skeletal muscle, force is regulated largely by recruiting different numbers of motor units. Because cardiac muscle contraction recruits all the myocytes at once, force produced by the heart must be regulated by changing the contractility of all of the cells because the number of cells participating in a contraction cannot be regulated.

During a ventricular cell action potential, calcium ions enter the cell through calcium ion channels that open during the plateau phase (phase 2). The calcium entering the cell via calcium channels stimulates the release of calcium from the sarcoplasmic reticulum (SR). This process of using calcium as a second messenger for the SR is called calcium-induced calcium release. Cross-bridge cycling is the same in cardiac muscle, although slower and more energy efficient due to the slow myosin ATPase of cardiac muscle. Cross-bridge cycling is ended by the removal of calcium around the myofilaments in cardiac muscle, but the process is more involved than it is in skeletal muscle. Calcium is removed by three energy-using processes. One is the same as that of the skeletal myocyte by active transport into the sarcoplasmic reticulum. Calcium is also removed by primary active transport across the cell membrane as shown in Figure 20-1. A third process is the secondary active transport that co-transports three sodium ions into the cell in exchange for one calcium ion transported out of the cell. The energy for the secondary active process comes from

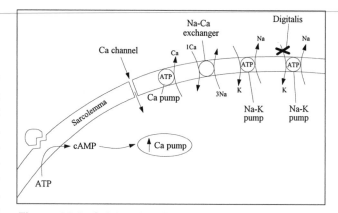

Figure 20-1. Calcium ion flux across cardiac ventricular myocyte membranes. During a ventricular cell action potential, calcium ions enter through specific calcium ion channels as well as being released by the sarcoplasmic reticulum. Calcium ions are then extruded by active transport using ATP directly, by secondary active transport in co-transport with sodium, and are pumped into the sarcoplasmic reticulum. Secondary active transport is dependent on the concentration of sodium ions in the cell, which is increased by the effect of digitalis on the Na-K pump. Accumulation of sodium in the cell results in calcium ion accumulation and increased ventricular contractility.

the sodium/potassium pump, which uses ATP directly. Failure to pump sodium out of the cell by the Na-K pump not only causes sodium to accumulate in the cell, but, by decreasing the concentration difference for sodium across the cell membrane, decreases the transport of calcium out of the cell by secondary active transport.

INNERVATION OF THE HEART

The heart is innervated by both divisions of the autonomic nervous system. Sympathetic innervation originates from the right and left stellate ganglia. Sympathetic neurons release norepinephrine, leading to production of cAMP through stimulation of β receptors. For the most part, stimulation of the right stellate ganglion, which sends neurons to the sinoatrial (SA) node, atrioventricular (AV) node, and atria, increases heart rate and conduction through the AV node. Stimulation of the left stellate ganglion, which sends sympathetic neurons to the ventricular mass, increases contractility. However, some overlap in function does occur; stimulation of the right stellate ganglion can produce a smaller increase in contractility than the left stellate ganglion. Parasympathetic innervation originates from the right and left vagus nerves (CN X). The vagus nerves release acetylcholine onto muscarinic receptors mainly on the SA and AV nodes. Stimulation of the right vagus decreases heart rate by its effect on the SA node,

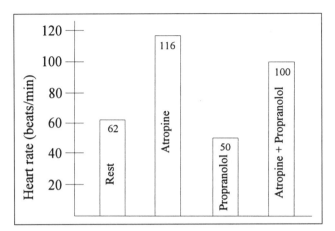

Figure 20-2. The effect of the autonomic nervous system on heart rate. At rest, heart rate is dominated by the slowing effect of the vagus nerve. Administration of anticholinergic and beta-blocking drugs increases heart rate to about 100 beats per minute. Blocking the effect of sympathetic stimulation of the heart produces a smaller decrease in heart rate than blocking the effect of the vagus increases heart rate. Also, note that blocking the sympathetic effect when the cholinergic effect is already blocked produces a small decrease in heart rate.

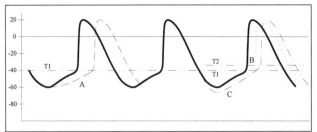

Figure 20-3. The effect of sympathetic and parasympathetic stimulation of SA nodal cells. A: Normal SA node action potential. B: Stimulation of the sympathetic input to the SA node increases the rate of spontaneous depolarization and increases heart rate. C: Stimulation of the vagal input to the SA node hyperpolarizes SA node cells and slows the rate of spontaneous depolarization, thereby decreasing heart rate.

and stimulation of the left vagus slows conduction through the AV node, thereby delaying ventricular contraction (Figure 20-2). The effect on the AV node can become strong enough to produce third-degree AV block, in which no conduction occurs through the AV node.

Acetylcholine slows phase 4 depolarization, thereby decreasing heart rate. In contrast, norepinephrine and other agents that bind to β receptors on the SA node cells increase the rate of spontaneous depolarization to increase heart rate (Figure 20-3). Heart rate can also be increased via release of epinephrine from the adrenal medulla, by drugs that bind to β receptors, and by drugs that block muscarinic receptors. In a denervated heart, the heart rate is approximately 100 bpm, but the resting heart rate of most healthy individuals is usually lower. The medical definition is a bit broader, stating that a normal heart rate is 60 to 100. A heart rate below 60 is termed **bradycardia**, and a heart rate greater than 100 is called **tachycardia**. At rest, the heart rate is determined primarily by the rate of parasympathetic stimulation, with a small contribution by sympathetic stimulation. A combination of both muscarinic and β receptor blockade produces a heart rate of approximately 100 bpm, the same as that of a denervated heart. β blockade using the drug propranolol alone produces a small decrease in heart rate, whereas atropine, a muscarinic blocker, produces a large increase in heart rate (see Figure 20-2). The low resting heart rate in highly

trained aerobic athletes is due to a high rate of vagal stimulation of the heart. Therapeutically, rapid heart rates can be slowed by maneuvers that stimulate the vagus, including carotid massage, and pressing on eyes.

CARDIAC PERFORMANCE

The same factors that determine skeletal muscle performance also determine the force of contraction, the velocity and extent of shortening of cardiac muscle: size of the heart, preload, afterload, and contractility. Preload is similar to that in skeletal muscle but is applied to a muscular chamber. Preload may be expressed either in terms of the pressure or volume that alters sarcomere length prior to contraction. Either end diastolic volume (EDV) or end diastolic pressure (EDP) may be used to quantify preload. The pressure-volume curve is similar to the active length-tension curve in muscle. As EDV and, therefore, preload and sarcomere length are increased, the heart can develop more pressure on the volume of blood within the ventricle. The length-tension curve differs somewhat from that of skeletal muscle in that stretching cardiac muscle beyond its optimum length is very difficult to accomplish. Over a physiologic range of preload, optimum length is not exceeded. The increased performance of the heart secondary to an increase in preload is the Frank-Starling effect, named for Otto Frank and Ernest Starling. This mechanism is useful for correcting small changes in afterload and preload that may occur over a short time, such as the effects of postural changes and effects of ventilation. With an increase in afterload, less blood will be ejected, leaving more blood in the ventricle as filling occurs. If the heart fills by the same amount before the next beat, the heart will have a greater preload and will produce more force. The heart, under these circumstances, can eject an amount that compensates for the decreased amount ejected in the previous beat. Another consequence of the Frank-Starling mechanism is a compensation for a decreased heart rate. To produce the same cardiac output, the heart can have a lower heart rate and greater stroke volume or a greater heart rate and smaller stroke volume. A decrease in heart rate increases the amount of filling of the ventricle and, therefore, increases preload and strength of contraction, which may increase the stroke volume sufficiently to compensate for the decreased heart rate.

The performance of the heart as a muscle also depends on its afterload, which is the load against which the muscle's sarcomeres are shortening. As discussed with skeletal muscle, as afterload increases, less sarcomere shortening is available for moving a load, latency before movement occurs increases, and movement is slower. In the case of the heart, afterload on the heart is quantified in terms of the pressure that the ventricle must overcome to eject blood. Afterload may be considered as either left ventricular systolic pressure or as aortic pressure. A higher aortic pressure leads to ejection of less blood, a longer delay between the onset of contraction and ejection, and slower ejection of the blood.

A more sophisticated and accurate method to quantify afterload is to compute wall stress using the law of LaPlace. Wall stress indicates the stress on each sarcomere as it shortens against a load. Mathematically, $(\tau) = P \times r/\text{thickness}$. The three components of wall stress relate to general principles of muscle performance. Sarcomeres are arranged around the chamber with a given pressure inside. As the sarcomeres shorten, the wall becomes stiffer and, thus, generates more pressure against the blood until the aortic valve opens. More energy must be used in sarcomere shortening if a greater pressure is needed to open the aortic valve. If the diameter across the chamber is greater, the ventricular wall is stretched such that fewer sarcomeres are operating in parallel. A thicker ventricular wall also has more sarcomeres operating in parallel than a thin wall. Wall stress (t) is the most accurate determinant of oxygen demand by the ventricle, and it can also be computed for the end of diastole as an index of preload. The anatomy of the ventricular chambers indicates the effects of wall stress. Where the radius of the ventricle is greatest, the wall is the thickest, and at the apex, where the radius is small, the ventricular wall is very thin. Moreover, the right ventricle, which experiences less wall stress, is very thin compared with the left ventricular wall thickness. Below, the effects of changing different components of wall stress on oxygen consumption of the heart will be described.

Contractility refers to strength of muscle independent of sarcomere length in skeletal muscle and in cardiac muscle as well. Whereas contractility in skeletal muscle does not change and muscle performance is altered by recruitment of motor units, performance of cardiac muscle depends on changes in contractility because no motor units exist in the heart—the whole of the muscle mass contracts with every beat. Contractility of the heart is determined by the amount of calcium available to the myofibrils following depolarization. Drugs, hormones, and neurotransmitters that increase the developed pressure at any given volume present in the ventricle just before ejection are called positive inotropic agents. Positive inotropic agents increase the calcium available to the myofibrils. These agents include norepinephrine released by sympathetic nerves, epinephrine released by the adrenal medulla, and other ligands that stimulate the β receptors. Stimulation of β receptors produces several effects that increase contractility. As shown in Figure 20-1, production of cAMP causes greater uptake of calcium by the sarcoplasmic reticulum, which makes more calcium available following the next action potential. Troponin is covalently modulated due to cAMP so that its affinity for calcium is increased, which increases the number of available binding sites for myosin on actin. A third effect is a greater number of open calcium channels due to covalent modulation secondary to cAMP. The net results of increased cAMP concentration are:

1. Stronger contraction due to more cross-bridges being formed
2. Faster development of force
3. Faster relaxation
4. Greater expenditure of ATP
5. Less energy efficient

The faster development of force shortens the length of systole during β adrenergic stimulation. The importance of shortening systole lies in the second effect of β stimulation, which is an increased heart rate. At an increased heart rate, the time between beats is decreased, and less time is available to fill the ventricles. The diminished filling time for the ventricles is partially offset by also decreasing the time necessary for systole. Some individuals take drugs that block β-adrenergic receptors (β-blockers). These drugs are used for several purposes including decreasing the contractility of the heart to reduce blood pressure, decreasing oxygen consumption by the heart if blood supply is impaired, and decreasing the automaticity of ventricular cells to prevent arrhythmias.

Other drugs have positive inotropic properties. Digitalis is a drug derived from a plant called foxglove. It was isolated from a preparation of "natural ingredients" used successfully to treat congestive heart failure. Digitalis decreases the activity of the Na-K pump, causing sodium to accumulate in the ventricular (and other) cells. Because calcium is removed by secondary active transport in addition to primary active transport, the accumulation of sodium in the cells decreases the co-transport of calcium and sodium out of the cell in the secondary transport mechanism. Therefore, the accumulation of sodium in the cell causes higher levels of calcium to accumulate in the cell, thus, enhancing the force of contraction of the heart. Digitalis, a drug frequently used for congestive heart failure, also slows conduction through cardiac cells, especially through the AV node, and can cause serious arrhythmias. Because the toxic dose of digitalis is only about double what the therapeutic dose is, people with congestive heart failure who use digitalis must be monitored carefully.

In end-stage congestive heart failure and certain individuals expected to recover from insults to the heart, such as surgery, the drugs dopamine, dobutamine, and either amrinone or milrinone are given to support contractility. This combination of drugs is termed "triple pressors" because they maintain blood pressure by increasing contractility in a weak heart. Dopamine and dobutamine bind specifically to the β-receptors of the left ventricle to increase cAMP in the ventricular cells. Amrinone and milrinone both inhibit phosphodiesterase, the enzyme that breaks down cAMP. Inhibition of phosphodiesterase increases the concentration of cAMP generated by β-receptor stimulation.

In the heart, summation, as observed in skeletal muscle with increasing action potential frequency, does not occur. Summation can occur in skeletal muscle because the action potential (1 to 2 ms) is much shorter than the twitch time (100 to 200 ms). In cardiac muscle, however, the action potential is almost as long as the twitch time (about 300 ms). Therefore, a second action potential cannot be introduced until the ventricular cells have completely or nearly completely relaxed. Under normal conditions, another action potential is not initiated during this time anyway. Even at a heart rate of 180 beats per minute, action potentials are developed every 333 ms. Instead of summation, however, contractility of the heart increases with increasing heart rate. As heart rate increases, less time is available for removal of calcium from the sarcoplasm, causing calcium to accumulate in the cell. Increased calcium concentration results in an increase in contractility. Secondly, the sympathetic nerves innervating the heart produce both an increase in heart rate and contractility under the same conditions (eg, exercise).

Heart size is usually quantified as the thickness of the ventricular wall. A heart with a thicker wall generates greater pressure for a given preload and contractility.

Wall thickness increases in individuals who undergo physical training that is either aerobic or anaerobic. Weight lifters have been shown to have significantly thicker ventricular walls than other athletes or untrained individuals. Increased wall thickness also occurs in certain types of cardiomyopathy (disease of the heart muscle) or diseases in which the afterload is increased (eg, aortic valve stenosis). Increased heart size due to increased thickness of the ventricular walls with training is a very different situation from a heart that increases in size due to an increase in the radius of the ventricle. Increased ventricular radius increases force of contraction by increasing preload. This dilation of the heart is a response to a pathologic condition such as congestive heart failure in which the inherent contractility of the heart is diminished and cardiac performance is initially maintained by increased preload. Whereas the heart of a normal person can be approximated as the size of a fist, a dilated heart in severe congestive heart failure can be the size of a softball or larger.

THE CARDIAC CYCLE

The cardiac cycle is the combination of electrical, pressure, volume, flow, and acoustical events that occur during each heartbeat. Each cardiac cycle begins with the production of an action potential by the SA node and ends with production of the next action potential. The duration of the cardiac cycle is determined by the heart rate. Cycle duration (s) = 60/HR (bpm). The cardiac cycle is divided into two parts, known as systole and diastole, that roughly correspond to contractile and resting phases. The duration of systole is about one-third of the total duration of the cardiac cycle, and it is the period during which the ventricle is developing force and the time during which ejection of blood from the ventricle occurs. Diastole is the period during which the ventricles are relaxing, or relaxed, and the phase during which ventricular filling occurs. The duration of diastole is about two-thirds of the total duration of the cardiac cycle.

Because the heart consists of two pumps in series, the events in the cardiac cycle are performed on both sides at approximately the same time. Averaged over a short period, blood flow through the left and right hearts is equal, although, for a few beats, a small difference can occur. In spite of the same cardiac output occurring from both ventricles, the pressures on the right side are approximately 20% to 25% of the left side, due to the greater conductance (lower resistance) of the pulmonary circulation compared with the systemic circulation.

The events of the cardiac cycle will be described initially for the left ventricle, and differences between the left and right will be described. Systole is divided into two phases called isovolumic (isovolumetric) contraction and ejection. Isovolumic contraction is analogous to the initial isometric portion of skeletal muscle contraction during which sarcomere shortening produces tension but no net movement occurs. It represents the latency between initiation of sarcomere shortening and the movement of the load (a volume of blood). Ejection is analogous to the isotonic portion of skeletal muscle contraction. Once the tension developed by the muscle exceeds the afterload, shortening (ejection) can occur. The isovolumic contraction phase begins with mitral valve closure that occurs when left ventricular pressure exceeds left atrial pressure. The end-diastolic pressure (EDP) is the pressure within the ventricle at the end of diastole and the start of systole, while the end-diastolic volume (EDV) is the volume of blood within the ventricle at the end of diastole and the start of systole. This pressure and volume serve as the preload to stretch the cardiac sarcomeres prior to contraction. The mitral and aortic valves are closed (the ventricular volume remains the same throughout), and intraventricular pressure rises rapidly from 2 to 12 mm Hg up to the diastolic aortic pressure of approximately 80 mm Hg. Isovolumic contraction ends when pressure in the ventricle becomes great enough to open the aortic valve.

The ejection phase begins when the aortic valve opens. At the start of ejection, the left ventricular pressure exceeds aortic pressure causing blood to flow out of the ventricle and pushing the aortic valve leaflets open. Under healthy conditions, the pressure gradient across the aortic valve is only 1 to 3 mm Hg. A valve that requires a greater pressure gradient to be opened is termed stenotic. A stenotic valve causes the ventricle to produce a pressure significantly greater than aortic pressure to produce ejection, thereby increasing the afterload on the ventricle. The volume of blood ejected from the ventricle is called the stroke volume (SV). In an average healthy heart, greater than 60% of the EDV is ejected. The volume of blood remaining in the ventricle at the end of ejection is called the end-systolic volume (ESV). Stated mathematically, SV = EDV–ESV. The fraction of the EDV ejected is called the ejection fraction (EF). Ejection fraction is often used as a simple index of the heart's strength. Stated mathematically, EF = SV/EDV.

As the ventricular cells begin to relax, pressure in the ventricle drops more rapidly than aortic pressure. When aortic pressure again exceeds ventricular pressure, the aortic valve begins to close. A small additional amount of blood will be ejected due to the inertia of the

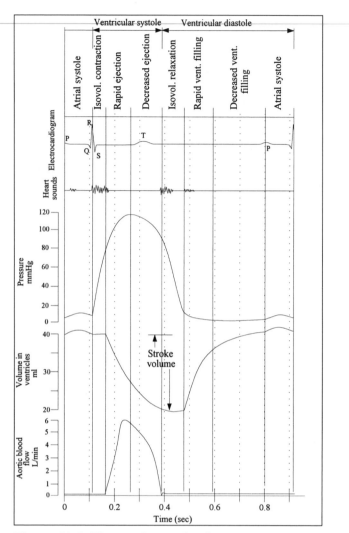

Figure 20-4. The cardiac cycle. Shown are electrical, acoustic, pressure, volume, and flow changes through the cycle.

blood, though aortic pressure slightly exceeds ventricular pressure (Figure 20-4). The ejection phase ends when a small volume (1 to 5 ml) of blood flows back toward the heart and closes the aortic valve. This backward flow appears on the arterial pressure trace as a momentary drop and rise in arterial pressure. This notch is termed the **incisura** and can be used as a marker for the end of systole.

Diastole also consists of two phases: isovolumic (isovolumetric) relaxation and filling. Isovolumic relaxation is the period when aortic pressure exceeds ventricular pressure, but ventricular pressure exceeds atrial pressure. Thus, both valves guarding the ventricle are closed, and volume cannot change. Filling is the period during which the preload is placed on the ventricles due to venous pressure and atrial contraction. Isovolumic relaxation begins when the aortic valve closes. No change in

TABLE 20-1
Summary of Events in the Cardiac Cycle

	MITRAL VALVE	AORTIC VALVE	LV PRESSURE	AORTIC PRESSURE	LV VOLUME
Isovolumic contraction	C	C	I	D	NC
Ejection	C	O	I	I	D
Isovolumic relaxation	C	C	D	D	NC
Filling	O	C	I	D	I

C = closed, O = open, I = increasing, D = decreasing, NC = no change, LV = left ventricular

left ventricular volume occurs because both the aortic and mitral valves are closed. Left ventricular pressure drops rapidly because the myocardium is relaxing, and pressure falls from approximately 100 mm Hg to a few mm Hg. Though a large pressure gradient favoring movement of blood from the aorta into the left ventricle exists, the aortic valve forms a tight seal, preventing blood from leaking back in. A valve that fails to resist backflow is called insufficient or incompetent. The backward flow through an insufficient valve is called regurgitation. Isovolumic relaxation ends when the mitral valve opens and filling can begin.

Filling begins when the mitral valve opens. Flow from the left atrium to the left ventricle begins when left ventricular pressure falls below left atrial pressure. At this time, the ventricle is still relaxing, and pressure in the ventricle falls in the early part of filling. A normal pressure gradient across the mitral valve is only 1 to 3 mmHg. A stenotic mitral valve causes blood to back up in the pulmonary circulation until pulmonary venous pressure is great enough to drive flow into the left ventricle at the same rate that the ventricle pumps it out. Flow across the mitral valve from the left atrium to the left ventricle is initially rapid and decreases later in diastole. Late in diastole, the left atrium contracts, forcing blood into the left ventricle. Left atrial contraction briefly increases the left atrium-left ventricle pressure gradient and contributes 15% to 20% of the volume of blood that fills the ventricle. There are no valves between the atria and veins; therefore, some of the pressure generated by atrial contraction forces blood into the ventricle to increase preload, but blood is also forced backward into the veins, producing a venous pulse. This can be detected in the jugular vein, especially in a person who is reclining. The delay in propagation of the action potential from the atria through the AV node to the ventricles allows time for atrial contraction to complete preloading of the ventricle. The duration of filling is a major determinant of the volume of blood that fills the ventricle. At very high heart rates, filling of the heart

may become compromised, resulting in a decrease in arterial pressure. Events of the cardiac cycle are summarized in Table 20-1.

EVENTS OCCURRING IN THE RIGHT VENTRICLE

The right ventricle has the same phases as the left ventricle, though the timing of the phases is slightly different. Due to the higher pressure in the aorta than the pulmonary artery, the pulmonary valve opens before the aortic valve, and, for the same reason, the aortic valve closes before the pulmonary valve. The pressure traces recorded from the right atrium, the right ventricle, and the pulmonary artery are similar in form to the traces in the left heart, except that they are 20% to 25% of the magnitude.

The function of the valves is to produce unidirectional blood flow. The cardiac valve leaflets are passive structures moved primarily by the motion of the blood adjacent to their cusps. The valves open only after a pressure gradient is established across them. Normal valves offer little resistance to forward flow of blood (1 to 3 mmHg). Valves that have a large pressure gradient (more than 5 mmHg) are stenotic. The leaflets begin to close when vortices behind the leaflets begin to swing them closed. Abnormal valves and valves subject to turbulent blood flow are prone to calcification and infection. The final closing motions of the valves are due to a small retrograde flow of blood. When closed, the atrioventricular valves are supported by the chordae tendineae and papillary muscles. Rupture of the chordae tendineae or papillary muscles can produce acute heart failure in which the normal arterial and venous pressure changes do not occur with cardiac pumping.

HEART SOUNDS

The first heart sound (S_1) marks the start of systole.

Heart sounds occur because of the vibrations of the blood, the myocardium, and the valves produced by cardiac contraction. The acceleration of blood against the atrioventricular valves and the subsequent deceleration caused by closing of the mitral and tricuspid valves creates the vibrations of the first heart sound, just as rapidly turning off a faucet running at full speed often creates a sound. The second heart sound (S_2) marks the end of systole. S_2 occurs because of vibrations associated with the closure of the aortic and pulmonic valves. There are two components of the second heart sound: A_2 is the aortic component of S_2 associated with aortic valve closure, and P_2 is the pulmonic component of S_2 associated with pulmonic valve closure. The interval between A_2 and P_2 varies with ventilation. Normally, A_2 precedes P_2 because the aortic pressure is greater than the pressure in the pulmonary artery. During inspiration, decreased thoracic pressure causes the pulmonary valve to close even later and the A_2-P_2 interval may increase to greater than 20 ms so that two second heart sound components can be discriminated. This phenomenon is called physiological splitting of the second heart sound.

Murmurs are abnormal heart sounds. They may be classified as either systolic or diastolic murmurs. Murmurs may be considered normal in very thin and young individuals. Systolic murmurs occur because of abnormal valve function during systole. During systole, blood should pass freely from the ventricle to the aorta and should not leak back into the left atrium. Aortic stenosis and mitral regurgitation will produce resistance to forward flow and backflow into the left atrium, respectively, during systole. Systolic murmurs, therefore, are caused by either aortic stenosis or mitral valve regurgitation. During diastole, blood should be able to flow freely across the mitral valve from the left atrium into the left ventricle during the filling phase, and the aortic valve should prevent backflow from the aorta into the left ventricle. A stenotic mitral valve and an insufficient aortic valve would, therefore, produce abnormal sounds during diastole. Valvular problems are infrequently found in the right heart, except for intravenous drug abusers who may have damage to right heart valves. Valve disease may occur due to congenital abnormalities, certain infections (rheumatic fever), septicemia (bacteria or other infectious agents in the blood), or aging. Valvular disease increases the workload on the heart and can lead to congestive heart failure if severe.

EFFECTS OF RESPIRATION

Inspiration decreases the intrathoracic pressure, enhancing movement of blood from veins to cardiac

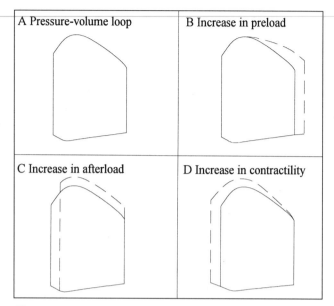

Figure 20-5. Pressure-volume loops. The area within a pressure-volume loop demonstrates the work done by the heart to move volume against a pressure, whereas the area below the loop demonstrates the work done on the heart by filling. A: Normal loop. B: Increasing preload by increasing ventricular filling and pressure during diastole. C: Increasing afterload on the heart requires a greater development of tension by the ventricular cells and diminishes emptying. D: Increasing contractility increases the pressure generated by the heart on the blood within the ventricles and enhances emptying of the ventricles.

chambers to arteries, and causes the pulmonary valve to open even sooner and close even later compared with the aortic valve. Expiration, especially forced expiration, impedes movement of blood through the heart. Forced expiration against a closed glottis is termed the Valsalva maneuver and increases intrathoracic pressure sufficiently to reduce cardiac output to the point of impairing cerebral and myocardial blood flow. The normal changes in preload and afterload caused by ventilation of the lungs are managed by the Frank-Starling effect to maintain cardiac output equal from the two ventricles.

WORK OF THE HEART

Mechanical work can be quantified as the mathematic product of pressure and volume. Force (N) per area (cm^2) times volume (cm^3) = force (N) times distance (cm). A way of examining the cardiac cycle that also displays cardiac work is the pressure-volume loop (Figure 20-5). The changes in pressure and volume are plotted with volume as the independent variable and pressure as the dependent variable. Time is not an element of this plot. Contractility is represented as the pressure generated by the heart for a given preload. Measuring the area within the pressure-volume loop demonstrates work done by the heart during the cardiac cycle, whereas measuring the area under the loop demonstrates the work done on the heart to preload it. Experiments using this type of visual aid show that as preload is increased, the stroke volume increases, whereas stroke volume decreases as afterload increases. Stroke volume also increases as the contractile state increases due to sympathetic stimulation, increased heart rate, digitalis, or some other mechanism for increasing intracellular calcium.

Hypertension, a form of pressure overload on the heart, will decrease stroke volume as will aortic stenosis, which is another form of pressure overload. Aortic and mitral regurgitation produce a volume overload, which implies that the heart is required to pump an excessive volume of blood to produce a normal forward or net cardiac output. Because some of the blood pumped by the ventricle leaks backward, the heart is obligated to pump a greater than normal volume.

Cardiac work can also be quantified by computing stroke work (SW), which can be used as an index of myocardial oxygen consumption. Stroke work is the work done when the stroke volume (SV) is ejected against the aortic pressure (SW = SV x mean arterial pressure or mean systolic left ventricular pressure). Several factors influence myocardial energy consumption and efficiency. An increased amount of work is performed when the heart is either pressure or volume overloaded. However, pressure overloading is energetically more expensive, and, therefore, this type of increased work is performed less efficiently.

Computation of wall stress can also be used to predict oxygen consumption. An important example is that of a dilated heart. With a large diameter and thin-walled ventricle, oxygen consumption is greater than the same amount of work performed in a normal size heart. Myocardial oxygen demand is increased with an increase in contractility caused by increased concentration of cAMP, but in a failing heart, increased contractility is more energy efficient than dilation. A new alternative to either inotropic drugs or heart transplant is called reduction ventriculoplasty. In this procedure, a piece of the left ventricle is removed to decrease the radius.

For any given individual, a certain combination of heart rate and stroke volume produces the greatest myocardial oxygen consumption efficiency. Increased heart rate increases myocardial oxygen demand but may be more efficient than increased pressure work, depending on other factors. This optimum heart rate, in terms of oxygen demand, depends on several factors, especially stroke volume, arterial pressure, and compliance of the arterial system. If blood vessels are stiff, as occurs in atherosclerosis, it is more efficient to increase heart rate and decrease stroke volume. With young, healthy arteries, a more efficient myocardial oxygen demand occurs with a lower heart rate and greater stroke volume.

SUMMARY

The processes of excitation-contraction coupling are the same in skeletal muscle and cardiac muscle, except for the signal for contraction and the ability to saturate troponin. All cardiac muscle cells are recruited for every heartbeat, and contractility is regulated to regulate muscle strength. Extracellular calcium that enters the cardiac myocyte during phase 2 of the action potential causes the sarcoplasmic reticulum to release calcium for binding to troponin. Relaxation is caused by uptake of calcium by the sarcoplasmic reticulum, but also by primary and secondary active transport of calcium out of the myocyte. Increasing the quantity of calcium that enters the cell during the action potential and that stored in the sarcoplasmic reticulum due to increased cAMP concentration increases contractility. The volume of blood that exists in the ventricle at the end of diastole and the pressure created by that volume stretch the sarcomeres, acting as a preload on the heart. Increasing the preload increases the force of contraction. Transient alterations in cardiac volume due to posture, ventilation, or other causes alter the force of contraction to compensate for the change. This phenomenon is called the Frank-Starling mechanism.

Afterload is the pressure against which the heart ejects blood. This is quantified by either peak ventricular or aortic blood pressure. Wall stress is the product of pressure and radius of the ventricle divided by wall thickness. Wall stress is the best predictor of oxygen demand or afterload on the heart. The sympathetic division of the autonomic nervous system increases heart rate via the right stellate ganglion and increases contractility via the left stellate ganglion. The heart rate increase is caused by faster phase 4 depolarization. The increased contractility is caused by binding of norepinephrine to β-adrenergic receptors and the production of cAMP. The vagus nerves provide the parasympathetic innervation of the heart. The right vagus nerve decreases heart rate by slowing phase 4 depolarization of the SA node. The left vagus slows conduction through the AV node. Digitalis increases contractility by slowing the sodium/potassium pump, which allows sodium to accumulate in the cell, which, in turn, slows secondary active transport of calcium out of the cell. Increased heart rate decreases the time available for transport of calcium out of the ventricular cells, allowing the accumulation of calcium in the cell. Normal heart rate is defined as 60 to 100 beats per minutes. Bradycardia is less than 60; tachycardia is greater than 100. Isovolumic contraction is analogous to the initial isometric component of an isotonic skeletal muscle contraction, in which sarcomere shortening results in sufficient tension to move the load. Isovolumic contraction begins when the ventricle begins to contract and closes the mitral valve and ends when pressure exceeds aortic pressure to cause the aortic valve to open. Ejection occurs when the aortic valve opens and ends when the ventricle relaxes sufficiently for aortic pressure to exceed ventricular pressure to close the aortic valve. As the ventricle relaxes and pressure decreases such that both the mitral and aortic valves are closed, the heart is in the phase of isovolumic relaxation. When pressure in the ventricle drops below atrial pressure, the mitral valve opens and filling begins. Filling ends when the ventricle begins to contract and causes the mitral valve to close and isovolumic contraction to begin again.

The first heart sound corresponds to the initiation of isovolumic contraction as the blood in the ventricle is accelerated and rapidly decelerated during mitral valve closure. The closure of the aortic and pulmonic valve cause blood to decelerate rapidly and the second heart sound to be generated. Systolic murmurs are caused by either aortic valve stenosis or mitral valve regurgitation. Diastolic murmurs are caused by either aortic valve regurgitation or mitral valve stenosis. Stenosis increases the afterload on the heart because a greater pressure must be generated to produce normal flow across the valve. Regurgitation causes a volume overload and an increased preload because of the greater volume that must be pumped to produce a normal net flow in the peripheral circulation. A pressure volume loop demonstrates the phases of the cardiac cycle in terms of changes in pressure and volume. The pressure for a given volume demonstrates contractility. The area within the loop shows the mechanical work done by the heart, and the area below the loop shows the work done on the heart by the preload. Ejection fraction is the proportion of the end diastolic volume ejected during systole. It is computed as SV/EDV and is a simple index of strength of the heart. An increased preload increases stroke volume, increased afterload decreases stroke volume, and increased contractility increases stroke volume. The law of LaPlace, using the equation for wall stress, is the most accurate predictor of myocardial oxygen demand. Wall stress equals pressure times radius divided by wall thickness. A thin-walled dilated ventricle has a greater demand for oxygen than a smaller diameter, thicker-walled ventricle. Stroke work is the product of stroke volume and pressure. For a given stroke work, oxygen consumption is greater if pressure is increased than if volume is increased. Increases in preload, afterload, contractility, and heart rate all increase myocardial oxygen demand. The most efficient combination of preload, afterload, contractility, and heart rate varies with the condition of the vascular system and health of the heart. For compliant vessels, a low heart rate and high stroke volume is most efficient, but for stiff vessels, a high heart rate and low stroke volume is more efficient.

BIBLIOGRAPHY

Berne RM, Levy MN. *Physiology*. St. Louis, Mo: Mosby-Year Book; 1998.

Ganong WF. *Review of Medical Physiology*. Norwalk, Conn: Appleton & Lange; 1995.

Guyton AC, Hall JE, Schmitt W. *Human Physiology and Mechanisms of Disease*. Philadelphia, Pa: WB Saunders; 1997.

Jean-Louis B. Information networks in the arterial wall. *News in Physiological Sciences.* 1999;14:68-73.

Melkumyants AM, Balashov SA, Khayutin VM. Control of arterial lumen by shear and stress endothelium. *News in Physiological Sciences.* 1995;10:204-210.

STUDY QUESTIONS

1. Why must contractility be adjustable in cardiac myocytes, as opposed to skeletal myocytes?

2. Why do cardiac cells need multiple controls over intracellular calcium concentration?

3. What would happen to contractility if the active transport of calcium out of cells was reduced?

4. Explain why contractility of cardiac myocytes increases as heart rate increases.

5. How does the heart compensate for transient changes in preload or afterload that occur with breathing?

6. How do β-adrenergic agents increase contractility? Heart rate? Afterload?

7. What valves are open during each phase of the cardiac cycle? How do the names of the four phases of the cardiac cycle relate to the valves that are open or closed?

8. How can one determine the beginning and end of systole by auscultation of the heart?

9. In terms of ventricular volume, define stroke volume and ejection fraction.

10. Explain why the minimum value of arterial pressure during the cardiac cycle occurs during systole.

11. What two possibilities exist for producing a systolic murmur?

12. In terms of ventricular and aortic pressures, why does an increase in afterload cause stroke volume to fall?

13. How does aortic insufficiency affect preload on the left ventricle? On the right ventricle?

14. Why does ventricular pressure fall during the initial portion of ventricular filling?

15. Why is the apex of the left ventricular so much thinner than the walls near the base of the heart?

LABORATORY EXERCISE

LABORATORY EXERCISE 20-1

CARDIAC CYCLE

Objectives:
1. Review the normal electrical activity of the heart.
2. Demonstrate procedures for recording an electrocardiogram.
3. Correlate mechanical and electrical functions of the heart.
4. Demonstrate how the EKG changes under physiologic conditions.
5. Recognize abnormal EKG patterns.

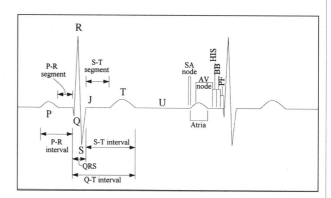

Figure 20-6. The named parts of the electrocardiogram (left). On the right, the sequence of activation of the heart occurring as the EKG is recorded is depicted.

Review of the electrocardiogram:
Similar to the EMG, the EKG is a recording of an electrical signal from muscle at the surface of the skin. Unlike the EMG, the EKG is a clear signal with a standard waveform. Because of the strength and uniformity of the signal, interpretation of the EKG is a useful way of determining if the electrical properties of the heart are normal. Damage to the myocardium, including ischemia, infarction, or abnormalities in the conducting system of the heart can be detected by standard EKG interpretation. In addition, the EKG can be used to determine if the heart has a proper rate and rhythm, or if changes in the size or position of the heart have occurred.

Because the heart has its own pacemaker and conduction system, the myocardium does not depolarize or repolarize all at once. The myocardium depolarizes and repolarizes in a predictable pattern. The signal picked up from electrodes will depend on the size of the signal (determined primarily by the mass of the myocardium) and the distance of the signal from the electrodes. By recording from different sites, one can determine if conduction is normal and where in the heart electrical abnormalities may originate. The EKG is recorded from several electrodes at once. Four electrodes are attached to the limbs (limb leads) from which six different recordings are made. In addition, there are six standard positions on the chest (precordial leads) from which a series of waveforms is recorded.

By convention, the EKG waveform has been broken down into six waves (noted as P, Q, R, S, T, and U waves) (Figure 20-6) and various intervals and segments have been defined. Standard interpretation of a twelve-lead EKG uses measurements of the size of these waves, intervals and segments to determine if an EKG is within normal limits (the term used for a normal EKG).

Materials:
Recorder with EKG selector switch
Lead cables:
  black: left arm
  white: right arm
  red: left leg
  green: right leg
Chest lead (moved to six different sites, some cables will have six separate wires)
Electrode paste, alcohol, gauze, centimeter rule

LABORATORY EXERCISE

Methods:

A. Recording resting EKG (at 25 cm/sec)

1. Examine the EKG with the following in mind:

    Rate: Is the rate between 60 and 100 bpm, or is there tachycardia or bradycardia?

    Rhythm: Does depolarization begin at the SA node, progress normally through the AV node and ventricular conduction system? Are atrial and ventricular rates the same? Is the P-R interval normal (<0.20 seconds)? Is the QRS complex normal (<0.12 seconds)?

    Integrity: Ischemia, injury, and infarction all alter the normal balance of depolarization across the myocardium, resulting in predictable changes in the EKG, depending on the area of the heart affected. Ischemia produces T wave inversion or ST segment depression, and sometimes both will be seen at once. T wave inversion suggests slowed repolarization and ST segment depression is indicative of an area of myocardium that is depolarized compared with other areas of the heart. Acute infarction is associated with ST segment elevation (the waveform resembles the cardiac membrane action potential) that persists for five days or so. Following a myocardial infarction, a Q wave will appear in the leads closest to the infarction. Unlike the temporary ST segment that elevates, Q waves become permanent indicators that an infarction occurred.

Questions:

1. What electrical events occur (which cells are depolarizing or repolarizing) during the P wave, PR interval, QRS complex, and T wave?

2. During what portion of the EKG are the atria contracting? The ventricles?

3. During what portion of the EKG does ischemia produce an alteration?

B. Physiologic changes in EKG

1. Record the EKG from lead II in the supine position. Have the subject stand up rapidly while recording the EKG. What happens to heart rate? What is the function of the sympathetic innervation to the heart?

2. Record the EKG while pressing on the eyeballs or massaging the carotid arteries. What happens to heart rate? What is the function of the parasympathetic innervation (vagus) to the heart?

C. Recording of phonocardiogram and carotid pulse

1. With a subject in supine, place a heart microphone where the best record can be obtained. This is most easily done by placing the microphone under the shirt near the second or third interspace (near the heart valves). A moderately heavy shirt will improve the quality of the recording. Then place the crystal pickup over a carotid artery.

2. Record the EKG (lead II), carotid pulse and phonocardiogram simultaneously for several cardiac cycles. Note: if you are using a two-channel machine, you will need to make three recordings to obtain all of the information. Record at a slow speed until you obtain a good recording. Then record at 50 mm/s for a short time to spread the record enough to analyze. By plugging stereo headphones into the output jack of the channel in which the heart sounds are being recorded, you can actually hear the heart sounds.

3. From this record make measurements described on the next page and correlate mechanical and electrical events.

LABORATORY EXERCISE

a. Total duration of the cardiac cycle (R to next R).

b. Duration of systole (from beginning of S_1 to beginning of S_2).

c. Duration of isovolumic contraction (from S_1 to rise of carotid pulse).

d. Ejection time (beginning of rise of carotid pulse to incisura).

e. Total duration of diastole (duration of cardiac cycle—duration of systole or beginning of S_2 to beginning of S_1).

f. Percent of cardiac cycle spent in systole and diastole.

g. What error have we made in measuring ejection time? Is this error large?

4. Repeat after having subject lift weights for 1 minute. With increasing heart rate, what happens to duration of systole? What happens to the percentage of the cardiac cycle spent in systole vs diastole? With an increase in afterload on the heart, what happens to duration of systole? Which phase of systole should be affected most when afterload is increased (same phenomenon as in skeletal muscle)?

D. Interpretation of EKG

The following six EKG tracings demonstrate the five following abnormalities: acute myocardial infarction, atrial fibrillation, premature ventricular contractions, and right bundle branch block. Systematically analyze the six EKGs to determine which tracing has which abnormality. What do the other two EKGs show?

Review of cardiac cycle lab and answers

1. P wave-avid depolarization, PR interval-AV node depolarization, QRS complex-ventricular depolarization, T wave-ventricular repolarization.

2. Atria contract during P wave and finish near beginning of QRS. Ventricles contract during QRS and relax at end of T wave.

3. EKG change with ischemia: inverted T wave or ST segment depression, also acute MI: ST segment elevation.

4. Increased heart rate is mediated by sympathetic stimulation to the heart as part of the baroreceptor reflex to compensate for postural change. This also includes increased contractility and faster conduction through AV node.

5. Pressing eyes or massaging carotid arteries decreases heart rate by stimulating parasympathetic (vagal) input to the heart. Vagus also slows conduction through the AV node. These maneuvers are useful for stopping supraventricular tachycardia (fast rate originating above the AV node), but could also cause AV block!

6. The length of the cardiac cycle includes four phases: isovolumic contraction in which the ventricles are contracting but have not developed enough pressure to open the aortic valve, ejection is the time during which blood moves from the left ventricle into the aorta, isovolumic relaxation is the time between closure of the aortic valve at the end of ejection until filling of the ventricles from the atria can begin again, and filling occurs between the opening of the atrioventricular valves and isovolumic contraction.

7. Total duration of the cardiac cycle is measured from any point on the EKG to the same point on the next cycle; the top of an R wave is a convenient point to use.

8. The first heart sound (S1) occurs during the latter part of the QRS complex and signals the onset of systole as blood accelerates against closed valves. The second heart sound is generated when the aortic and pulmonary valves are closed and blood "bounces" against the closed valves; therefore the beginning of the second heart sound (S2) marks the end of systole.

LABORATORY EXERCISE

9.   Systole consists of two phases: isovolumic contraction and ejection. The first heart sound is the beginning of systole and the beginning of isovolumic contraction. The second heart sound is the end of systole and the end of ejection. The end of isovolumic contraction and beginning of ejection can only be determined by recording the movement of blood into the aorta (using the carotid artery introduces a small error in the determination). The beginning of the upstroke on the carotid pulse waveform shows the beginning of ejection, which is also the end of isovolumic contraction. The incisura (the dip on the carotid pulse waveform marks the end of ejection and should occur at the same time as the second heart sound, which also marks the end of ejection and systole).

10. We can determine the total duration of diastole, but cannot determine how much is isovolumic relaxation and how much is filling. We would need something to tell us when the mitral valve opens. Opening of the mitral valve does not show on the EKG, carotid pulse, or heart sounds.

11. Typical values for the phases:
     a. Cardiac cycle: 800 ms (heart rate = 75)
     b. Systole: 270 ms
     c. Isovolumic contraction: 50 ms
     d. Ejection: 220 ms
     e. Diastole: 530 ms
     f. Isovolumic relaxation: 90 ms
     g. Ventricular filling: 440 ms

12. Percentage of cardiac cycle in systole = 270/800 ms = 34% (1/3)

13. Percentage of cardiac cycle in diastole = 530/800 ms = 66% (2/3)

14. With increasing heart rate, the decreased time available for the cardiac cycle is taken primarily from diastole. Systole becomes somewhat shorter due to sympathetic stimulation, but diastole is shortened more than systole with the result that systole becomes a greater percentage of the cardiac cycle.

15. Interpretation of EKG: be able to identify ischemia (ST segment depression), acute MI (ST segment elevation, looks like the ventricular action potential), and premature ventricular contractions (wide, large amplitude, T wave, and QRS go in opposite directions). These three will be the most likely to be tested on a board exam.

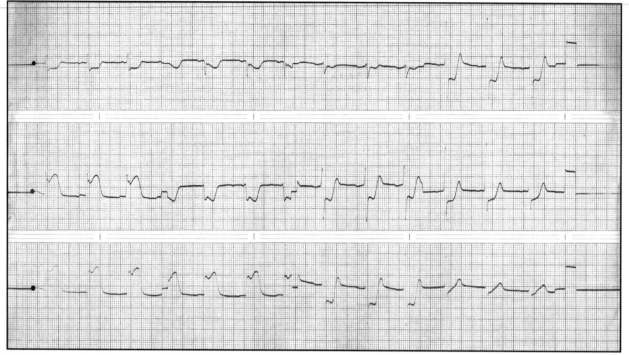

EKG 1

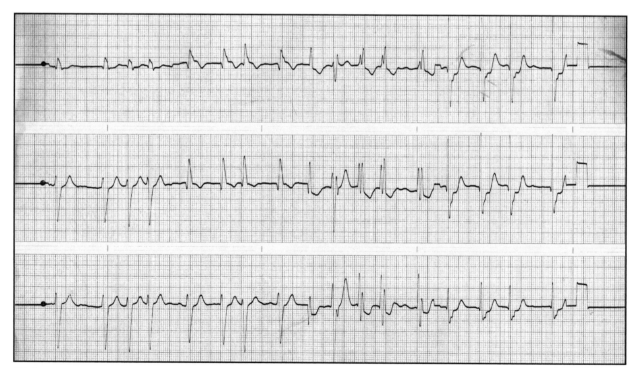

EKG 2

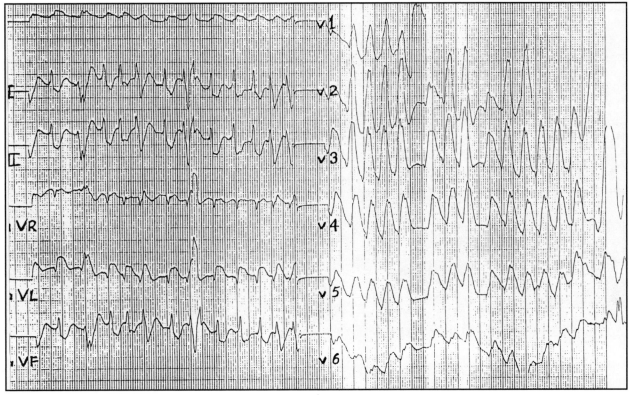

EKG 3

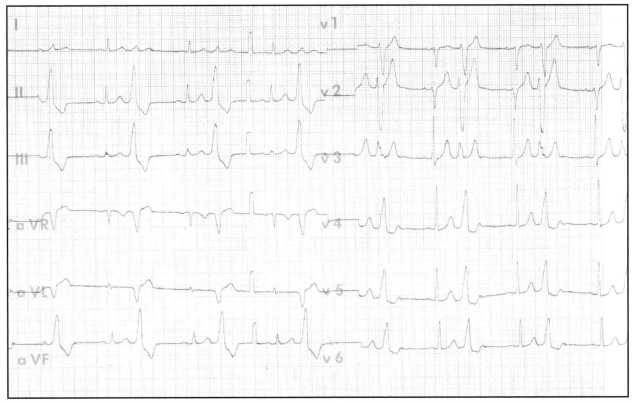

EKG 4

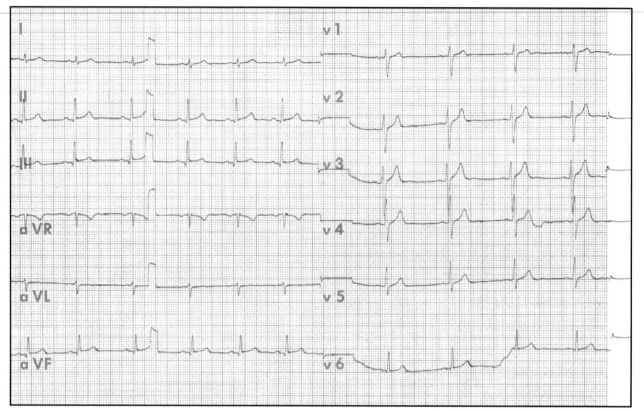

EKG 5

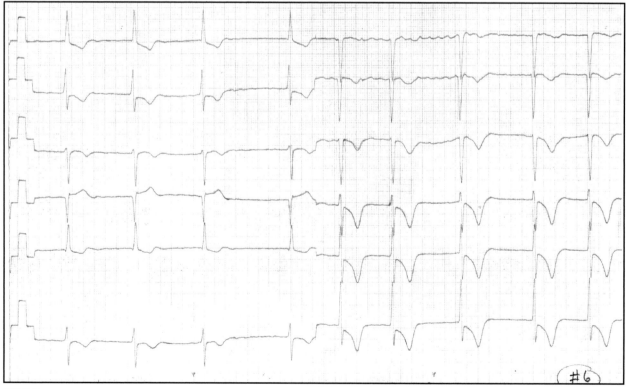

EKG 6

TWENTY-ONE

Hemodynamics

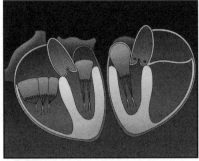

OBJECTIVES

1. Describe the relationships among bulk flow (Q), velocity (v), and cross-sectional area (A) in blood vessels.

2. List the factors determining blood flow and their effects: ΔP, length, viscosity, and radius.

3. Describe how resistance and conductance change with blood vessel arrangements of parallel vs. series and how blood pressure changes as it flows through vessels.

4. Describe the relationship among mean arterial pressure, cardiac output, and total peripheral resistance.

5. Explain how the compliance of the arterial wall influences pressure development.

6. Define wall stress and the factors that influence wall stress.

7. Define mean arterial pressure (MAP), and compute it from systolic and diastolic pressure.

8. Explain the role of elastic large arteries in transforming pulsatile flow to nearly continuous flow.

9. Explain the interaction between arterial compliance and optimum heart rate.

10. Describe how changes in stroke volume and arterial compliance influence pulse pressure.

11. Describe the production and destruction of red blood cells:
    a. life span
    b. stimulus for production of red cells
    c. other blood cells and their functions
    d. breakdown products of red cells
    e. types of anemia: hemolytic, macrocytosis, microcytosis, bleeding
    f. define hematocrit and normal values for men and women and the consequences of elevated hematocrit

12. Describe the functions of the plasma proteins.

The behavior of blood within vessels can be predicted by principles of physics. This chapter describes how blood flow is affected in individual vessels, then in a network of vessels. The same principles can then be applied to the systemic circulation as a whole to predict how blood pressure and cardiac output will change under various conditions. Properties of the blood will be described at the end of the chapter.

HEMODYNAMICS

Hemodynamics is the study of the physical principles governing the flow of blood through the cardiovascular system. Geometric, electric circuit, and fluid dynamic principles may be applied to predict the behavior of blood flow. The relationship between blood flow linear velocity in cm/s and bulk flow in cm^3/s (equivalent to ml/s) is a direct consequence of blood vessel geometry. Velocity is a linear measure of blood cell movement over time in units of cm/sec, whereas flow is the volume of blood moved over time in units of cm^3/s. Velocity (v) and flow (Q) are related by the equation: Q (cm^3/sec) = v (cm/sec) x A (cm^2) in which A = cross-sectional area (πr^2 or $\pi d^2/4$). A second application of this relationship among velocity, flow, and cross-sectional area is in the comparison of velocity through different vascular segments of the circulatory system. In all serial segments of a closed vascular circuit, the volume of blood flowing through each segment is constant, regardless of the cross-sectional area of any particular segment (Figure 21-1).

This means that, if the circulation is in a steady state, blood flow in liters/minute through the aorta equals blood flow through all of the branches that come off it and equals the sum of the blood flow through all the capillaries and the sum of the flow through the veins. As blood vessels branch, the sum of the cross-sectional area increases. As a result, the cross-sectional area of all the arteries that branch from the aorta is much greater than the cross-sectional area of the aorta itself. The many capillaries that branch from arterioles have a collective cross-sectional area that becomes enormous relative to the aorta. Veins, which are more numerous and have a larger cross-sectional area, have a greater collective cross-sectional area than their corresponding arteries (Figure 21-2). Given this information, we can explain why the velocity of blood flowing through an artery is greater than its paired vein and why blood flow velocity is extremely slow in capillaries. Velocity is so slow that one can distinguish single cells moving through capillaries under a microscope. It is also easy to distinguish an

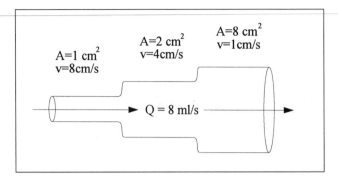

Figure 21-1. The relationships among velocity, cross-sectional area, and bulk flow in contiguous segments of blood vessels. Flow must be equal in contiguous segments, and, because the product of velocity and cross-sectional area equals flow, the product of velocity and cross-sectional area must be equal in contiguous segments. As cross-sectional area increases from 1 cm^2 in the first to 2 cm^2 in the second segment, velocity must decrease in proportion from 8 cm/s to 4 cm/s, and in the third segment with a cross-sectional area of 8 cm^2, velocity decreases to 1 cm/s.

arteriole feeding a capillary bed with its thicker wall, smaller diameter, and greater velocity from its paired venule draining the capillaries.

The factors that determine the bulk flow through a blood vessel are the same as those discussed in Chapter Two for any hydraulic system with the additional factors that result from having cellular components in the fluid. Flow, as the dependent variable, is directly proportional to pressure and conductance (Q = gΔP). Because of the way Ohm's law is written, blood flow is sometimes analyzed in terms of a DC circuit as P = Q x R (Figure 21-3). Flow is directly proportional to conductance and inversely proportional to resistance. The primary determinants of conductance are cross-sectional area and length. Conductance increases with cross-sectional area and decreases with the length of the pathway over which flow occurs as energy is lost. Energy, in this case pressure, is lost in interactions of the blood with the vessel wall and, as discussed below, with itself. With increasing radius, the energy lost interacting with the vessel wall decreases rapidly because the circumference of a vessel in contact with blood increases linearly with increasing radius (circumference = $2\pi r$), whereas cross-sectional area increases as the square of the radius (CSA = πr^2). Conductance increases in proportion to the fourth power of the radius. If radius is doubled, conductance and, therefore, flow for a given pressure increases 2^4 or 16 times. In terms of resistance, doubling radius decreases resistance to 1/16. The relationship between vessel length and conductance is linear; conductance decreases and resistance increases with length (Figure 21-4).

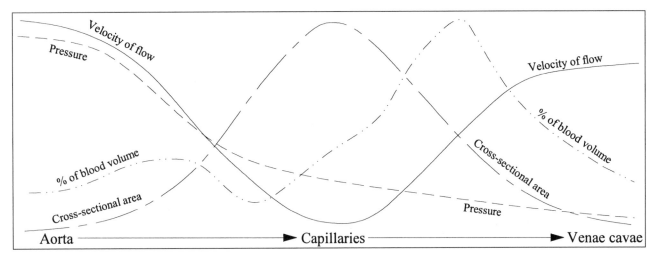

Figure 21-2. Hemodynamics in the different segments of the systemic circulation: flow velocity, pressure, cross-sectional area, and percentage of blood volume contained within each segment. Note the loss of pressure as blood is driven through vessels from the aorta to the vena cava. The greatest drop occurs in arterioles that distribute blood flow within organs. An inverse relationship exists between cross-sectional area and velocity as explained previously. Within the capillaries, cross-sectional area becomes tremendous due to the extent of branching of vessels, which causes velocity to be very slow. Slow velocity allows greater time for exchange of substance and thermal energy. Also note the fraction of blood volume in small venous vessels. With a high cardiac output, much of this volume can be mobilized to the arterial side of the circulation.

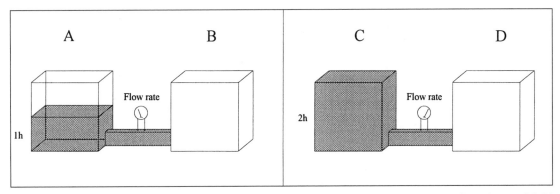

Figure 21-3. Effect of pressure on flow of blood. Pressure is determined by the height of a column of fluid in the formula $P = \rho gh$, where ρ is the density of a fluid, g is the acceleration of gravity, and h is the height of a column of fluid. In this example, flow from C to D is twice that of the flow from A to B because the difference in pressure from C to D is twice that between A and B. In the cardiovascular system, the pressure to drive flow comes from the pumping of blood by the heart from veins into arteries. Pumping of blood decreases venous pressure and increases arterial pressure to create the pressure difference that drives blood flow through the circulation. If the difference between arterial and venous pressure doubles with the same resistance in the circulation, flow will double.

VISCOSITY

Because of the presence of blood cells, viscosity of the blood must be taken into account. Viscosity is created by the interaction of the fluid with itself, rather than with the vessel wall. To describe viscosity, we need to picture blood flow in concentric layers around the longitudinal axis of the vessel. If viscosity is low, the layers of blood slip easily past each other. In a viscous fluid, the layers interact more and need more energy to be dragged across each other. A viscous fluid, such as maple syrup, clings to itself and flows slowly for this reason. On the other hand, too little viscosity requires greater energy to produce the flow predicted by conductance and pressure. Viscosity prevents turbulence and keeps the flow of blood in layers. Turbulent flow (Figure 21-5) causes energy to be lost from interaction of the blood with itself, which dissipates the pressure-driving flow. Viscosity is measured in such a way that conductance decreases and resistance increases linearly with viscosity

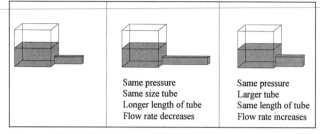

Figure 21-4. Effect of conduit size on flow. In the middle panel, the same pressure drives flow through the conduit, and the conduit has the same cross-sectional area, but twice the length. Resistance of the conduit doubles (conductance is halved), and blood flow is halved. On the panel on the right, pressure is the same, the length of the conduit is the same as the panel on the left, but the conduit has twice the cross-sectional area as that on the left. Flow increases with the fourth power of the cross-sectional area; therefore, with twice the cross-sectional area, blood flow increases 2^4, or 16 times. In the circulation, conduit size is altered primarily by control of smooth muscle of the arterioles, which, in turn, increases or decreases cross-sectional area of individual vessels.

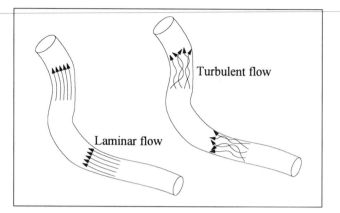

Figure 21-5. Laminar and turbulent blood flow. In laminar flow, the blood travels in concentric layers with little interaction between layers and loss of energy, with the inner layers traveling faster than the outer layers. In turbulent flow, the layers interact with each other and with the vessel walls. Energy is lost, resulting in decreased blood flow for a given arterial pressure, blood vessels are damaged, and atherosclerosis may occur.

(η). Viscosity of blood is determined primarily by hematocrit (the fraction of blood volume occupied by red blood cells). The relationship between hematocrit and viscosity is not linear; viscosity increases more rapidly than hematocrit. At hematocrit values greater than normal, viscosity increases to unmanageable levels (Figure 21-6).

POISEUILLE'S LAW

Poiseuille is credited for performing experiments to demonstrate the relationships among geometry, viscosity, and flow through glass tubes with an equation now named after him, which incorporates the elements described above: $Q = (\pi\, r^4\, \Delta P)/(8\, L\eta)$. Pressure and the one term that increases conductance (radius) are placed in the numerator, and the terms that decrease conductance (length and viscosity) are placed in the denominator. The constants of π and 8 exist to convert the proportionality into an equation due to the geometric considerations of conductance. Conductance can be predicted as $\pi r^4/8L\eta$ and resistance as its reciprocal, $R = (8L\eta)/(\pi\, r^4)$. Poiseuille's equation is a rearrangement Ohm's law applied to the vascular system ($Q = g\Delta P$) and substituting for g as above.

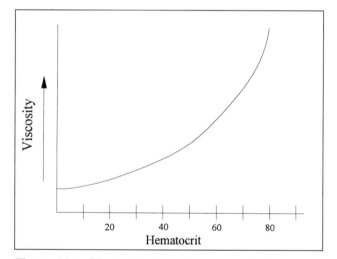

Figure 21-6. Effect of hematocrit on viscosity. Blood flow decreases in proportion to viscosity, which is determined chiefly by the ability of plasma and cellular elements to slip past each other. An increase in the fraction of blood volume occupied by red cells (hematocrit) does not increase viscosity linearly. An increase in viscosity above 60% (normal is mid 40s for men) can increase blood viscosity to a lethal value.

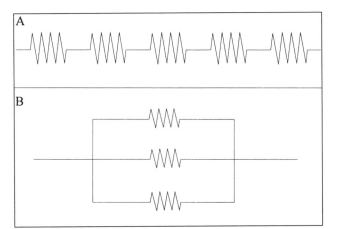

Figure 21-7. Resistance in series (top) and in parallel (bottom panel). Resistances in series are seen in the circulatory system as the different vessel segments (ie, arteries, arterioles, capillaries, venules, and veins). As blood travels through resistances in series, pressure is dissipated. Resistances in parallel are seen within each segment of the circulation (ie, the hepatic artery, mesenteric arteries, renal arteries, etc, are in parallel). The greater the number of resistances that exist in parallel, the lower the resistance of the segment as a whole. Stated in terms of conductance, the more conductors in parallel, the greater the conductance of the entire segment. This characteristic is most evident in the capillaries. Individual capillaries have a very low conductance (high resistance), but the large number of them in parallel results in a much lower aggregate resistance than one might anticipate.

HEMODYNAMIC CONSEQUENCES OF SERIES AND PARALLEL ARRANGEMENTS OF BLOOD VESSELS

The conductance of an entire vascular bed within a tissue depends on the geometrical arrangement of the vessels. The different vessel types (ie, arteries vs. arterioles) in the cardiovascular system are arranged in series, and the individual members of each vessel type, such as the arterioles or the capillaries, are usually arranged in parallel to each other.

The conductance of a series of vessels decreases with the length, or, in terms of resistance, the total resistance equals the sum of the resistances in series. As vessels are added in series (increasing length by adding arterioles to arteries and capillaries to arterioles), the conductance decreases, and the resistance increases. For conductance in parallel, total conductance equals the sum of the individual conductances. For parallel resistors, the inverse of the total resistance equals the sum of the inverses of the resistances. As vessels are added in parallel, the conduc-

tance increases, and the resistance decreases. No matter how small the conductance or how great the resistance of the blood vessels added in parallel, adding another pathway for blood flow will increase flow for a given pressure difference across the vascular bed. This concept explains the relationship between number of capillaries in a bed and the resistance to flow. Although individual capillaries have high resistance, the large number of capillaries arranged in parallel causes little dissipation of pressure during flow through them. Most of the resistance in the systemic circulation occurs at the level of arterioles, not capillaries (Figure 21-7).

HEMODYNAMIC PRINCIPLES APPLIED TO THE SYSTEMIC CIRCULATION

The sum of all resistances within the systemic circulation is termed the total peripheral resistance (TPR), but we do not have a corresponding term for conductance for historical reasons. The term TPR allows us to create an equation to predict changes in pressure and flow for the entire systemic circulation just as we can examine individual vessels using the terms ΔP, R, and Q. Because blood flow through the circulation is in steady state with the pumping of blood from the left ventricle, the sum of all regional systemic blood flows is equal to the cardiac output (CO). The driving force for bulk flow through the entire systemic circulation is aortic pressure - right atrial pressure. We will neglect the small right atrial pressure and assume that mean arterial pressure computed from systolic and diastolic pressure measured from a large artery is equal to aortic pressure averaged over the cardiac cycle. With these assumptions, we can state that the average pressure driving the cardiac output through the TPR is the mean arterial blood pressure (MAP). If we then apply Ohm's law to the systemic circulation (MAP = CO x TPR), the value of TPR is dependent on the resistance of many vascular beds arranged in parallel. By altering the resistance of individual vascular beds relative to the TPR, the distribution of the cardiac output can be changed. Depending on the degree of local changes in resistance, TPR may be affected sufficiently to alter mean arterial pressure for a given cardiac output. Therefore, a change in the needs for blood flow to one organ or tissue may require either a change in cardiac output or a compensatory change in resistance to blood flow in other tissues to maintain blood pressure at its regulated value. Large, sudden changes in peripheral resistance will produce changes in cardiac output and arterial pressure. A decreased TPR will produce a transient decrease in MAP and CO, and may redistribute blood flow away from organs such as the brain that previously had a low resistance compared with other tissues.

Blood vessel compliance also determines the flow of blood from the heart and through the circulation. Compliance is a measure of distensibility of an object and is defined as compliance = $\Delta V/\Delta P$. The more compliant an object is, the greater the change in volume is for any increment in pressure. Stiffness is the inverse of compliance ($\Delta P/\Delta V$), and the stiffer an object is, the greater the change in pressure is for any increment in volume. For example, aortic pressure increases more in a stiff, atherosclerotic aorta for a given stroke volume than in a healthy, compliant aorta.

The law of LaPlace ($\tau = P \times r$) was introduced as part of the discussion of wall tension in the ventricle (τ = tension in the vessel wall, P = transmural pressure, r = radius of a vessel). Wall tension can be visualized as a force tending to pull apart the cells that make up the vessel wall, which could rupture the vessel if it becomes great enough or if the wall is weak (Figure 21-8). Due to the phenomenon described by the law of LaPlace, vessels with a small radius develop very little tension in their walls even with high pressure. Therefore, a capillary subjected to a pressure of 20 to 30 mmHg and composed of only a single layer of endothelium will not rupture, whereas the aorta, with an average pressure during the cardiac cycle that is only about three times as much, requires a thick layer of fibrous tissue to prevent rupture due to its greater radius. The danger of an aneurysm is that, as the wall weakens, the radius increases, producing a positive feedback between wall tension and radius that can lead to rupture and a rapid, potentially fatal loss of blood volume.

ARTERIAL BLOOD PRESSURE

The large arteries offer very little resistance to blood flow; therefore, arterial pressure measured at either brachial artery with a sphygmomanometer usually gives a reliable estimate of arterial pressure. By definition, systolic arterial pressure is the maximum pressure during a cardiac cycle. The maximum pressure of the cardiac cycle occurs shortly after ejection begins. Diastolic pressure is defined as the minimum pressure during the cardiac cycle. Because blood pressure decreases near the end of ejection and continues to fall until ejection occurs again, the minimum pressure in the arteries occurs immediately before ejection, which is at the end of isovolumic contraction. Technically, therefore, diastolic pressure does not occur during diastole but during the

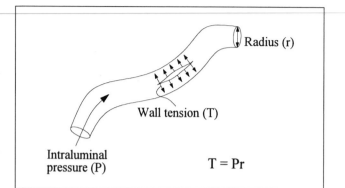

Figure 21-8. Wall stress in a blood vessel. Wall stress (τ) is the product of radius and pressure within the vessel. Wall stress acts to pull a vessel apart. Collagen fibers and other elements act in opposition to wall stress. In general, vessels are constructed with a thickness proportional to wall stress. Capillaries have a very small radius and can be only one cell thick, whereas the aorta has a very thick muscular and fibrous wall to withstand its wall stress.

first phase of systole. Pulse pressure is defined as the difference between systolic and diastolic pressure (SP - DP). The name implies that it is the change in pressure that occurs with a pulse. Mean arterial pressure is the average pressure in the large arteries integrated over an entire cardiac cycle. The contributions of systolic and diastolic pressures are dependent on heart rate with diastole lasting approximately twice as long as systole. Therefore, a reasonable estimate for MAP is one-third of the pulse pressure above diastolic (ie, MAP = DP + PP/3). A mathematically equivalent equation is MAP = (SP + 2 x DP)/3. This computed value for MAP is close to what is derived electronically from direct measurement of arterial pressure with an arterial line and transducer with integration over the cardiac cycle.

Arterial pressure varies with time of day and activity. Both systolic and diastolic pressure increase with age. The large arteries convert the intermittent ejection of blood into the aorta into a nearly steady flow of blood in the microcirculation. Although flow in an individual blood vessel within the microcirculation changes intermittently, this fluctuation is due to changes in the smooth muscle tone of the vessels, producing alterations in the conductance of blood into the individual vessel. The elasticity of the arterial system, by converting pulsatile pumping into steady flow, minimizes the work of the heart. Large vessels are compliant and are stretched when blood is ejected from the heart. Normal arterial vessels are elastic and recoil during diastole to maintain flow into the circulation after ejection ceases. A vessel with a relatively high compliance will develop less pressure when a given stroke volume is ejected compared with a stiff vessel having a relatively low compliance. An aorta with a high compliance allows a greater stroke volume. This allows an individual to have a lower heart rate. The compliant aorta also maintains a suitable diastolic pressure for a longer time than a stiff aorta, due to the greater volume ejected into the aorta. For this reason, a stiff aorta requires a higher heart rate and lower stroke volume to maintain systolic and diastolic pressures at normal levels, which also increases the work of the heart.

Systolic pressure is determined by the volume of blood present and the compliance of the vessels in the arterial system at the peak of ejection. Diastolic pressure is determined by the volume of blood and the compliance of the vessels present in the arterial system just before ejection. Pulse pressure is the result of the change in the volume of the arterial system that occurs over one cardiac cycle (PP = SP − DP). Pulse pressure is, therefore, determined by the increase in volume with ejection. Because blood is ejected into the aorta more rapidly than it can flow through the systemic circulation, the aortic volume increment during ejection is the stroke volume ejected less the peripheral run-off during ejection. The second factor influencing pressure in the aorta at any time is the compliance of the vessels. With all other factors kept constant, increasing stroke volume increases systolic and pulse pressure. Compliance can decrease because of a change in the inherent properties of the blood vessels or because of an elevation in mean pressure distending the vessels. Decreased compliance increases pulse pressure because systolic pressure increases more with ejection into a stiff vessel and blood runs off more rapidly decreasing diastolic pressure. During exercise, which increases contractility of the heart, the rate of ejection will increase relative to the rate at which blood flows out of the aorta and systolic pressure and pulse pressure will increase. Pulse pressure rises with exercise, arteriosclerosis, and hypertension. In aortic insufficiency with leakage of blood back into the ventricle, pulse pressure increases as blood runs off both into the systemic circulation and into the left ventricle, thereby decreasing diastolic pressure. Pulse pressure decreases in aortic stenosis because of the small stroke volume caused by the resistance of the aortic valve.

BLOOD

The medium that carries nutrients, wastes, and body heat by convective transport is the blood. In addition to serving as a medium for transport, blood has many other important functions that may be carried out by its cells as well as the noncellular elements or humoral factors. Blood consists of several important components that can

be observed following centrifugation. Plasma, the buffy coat, and packed red cells are observable with the unaided eye. Centrifugation allows us to determine the hematocrit of the blood. Hematocrit is an important value to know, especially in the person who may have experienced significant blood loss following surgery or is undergoing cancer chemotherapy. It is defined as the fraction of blood that consists of red cells, expressed as a percent. Normal values are higher for men than for women, presumably due to the effect of testosterone. For men, hematocrit is expected to be in the range of 43% to 49% and for women, 38% to 44%. A decrease in hematocrit reduces the ability to perform activities as the oxygen-carrying capacity of the blood is decreased. Regulation of hematocrit will be discussed later in this chapter.

ERYTHROCYTES

Red blood cells, also called erythrocytes or, more simply, red cells, represent 99% of blood cells. Their size varies somewhat, averaging 8 μm in diameter. Red cells are very deformable and can pass easily through capillaries that may be smaller in diameter. Red cells perform basically as hemoglobin containers that carry oxygen around the circulation. Hemoglobin consists of globin plus four units of heme. An iron atom in the center of each heme subunit can bind O_2; therefore, each hemoglobin molecule can carry up to four molecules of O_2. Red cells, as well as white cells and platelets, are produced in the bone marrow. As the cells develop, they begin to produce Hb and lose their nuclei and other organelles to become flexible hemoglobin packages. The red cells are released into blood as immature cells called reticulocytes that can be distinguished from mature red cells under the microscope. They mature within a few days into erythrocytes where they have a life span of approximately 120 days in the circulation. We must replace approximately 1% or 100 billion red cells every day. Old red cells are recognized and destroyed in the spleen.

Iron is required for red cell synthesis, but some is lost when the red cells are destroyed. This amount of iron lost each day is replaced by ingestion. In contrast to most electrolytes, which are controlled by the kidneys, the amount of iron absorbed is controlled by intestinal epithelium. Sixty-five percent of body iron is in the form of Hb, 0.1% is in a transport form called transferrin in plasma, and 15% to 30% of the body's iron is stored in liver as ferritin or accumulations of ferritin called hemosiderin (Figure 21-9). Hemosiderin produces the yellow-brown color of old bruises. Blood that accumulates in the tissue is broken down into different pigments called bilirubin and biliverdin that initially color a bruise. Removal of these substances allows the accumulated iron in the form of hemosiderin to be seen later. Eventually, the hemosiderin is removed from the tissue by macrophages. Destruction of red cells by the spleen releases iron into plasma. In the plasma, iron binds to transferrin, which carries iron to bone marrow for recycling.

RED CELL PRODUCTION (ERYTHROPOIESIS)

The production of red cells or erythrocytes is known as erythropoiesis. Iron, folic acid, and vitamin B_{12} are required to synthesize red cells. Iron is required for hemoglobin (Hb). Folic acid is essential for synthesis of DNA, and vitamin B_{12}, a cobalt-containing molecule, is necessary for folic acid action. Vitamin B_{12} is found only in animal products, and, consequently, a strict vegetarian diet can lead to anemia, which is the term for a decreased oxygen-carrying capacity of the blood. The hormone erythropoietin (EPO) is secreted by the kidney in response to a decreased O_2 delivery to kidney. EPO acts on bone marrow to stimulate red cell production. Testosterone also stimulates EPO, thus causing men to have a greater hematocrit than women following puberty. Before puberty, hematocrit is approximately equal in boys and girls and similar to that of women. Synthetic EPO has been developed to aid individuals with anemia due to cancer chemotherapy or other diseases. However, aerobic athletes, especially cyclists, have been using this to elevate hematocrit artificially in an effort to enhance their performance by increasing the oxygen-carrying capacity of their blood. Unfortunately, the increase in hematocrit may elevate viscosity of the blood to life-threatening levels, and some cyclists have expired this way.

ANEMIA

A decreased capacity of the blood to carry oxygen is called anemia. Anemia may be caused by a decreased number of red cells, Hb, or both and may also be caused by carbon monoxide poisoning because hemoglobin has a much greater affinity for carbon monoxide than for oxygen. Causes of anemia are decreased iron, folic acid, and vitamin B_{12}, which are required for red cell synthesis, bone marrow toxicity or cancer (leukemias and related diseases), decreased EPO, and increased destruction (hemolytic anemias). The most common cause of ane-

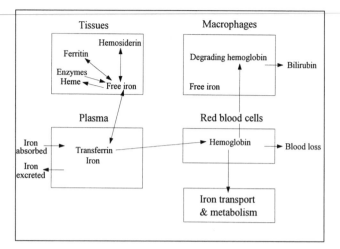

Figure 21-9. Iron transport and metabolism. Iron is a major constituent of red blood cells and is constantly replaced and recycled as old red cells are destroyed and new cells are made.

mia, however, is bleeding, especially gastrointestinal bleeding and blood loss during surgery. Lack of iron causes red cells to be smaller than normal (microcytic anemia), whereas deficiency of either folic acid or vitamin B_{12} results in large, immature red cells being released into the circulation (macrocytic anemia).

Sickle cell anemia is caused by a genetic mutation in which one amino acid that is hydrophobic is substituted for a hydrophilic amino acid. At a physiologic, high PO_2, the hemoglobin behaves normally; however, at a low PO_2, hemoglobin precipitates and deforms, resulting in "sickled" red cells. The anemia results from a shortened life span of the deformed cells. In addition, deformed red cells occlude the capillaries, resulting in tissue death in many locations throughout the body. Individuals with sickle cell disease may periodically experience sickle cell crises that are painful and may result in a further accumulation of organ damage. Health care professionals may intervene because of joint replacements necessitated by aseptic necrosis of joints, especially the heads of the femur and humerus.

In addition to the red cells packed at the bottom of a tube of centrifuged blood, one may observe a thin intermediate layer called the buffy coat and a straw-colored fluid at the top of the tube called plasma. The buffy coat consists of platelets and white blood cells (WBCs, leukocytes). Plasma contains numerous proteins, nutrients such as glucose, waste products, and electrolytes (mainly NaCl). Serum is the name given to plasma with its clotting factors removed. Some of the important proteins include both pro- and anticoagulant proteins, the complement system proteins, and immunoglobulins (antibodies). The complement system consists of a group of about 20 proteins that can be activated to combat infection. Important effects of the complement system are opsonization, which is a process of "labeling" a foreign particle for destruction, and chemotaxis. This signaling process attracts immune cells to the site of complement, thus promoting the effects of inflammation. Immunoglobins constitute about 20% of the plasma proteins. There are five general classes of immunoglobulins termed IgM, IgG, IgA, IgD, and IgE, which are associated with certain immune functions.

IMMUNE SYSTEM

White cells are larger than red cells and are less deformable, so they move slowly through blood vessels. The primary function of white cells is inflammation in response to tissue injury or foreign particles. The basic types of white blood cells are monocytes, lymphocytes, neutrophils, basophils, and eosinophils. Monocytes act as scavengers, but also produce important chemical signals. The name given to these chemical signals has changed over the years. In tissues, monocytes are called macrophages. The terms monokine and lymphokine were once used to express the idea that different chemical messengers were produced by monocytes and lymphocytes. Later, this idea was abandoned when overlap of chemical messengers was discovered and the term cytokine was used. Today, the term chemokine is also used for chemical messengers involved in inflammation and repair.

Lymphocytes include B cells, T cells, and some less common lymphocytes. B cells are involved in antibody-mediated immunity. Several subtypes of T cells have been described in the literature and most pathology texts. Cytotoxic or killer T cells destroy pathogens more directly in what is called cell-mediated immunity. In cell-mediated immunity, the interplay of several types of cells is required. Macrophages present antigens to appropriate T cells to activate a response against a specific type of pathogen, cancer cell, or virally infected cell. Helper T cells release cytokines that stimulate proliferation of killer T cells specific to the antigen presented by the macrophage. Specific B cells are selected for transformation into plasma cells, which produce quantities of antibodies against a specific antigen. Binding of antibodies to antigens activates components of the immune system, especially the complement system, which leads to the destruction of the labeled cells.

Neutrophils, basophils, and eosinophils as a group are referred to as granulocytes. The particular cell is named for type of stain that it takes up. Neutrophils are the most prevalent white cell. They produce most of the initial inflammatory response to bacterial infections and tissue injury and represent a large contribution to the collection of fluid that we call pus or purulent exudate. Basophils are histamine-releasing cells found in the blood. Mast cells have a similar function as basophils in tissue. Histamine is an early chemical signal of tissue injury and produces many of the early responses to injury that are commonly seen as acute inflammation. Opening of gaps between endothelial cells in venules helps neutrophils reach the site of injury or infection and causes pain, heat, swelling, and redness associated with inflammation. Eosinophils are involved in allergic responses and worm infections. Certain conditions, including cancer chemotherapy, leukemia, bone marrow diseases, and whole body radiation, can cause the white blood cell count to reach levels that are so low that reverse isolation precautions must be observed. Reverse isolation is also used when the immune system is suppressed to prevent rejection of organ transplants. The health care professional must wear a face mask, gown, and gloves, and sanitize equipment, such as walkers, stethoscopes, or anything else that may have been touched by others.

PLATELETS

Megakaryocytes developed from myeloid stem cells fragment into platelets. The major role of platelets is hemostasis, the sequence of events that forms a thrombus and stops blood from leaking from damaged vessels. Platelets adhere to collagen located in the walls of damaged blood vessels. In addition, they release secretory granules containing molecules that aid in the process. The platelets change shape and adhere to one another to form a platelet plug. One molecule, called thromboxane A_2, is derived from the prostaglandin pathway, and its production is inhibited by aspirin. Thromboxane A_2 released by platelets enhances further platelet aggregation and helps to decrease blood loss by causing vasoconstriction. Thromboxane A_2 has been implicated in abnormal hemostasis that may lead to myocardial infarctions and strokes. Therefore, many physicians have been advocating the use of daily doses of aspirin to reduce the risk of these diseases. Diseases that reduce platelet count, including bone marrow disease and suppression of the bone marrow by cancer chemotherapy, can cause severe bleeding. One should always check the platelet count in these individuals before engaging in activity. Resistance exercise may not be allowed if platelet counts are low because of the potential for damaging blood vessels. Platelets are often transfused in these cases.

PRODUCTION OF BLOOD CELLS

All blood cells come from a common cell type, the pluripotent stem cell located in bone marrow. The first branch in production is to form either lymphoid or myeloid stem cell. Lymphoid stem cells give rise to the lymphocytes. The B cells develop in the bone marrow, leave into the blood, and migrate to lymphoid tissue found in lymph nodes and other tissues. T cells first migrate to the thymus gland where they mature into cells that will respond to different types of foreign materials. Myeloid stem cells give rise to all other blood cells, including monocytes, granulocytes, red cells, and platelets (Figure 21-10).

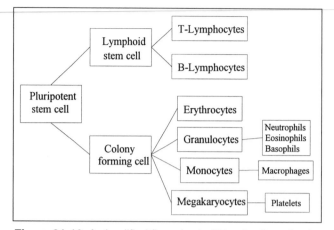

Figure 21-10. A simplified flow chart of blood cell synthesis. Different growth factors are now available pharmacologically that stimulate specific pathways for individuals with cancer or kidney disease.

SUMMARY

Velocity, cross-sectional area, and bulk flow through a vessel are related by the equation velocity times cross-sectional area equals flow. Larger diameter vessels with the same flow as a smaller vessel, such as a paired vein and artery, have a slower velocity. Conductance of a vessel increases with radius and decreases with length of the vessel and the viscosity of blood according to Poiseuille's law: $Q = \Delta P \; \pi r^4 / 8 \; l\eta$. Viscosity is determined by hematocrit, the fraction of blood consisting of red blood cells. At high levels of hematocrit, viscosity increases to life-threatening values. The addition of blood vessels in parallel increases the conductance and decreases the resistance of a vascular bed. Hemodynamic principles can be applied to the entire circulation using the equation MAP = CO x TPR. Local changes in resistance, if great enough, require central control of cardiac output and TPR to maintain MAP.

The optimum heart rate is determined by the compliance of the large arteries. With a high compliance, a low heart rate and high stroke volume is more energy efficient. With low compliance, a high heart rate and low stroke volume is more efficient. The law of LaPlace explains the required thickness for different types of blood vessels. Because tension = pressure x radius, small radius vessels such as capillaries are not at risk for rupturing in spite of having a thin wall. Arteries with large radii and higher pressure require a thick layer of fibrous tissue to prevent rupture. An aneurysm is a bulging of an artery that promotes a positive feedback between wall tension and radius. The increased radius increases wall tension, and increased wall tension increases radius with the increasing risk of rupture.

Systolic pressure is defined as the maximum pressure during the cardiac cycle, which occurs at the peak of ejection. Diastolic pressure is defined as the minimum pressure in the arteries during the cardiac cycle, which occurs just prior to ejection, which is at the end of isovolumic contraction (the first phase of systole). Mean arterial pressure is one-third of the way between diastolic pressure and systolic pressure. Pulse pressure is the increase from diastolic pressure to systolic pressure with ejection. Mean arterial pressure may be computed as diastolic pressure plus one-third pulse pressure or (2DP + SP)/3. Pulse pressure is determined by stroke volume, rate of ejection, and the compliance of the aorta and large arteries. Pulse pressure is increased during exercise, in arteriosclerosis, in hypertension, and in aortic insufficiency. Aortic stenosis decreases pulse pressure.

The blood can be centrifuged into three layers: plasma, buffy coat, and packed red cells. Hematocrit is determined as the percentage of blood volume occupied by red blood cells. The functions of the cellular and humoral components of the blood and the production of red blood cells and the other cells are described.

BIBLIOGRAPHY

Cowley AW Jr. Long term control of arterial blood pressure. *Physiological Reviews.* 1992;72:231-300.

Dampney RAL. Functional organization of central pathways regulating the cardiovascular system. *Physiological Reviews.* 1994;74:323-364.

Faraci FM, Heistad DP. Regulation of cerebral circulation: role of endothelium and potassium channels. *Physiological Reviews.* 1998;78:53-97.

Folkow B, Svanborg A. Physiology of cardiovascular aging. *Physiological Reviews.* 1993;73:725-764.

Gonzalez C, Almaraz L, Obeso A, Rigual R. Carotid body

chemoreceptors from natural stimuli to sensory discharge. *Physiological Reviews*. 1994;74:829-898.

Lakatta EG. Cardiovascular regulation mechanisms in advanced age. *Physiological Reviews*. 1993;73:413-467.

Marshal JM. Peripheral chemoreceptors and cardiovascular regulation. *Physiological Reviews*. 1994;74:543-594.

Monos E. How does the vein wall respond to pressure? *News in Physiological Sciences*. 1993;8:124-128.

Monos E, Bérczi V, Nádasy G. Local control of veins: biomechanical, metabolic, and humoral aspects. *Physiological Reviews*. 1995;75:611-666.

Persson PB. Modulation of cardiovascular control mechanism. *Physiological Reviews*. 1996;76:193-244.

STUDY QUESTIONS

1. Why is the velocity greater in a paired artery than vein?

2. What occurs to pressure as blood flows along a vessel?

3. What happens to this change in pressure in a narrow vessel compared with a wide vessel?

4. Why can we get reasonable estimates of arterial pressure from the brachial artery? Why is the value not significantly lower there than in the aorta?

5. What is the advantage of having short, wide renal arteries in terms of renal function?

6. Why does mean arterial pressure fall if cardiac output does not change when TPR decreases?

7. Why do large arteries need a thick connective tissue layer, but capillaries do not burst with a single cell thickness?

8. What is mean arterial pressure if blood pressure is 120/80? State in words what the formula for mean arterial pressure means in terms of pulse pressure.

9. Why is a high heart rate more energetically efficient with a stiff aorta?

10. Why is blood flow nearly steady in blood vessels of end organs if blood is pumped by the heart intermittently?

11. What would happen to plasma volume if production of plasma proteins fell?

12. What are the consequences of decreased production of blood cells with cancer chemotherapy?

LABORATORY EXERCISE

LABORATORY EXERCISE 21-1

BLOOD PRESSURE

Objectives:
1. Demonstrate procedure for determination of arterial blood pressure.
2. Describe use of the palpatory and auscultatory methods in measuring blood pressure.
3. Discuss interrelationships between the cardiac cycle and peripheral regulation of blood flow.
4. Calculate mean arterial pressure and pulse pressure.
5. Observe the effects of gravity and exercise on blood pressure.

Review of blood pressure:
Over short distances, diffusion and mediated transport work well to exchange substances. To maintain exchange necessary for cell survival, substances must be brought near the cell by blood flow. Blood flow through the vascular system is created by a difference in pressure caused by myocardial contraction. The role of the heart is to move sufficient blood from the venous side of the circulation to the arterial side to maintain the cardiac output demanded by the tissues. Arterial pressure is determined by the volume of blood in the arterial system and the compliance of the arteries (how easily the arterial vessels can be stretched). Because pressure in the right atrium is approximately zero, and the resistance of large arteries is very small, the driving force determining blood flow can be estimated by measuring arterial pressure in a peripheral artery, such as the brachial artery. For a given pressure gradient across a vascular bed, the blood flow rate is determined by the resistance to flow in that bed. The sum of blood flow throughout the body is called the cardiac output and the sum of all vascular resistances is called the total peripheral resistance (TPR).

When the left ventricle contracts, it moves a volume of blood (stroke volume) from the ventricle into the aorta against the pressure that exists in the aorta. All of the blood ejected cannot move instantaneously into and out of the arterial system during ventricular ejection; more blood moves into the arteries from the ventricle than moves out into the rest of the circulation. Therefore, the volume of the arteries is increased, which in turn increases pressure in the arteries. As ventricular ejection ceases (the heart enters the phase called diastole), blood continues to leave the arteries and move through the rest of the vascular system, which causes pressure in the arteries to decrease. Pressure continues to decrease until more blood is ejected from the heart into the aorta. Therefore, arterial pressure is at its minimum just before ventricular ejection during the phase of systole called isovolumic contraction. Arterial pressure at this time is called the diastolic pressure, although it technically occurs during the first phase of ventricular systole. The normal value is about 80 mmHg.

As the heart contracts, entering the phase called systole, pressure increases in the left ventricle until the aortic valve opens and blood is ejected. The ejection of blood during systole suddenly increases pressure and continues to raise pressure in the arteries until the heart relaxes. The maximum pressure in the arterial system during systole is termed systolic pressure and has a value of about 120 mmHg.

Arterial pressure changes throughout the cardiac cycle. For purposes of analyzing the cardiovascular system, we are interested in determining an average value of arterial pressure throughout the cardiac cycle. This value is called mean arterial pressure (MAP). One may then use this value to describe the relationships among cardiac output (CO), TPR and arterial pressure as: MAP = CO x TPR in analogy with Ohm's law for direct electrical current of V = I x R. If systole and diastole

LABORATORY EXERCISE

were to occupy the same proportion of the cardiac output, we could simply average the two values of 120 and 80 and say that MAP = 100 mmHg. The proportion of cardiac output spent in systole and diastole is determined by the heart rate. As heart rate decreases, there is more time for arterial pressure to fall, and for a given systolic pressure, MAP becomes less. One approach to determining MAP would be to record arterial pressure throughout the cardiac cycle and to integrate pressure. This can only be done by directly measuring arterial pressure with a catheter in an artery. A simpler approach is to determine for the normal range of human heart rates what the relative contributions of the maximum and minimum pressures are to the average pressure throughout the cardiac cycle. We estimate mean arterial pressure as one-third of the way between diastolic and systolic pressure and can be computed as: diastolic + 1/3 x (systolic - diastolic) or if you prefer: (systolic + 2 x diastolic)/3. The equations are algebraically identical. Using the values of 120 and 80 mmHg, we can compute MAP as 93 mmHg.

Another concept one may use is that of pulse pressure. Pulse pressure is simply the difference between systolic and diastolic pressure. The greater the volume ejected into the aorta, the greater the increase in pressure will be. In addition, the faster the stroke volume is ejected, the greater is the difference between the amount of blood entering and leaving the aorta and the greater the increment in pressure during ejection will be. As implied above, the greater the compliance of a vessel, the less pressure will increase for a given volume of blood moved into the vessel. On the other hand, a stiff vessel will demonstrate a large increase in pressure during ejection and pressure will decrease rapidly at the end of ejection. A stiff vessel will therefore have a high pulse pressure. Thus, three factors determine pulse pressure: stroke volume, rate of increase in arterial volume, and vessel compliance.

Blood pressure is typically measured with a sphygmomanometer. This device includes a cuff to surround the arm with an inflatable bladder inside and a device (a manometer) to measure pressure inside the cuff. The cuff is inflated to a pressure that exceeds systolic pressure, occluding blood flow below the cuff. Palpation of the pulse at the wrist will confirm this. By slowly allowing air out of the cuff, pressure inside the cuff will decrease, allowing blood to flow through the brachial artery. The pressure recorded from the cuff at the moment blood can first flow through the artery will occur only at the peak arterial pressure of the cardiac cycle, creating a high pitched sound as blood accelerates and decelerates. Although this number is somewhat lower and not equal to peak pressure in the artery, it is used as our estimate of systolic pressure. We can palpate the pulse at the wrist to determine what cuff pressure is just below systolic pressure. However, we cannot determine diastolic pressure by palpating the radial pulse. When cuff pressure is just below diastolic pressure, blood should flow freely through the brachial artery; therefore, sounds will not be made as blood flow starts and stops any more. In practice, one uses a stethoscope to listen for the sounds that indicate systolic and diastolic pressure. While allowing the cuff to deflate (slowly but not so slowly that it becomes uncomfortable for the patient), the observer places a stethoscope over the brachial artery just below the cuff to listen for the Korotkoff sounds. When pressure in the cuff becomes less than systolic pressure, a soft, tapping, intermittent sound can be heard as blood can get by the cuff at the very peak of systole. One then records the cuff pressure at this moment as systolic pressure. As pressure continues to fall in the cuff, more blood can pass the cuff and the intermittent tapping sounds become louder. As pressure continues to fall, blood can flow throughout more of the cardiac cycle, and a lower, muffled sound can be heard. Cuff pressure at this point was once commonly used as the value for diastolic pressure. However, when cuff pressure is just less than diastolic pressure, no more sounds are heard. Pressure at this point is now most commonly recorded as the diastolic pressure. We will first use the palpatory method of determining systolic pressure and then use the auscultatory method to determine both systolic and diastolic pressure.

LABORATORY EXERCISE

Materials:
Sphygmomanometer
Stethoscope
Meter stick
Bicycle ergometer

Methods:
A. Determination of systemic arterial pressure by the palpatory method
1. Ask the patient to sit quietly for several minutes to allow blood pressure to stabilize. Apply the cuff snugly to the upper arm and rest the arm on a flat surface at approximately heart level. While palpating the radial artery, rapidly inflate the cuff until the radial arterial pulse can no longer be detected. Slowly release the air in the cuff and note the pressure at which the radial pulse reappears.Repeat as necessary.

2. Write down the value here: _____ mmHg (palpatory method)

B. Auscultatory method
1. Have the patient assume the same position as above. Palpate the brachial artery and place the stethoscope diaphragm over the artery below the cuff. Be sure that the stethoscope does not touch the cuff and that there is no air space between the stethoscope and the skin. Inflate the cuff approximately 30 mmHg above the level determined by the palpatory method. Slowly release the air in the cuff while listening for the sounds described above.

2. Record systolic pressure as that cuff pressure at which the appearance of faint, clear tapping sounds are heard.

3. Record diastolic pressure as that cuff pressure at which sounds are no longer heard. Listen for the muffling sounds just prior to the disappearance of sound.

4. Blood pressure = _____/_____ mmHg (auscultatory method).

5. Determine the systolic and diastolic blood pressures in both arms with the person sitting. Make one determination of the blood pressure with the person supine and three after the patient stands up. Each student should make several determinations of blood pressure using the auscultatory method.

6. Compute pulse pressure and mean arterial pressure.
    Pulse pressure = _____ mmHg
    MAP = diastolic + 1/3 pulse pressure = _____ mmHg

C. Questions:
1. Is the pressure determined by the palpatory method more nearly equal to the systolic or diastolic pressure determined by the auscultatory method?

2. What is one possible explanation of the Korotkoff sounds?

3. Why is the palpatory method useful?

LABORATORY EXERCISE

D. Effect of gravity

1. Have the subject assume the supine position on a table top. Measure blood pressure.
    BP = _____/_____   MAP = _____ mmHg

2. Have the subject turn onto the side opposite of the cuff and raise the arm toward the ceiling. Measure blood pressure again. Estimate the distance in centimeters between the cuff and the middle of the subject's heart with a meter stick.
    BP = _____/_____   MAP = _____ mmHg Distance = _____ cm

3. Instruct the subject to allow the arm with the cuff to hang off the edge of the table. Measure blood pressure and estimate the distance between the cuff and middle of the subject's heart. The pressure exerted by 1 cm of water equals that of a column of 0.74 mmHg.
    BP = _____/_____   MAP = _____ mmHg   Distance = _____ cm

4. Compare the pressures and distances from the heart measured in the three positions.
    Supine MAP   = _____
    Arm up MAP + (.74 x distance up [cm])   = _____
    Arm down MAP - (.74 x distance down [cm])   = _____

5. The three results above should be within 5 to 10 mmHg of each other. If not, check for error in measuring distance from the center of the heart, or repeat blood pressure measurements. Why should the numbers be equal? Your answer should be much more specific than "Gravity."

E. Blood pressure during exercise

1. Determine resting blood pressure while sitting on a bicycle ergometer. It is much easier to hear if the arm in the cuff is not touching the ergometer. The person measuring blood pressure should support the arm away from the subject's body.

2. Have the subject pedal against an unloaded ergometer. Measure blood pressure after 3 minutes.

3. Increase load to 25 watts. After 3 minutes, determine blood pressure.

4. Continue increasing load in 25-watt increments, measuring blood pressure at each load until the subject begins to tire.

5. What happens to blood pressure with increasing work load? Do systolic and diastolic pressure change the same way?

6. What happens to pulse pressure? Why should it change this way? Note: remember what factors determine pulse pressure and why.

TWENTY-TWO

Control of the Cardiovascular System

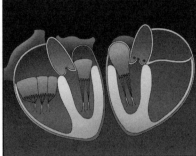

OBJECTIVES

1. Define capillary density.

2. Describe intrinsic (local) regulation of blood vessel diameter:
   a. define autoregulation
   b. describe myogenic regulation
   c. describe effect of increased flow rate on arterial tone
   d. describe metabolic regulation of flow (active hyperemia)
   e. describe reactive hyperemia

3. Describe extrinsic regulation of blood vessel diameter.

4. List the primary factors that determine blood flow to the heart, skeletal muscle, and the brain.

5. Describe factors influencing exchange of fluid across capillaries:
   a. vasodilation, vasoconstriction, muscle pump
   b. malnutrition, liver disease, kidney disease
   c. histamine, bacterial toxins, immune response
   d. heart failure

6. Describe structure and function of the lymphatic system and the effect of blockage or damage to lymphatic vessels.

7. Explain the effects of an upright posture on the venous system and cardiac output.

8. Describe factors that enhance venous flow from a dependent position: muscle pump, venous valves, respiratory activity.

9. Describe the interrelationship between venous pressure and cardiac output.

10. Describe the baroreceptor reflex.

The cardiovascular system is controlled at two levels simultaneously. Centrally, mean arterial pressure must be regulated to ensure sufficient pressure to drive flow through all tissues. Blood flow must be regulated within each tissue to ensure adequate convective transport of nutrients and wastes. Because arterial pressure falls minimally through large vessels, the term MAP (mean arterial pressure) minus (venous pressure in the tissue) represents the driving force for flow to all tissues. Within organs, arterioles regulate the distribution of flow by altering the conductance of the vessels. When demand for blood flow increases, arterioles dilate, resulting in an enhanced conductance in the presence of a regulated arterial pressure.

The equation MAP = CO x TPR may be used to analyze function of the cardiovascular system as a whole. MAP is regulated at approximately 93 mmHg, and approximately 5000 ml of blood flow are demanded by the tissues of the body each minute. As discussed in Chapter Twenty, the cardiovascular system is in a steady state produced by the energy used in pumping blood from the veins into the arteries. The cardiac output is, therefore, equal to the sum of local tissue blood flow throughout the body. If arterial pressure is kept constant, tissues simply increase or decrease their blood flow supply by producing paracrine signals to alter conductance. This process by which tissues control their own blood flow is known as autoregulation. The reciprocal of the sum of all the conductances of the systemic circulation is the total peripheral resistance (TPR).

The heart and blood vessels are regulated so that the 5000 ml/min demanded by the tissues are delivered at a MAP of 93 mmHg. TPR is regulated centrally, while it is also determined locally by autoregulation. At times, these two types of regulation may work together easily, or they may be in conflict. Central and local control of hemodynamics and their interrelationships are described in this chapter. In addition, the active nature of the veins in resolving the conflicting central and local regulatory demands is described.

LOCAL CONTROL OF BLOOD FLOW

Within each tissue, the structure of the microvascular bed varies according to the specific needs of the tissue. The density of exchange vessels (capillary density) is generally proportional to the metabolic requirements of the tissue. An example already encountered was the difference in the number of capillaries per square millimeter in the heart compared to that of skeletal muscle. The

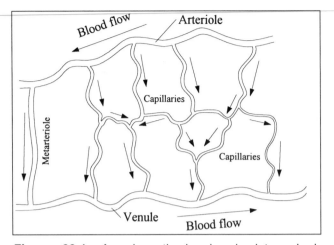

Figure 22-1. A schematized microcirculatory bed. Capillaries branch from terminal arterioles, and the capillaries are drained by venules. Blood flow in the arterioles and venules occur in opposite directions. In some beds, metarterioles that bypass the capillary bed may be observed. Within individual capillaries, intermittent flow and reversal of flow can be periodically observed.

small blood vessels within the tissue constitute the microcirculation. These vessels include arterioles, terminal arterioles that give rise to capillaries, capillaries, and the venules that collect blood from the capillaries. In some vascular beds, a precapillary sphincter consisting of an area preceding the capillary that permits flow into specific capillaries can be observed. In most vascular beds, changes in the vascular tone of the terminal arteriole alter the pressure of the blood entering the capillaries. Should sufficient pressure be available at the entrance of the capillary, forward flow will result. Red blood cells pass in single file through the capillaries from high pressure in the terminal arteriole toward low pressure in the venule. In many capillaries, the pressure is not great enough, and red cells can be observed to oscillate or even flow backwards intermittently. Cyclic changes in vascular tone with demands from both central control of blood pressure and local demands for blood flow produce intermittent fluctuations in flow through the capillaries (Figure 22-1).

The factors that influence the diameters of the arterial vessels can be divided into five general categories: neural, humoral (hormonal), metabolic, myogenic, and endothelial (Table 22-1). The neural input is primarily innervation by sympathetic nerves. The greatest effect of the sympathetic nerves is on the small arteries and arterioles. Neural regulation of smooth muscle tone is involved primarily in the rapid and short-term control of systemic blood pressure. The sympathetic neurons appear to have little influence over the terminal arterioles and precapillary sphincters.

TABLE 22-1

Types of Vascular Control

TYPE	EFFECTOR	LOCAL OR CENTRAL	FUNCTION
Neural	Sympathetic nerves	Central	Rapid, short-term control of arterial pressure
Humoral	Hormones: epinephrine, angiotensin II act directly on vessels; aldosterone, antidiuretic hormone, atrial natriuretic factor influence volume within vessels	Central	Regulation of extracellular and intravascular volume for long-term control of arterial pressure
Metabolic	Paracrine: CO_2, O_2, adenosine, others	Local	Couple blood flow and metabolism
Myogenic	Smooth muscle cells	Local	Maintain transmural pressure
Endothelial	Endothelial cells, NO	Local	Couple flow and metabolism, propagate vasodilation

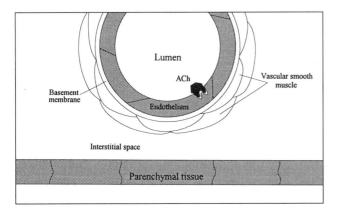

Figure 22-2. Sites of control of vascular tone. Endothelial cells may generate vasodilatory signals either through production of prostacyclin in response to shear stress or by binding of specific ligand, such as acetylcholine. Prostacyclin produces a propagation of vasodilation along a vessel as flow rate increases. Binding of acetylcholine leads to the generation of nitric oxide and cyclic guanosine monophosphate (GMP), which, in turn, cause vasodilation. Substances within either the lumen of the blood vessel, such as hemoglobin, or in the interstitial space surrounding vascular smooth muscle may change vascular smooth muscle tone.

A number of vasoactive hormones affect the smooth muscle tone in the arterial vessels and are responsible for long-term control of blood pressure. One discussed earlier in the context of the kidney is angiotensin II. Several commonly used drugs for controlling hypertension involve blocking the effect of angiotensin II. Vasopressin, also known as ADH or antidiuretic hormone, also increases the tone of vascular smooth mus-

cle. Other known vasoactive substances include histamine, serotonin, thromboxane A_2, which is released by platelets, and prostacyclin, which is released by endothelial cells.

Metabolic control of vascular smooth muscle involves the production of vasodilator metabolites produced during tissue metabolism. As their name implies, these metabolites link metabolic rate to blood flow by causing the vascular smooth muscle to relax with resultant vessel dilation. This provides a coupling mechanism between local tissue need and local blood flow.

Myogenic control refers to the influence of pressure within the vessel on smooth muscle tone in the vessel wall. The difference in pressure across the vessel wall is called the transmural pressure. Increasing the transmural pressure causes the vessels to constrict, whereas decreasing the transmural pressure causes them to dilate. Most commonly, transmural pressure rises when there is an increase in pressure within the vessel. Experimentally, the same phenomenon can be observed by decreasing the pressure outside the vessel.

Historically, the endothelial cells that line the vessels have been assigned a passive role as a barrier between blood cells and the fibrous tissue below. The importance of this barrier function is noted when the fibrous tissue comes in direct contact with the blood to initiate the clotting mechanism. Endothelial control of the vascular smooth muscle occurs by paracrine influence. Endothelial-derived relaxing factor (EDRF) is released by endothelial cells when specific humoral vasodilating substances bind to receptors on the endothelial cells (Figure 22-2). EDRF, which appears to be nitric oxide

(NO) and perhaps other substances, has the direct smooth muscle relaxing effect. Recently, hemoglobin has been shown to be a potential source of nitric oxide when oxygen saturation of hemoglobin is decreased, and it has been speculated that hemoglobin acts to couple metabolism and blood flow. Prostacyclin (PGI_2), a prostaglandin released from endothelial cells, causes vasodilation and inhibits platelet adhesion, which are effects directly opposite those of thromboxane A_2 released by platelets. Prostacyclin release is stimulated by the shear stress on endothelial cells that occurs with the flow of blood. As blood flow velocity increases with vasodilation downstream due local control, increased shearing on the endothelial cells causes release of prostacyclin, which causes larger, upstream vessels to dilate also and further increase the blood flow to the active tissue.

The sum of all the factors described above determines the diameter of the precapillary resistance vessels. These factors may work together or, often, in opposition. The sensitivity of a given vessel to each factor described above varies with the type of vessel (artery, arteriole, venule, etc.) and among the various tissues. For example, skeletal muscle and kidney are very sensitive to sympathetic stimulation, while the heart and brain are not. Therefore, in an emergency, pressure can be maintained by generalized vasoconstriction, but blood flow to the heart and brain is maintained. Unfortunately, vasoconstriction of renal vessels can cause the kidneys to fail after the emergency has been rectified and, in some cases, require kidney transplant or hemodialysis to replace kidney function. The signals responsible for regulation of blood flow to skeletal muscle, the heart, and the brain will be discussed below. In general, the sympathetic nervous system produces the degree of vasoconstriction needed to maintain MAP. Local metabolism in a specific tissue may cause enough of a paracrine signal to produce complete relaxation in spite of a strong central neural signal for vasoconstriction, or, in other tissues, vasoconstriction cannot be overcome, and ischemic damage results, especially in the kidneys.

The types of local regulation include active hyperemia, pressure autoregulation, and reactive hyperemia. Active hyperemia refers to the situation in which blood flow is increased in response to an increase in tissue metabolism. It is generally due to paracrine signaling, in which accumulation of a metabolite acting as a paracrine signal for relaxation of vascular smooth muscle couples metabolism and blood flow. When metabolic rate decreases, the increased blood flow washes the metabolite from the tissue, and the vessel diameter returns to normal. In pressure autoregulation blood flow is kept

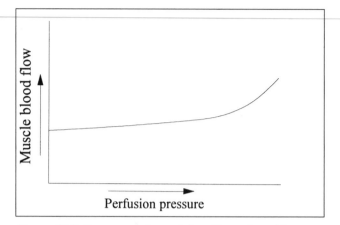

Figure 22-3. Pressure autoregulation. Through a wide range of perfusion pressure, systemic blood vessels respond to a change in the transmural pressure to maintain a constant flow. In response to increased pressure, vascular smooth muscle constricts to increase resistance in proportion to pressure. Conversely, decreased pressure (and, therefore, transmural pressure) results in decreased resistance in proportion to the increased pressure to maintain flow.

constant in the face of changing arterial pressure. Increased pressure is matched by an increase in resistance that returns blood flow to normal. Decreased pressure leads to decreased resistance. Pressure autoregulation works well over a large range of arterial pressure (Figure 22-3). When this range is exceeded, blood flow will fail to be regulated. Reactive hyperemia is a response to a diminished blood flow that results from occlusion of vessels, followed by release of the occlusion. Occlusion may be mechanical, including placing a leg over the edge of a chair or it may be pathologic occlusion, as seen in Raynaud's disease. Accumulation of metabolites during occlusion results in a tremendous increase in the conductance of the vessels of the tissue. When the occlusion is removed, blood flow may reach its maximal level in the tissue for a time until the paracrine signal is carried out of the tissue by the increased blood flow. Raynaud's disease (idiopathic) and Raynaud's phenomenon (secondary to another disease process) produce vasospasm of small arterial vessels in the fingers and related areas. Vasospasm causes the skin to turn white initially due to lack of circulating hemoglobin in the skin and may proceed to a bluish hue (cyanosis). As the vasospasm subsides, reactive hyperemia changes skin color to red.

REGULATION OF SKELETAL MUSCLE BLOOD FLOW

The amount of blood flow supplied depends on the muscle type and its activity. Slow twitch muscle has twice

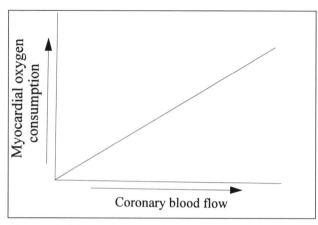

Figure 22-4. The relationship between coronary blood flow and myocardial oxygen consumption. Note the nearly linear relationship in the heart. In contrast, most other organs do not demonstrate such a linear relationship. The heart has a nearly maximal a-v O_2 difference at rest and must increase coronary blood flow in proportion to increased metabolic rate, whereas other tissues experience increases in both blood flow and a-v O_2 difference to meet the increased demand for oxygen.

the resting flow of fast twitch muscle. At rest, skeletal muscle, which contributes approximately 40% of body mass, receives only 15% of the cardiac output. Blood flow in many capillaries of resting skeletal muscle may be near zero at any given moment due to the high resistance of skeletal muscle arterioles produced by high resting sympathetic tone. The decreased pressure of blood entering capillaries in this case can be insufficient to drive red blood cells through capillaries until either arteriolar pressure increases or venular pressure decreases. When skeletal muscle metabolic rate is low, high sympathetic tone creates a high total peripheral resistance at rest, which produces the benefit of decreasing the cardiac output necessary for the heart to maintain arterial pressure. During exercise, dilation of skeletal muscle arterioles can decrease total peripheral resistance dramatically as skeletal muscle blood flow and oxygen consumption can increase 10 to 20 times during exercise, and cardiac output must increase profoundly to maintain arterial pressure. Blood flow to oxidative muscles may be five times greater than that of glycolytic muscles during exercise, and the total skeletal muscle blood flow can increase from 15% to as much as 85% of cardiac output. The signal for active hyperemia is not clear, but possibilities include decreased oxygen, increased CO_2, and, as described above, the desaturation of hemoglobin. Experimentally, many substances have been shown to produce vasodilation of skeletal muscle arterioles, but linking their presence to increased metabolic rate and increased blood flow has been difficult to demonstrate.

Blood flow is also dependent upon the force that

muscle contraction places on vessel walls. During rhythmic, low-intensity activity, such as aerobic exercise, muscle contraction produces little disruption of muscle blood flow. Prolonged, forceful contractions can completely occlude blood flow. These anaerobic activities, however, are not sustainable or dependent on blood flow for their performance.

REGULATION OF THE CORONARY CIRCULATION

Capillary density in the heart is greater than in skeletal muscle because the cardiac muscle fibers are smaller in diameter than skeletal muscle fibers and a larger number of capillaries surrounds each cardiac myocyte compared with skeletal muscle cells. This difference in capillary density makes myocardial capillaries about 15 times more effective in exchanging substances than skeletal muscle capillaries because the distance for diffusion is less. Myocardial blood flow is high under resting conditions, and the arteriovenous O_2 difference (amount of oxygen extracted from the flowing blood) is high compared with other tissues (Figure 22-4). The right and left coronary arteries and their branches provide the entire blood supply to the myocardium. Coronary circulation, because of its proximity to the aortic valve, differs from other organs in one particularly important way. In other organs, flow is nearly steady and does not change substantially with the cardiac cycle due to the filtering effect of the large arteries. In organs distal to the aorta, expansion of arteries during systole and recoil during diastole keep flow nearly constant over the cardiac output. In contrast, pressure within the root of the aorta drives flow through the coronary arteries because they branch directly behind the right and left cusps of the aortic valve. Coronary blood flow, therefore, varies with the cardiac cycle (Figure 22-5). Flow measured in the right coronary artery follows the changes in aortic pressure during the cardiac cycle. In the left ventricle, flow is also dependent on the contractile activity. Just as compression of blood vessels of skeletal muscle can temporarily diminish blood flow, myocardial compression of the left ventricle reduces blood flow to zero for part of systole. Although systole accounts for 33% of the cardiac cycle, only 20% to 25% of left ventricular blood flow occurs during systole. In the right ventricle, pressure is lower, and flow is more uniform through the cardiac cycle. Left ventricular muscle is at a greater risk for insufficient blood flow for these reasons; therefore, death of myocardial tissue secondary to ischemia (myocardial infarction) occurs almost exclusively in the left ventricle. Coronary vessels are also prone to development of atherosclerotic plaque due to the high pressure and multiple, short branches of the coronary vessels that create shearing stress on the coronary vessel walls.

The rate of coronary blood flow is determined primarily by metabolism of the cardiac muscle. Adenosine, a product of metabolism of the myocytes, has been suggested to be the primary factor in controlling coronary blood flow. Although α-adrenergic receptors have been located on coronary vessels, these do not appear to produce vasoconstriction under normal conditions, but may contribute to pathologic conditions.

REGULATION OF THE CEREBRAL CIRCULATION

The arterial supply of the brain originates from the internal carotid and the vertebral arteries. Communications between arteries (including the circle of Willis) help protect the brain from occlusion of one vessel. Because the cranial contents are surrounded by a rigid structure, the overall volume cannot change. Increases in blood volume, whether inside vessels or hemorrhage, can cause severe headache.

Normal cerebral blood flow is 56 ml/min per 100 g of tissue, accounting for 14% of cardiac output. Regional blood flow in the brain varies with the tissue being supplied and the activity of the tissue. Average blood flow to gray matter, which consists primarily of cell bodies and synapses, is 77 ml/min per 100 g, whereas average blood flow to white matter, which has a lower metabolic rate, is 20 ml/min per 100 g. When specific areas of the brain increase activity, blood flow to those areas increases. The brain is intolerant of ischemia; if flow is interrupted for only 5 seconds, there is loss of consciousness. Blood flow and metabolism are linked clearly in the brain. Increasing blood or cerebrospinal fluid CO_2 produces vasodilation. Breathing is indirectly controlled by cerebrospinal fluid CO_2, which alters the pH of cells that regulate ventilation. Changes in blood CO_2 because of altered respiratory function change brain blood flow and have predictable consequences. Moreover, CO_2 has a depressant effect on the brain. If a person hyperventilates, blood flow decreases to the brain, resulting in dizziness and diminished cerebral function. Often, a person who has a high intracerebral pressure secondary to injury or stroke is placed on a ventilator to cause hyperventilation deliberately, which decreases the volume of blood in the brain and intracerebral pressure to prevent further injury to the brain. Hypoventilation, by definition, results in an increase in

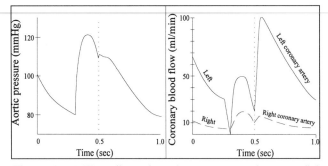

Figure 22-5. The effect of aortic pressure and myocardial contraction on coronary blood flow. On the left, aortic pressure is shown. Because coronary vessels arise directly from the aorta, the filtering action of the aorta and large arteries is not available to smooth the pressure pulse. This pressure pulse creates a flow within the coronary vessels that varies with aortic pressure. This phenomenon is observed in the right coronary vessel. Flow in the left coronary artery is further complicated by the forceful contraction of the myocardium. At the peak of systole, the force of contraction nearly stops left coronary flow. During diastole, a tremendous increase in left coronary flow is observed.

CO_2, which increases brain blood flow. In the short term, a hypoventilating person will complain of a headache due to the increased blood volume in the skull. In the long term, the depressant effect of CO_2 causes a person to become giddy, then somnolent, and may lead to coma if CO_2 rises high enough and long enough. Some individuals with chronic lung disease can tolerate a high level of CO_2 that would be lethal if it occurred acutely. Cerebral blood flow is well regulated between systemic arterial pressures of 60 to 160 mmHg (pressure autoregulation) when blood arterial carbon dioxide is kept constant.

EFFECT OF REGULATION OF BLOOD FLOW ON CAPILLARY FILTRATION AND ABSORPTION

Under resting conditions, only a small fraction (1% to 2%) of the plasma passing through the capillaries leaks into the interstitium (is filtered). As discussed in the chapter on body fluids, the amount of fluid filtered is important in the regulation of blood and interstitial fluid volume. The magnitude of filtration and absorption by the capillaries is determined by the hydrostatic and osmotic pressures existing across the capillary wall. Factors favoring filtration (loss of fluid into the interstitial space) include capillary hydrostatic pressure and tissue osmotic pressure. Factors favoring absorption (gain of fluid from the interstitial space) are plasma protein osmotic pressure (colloid osmotic pressure) and tissue

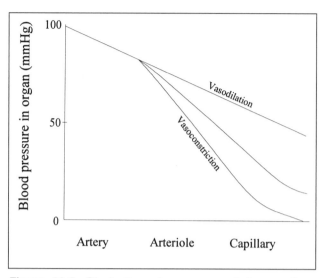

Figure 22-6. Dissipation of pressure entering capillary beds. Under normal, resting conditions, the greatest loss of pressure occurs in arterioles. During exercise, for example, dilation of arterioles reduces the dissipation of pressure entering the capillaries, and pressure within capillaries increases, which may lead to leakage of fluid in muscle capillaries during exercise. Vasoconstriction of arterioles creates a greater than normal dissipation of pressure along them with a consequence of lower-than-normal capillary pressure and net absorption of fluid from the interstitial space into capillaries.

hydrostatic pressure. Because capillaries are relatively impermeable to proteins, the concentration of protein in the plasma is greater than the concentration in the interstitial fluid. The greater concentration of protein molecules in the plasma causes plasma osmotic pressure to be approximately 23 mmHg higher than interstitial fluid osmotic pressure. Tissue hydrostatic pressure under normal circumstances is zero or less due to the presence of glycoproteins in the interstitial space. These glycoproteins absorb water in a manner similar to gelatin, thereby preventing bulk flow of interstitial fluid. Only when the ability of the glycoproteins to form a gel is overwhelmed by interstitial fluid will free movement of fluid occur. This condition, known as pitting edema, can be demonstrated by pushing fluid about under the skin.

The Starling-Landis equation describes the movement of fluid from capillaries to the interstitial space mathematically. Starling developed the theory, and Landis, at a much later date, confirmed Starling's ideas by measuring pressures in the microcirculation. The equation is as follows: fluid movement = k [$(P_c + \pi_i) - (P_i + \pi_p)$], in which P_c = capillary hydrostatic pressure, P_i = interstitial fluid hydrostatic pressure, π_p = plasma oncotic pressure, and π_i = interstitial fluid oncotic pressure. The term k is the capillary filtration constant and expresses the idea that capillaries in different tissues are

tighter or leakier. In tissues such as the spleen and liver, large molecules are free to cross the capillaries, and k is high. In the brain, with its blood-brain barrier, k is extremely low. Because other solutes freely cross capillary walls, the osmotic pressure gradient across the capillary depends upon the difference between plasma protein concentration and tissue protein concentration. This difference, under resting conditions, produces nearly equal and opposite flow of water as the hydrostatic pressure within the capillary. Severe imbalance between the forces causing filtration and those causing absorption results in edema. A loss of plasma proteins due to kidney disease, liver disease, or malnutrition can produce severe edema. The permeability of the microcirculation, especially venules, is increased during the process of inflammation, and swelling occurs, which accounts for much of the pain associated with inflammation. Histamine is the compound most associated with the increased permeability. Certain bacterial toxins and components of the complement system activated during infection also increase vessel permeability.

Because of anatomic and physiologic differences, all capillaries do not have the same hydrostatic pressure. For example, the capillaries of the glomerulus have a very high hydrostatic pressure, which leads to large fluid loss into the proximal tubule. Even within the same tissue, some capillaries filter fluid along their entire length, and other capillaries may reabsorb along their entire length. In areas where capillaries have low hydrostatic pressure, interstitial fluid pressure may actually be negative.

Capillary hydrostatic pressure is influenced by several related factors, including systemic arterial pressure, precapillary resistance, postcapillary resistance, and venous pressure. From the input end of the capillary, pressure produced by the beating of the heart is dissipated as blood travels through the arterial vessels (Figure 22-6). A low conductance (or high resistance) of the arteries and arterioles feeding the capillary decreases capillary hydrostatic pressure as more of the arterial pressure is dissipated through constricted arterial vessels, which may cause capillaries to absorb fluid from the interstitial space. Increasing conductance of arterioles, on the other hand, leads to temporary edema that lasts as long as the arterioles are dilated. Increased capillary pressure overcomes the plasma oncotic pressure, resulting in net filtration. The process of creating swelling of muscles during exercise is called "pumping up" and is accomplished by body builders just before going on stage by lifting weights. This swelling resolves rapidly as exercise ceases and capillary hydrostatic pressure returns to its resting value.

Increased venous pressure at the other end of the

capillary reduces the outflow of blood from the capillary to the venule and increases the volume and pressure in the capillary until a new steady state results in which the increased capillary pressure drives blood into the venules at the same rate that arteriolar pressure drives flow into the capillary. Elevated venous pressure, which leads to increased capillary pressure, not only causes edema, but also causes leakage of large molecules, such as fibrinogen, which is converted to fibrin in the interstitial space around the capillaries. This layer of fibrin, along with excess fluid surrounding the capillaries, causes malnutrition of the tissues and venous insufficiency ulcers. The elevated venous pressure in the lower extremities responsible for venous insufficiency ulcers usually results from failure of the muscle pump mechanism.

The muscle pump, just like any pump mechanism, requires a source of compression of fluid, one-way valves to drive flow in the forward direction, and an unobstructed outflow conduit. The muscle pump can fail due to a problem with any of the three components. Lack of muscle activity because of prolonged inactivity of the muscle, especially standing or neurologic injury or disease, prevents venous blood from being pumped forward beyond the venous valves. Incompetent venous valves allow blood to flow backwards with gravity increasing the volume and pressure in veins and, therefore, in capillaries. Outflow obstruction can be caused by pregnancy, obesity, or tumors. Health-care professionals can inadvertently create obstruction of venous outflow by inappropriate application of compression garments.

Increased venous pressure and edema also occur as a consequence of increased venous blood volume. In congestive heart failure, decreased blood flow to the kidneys results in aldosterone production, retention of sodium and water, and increased blood volume. In addition, the inability of the heart to pump blood from the veins into the arteries results in a large venous volume and pressure. Increased venous pressure, at least initially, increases preload on the heart and improves pumping. However, the elevated venous pressure also causes leakage of fluid into tissues. The edema that occurs in the lung secondary to congestive heart failure may lead to acute episodes of dyspnea and even death. A person with failure of the left ventricle may have orthopnea, a condition in which the person must be in an upright position to breathe normally because a horizontal position allows fluid to accumulate in the lungs.

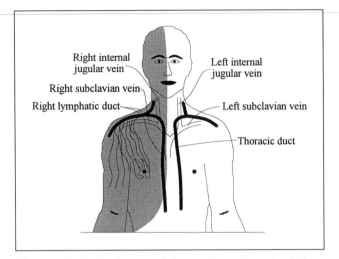

Figure 22-7. Drainage of lymph into the circulation. Lymphatic vessels from the right upper quadrant, head, and neck drain into the right lymphatic duct, which drains into the right subclavian vein. Other lymphatic vessels drain into the thoracic duct, which drains into the left subclavian vein.

LYMPHATICS

The major function of the lymphatic system is to return interstitial fluid and plasma proteins to the blood. The lymphatic system is the only mechanism for a net transport of plasma proteins into the blood. Lymph flow can be increased 20-fold in order to compensate for an increase in filtration. Interstitial fluid is collected by terminal lymphatic capillaries and is then called lymph. Lymph is propelled through the lymphatic system by spontaneous contractile activity of the lymphatic vessels and by intermittent skeletal muscle contractions. This process is facilitated by the presence of one-way valves. The movement of fluid beyond the valves, followed by relaxation, produces a negative pressure within the lymphatic capillaries. Interstitial fluid and debris then driven into the lymphatic vessels during relaxation. Closure of the one-way valve at the opening of the lymphatic capillaries during contraction drives flow forward into the vessels. Lymphatic vessels converge into either the right lymphatic duct or the thoracic lymphatic duct (Figure 22-7). The right lymphatic duct collects lymph from the right side of the head, neck, upper thorax, and the right upper extremity and drains into the right subclavian vein. The thoracic duct collects lymph from the rest of the body and drains into the left subclavian vein. Failure of the lymphatic vessels to remove excess fluid from the interstitial space causes swelling. Lymphedema is the

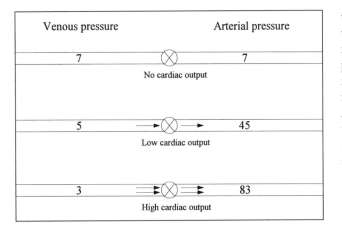

Venous pressure		Arterial pressure
7	⊗	7
	No cardiac output	
5	→⊗→	45
	Low cardiac output	
3	⇒⊗⇒	83
	High cardiac output	

Figure 22-8. The effect of cardiac pumping on arterial and venous pressure. The translocation of blood from veins to arteries reduces venous pressure and increases arterial pressure. Without any cardiac pumping, blood pressure is identical throughout the circulation. Note that the movement of blood from veins to arteries has approximately 19 times the effect on arterial pressure as it has on venous pressure. A cardiac output that reduces venous pressure by 2 mmHg increases arterial pressure by 38 mmHg due to the greater compliance of venous vessels compared to arterial vessels. This phenomenon generates sufficient arterial pressure to drive flow through the systemic circulation.

term used to describe edema secondary to lymphatic obstruction. Lymphatic vessels may be damaged by surgery or radiation therapy used to treat cancer. Infestation by worms is called filariasis and produces the condition called elephantiasis because of the hard, thickened, skin with the texture of an orange peel that resembles the skin of an elephant. Techniques for treating lymphedema are collectively known as comprehensive decongestion therapy. This therapy consists of a specialized massage using light pressure and continual contact, compression bandaging, and exercise. The massage is done proximally, starting at the neck and progressing distally to empty the proximal lymphatic vessels ahead of the distal vessels. Exercises done with compression bandaging can promote cyclic compression of the affected extremity to encourage proximal pumping of lymph toward the subclavian veins.

The lymphatic system also has an immune function. Foreign material, bacteria, fungi, viruses, and cancer cells can be taken up by the lymphatic vessels and transported to lymph nodes where immune cells are located. If the lymph nodes are overwhelmed by an infectious agent, they swell and produce lymphadenitis (inflammation of the lymph "glands"). Infection of the lymphatic vessels produces red streaks in the condition called lymphangitis. Unfortunately, lymphatic vessels also provide cancer cells with a pathway for metastasis (spread to areas distant from the tumor). Metastasis also occurs

through blood vessels (hematogenous spread) and through body cavities (seeding). Lymph nodes are often removed in the area of a tumor, which damages the pathway for lymphatic drainage. Moreover, the use of radiation to treat cancer damages lymphatic vessels. This is particularly a problem with breast cancer. Approximately 50% of breast cancer occurs in the area of the breast that drains through axillary lymph nodes. Removal of lymph nodes in this area and radiation to the axillary region can cause lymphedema to occur.

CENTRAL VENOUS PRESSURE AND HEART FUNCTION

Veins are much more distensible than arteries, and they have what is called a capacitance function in contrast to the distributing function of arteries. Alteration of the diameter of arterial vessels affects the heart by changing the resistance against which the heart must pump (afterload). In contrast, changes in the diameter of the venous vessels influence the ventricular volume and pressure produced during the filling phase of the cardiac cycle (preload). To regulate cardiac function, both preload and afterload need to be appropriate for a given demand for cardiac function. The heart functions as a pump to translocate blood from the very compliant central veins to the arteries, which have 5% the compliance of the veins. Moving a volume of blood from the compliant veins to the stiffer arteries produces a small decrease in venous pressure. Adding this volume of blood to the arteries, however, produces an increase in arterial pressure that is 19 times greater than the decrease created in venous pressure by removing this volume (Figure 22-8). This difference in arterial and venous compliance allows the heart to pump blood through the systemic circulation. Venous pressure is needed to create sufficient preload on the heart to pump blood forcefully into the arteries. Because the increased arterial pressure needed to drive flow through the circulation can be produced with only a small decrease in venous pressure, preload on the heart is not reduced in proportion to the increase in arterial pressure produced by pumping of blood from veins to arteries. Secondly, the low pressure in veins creates a pressure difference to drive the flow of blood from arteries, through capillaries, to veins, and back to the heart.

EFFECTS OF GRAVITY ON VEINS

If the blood vessels of the body were rigid tubes, gravity would have no net effect on the flow of blood through veins and, therefore, venous return to the

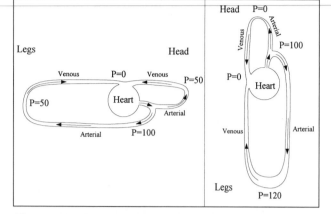

Figure 22-9. Effect of gravity on veins. In a horizontal position, the pressure generated by a column of fluid (ρgh) has no effect at the feet or head. Vascular pressure is determined simply by cardiac pumping and local resistance. In the fully upright position, pressure is determined both by cardiac pumping and by the effect of a column of fluid, with increased pressure in the feet and decreased pressure in the head. Venous function is maintained in the feet by the presence of venous valves and muscle pumping action to prevent excessive pressure and leakage of fluid into the interstitial space. In the head, veins would collapse if they were not tethered to surrounding tissues, forming the venous sinuses observed in the brain.

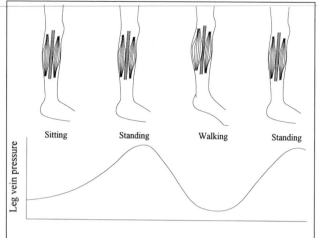

Figure 22-10. The muscle pump of the lower extremity. Going from sitting to standing, venous pressure increases as the column of fluid from the heart to the legs and feet increases. The muscle pump becomes active during walking and serves to decrease venous pressure. Static standing allows venous pressure to increase again. Venous volume may become great enough with prolonged static standing to cause fainting due to decreased preload on the heart.

heart. If this were the case, the influence of gravity on one side of the tube would be negated by an equal and opposite force on the other side in the same way that a siphon moves fluid from an area of high to low pressure, regardless of the path (Figure 22-9). However, gravity does affect venous return because the cardiovascular system is composed of distensible vessels instead of rigid tubes. Below the heart, and especially in the legs and feet, veins become distended by the increased pressure resulting from the height of the fluid column. Distention of the venous vessels due to gravity can cause pooling of blood in the vessels of the dependent parts of the body. Standing rapidly can cause a transient decrease in preload on the heart, leading to dizziness, "seeing stars," and even fainting caused by distention of veins in the lower extremity. Fainting may also occur due to prolonged standing with lack of muscle pumping to move venous volume back toward the heart, especially in the heat when venous volume is increased to dissipate heat.

In veins above the heart, collapse can occur due to the negative pressure within the vein. Collapse of veins within the skull is prevented by the firm attachment of venous vessels called sinuses to other structures within the skull. Unfortunately, because of the rigid attachment of venous sinuses to the skull, a sudden acceleration of the head due to trauma can tear veins from the sinuses and can cause slow bleeding into the skull, resulting in a

subdural hematoma. The slow increase in pressure within the skull can produce temporary or permanent neurologic damage and even death if untreated.

VENOUS VALVES

The pressure produced by a column of fluid is defined as $P = \rho \, g \, h$, where ρ is density (kg/m^3), g is acceleration of gravity (9.8 m/sec^2), and h is the height of the column. This equation reduces to (kg x m/sec^2)/m^2 or force per area (pressure). As discussed above, the vertical position can result in a tremendous pressure in the dependent lower extremities, which would tend to distend the veins, decrease central venous pressure, and decrease preload on the heart. Closure of venous valves breaks up the fluid into smaller columns supported by the venous valve leaflets, which decreases the pressure below each venous valve. Because of the presence of venous valves, intermittent contraction of muscle functions as a pump to lower venous pressure and assist in venous return (Figure 22-10). Lack of muscle pumping due to paralysis of the muscles of the leg results in increased venous pressure and may cause venous insufficiency ulcers by the mechanism described earlier. The negative pressure generated in the thorax by breathing, combined with the presence of venous valves, aids in the flow of venous blood in a manner similar to

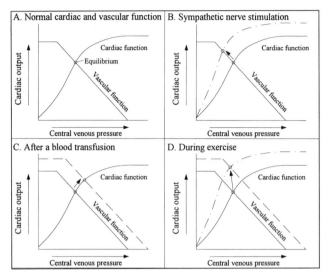

Figure 22-11. Interdependence of CVP and cardiac output. Cardiac output increases with central venous pressure due to the effect of ventricular preload (cardiac function curve). However, increased cardiac output decreases central venous pressure (vascular function curve). If only these two factors determined cardiac function, cardiac output and central venous pressure would be constrained to the values that allow them to determine each other as shown in panel A. Other factors can alter the relationship between CVP and cardiac output. In panel B, an increase in sympathetic input to the heart increases cardiac output for a given central venous pressure. This change causes both an increase in cardiac output and a decrease in central venous pressure. In panel C, the results of increased vascular volume are depicted. Transfusion allows a greater central venous pressure for a given cardiac output, with the result of a greater cardiac output and CVP. In panel D, the effects of sympathetic input to the heart and large veins are depicted. As in panel B, sympathetic input to the heart increases cardiac output for a given CVP. In addition, venoconstriction increases CVP for a given venous volume, which allows CVP to be maintained in the face of increased pumping of blood out of veins into arteries. The combination of sympathetic input to the heart and veins allows cardiac output to increase to five times its resting value during exercise.

the muscle pump. These mechanisms also aid the movement of lymph toward the lymphatic ducts.

INTERRELATIONSHIP BETWEEN CARDIAC OUTPUT AND VENOUS PRESSURE

Because the cardiovascular system is a closed circuit, the rate of venous return to the heart must equal the cardiac output over any prolonged period. With no flow, pressure anywhere in the circulatory system would be strictly a function of blood volume and capacitance.

Pressure eventually becomes equal throughout the circulatory system and, in this case, is called mean circulatory pressure. As discussed earlier, blood is made to flow through the cardiovascular system by the heart pumping blood from the venous system into the arterial system. This increase in arterial volume produces the pressure that drives blood flow. The removal of blood from the venous vessels results in a decrease in venous pressure, which also contributes to peripheral blood flow by increasing the difference in pressure between the aorta and vena cava. The strength of the heart is dependent on its preload, which is determined by the venous pressure. Therefore, cardiac output is dependent upon venous pressure.

Pressure in the large veins just outside of the heart is called central venous pressure (CVP). Because CVP acts to preload the heart and cardiac output is dependent on preload, cardiac output increases as a function of CVP. Cardiac output in this case is the dependent variable. However, as described above, removal of blood volume from the veins decreases venous pressure. As cardiac output increases and decreases venous volume, CVP falls; therefore, CVP decreases as a function of cardiac output. CVP in this case is the dependent variable. This creates the potential for conflict because cardiac output is dependent on CVP and CVP is dependent on cardiac output. These two functions are therefore mutually dependent in the body.

In the absence of any other controls over the cardiovascular system, cardiac output and CVP could never change from the unique values that generate each other. If cardiac output were to increase, CVP would decrease, which in turn would decrease cardiac output to its previous value and bring CVP back to its starting value before cardiac output changed. Therefore, if nothing else changes in the cardiovascular system, cardiac output cannot be changed. Although we can plot the two relationships separately to see the effect of cardiac output on CVP and the effect of CVP on cardiac output, plotting the effects of each on the other on the same graph demonstrates a unique point where the two graphs intersect (Figure 22-11). At this point on the graph, the value of CVP produces the value of cardiac output plotted at the intersection, and the value of cardiac output at the intersection produces the value of CVP that produces this value cardiac output. No other values of CVP or cardiac output can exist in a steady state unless the relationships between cardiac output as a function of preload is changed or venous pressure as a function of venous volume is changed.

Central venous pressure must be regulated to allow cardiac output to respond to changes in local demand for blood flow. Three factors allow cardiac output to increase when needed:

- Sympathetic stimulation to the heart
- Sympathetic stimulation to the great veins
- Sympathetic stimulation to arterioles

When the conductance of vessels increases during exercise, a greater cardiac output must occur to maintain the relationships among mean arterial pressure, cardiac output and total peripheral resistance. If total peripheral resistance falls, mean arterial pressure will also decrease unless cardiac output increases (MAP = CO x TPR). Sympathetic stimulation to the heart increases contractility, which increases the cardiac output at any given CVP. Therefore, stroke volume and heart rate can increase to meet the increased need for blood flow to the tissues.

Central venous pressure is maintained in the face of an increased cardiac output by sympathetic stimulation of the smooth muscle of the large, central veins. As cardiac output increases, more of the blood volume is shifted to the arteries. Because pressure in the veins is the product of volume and compliance, a decrease in venous volume would result in a decrease in venous pressure and preload on the heart. Decreased preload on the heart would then prevent cardiac output from changing. Constriction of the large veins decreases their compliance and maintains CVP in spite of an increase in cardiac output from a resting value of 5 liters per minutes to as high as 25 liters per minute.

Mean arterial pressure can also be maintained during exercise by increasing the vascular resistance in less active tissues. Generalized increased sympathetic stimulation to arterioles prevents TPR from falling as much it might with exercise, which has the effect of decreasing blood flow to less active tissues. Because TPR does not fall as much, cardiac output is not required to increase as much to maintain mean arterial pressure. Generalized vasoconstriction extends cardiac output reserve by allowing a greater intensity of work before maximum cardiac output is reached. Without this vasoconstriction, blood flow would be maintained to less active tissues, diverting cardiac output from the working muscles. Sympathetic stimulation allows cardiac output to increase markedly by increasing how much blood can be pumped into arteries for a given preload and by maintaining venous pressure in the face of decreased venous volume. In addition, sympathetic stimulation of blood vessels redistributes blood flow to tissues with greater demand for blood flow and decreases the amount of blood that needs to be pumped to maintain arterial pressure.

FACTORS INFLUENCING CENTRAL VENOUS PRESSURE AND CARDIAC OUTPUT

Cardiac output and CVP are influenced by a number of factors related to the determinants of pressure (volume and compliance) and the determinants of cardiac performance (preload, afterload, contractility, and heart rate). With increased blood volume, as might occur with a transfusion, more blood is present in the venous vessels and, for any given cardiac output, CVP is greater and due to the increase in CVP cardiac output increases. The result of transfusion is an increase in both the cardiac output and central venous pressure. Blood loss, as in hemorrhage, has the opposite effects of a transfusion. Both CVP and cardiac output are decreased. Blood pressure is maintained, at least initially, by sympathetic stimulation to the heart and arterial and venous vessels. Heart rate and contractility are increased, TPR is increased, and venous compliance decreases. Decreasing venous compliance increases CVP toward normal and, as a result of the increase in CVP, cardiac output and arterial pressure are increased toward normal. If hemorrhage is not stopped, blood pressure falls in spite of an increased heart rate, and a weak, rapid (thready) pulse can be detected.

With an increase in afterload or peripheral resistance, more arterial pressure is required to drive the same cardiac output across the arteriolar resistance vessels. This requires more volume to be placed in the arterial vessels. As a result of increased afterload on the heart, CVP decreases. Increasing myocardial contractility results in a greater cardiac output for any given CVP (greater stroke volume [SV] for the same preload). More blood will be translocated into the arterial side due to the increased force of contraction of the heart, resulting in less blood on the venous side and decreased CVP. In congestive heart failure (CHF), contractility is decreased. Cardiac output falls, and CVP increases. The elevated CVP increases preload to help maintain the force of contraction. Initially, cardiac output is close to normal, but at a higher energy cost due to the greater wall stress on the ventricle. The increased blood volume due to hormonal influences described earlier also helps to maintain a more nearly normal CO, but at the expense of a dilated heart and increased blood volume. Eventually, the increased volume with its accompanying edema and the increased metabolic demands on the heart will lead to loss of compensation. Treatment with digitalis to increase contractility by increasing intracellular calcium concentration reduces the dilation and edema. Other approaches to congestive heart failure include diuretics to decrease preload and vasodilator drugs to decrease afterload. Drugs that prevent the conversion of angiotensin I to angiotensin II, called angiotensin-converting enzyme (ACE) inhibitors, improve cardiac function in many individuals with congestive heart failure, which allows the person to avoid the side effects of digitalis and diuretics.

CONTROL OF ARTERIAL PRESSURE

The body has a number of mechanisms that contribute to long-term maintenance of blood pressure at the proper level. Endocrine signaling mechanisms are useful for long-term controls, and the nervous system is useful for making rapid changes. Long-term regulation of blood pressure is under the influence of hormones including atrial natriuretic factor (ANF), antidiuretic hormone (ADH, vasopressin), aldosterone, angiotensin II, and epinephrine. These hormones determine the volume of blood vessels, which, in turn, determines blood pressure in the long-term. Other mechanisms include physical mechanisms such as pressure (cold) diuresis, in which the increased central blood volume caused by peripheral vasoconstriction increases glomerular filtration rate and loss of fluid into the urine.

The nervous system is capable of regulating blood pressure rapidly through alterations in cardiac output and total peripheral resistance. The CNS controls blood pressure via autonomic outflow to the heart and blood vessels (both arterial and venous). The most important reflex for acute control of blood pressure is the baroreceptor reflex. Baroreceptors are stretch receptors located principally in the walls of the carotid sinus and aortic arch. The baroreceptors respond to stretch and deformation of vessels produced by the arterial pressure. Increasing arterial pressure increases the number of action potentials going from the baroreceptors to the CNS. Carotid baroreceptors respond to pressures as low as 50 mmHg and as high as 200 mmHg. Below 50 mm Hg, no greater effector response to increase blood pressure occurs, and, above 200 mmHg, no greater effector response to lower blood pressure occurs. Control centers in the brain stem are not discrete anatomical nuclei, but are dispersed through the medulla and lower pons. The vasomotor area is a collection of neurons responsible for the tonic activity of sympathetic nerves innervating the blood vessels. Pressor neurons cause vasoconstriction, and depressor neurons inhibit the pressor area. Located in the same region are neurons that produce increased heart rate and contractility via the sympathetic output. This area is called the cardioexcitatory area. Parasympathetic neurons with their origin in the dorsal motor nucleus of the vagus or nucleus ambiguous decrease heart rate.

The carotid baroreceptors are tonically active at normal blood pressures. Stimulation of the carotid and aortic baroreceptors causes inhibition of the pressor area of the vasomotor center and cardioexcitatory area. Increased pressure causes stimulation of the depressor area of the vasomotor center and the cardioinhibitory center. In response to increased pressure, the central integrating regions produce vasodilation and a decrease in heart rate and contractility, which bring blood pressure back toward its regulated value. A decrease in blood pressure, such as assuming an upright posture from lying, causes a decrease in the activity of the carotid baroreceptors, which results in peripheral vasoconstriction, increased heart rate, and contractility, which will bring blood pressure back up toward normal.

Whereas the carotid baroreceptors can respond to maintain blood pressure during rapid changes in cardiovascular conditions, such as standing rapidly, cardiac stretch receptors located in the atria are sensitive to changes in blood volume and behave as more slowly acting baroreceptors. One type of atrial receptor can compensate for decreased blood volume via sympathetic vasoconstrictor fibers and ADH secretion, and a second type causes release of a hormone (atrial natriuretic factor) that increases Na excretion in the urine (natriuresis) when atrial volume increases. The loss of sodium then acts to lower vascular volume and pressure. Peripheral chemoreceptors that will be discussed in the respiratory unit also have an effect on blood pressure. Extremely low levels of oxygen in the blood produce an increase in arterial pressure, as well as stimulating ventilation.

SUMMARY

The cardiovascular system is regulated both centrally to maintain MAP and locally to maintain adequate flow to tissues. MAP is regulated by sympathetic nerves to increase heart rate, increase contractility, and increase TPR by generalized vasoconstriction in the face of decreased MAP. With increased MAP, decreased sympathetic stimulation and increased vagal (parasympathetic) stimulation produce decreased heart rate, decreased contractility, and decreased TPR. Locally, active hyperemia, pressure autoregulation, and reactive hyperemia are used to match blood flow to local needs. Active hyperemia is an increased blood flow in response to increased metabolic rate.

Pressure autoregulation is an alteration in vessel conductance that compensates for a change in pressure to maintain flow constant. The myogenic response is mediated by the smooth muscle cells themselves to maintain flow. Reactive hyperemia is a compensatory increase in flow to make up for decreased flow during vessel occlusion. Both paracrine signals in the form of metabolite accumulation and the myogenic response contribute to active and reactive hyperemia and pressure autoregulation. Skeletal muscle blood flow can increase 15 to 20 times during activity due to high sympathetic tone at rest and active hyperemia during exercise. The heart displays active hyperemia, and its flow pattern is complicated by the pressure generated by its contraction.

Regions of the brain display changes in flow consistent with the functions of the area of the brain being used. Capillary filtration is due to an imbalance in forces, tending to drive water across blood vessels. Under normal, resting conditions, little filtration occurs. Increased pressure due to active hyperemia, loss of plasma proteins, or leakage in inflammation causes edema. Following exercise, the edema resolves. In congestive heart failure, edema results from the combination of increased blood volume and the inadequate pumping of the heart failing to decrease venous pressure sufficiently.

Lymphatic vessels return plasma proteins and excess interstitial fluid to the subclavian veins. The compliance of veins is physiologically regulated to maintain central venous pressure to preload the heart. Distensibility of veins causes gravity to have an effect on blood flow through veins. Collapse of veins can occur above the heart, and veins below the heart can become distended, resulting in a transient decrease in central venous pressure upon assuming an upright position. The muscle pump and ventilation, in conjunction with the venous valves, diminish the effects of gravity on venous flow. Central venous pressure and cardiac output are interdependent.

Cardiac output decreases central venous pressure, and central venous pressure increases cardiac output. CVP and cardiac output must exist at values that allow CVP and cardiac output to produce one another. Alterations in cardiac output, TPR, and blood volume, accompanied by changes in CVP, allow cardiac output to meet local tissue needs. Increased contractility decreases the need for CVP by producing a greater cardiac output for a given CVP. Short-term regulation of blood pressure uses the baroreceptor reflex, whereas long-term regulation of blood pressure is dependent on maintaining the fluid volume of the circulatory system.

BIBLIOGRAPHY

Berne RM, Levy MN. *Physiology*. St. Louis, Mo: Mosby-Year Book; 1998.

Hole JW Jr. *Essentials of Human Anatomy and Physiology*. 4th ed. Dubuque, Iowa: Wm. C. Brown Publishers; 1992.

Irisawa H, Brown HF, Giles W. Cardiac pacemaking in the sinoatrial node. *Physiological Reviews*. 1993;73:197-227.

Schauf C, Moffett D, Moffett S. *Human Physiology: Foundation and Frontiers*. St. Louis, Mo: Times Mirror/Mosby College Publishing; 1990.

STUDY QUESTIONS

1. How does the accumulation of metabolites produce both active hyperemia and pressure autoregulation? What other factor contributes to pressure autoregulation?

2. If peripheral resistance falls in the absence of an increase in cardiac output, how would mean arterial pressure change? How does cardiac output change to maintain mean arterial pressure?

3. What does a change in arteriolar diameter do locally?

4. What does changing arteriolar diameter do centrally?

5. How is the blood flow through coronary vessels different from that of other organs?

6. Why is the left ventricle at a much greater risk of ischemia than the right ventricle?

7. Explain how malnutrition or liver disease causes edema.

8. Why can't cardiac output change if the volume and compliance of central veins does not change?

9. Why must venous vessels within the skull be attached in the form of venous sinuses?

10. Explain why heart rate and contractility of the heart increase when we stand up rapidly.

TWENTY-THREE

Function of the Lungs

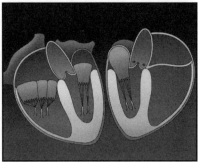

Sustained metabolic activity of most cells is supported by oxidative metabolism. The oxygen removed from the blood is replaced by ventilation. CO_2 produced by oxidative metabolism diffuses out of cells and is eliminated by ventilation. Ventilation is regulated to maintain the concentration of CO_2; replacement of oxygen occurs as a byproduct of ventilation. Ventilation is also an important way of maintaining acid-base balance. Carbon dioxide produced by metabolism behaves as an acid due to the chemical reaction: $H_2O + CO_2 \rightleftharpoons H_2CO_3 \rightleftharpoons H^+ + HCO_3^-$ in which carbon dioxide combines with water due to the enzyme carbonic anhydrase to form carbonic acid. One carbonic acid molecule forms a hydrogen ion and a bicarbonate ion. Bicarbonate ion is the major extracellular buffer, absorbing excess hydrogen ions and ridding the body of acid by the elimination of CO_2 by ventilation. The processes involved in acid-base balance will be described further in Chapter Twenty-Six. By increasing or decreasing CO_2 elimination via ventilation, the carbonic anhydrase reaction is shifted away from or toward H^+ production. Increased ventilation decreases plasma $[CO_2]$ and decreases plasma $[H^+]$, thereby increasing plasma pH. Decreased ventilation, on the other hand, increases plasma $[CO_2]$ and increases plasma $[H^+]$, which decreases plasma pH.

The lungs represent a large surface area in contact with the external environment. Several mechanisms described below work to protect against foreign matter. Activation of chemical messengers, especially angiotensin II from angiotensin I, also occurs in the lungs. Converting enzyme is located on the epithelium of blood vessels in the lungs. Another important function of the lungs is to trap emboli that result from thrombi from systemic veins and dissolve them. All blood returning from the systemic circulation first passes through lungs before returning to the systemic circulation. Thrombi are most likely to develop in systemic veins in which blood flow is sluggish, especially in the lower extremities. Mast cells within the lung release heparin, allowing the emboli to be degraded. Most emboli are asymptomatic because they occlude a small area of lung and can be degraded before any damage occurs. Larger emboli can cause infarction of a portion of a lung and hemoptysis (coughing up blood). Very large pulmonary emboli may occlude the pulmonary circulation completely, producing acute heart failure and death rapidly.

GAS LAWS

When discussing the movement of gases required for ventilation, rules governing both bulk flow and dif-fusion must be used. The principles discussed in Chapter Twenty-One on hemodynamics apply equally to airflow through the airways by bulk flow in which pressure is the driving force. Movement of gas by diffusion occurs across the alveoli of the lung between the blood and alveolar air and across the blood vessel walls between blood and peripheral tissues. The driving force for movement of gases through the respiratory system and blood by diffusion is partial pressure. This concept can be used for a mixture of gas if we assume that the gas molecules are far enough apart that they do not interact. Put another way, we assume that the probability of an oxygen molecule moving across a barrier is unrelated to the other gases present in the mixture; it is determined only by the pressure exerted by oxygen molecules on the two sides of the barrier. Partial pressure is computed as the fraction of the gas mixture that is composed of a particular gas times the pressure exerted by the entire mixture. For example, with an atmospheric pressure of 760 mmHg and with 21% of the atmosphere composed of oxygen, the partial pressure of oxygen (PO_2) is 21% of 760 mmHg or 160 mmHg. Nitrogen makes up almost all of the remaining 79%, so PN_2 equals 600 mmHg. Only about 0.3% of the atmosphere is composed of CO_2, but about 5% of the gas dissolved in blood is CO_2, so the PCO_2 of blood is about 40 mmHg. The purpose of using partial pressures instead of concentrations is to simplify discussion of movement of the gases between different fluids. Because gases equilibrate in volume in proportion to their solubility in the different fluids, concentration of gases does not provide us with meaningful information in terms of the driving force for gas movement. However, if the solubility of oxygen in one fluid is greater than another and the two are exposed to each other, the partial pressure will become identical over time; the concentration of oxygen in ml of oxygen per ml of fluid will be greater in the solution with greater oxygen solubility.

The gas laws used in chemistry are also useful in physiology. They include the general gas law, Charles' law, Boyle's law, Dalton's law, Avogadro's law, also used in the discussion above, and Henry's law. Boyle's law is stated as $P_1 V_1 = P_2 V_2$ with temperature constant. Boyle's law can be used to explain how bulk flow is generated by the muscles of inspiration. Using the muscles of inspiration to increase the volume of the thorax produces the subatmospheric (negative) pressure in the thorax needed for bulk flow of air from the atmosphere into the lungs. Charles' law, which is stated as $V_1/V_2 = T_1/T_2$ with pressure constant, is needed to account for the difference in the volume occupied by a number of molecules taken from the atmosphere compared with the volume that the same number of gas molecules occupies in the body, where temperature is usually greater. Charles' law is used in the conversion factor for STPD (standard temperature and pressure, dry). Converting a volume of gas to what a volume would occupy at a standard for temperature and pressure is an indirect way to deal with a number of molecules of gas. Variations in conditions of pressure and temperature would reduce the meaningfulness of stating that a certain volume of oxygen is consumed if that volume varied with atmospheric pressure, air temperature, presence of water vapor, and body temperature. By converting to STPD, everyone who reports a given value for gas volume is discussing the same number of molecules of gas.

The general gas law is stated $PV = nRT$ and describes the relationship between pressure, volume, number of molecules, and temperature. This equation takes into account both Boyle's law and Charles' law. In this equation, P is pressure, V is volume, n is the number of gas molecules, R is the universal gas constant, and T is temperature. This equation allows us to discuss gases in terms of volume occupied, instead of molar concentrations. This equation can be used to standardize the number of molecules that occupy a given volume using the standards described in the paragraph below with standard temperature of O°C or 273°K and 760 mmHg atmospheric pressure.

Two standards that use the general gas law are STPD and BTPS. STPD stands for standard temperature and pressure, dry. This number states the volume that a given number of O_2 or other gas molecules would occupy at a temperature of 273°K, a pressure of 760 mmHg, and 0% humidity. Because a given volume of a gas will contain a different number of molecules depending on temperature and pressure, volume corrected to STPD allows one to perform a simpler measurement of volume to express the number of oxygen molecules consumed by oxidative metabolism. BTPS stands for body temperature and pressure, saturated. This correction takes into account the body temperature, atmospheric pressure, and the space occupied in the gas mixture by water vapor at a given temperature. Water vapor is added to the inspired gas to its maximum concentration (the gas is saturated with water vapor) as the gas passes through the airways. The actual volume of gas occupied by water vapor depends on the temperature of the gas. Warmer gas holds more water vapor. At a normal body temperature of 37°C, water vapor contributes 47 mmHg of partial pressure. Ventilatory volumes are typically reported in terms of BTPS, whereas oxygen consumption is reported corrected for STPD. BTPS can be converted to STPD by multiplying the volume of gas by $(273/310) \times [(P_B - 47)/760]$ where 47 mmHg is the water vapor pressure at a temperature of

37°C and body temperature is 273 plus 37° to convert to absolute temperature in degrees Kelvin.

Avogadro's law states that equal volumes of different gases at the same temperature and pressure contain the same number of molecules. One mole of ideal gas occupies 22.4 L at STPD. Dalton's law states that the partial pressure of a gas in a mixture is the pressure that this gas would exert if it occupied the same volume in the absence of any other gases. Both Avogadro's law and Dalton's law were used at the beginning of this section. These laws allow us to use the idea of partial pressure as the driving force for gas movement by diffusion. Assuming these two laws to be true, the volume of gas in a fluid is proportional to its partial pressure and its solubility in the fluid for the gas.

The driving force for movement of gases between two fluid media (eg, between plasma and interstitial fluid or between alveolar air and pulmonary capillaries), can be described easily because of Henry's law, which states that the partial pressure of a gas in solution is equal to the partial pressure of that gas in the mixture of gases with which the liquid is in equilibrium. If the partial pressure of O_2 in a gas is 150 mm Hg and O_2 is moving equally into the solution and into the gas, then the PO_2 of the solution is also 150 mm Hg. According to Henry's law, the concentration of a gas dissolved in a liquid is **proportional** to its partial pressure (eg, $[O_2] = k \times PO_2$, where k is the solubility of O_2 in the solvent). By comparing partial pressures, we can understand the direction of gas movement between compartments without knowing concentration or solubility of the fluid for the gas. The rate at which a gas moves from one compartment in the body to another is directly proportional to the difference in partial pressure.

AIRWAY ANATOMY

The airways may be divided into upper airways, which are located in the head and neck, and lower airways located within the chest. The upper airways consist of the nose, pharynx, nasopharynx, oropharynx, and larynx. The larynx is the beginning of separate pathways for the respiratory and digestive systems. Above the larynx, both air and substances meant for the digestive system can mix. Swallowing, described in Chapter Twenty-Eight, must be coordinated to prevent aspiration of solids and liquids. The lower airways consist of the trachea, the left and right bronchus, bronchi, smaller airways called bronchioles, and terminal bronchioles. Terminal bronchioles are the smallest airways that only conduct gases and do not exchange gases with the blood. Airways distal to the terminal bronchioles have

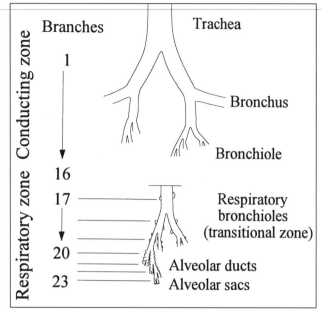

Figure 23-1. Branching in airways. Gas exchange occurs in the conducting zone by bulk flow from high to low pressure. In the respiratory zone (generations 17 to 23), gas exchange occurs by diffusion. The transitional zone represents an area in which both bulk flow and diffusion occur.

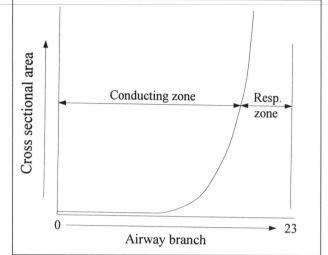

Figure 23-2. Airway cross-sectional area as a function of generation of airway branch. As airways branch into a new generation, the sum of the daughter airways increases. The increased cross-sectional area with each succeeding branch explains the decrease in aggregate resistance of each airway branch.

alveoli on their sides to provide exchange of gases between the blood and atmosphere. These airways are called respiratory bronchioles. Alveolar ducts consist of passages among groups of alveoli, which terminate with alveolar sacs. Alveolar ducts may be pictured as a hallway lined with rooms with the rooms being the alveoli.

The airways are produced by approximately 20 generations of branching (Figure 23-1). The first few generations have cartilage to protect them from changes in thoracic pressure. By branch #17, alveoli begin to appear on sides of respiratory bronchioles. The preceding branch, which has no alveoli, is called a terminal bronchiole. By branch #20, we have the alveolar ducts that are more like passages between groups of alveoli than airways. Alveolar sacs usually occur at the end of the 23rd branch, which represents the end of branching. With each successive generation of branching, a geometric increase in the number of branches and total cross-sectional area occurs. An average human lung has 60,000 terminal bronchioles, 500,000 respiratory bronchioles, and 8 million alveolar sacs, for a total of 300 million alveoli.

Based on the type of driving force for movement of gas molecules, the lower airways are divided into two zones called the conducting zone and the respiratory zone. The conducting zone consists of the branches from the trachea to the terminal bronchioles and functions to bring air to the respiratory zone by bulk flow.

The respiratory zone consists of the branches from the respiratory bronchioles to the alveolar sacs where gas exchange occurs by diffusion. In the conducting zone, gas moves from high pressure to low pressure by bulk flow, the same as blood in blood vessels, but in the respiratory zone, gas moves by diffusion from high partial pressure to low partial pressure. The respiratory bronchioles are sometimes called the transitional zone because both bulk flow into the airways and diffusion of gases across the alveoli occur at this level.

Because cross-sectional area of the daughter branches exceeds that of the preceding airway and the increasing number of airways with each generation of branching of the airways, total cross-sectional area increases sharply from the conducting zone to the respiratory zone (Figure 23-2). The same principle relating velocity, flow rate, and cross-sectional area discussed in hemodynamics applies to bronchioles. Because air flow is the same in each airway generation, velocity decreases as cross-sectional area increases with branching. Velocity approaches zero in the respiratory zone because of the enormous collective cross-sectional area of these airways. Although individual small airways have a high resistance, the large number of small airways in parallel has a very low resistance collectively. The highest resistance in the airways actually occurs in the larger airways entering the segments of the lung, and resistance decreases rapidly with each generation of branching

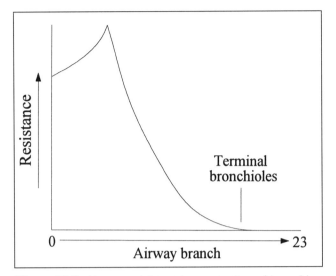

Figure 23-3. Airway resistance by generation of branching of airways. Note that with increased branching, resistance diminishes tremendously.

(Figure 23-3). Small airway disease is insidious because a large change in resistance of small airways must occur before a change in total airway resistance can be detected. Damage can occur for many years before disease is diagnosed clinically.

ANATOMY OF THE LUNGS

The normal individual has two lungs that occupy almost all of the chest volume. On the left side of the chest, however, the heart occupies a significant volume. The left lung gives the appearance of being shifted to the left and only has two true lobes compared to three lobes of the right lung. Within each lobe exist more than one segment served by segmental bronchi, which branch from the left and right main bronchi. Each segment can be drained of secretions using what is called postural drainage. One area of the left lung that outwardly resembles a smaller version of the right middle lobe is called the lingula. For the purpose of postural drainage, the lingula is treated as if it were a left middle lobe. Due to the presence of the heart, the left main bronchus is more horizontal than the right main bronchus, and aspiration is more likely to occur into the right lung. For this reason, the right middle and right lower lobes are more susceptible to pneumonia than other areas of the lungs. The lungs extend vertically more in the posterior of the chest than in the anterior, and corresponding lobes in the posterior chest are more caudal than in the anterior of the chest. This, too, impacts postural drainage and airway clearance techniques.

The volume occupied by airways is only about 150 ml. For a given individual, an estimate is 1 ml per pound of body weight. Although individual alveoli are very small, the large number of these makes the alveoli occupy a much larger volume of the lungs than the airways. The volume of the airways is called the anatomic dead space because this volume is ventilated but does not exchange gases with the blood. With each breath of 400 to 500 ml, only 250 to 350 ml of fresh air reaches alveoli.

Smooth muscle surrounding the walls of the airways regulates airway resistance and compliance, just as it does in blood vessels. Because large airways are subject

Postural Drainage

Postural drainage is a means of using the assistance of gravity to clear airways. Each segment of the lung has a particular position that allows secretions to drain from small airways into larger airways where the secretions can be coughed up or removed by suction. A person may be placed in a certain position for up to 15 minutes, or this time can be decreased by supplementing drainage with other airway clearance techniques (ACT). These include percussion, shaking, and vibration. Percussion is the use of cupped hands striking the chest at a frequency of about six times per second, usually alternating right and left hands over the same area of the chest that is being drained. Percussion is not coordinated with breathing, but shaking and vibration are. Shaking, as the name implies, is a forceful movement of the chest with the hands applied to the area of the chest to be drained. The person receiving airway clearance takes in a deep breath first, then exhales as the therapist creates large movements of the chest at a rate of twice per second. Air is forced out of the lung causing four to six audible sounds similar to a car trying to start with a dying battery. Vibration is a more gentle, but rapid movement of the hands in contact with the chest and may be more suitable for a person who cannot tolerate percussion or shaking. The hands are kept in contact, and rapid, small movement of the elbows and shoulders are made during expiration following a deep inspiration. A typical sequence consists of positioning, percussion, and shaking followed by coughing. Mechanical devices are also available to assist airway clearance.

to pressures of both the thorax and atmosphere, they can collapse under high flow conditions in a fashion similar to veins above the heart. By making the airways stiffer, increased smooth muscle tone reduces the influence of the difference in pressure across the walls of the airway and prevents collapse. Bronchoconstriction also reduces anatomic dead space by reducing the diameter of the airways. In contrast to these physiologic changes in bronchial smooth muscle tone, a pathological increase in airway resistance can occur in asthma and related conditions. Breathing through pursed lips causes pressure to remain positive in the airways and prevents airway collapse. A number of devices use positive expiratory pressure to help clear airways by preventing the trapping of secretions in airways that collapse with coughing. Mechanical ventilators can be set to produce positive end-expiratory pressure to prevent airways from collapsing.

FACTORS CONTROLLING AIRWAY RESISTANCE

Airway smooth muscle has both muscarinic and adrenergic receptors. Acetylcholine released by parasympathetic nerves and cholinergic drugs bind to muscarinic receptors to cause constriction. Epinephrine, a hormone produced by the adrenal medulla, binds to β_2 receptors, producing increased intracellular cAMP and relaxation of bronchial smooth muscle. Histamine is released by mast cells in the lungs and other tissues as a result of allergic reactions. The release of histamine can produce sufficient smooth muscle tone to interfere with breathing. Epinephrine or a drug that binds to β receptors is used to produce rapid relaxation of pathologic bronchoconstriction. Drugs specific for β_2 receptors have

much less effect on the heart, which has β_1 receptors. Theophylline and related drugs have been used to produce bronchodilation pharmacologically. The mechanism was once thought to be inhibition of the enzyme that degrades cAMP, called phosphodiesterase, which would allow cAMP to increase inside the cell. It is now thought that the primary effect of theophylline is blockage of purinergic receptors (receptors for ATP and related compounds).

Carbon dioxide also influences airway diameter. Decreased CO_2 in airways constricts airways, and increased CO_2 in airways relaxes airways. By decreasing the resistance of airways with an increase in CO_2, ventilation increases, bringing CO_2 concentration back to normal. Airway resistance is altered during exercise by parasympathetic nerves, which increase bronchial smooth muscle tone. Increased smooth muscle tone decreases compliance and prevents collapse during forced expiration. During forced expiration, increased abdominal pressure is transmitted to the thorax, which increases the pressure difference between the alveoli and the atmosphere to drive more air out of the lungs. This increased pressure surrounding small airways causes them to collapse. Large airways do not collapse because of the cartilage surrounding them in addition to the effect of the smooth muscle. During deep inspiration, airway resistance is decreased passively by a phenomenon called lateral traction. Because the airways are attached to the surrounding lung tissue, expansion of the lungs pulls the walls of the airways outward. Increased bronchial smooth muscle tone during exercise also decreases anatomic dead space. Because anatomic dead space is decreased, more of the inspired volume goes to the respiratory zone instead of the conducting zone. The ability to sigh, yawn, and laugh prevents collapse and infection of the lung. The loss of these abili-

Asthma

This disease is a chronic condition of airway inflammation with acute episodes of bronchoconstriction and mucus production. Before the basic condition was understood, asthma was treated strictly as an acute disease of increased airway resistance by rescue treatments of bronchodilator drugs. Later, corticosteroid drugs were used to control chronic airway inflammation. However, corticosteroids have potentially devastating side effects, especially on young children. Corticosteroids can suppress the immune response sufficiently to make chicken pox deadly. They can also produce growth retardation and aseptic necrosis of bones (also occurs with treatment of systemic lupus erythematosus). Aerosol delivery and newer formulations of corticosteroids for asthma have decreased the systemic side effects of corticosteroids. The latest advance in medical treatment has been the development of drugs that decrease the production of leukotrienes, which appear to be responsible for much of the airway inflammation of asthma. People with asthma use a device called a peak flow meter to measure maximum flow rates. Before overt symptoms of an acute attack can be observed, the peak flow will be diminished. Using peak flow information decreases the risk of a person being caught off guard for an acute episode of bronchoconstriction and mucus production.

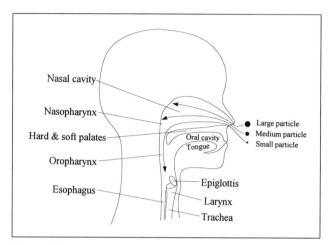

Figure 23-4. Management of inhaled particles by the upper airways. The heavier an object is, the more likely it is to continue in a straight path. Large particles inhaled through the nose strike the back of the nasopharynx and become trapped in the mucus. Only very small particles are capable of entering the lungs. Particles entering the lungs become trapped in mucus of the airways and are carried upward by ciliary action. Extremely small particles may enter the alveoli but then become exhaled. Remaining particles are handled by macrophages in the alveoli.

ties puts a person at risk for atelectasis (partial lung collapse) and pneumonia.

ALVEOLI

As stated above, airways make up a small proportion of the volume of the lungs. Lung volume ranges from 1200 to 6000 ml with breathing, compared to the 150 ml of anatomic dead space. The rest of the volume and most of the change in volume with ventilation occurs in the alveoli. This 150 ml of gas remains in the conducting zone and cannot participate in exchange of gases with the blood. Alveoli are found on the sides of respiratory bronchioles, on the ends of terminal bronchioles, and as pockets on the sides of alveolar ducts. The alveoli almost entirely fill the gaps among the airways. Alveoli communicate through pores of Kohn that act to stabilize this collection of small bubbles; otherwise, according to the law of LaPlace, the small bubbles would coalesce into progressively larger, more stable bubbles. Approximately 300 million alveoli, each with a diameter of about 0.33 mm in diameter, exist in the average human lung. The total surface area of the alveoli is approximately 75 m^2 or the size of a tennis court. Each alveolus is almost entirely covered with capillaries, with small areas between capillaries. This alveolar surface area, with its blood-covered surface, presents ample

opportunity for exchange of gases across the alveolar walls.

Two populations of cells are found in the alveolar walls. Type I cells are much more common than type II cells. Type I cells are the epithelial cells that line the air side of the alveolus. Air and blood are separated by type I cells, capillary endothelium, and interstitial space. Some connective tissue, including collagen and elastin fibers, is present to support lung structure. Type II cells produce a mixture of chemicals called surfactant. Without surfactant, lungs are too stiff to be compatible with normal breathing. The role of surfactant in breathing is described more thoroughly in the next chapter on the mechanics of ventilation.

REMOVAL OF INHALED PARTICLES

Other functions of the lungs include the removal of foreign material by the mucociliary mechanism and the warming and hydration of the atmospheric air that enters the lungs. As described earlier, airways normally lose sufficient water to saturate the inspired air with water vapor. Dehydration prevents proper humidification and leads to a thick mucus that may need to be removed by airway clearance techniques. Air reaching alveoli normally approaches core temperature except at high ventilatory rates in cold air. Warming and humidification of inspired air protect the lungs from the effects of cold, dry air that are quite evident on exposed skin in the winter.

Because the lungs have an enormous surface area exposed to the external environment, mechanisms are required to remove particulate matter that enters with the air. Three basic mechanisms operate on different sized particles (Figure 23-4). Large particles are removed in the nose due to their inertia. The greater the mass of a particle is, the more likely it will be to continue to move in a straight line into the back wall of the nasopharynx. Large particles will then stick to mucus and be removed by expectoration or swallowing. Medium-sized particles are deposited in small airways by the process termed sedimentation. Sedimentation occurs where velocity becomes low with increasing cross-sectional area in distal airways. The heavier particles settle proximally in airways, and the lighter particles settle more distally. Particles will typically settle out in the terminal and respiratory bronchioles. Particles adhering to mucus on bronchial walls are swept up by the mucociliary mechanism and are either expectorated or swallowed. Ciliary movement is paralyzed by inhaled irritants, especially tobacco smoke. Smoking also increases the quantity of mucus secreted due to inflammation, resulting in a condition in which copious quantities of mucus are produced, but not removed effectively. Chronic bronchitis produces a characteristic cough in which mucus is moved through the airways, but is not effectively removed. Small particles (less than 0.1 μm in diameter) reach alveoli, but most are simply exhaled. Particles remaining in the alveoli are removed by macrophages, then carried to lymphatics or blood. Some types of particles, such as asbestos, coal dust, beryllium, and silica, are not removed effectively and cause chronic inflammation of the lung and fibrosis. These diseases cause fibrosis of the lung and what are termed restrictive lung diseases. One of the dangers of wet alveoli, which occurs with pneumonia, is trapping of microbes in a warm, moist environment. Provided with a suitable environment, microbes may reproduce at a rate exceeding the ability of the immune system to destroy them.

SUMMARY

The lungs function primarily to rid the body of carbon dioxide generated by oxidative metabolism. The loss of carbon dioxide is important in maintaining pH of the body fluids. Accumulation of carbon dioxide decreases pH. Exchange of oxygen occurs as a by-product of ventilation. The lungs also convert angiotensin I to angiotensin II and trap emboli. Partial pressure is exerted by an individual gas within a mixture of gases. The partial pressure of oxygen in the air at 760 mmHg atmospheric pressure is 160 mmHg (21% of 760). Boyle's law explains the relationship between pressure and volume of a gas, and Charles' law explains the relationship between temperature and volume. The general gas law is written $PV = nRT$ and quantifies volume for a given pressure, temperature, and number of gas molecules. Avogadro's law and Dalton's law are convenient for us to view partial pressure as the driving force for diffusion of gas. Gases move from an area of high partial pressure to low. The concentration of gas in a liquid depends on both the partial pressure and the solubility of the gas in the liquid. Henry's law allows us to use partial pressure of a gas in both a mixture of gas and in a liquid in equilibrium with the gas. The diffusion of a gas across a membrane depends solely upon the difference in partial pressure of that gas across the membrane. STPD stands for standard temperature and pressure, dry

and allows us to measure a volume of a gas rather than having to compute the number of molecules in a volume based on the temperature, pressure, and quantity of water vapor. BTPS stands for body temperature and pressure, saturated and is used for volumes of gas within the lungs. The upper airways consist of those in the head and neck. The lower airways are further divided into the conducting zone and respiratory zone. The conducting zone allows bulk flow of air but does not exchange gases with the blood. Movement of gas through the respiratory zone is by diffusion from high partial pressure to low, and alveoli are found in the respiratory zone to allow exchange of gases with the blood. The branching of airways results in increased collective cross-sectional area with each generation of branching, with the result of decreased velocity and resistance to airflow. As velocity approaches zero in the respiratory zone, the mode of transport of gases switches from bulk flow to diffusion. Although individual small airways have a large resistance, the large number of small airways results in a very low collective resistance so that small airway disease may develop over many years before any change in resistance of the airways in general can be detected. The upper airways and conducting zone are ventilated with each breath but do not exchange air. These areas are called the anatomic dead space. Airway resistance and compliance are regulated physiologically by alterations in bronchial smooth muscle tone. Decreased diameter increases resistance but also decreases compliance, which reduces the possibility of small airways collapsing during high velocity flow. Parasympathetic nerves release acetylcholine onto muscarinic receptors to produce bronchoconstriction. Epinephrine binds to β_2 adrenergic receptors to produce relaxation via cAMP. Bronchodilator drugs work by either binding to β receptors or by inhibiting phosphodiesterase to increase cAMP concentration. Histamine released during allergic responses causes bronchoconstriction. Approximately 300 million alveoli with an average diameter of 0.33 mm have a collective surface area of 75 m^2 exposed to the external environment to exchange gases. The outside of the alveoli is virtually covered with capillaries. Large particulate matter, due to its inertia, impacts the back of the nasopharynx and is trapped in a layer of mucus. Medium-sized particles settle in small airways where the velocity of air flow approaches zero. This material is trapped in mucus and is moved up the airways toward the mouth by ciliary action. Small particulate matter is expired with the gas, and what is not removed is taken up by macrophages.

BIBLIOGRAPHY

Berne RM, Levy MN. *Physiology*. St. Louis, Mo: Mosby-Year Book; 1998.

Dectamer M. Respiratory muscle interaction. *News in Physiological Sciences*. 1993;8:121-124.

Ganong WF. *Review of Medical Physiology*. Norwalk, Conn: Appleton & Lange; 1995.

Guyton AC, Hall JE, Schmitt W. *Human Physiology and Mechanisms of Disease*. Philadelphia, Pa: WB Saunders; 1997.

West JB. *Respiratory Physiology: The Essentials*. 4th ed. Baltimore, Md: Williams & Wilkins; 1990.

STUDY QUESTIONS

1. Why is the concept of partial pressure useful in determining the direction and rate of gas movement by diffusion? If hemoglobin increases the solubility of oxygen in blood, how does hemoglobin affect the amount of oxygen in the blood at a given partial pressure?

2. Why is it necessary to report oxygen consumption in STPD?

3. How is oxygen transported through the conducting zone? How is it transported through the respiratory zone? What is unique about the transitional zone?

4. Where is airway resistance typically highest? Why does airway resistance decrease with each generation of airway branching?

5. What is anatomic dead space? How much is it in the average person? What would happen if a person breathed in this much with each breath?

6. How does the trapping of emboli by the lung benefit the organism? How can trapping of an embolus be lethal?

7. Why are large particles breathed in trapped in the nasopharynx? What would happen with mouth-breathing?

TWENTY-FOUR

Mechanics of Ventilation

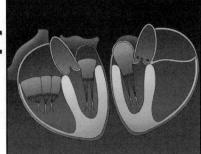

Ventilation is the process by which fresh air from the atmosphere is brought into the lungs to allow exchange of gases with the blood. Ventilation rids the body of carbon dioxide produced by aerobic metabolism as volatile acid. Oxygen is added to the blood during this process. Ventilation requires energy expenditure to maintain a steady state in which the carbon dioxide generated and the oxygen consumed by metabolism are eliminated and replaced, respectively. Muscles of ventilation disturb the equilibrium position of the chest wall to produce inspiration. In people with lung disease, a greater proportion of oxygen consumption is used to support breathing. Increasing lung volume produces a subatmospheric (negative) pressure within the lungs that drives bulk flow of air into the lungs. Similar to a spring, the energy used to stretch the elastic structures of the lung during inspiration creates elastic recoil that drives air out of the lungs. The mechanics of ventilation, the factors that determine the rate of bulk flow and the exchange of gas between the atmosphere and the alveoli, are described in this chapter.

MUSCLES OF VENTILATION

Several muscles can be used to produce the increased outward force on the chest wall that produces inspiration. The diaphragm, external intercostals, scalenes, sternocleidomastoid, and levator scapulae are all skeletal muscles and have all the properties of skeletal muscle including fatigue. The diaphragm is the principal muscle of inspiration, accounting for two-thirds to three-quarters of the increase in thoracic volume during inspiration. The diaphragm completely separates the thorax from the abdomen, surrounding the vertebral column, esophagus, and great vessels. Contraction of the dome-shaped diaphragm increases the vertical dimensions of the thorax. Moreover, using the abdominal contents as a fulcrum, the muscle fibers of the diaphragm pull the rib margins toward its central tendon, elevating the margins of the lower ribs and increasing the horizontal dimensions of the chest wall (Figure 24-1). During normal breathing, the diaphragm descends about 1 cm, increasing to 10 cm during forced breathing. Intercostals stabilize the ribs so they do not pull apart during inspiration. In a person with a spinal cord injury affecting the abdominal and intercostal muscles, reserve for breathing can become very limited in spite of complete innervation of the diaphragm. Without innervation of the abdominal muscles, the diaphragm compresses the abdominal contents and elongates the thorax, but insufficient abdominal pressure cannot support the central tendon and the rib mar-

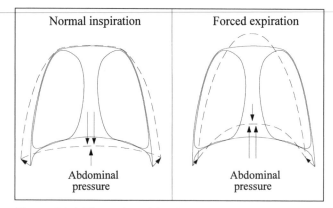

Figure 24-1. The action of the diaphragm during inspiration. The solid lines represent resting positions of the elements of the ventilatory pump. With sufficient abdominal pressure, contraction of the diaphragm pulls the lower rib margins toward the diaphragm's central tendon, resulting in an upward and outward movement of the lower ribs and a small descent of the diaphragm (left panel). Forced expiration is depicted in the right panel. Strong contraction of the abdominal muscles forces the diaphragm upward and decreases the size of the thorax to force air from the lungs.

gins are not pulled toward the central tendon. Because of loss of intercostal muscle function, the distance between ribs is increased, and the chest diameter retracts instead of expanding during inspiration.

Scalenes and the sternocleidomastoids are sometimes called accessory muscles of inspiration. These muscles are relatively inactive with quiet breathing but become markedly active and hypertrophy when the diaphragm alone cannot produce sufficient chest wall movement as in forceful breathing or lung disease. Scalenes aid the diaphragm by elevating the first two ribs, and sternocleidomastoids lift the sternum. Marked use of the scalenes and sternocleidomastoids can often be observed in individuals with emphysema. Other muscles attached to the rib cage and upper extremities, such as the latissimus dorsi, pectorals, and trapezius, can also assist inspiration by pulling the chest wall outward either directly or indirectly through scapular and humeral attachments when the upper extremities are stabilized distally. Breathing this way is common in diseases, such as emphysema or asthma. The tripod position describes the situation in which the forearms are stabilized to act as the origin and the upper extremity muscles aid in chest wall movement. Leaning forward to displace the abdominal contents reduces the effort required to move the diaphragm downward against abdominal pressure. Often, people with chronic lung disease use either three- or four-wheeled walkers with hand brakes and baskets to ambulate with the upper extremities stabilized on the walker and leaning forward.

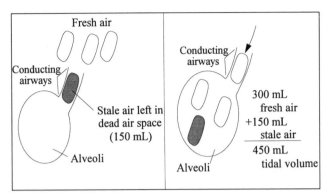

Figure 24-2. Mixing of fresh and stale air by the ventilatory pump. On the left, conditions existing before inspiration are depicted. Following expiration, about 150 ml of stale air remains in the airways. With inspiration (right), 450 ml of fresh air enters the lungs. The first 150 ml entering the alveoli are stale air, 300 ml is fresh air, and the last 150 ml of inspired air remains in the airways (anatomical dead space).

Forced expiration is accomplished by contraction of abdominal muscles, which increases abdominal pressure. Forced expiration occurs during heavy exercise and voluntary activity, such as inflating a balloon or blowing out candles. Increased abdominal pressure forces the contents of the abdomen into the thorax, thereby increasing pressure within the thorax and aiding in expiration. All of the volume of the lungs cannot be emptied under normal conditions. Forced expiration is limited by collapse of small airways as positive pressure is transmitted to the thorax. Greater effort cannot remove any more volume, because air is trapped behind the collapsed small airways. Abdominal muscle contraction is also important to produce coughing. Paralysis or weakness of these muscles in spinal cord injury or neurologic disease can produce an inability to cough effectively and clear the lungs of mucus, which increases the risk of lung infection.

VENTILATORY VOLUMES

Several volumes have been defined to aid discussion of the process of ventilation. These include tidal volume (V_T), minute ventilation, and alveolar ventilation. Tidal volume is the amount of air that enters the lungs with a normal inspiration or leaves with a normal expiration. The rate at which air enters the lungs is called minute ventilation. Minute ventilation (ml/min) is determined by the tidal volume and the frequency (f) of breathing as V_T x f. A typical example is 450 ml x 10/min = 4500 ml/min. However, minute ventilation is not a useful description of the potential for exchange of gases between the atmosphere and alveoli because not all of the air that passes from the atmosphere through the mouth reaches the alveoli. This is because of the dead space discussed in Chapter Twenty-Three. Dead space represents a volume of lung that is ventilated but does not exchange gas with the blood. The anatomic dead space, which consists of airway volume, is about 150 ml in a normal person (approximately 1 ml per pound of body weight). In addition, certain diseases cause a physiologic dead space to occur. Physiologic dead space represents alveolar volume that is ventilated but has no (or low) blood flow to allow exchange of gases between the alveoli and blood. Ventilation of these alveoli has the same effect in terms of gas exchange as enlarging the volume of the airways.

The term that describes the rate of bulk flow into areas that exchange gas is called alveolar ventilation (V_A), which is equal to (tidal volume – dead space) x f. An example is (450 – 150 ml) x 10/min = 3000 ml/min. Alveolar ventilation defines the amount of fresh air that enters alveoli each minute. Using our examples above, inspiration brings 450 ml of air into the lungs. The first air to enter alveoli, however, is the 150 ml of stale air left in the airways from the previous breath. An additional 300 ml of the 450 ml of fresh air entering the lungs also enters the alveoli, and the final 150 ml of fresh air remains in the airways where exchange cannot occur. During expiration, 150 ml of fresh air in the airways and 300 ml of stale air from the alveoli are expired, but 150 ml of stale alveolar air will remain in the airways to be brought back into the alveoli with the next breath. Therefore, each breath only brings 300 ml of fresh air into the alveoli and 150 ml of fresh air into the airways where it is wasted (Figure 24-2).

The effectiveness of ventilation is determined by a combination of three factors: tidal volume, dead space, and frequency. Two examples of breathing patterns with identical minute ventilation, but different alveolar ventilation should clarify the point. In one case, the individual breathes rapidly and shallowly because of an asthma attack that provokes panic. With a frequency of 30/min and a V_T of 200 ml, minute ventilation equals 6000 ml/min, compared with a normal pattern of 500 ml at a rate of 12/min, which also produces a minute ventilation of 6000 ml/min. In the first case, V_A = 200 – 150 ml x 40/min = 2000 ml/min, and in the second example, V_A = 500 – 150 ml x 12/min = 4200 ml/min. As the example shows, rapid, shallow breathing is ineffective in exchanging gases with the environment. Unfortunately, in a situation in which a person becomes short of breath (SOB), frequency often increases markedly, and V_T decreases, resulting in poor exchange of gases. A person with asthma or other breathing disorders must be taught to relax and slow the rate of ventilation to exchange gases effectively. Techniques include pursed lip breathing, diaphragmatic breathing, tripod position, and leaning forward. Pursed lip breathing has two benefits. Pursing the lips slows the rate of airflow during expiration, thereby decreasing frequency, and it also creates a back pressure or positive airway pressure during expiration that prevents airway collapse. Diaphragmatic breathing encourages the use of a greater number of muscles to pull the chest wall outward. A person is taught to feel the movement of the upper and lower chest by placing the hands over these two locations. The person consciously attempts to move the lower ribs up and out and decrease the upper chest movement.

The effectiveness of different breathing patterns can also be assessed by applying the Fick principle to the exchange of uptake of oxygen through the lungs. Knowing the consumption of oxygen, atmospheric PO_2 and alveolar ventilation allows the PO_2 of alveolar air to be estimated. In analogy of the Fick principle used to describe the cardiac output and PO_2 in the blood, we can state this idea applied to ventilation as $VO_2 = V_A \times$ (atm − alv O_2 difference). We can simplify the concentration of oxygen in the atmosphere and alveoli as $(PO_2 - P_AO_2)/P_{atm}$, where PO_2 is the partial pressure of oxygen in the atmosphere, P_AO_2 is the partial pressure of oxygen in the alveolus, and Patm is the barometric pressure. Rearranging the formulas, we can state that $P_AO_2 = PO_2 - (VO_2 \times P_{atm})/V_A$. Using examples in which we have a typical value of oxygen consumption of 250 ml/min with different degrees of alveolar ventilation, we can see how alveolar gas composition varies. With a typical value of V_A of 6000 ml/min, P_AO_2 is 118 mmHg. If VO_2 were to remain at 250 ml/min, but V_A were increased to 8000 ml/min, P_AO_2 would be increased to 126 mm Hg. However, if VO_2 were to remain at 250 ml/min, and VA were decreased to 2000 ml/min as in the example of panic breathing above, P_AO_2 would fall to 55 mmHg. As these examples demonstrate, the greater the rate of V_A relative to VO_2, the closer the alveolar PO_2 comes to atmospheric PO_2. This equation also makes the point that if we need to maintain alveolar PO_2 during increased oxygen consumption (eg, during exercise, we need to increase V_A in proportion to the increase in oxygen consumption). As we will see in the next chapter, PO_2 of the arterial blood will equilibrate with alveolar PO_2. Thus, poor alveolar ventilation results in low levels of oxygen in the arterial blood, and, because PO_2 is the driving force for diffusion of oxygen into tissues, tissue PO_2 would be decreased as well.

LUNG VOLUMES

Several lung volumes have been described that relate to lung function. Some of these volumes can be measured easily with a spirometer (respirometer), whereas others must be measured indirectly (Figure 24-3). Measurement of these lung volumes can distinguish clearly among different breathing disorders. Tidal volume (V_T) has already been defined above as the volume of air taken in with each normal inspiration or expired with normal expiration. Functional residual capacity (FRC) is an important volume both from the viewpoint of differential diagnosis of lung disease and to understand the mechanical processes of ventilation. FRC is the volume of air present in the lungs at the end of normal expiration. Because all respiratory muscles are relaxed, this volume represents the result of equilibrium between forces of the chest wall directed outwardly and those of the lung tissues directed inwardly. Residual volume (RV) is the volume of air that remains in the lungs after maximal expiration. Because muscles of forced expiration are used to create a positive pressure in the thorax, small airways collapse and trap a volume of air in the alveoli. A greater effort of forced expiration at this lung volume does not produce any greater removal of air from the lungs because of the collapse of the airways. Inspiratory reserve volume (IRV) is the volume of air that can be inspired beyond the normal tidal volume. Thus, it represents the reserve for increasing ventilatory volume with increased demand for ventilation. A similar concept applies to the expiratory reserve volume (ERV). This is the volume of air that can be expired beyond the normal tidal volume, and it represents our reserve for forced expiration. Using the volumes described above, the following relationships become apparent: FRC = ERV + RV, and FRC + V_T + IRV represents the total capacity of the lungs for air, which is called total lung capacity (TLC). Total lung capacity can be expressed as either TLC = RV + ERV + V_T + IRV or TLC = RV + vital capacity (VC). Vital capacity is measured as the volume of air that can be expired after a maximal inspiration or can be computed as IRV + V_T + ERV. Two other terms that are sometimes used are inspiratory capacity = IRV + V_T and expiratory capacity = ERV + V_T.

FUNCTIONAL RESIDUAL CAPACITY

An understanding of lung mechanics revolves around the concept of the functional residual capacity.

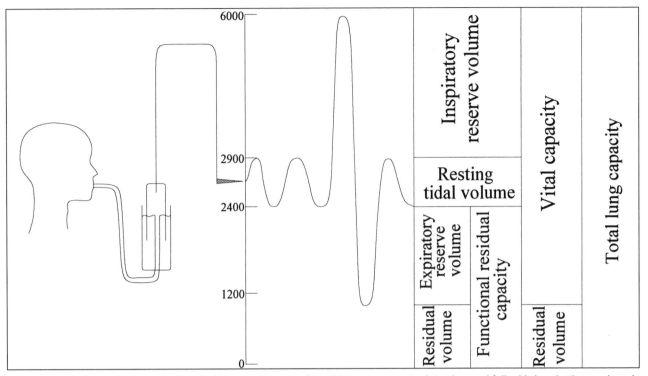

Figure 24-3. Lung volumes as recorded by a spirometer. Breathing causes a tank to rise and fall with inspiration and expiration. A pen records the movement of the tank on a revolving drum. Various maneuvers can be recorded. Vital capacity is recorded as the volume of air that can be maximally expired following a maximal inspiration. Inspiratory reserve volume is calculated as the volume increase above tidal volume, and expiratory reserve volume is calculated as the volume that can be expired beyond tidal volume. Note that, because residual volume cannot be directly measured with a spirometer, functional residual capacity and total lung volume cannot be determined by spirometry. These measurements require a dilution technique.

As described above, functional residual capacity is a static lung volume that exists when respiratory muscles are relaxed and is, therefore, created by the passive forces acting on the alveoli. Surface tension and elastic fibers surrounding alveoli tend to make the lungs collapse, whereas the elastic properties of the chest wall (ribs) tend to make the chest wall spring out. The alveolar forces and chest wall forces are not allowed to act independently due to the presence of the pleura. The pleura is a double-layered tissue that surrounds each lung. One layer, called the parietal pleura, attaches to the chest wall, and the other layer, called the visceral pleura, attaches to the surface of the lung. The two layers are separated by a small volume of pleural fluid that allows the two layers to slide across each other and, more importantly, opposes the tendency of the two layers of pleura to be pulled apart by the oppositely directed forces of the alveoli and chest wall, just as pulling two sheets of glass apart becomes difficult with water between them (Figure 24-4).

The chest wall pulls the parietal pleura outward as the lungs pull the visceral pleura inward. The oppositely directed forces produce a negative pressure between layers of pleura according to Boyle's law. Boyle's law states that pressure and volume are inversely related for a fixed number of molecules and temperature. An increased volume for a given number of molecules decreases pressure; therefore, the oppositely directed forces on the two layers of pleura create a subatmospheric pressure within the pleural space, which is called the intrapleural pressure. The greater the force pulling the two layers of pleura apart, the more negative the intrapleural pressure becomes. The elastic structures of the lungs and chest wall behave as springs in which the greater the structures are stretched, the greater their restoring forces become in accordance with Hooke's law. The behavior of the ribs can be likened to that of an archery bow and that of the alveoli to a party balloon (Figure 24-5).

Pressures within the respiratory system have historically been measured in cm H_2O because of the use of water-filled U-tube manometers. This allows small pressure changes to be read more easily than could be seen in millimeters of mercury. At equilibrium, intrapleural pressure is –5 cm H_2O. This negative pressure pulls the chest wall inward until the ribs have a restoring force of

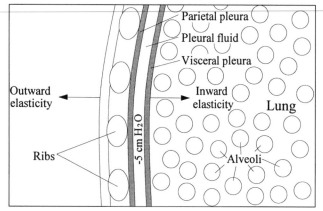

Figure 24-4. Factors determining functional residual capacity (FRC). The normal chest wall has elasticity directed outward, similar to an archery bow. Left to itself, the chest wall would spring out. Alveoli have elasticity directed inward, similar to an inflated balloon. Left to themselves, alveoli would collapse. The presence of the double-layered pleura with its pleural fluid creates a balance of forces across the chest. The lung volume at which the negative intrapleural pressure is equal and opposite to the pressure caused by the elasticity of the chest wall outward and equal and opposite to the pressure caused by elasticity of the alveoli inward is the FRC. For the lungs to assume any volume other than FRC requires another force to disturb the equilibrium of inward and outward forces. Inspiration is created when muscles of inspiration aid the movement of the chest wall outward. Forced expiration is created when abdominal muscles aid the movement of the alveoli inward.

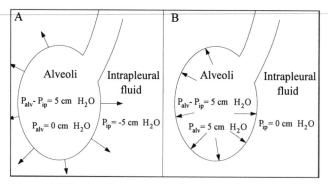

Figure 24-5. Alveolar movement with negative and positive pressure ventilation. In panel A, an alveolus increases in volume due to a negative pressure surrounding it. This situation is produced by a device such as an iron lung. This situation is also caused by the creation of a greater negative pressure in the intrapleural space caused by contraction of muscles of inspiration. In panel B, alveolar volume is increased by applying positive pressure through the airways. This situation is produced by modern ventilators. Note that the result, in terms of increased alveolar volume, is the same whether it is produced by a negative pressure outside the alveolus or a positive pressure inside the alveolus.

5 cm H_2O directly outwardly. At the same time, the negative intrapleural pressure pulls the alveoli open until the alveolar walls have a restoring force of 5 cm H_2O directed inwardly. The intrapleural pressure of -5 cm H_2O produces equilibrium at the volume called FRC.

The integrity of the pleura can be compromised by a wound through the chest wall due to a motor vehicle accident, stab wound, or other injury. When this occurs, intrapleural pressure equals atmospheric pressure, eliminating the ability of the chest wall and alveoli to influence each other. The inward recoil of the lungs unopposed by intrapleural pressure causes the lungs to collapse, and the outwardly directed recoil of the chest wall unopposed by any negative intrapleural pressure allows it to spring out. This condition is termed pneumothorax or collapsed lung (Figure 24-6). Pneumothorax is usually unilateral and is obvious to even the untrained observer as one side of the chest becomes much larger than the other. The defect in the chest wall must be repaired and the negative intrapleural pressure restored by removal of air and excess fluid from the intrapleural space via a chest tube attached to suction. The same problem occurs with blood accumulation in the pleural

space (hemothorax) or a combination of air and blood in the pleural space (hemopneumothorax), which can also be caused by trauma. Another type of trauma affecting lung mechanics is flail chest, in which multiple ribs are fractured at more than one place. Within the fractured segment, the ability of the chest wall to spring out is lost. In these areas, paradoxical chest wall movement occurs in which the chest moves inward during inspiration and outward during expiration similar to what happens with paralysis of the intercostal muscles.

Alteration of lung volume from the equilibrium position of FRC is accomplished by additional forces that either aid movement of the chest wall outwardly or collapse of the alveoli inwardly. At FRC, the intrapleural pressure equals -5 cm H_2O. Altering the lung volume requires altering the intrapleural pressure from this value. As intrapleural pressure becomes more negative, alveoli are pulled open more in accordance with Hooke's law, and air flows into the lungs. As intrapleural pressure returns to -5 cm H_2O, the restoring force of the stretched alveoli drives air out of the lungs until FRC is attained. Pulling the chest wall outward by the muscles of inspiration produces a more negative intrapleural pressure, whereas compressing the abdominal contents and displacing them upwards during forced expiration by contracting the abdominal wall muscles creates a positive intrapleural pressure to decrease lung volume below FRC and toward RV (Figure 24-7).

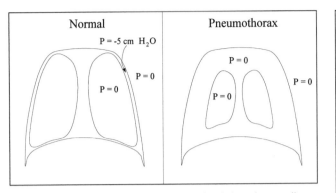

Figure 24-6. Pneumothorax. A breach of the pleura allows the natural elasticity of the chest wall to expand the chest and the natural elasticity of the lungs to collapse. Note that each lung has its own pleura so that a breach of one pleura still allows ventilation to occur. The effectiveness of breathing in oxygenating blood is diminished in unilateral pneumothorax, whereas bilateral pneumothorax prevents ventilation totally.

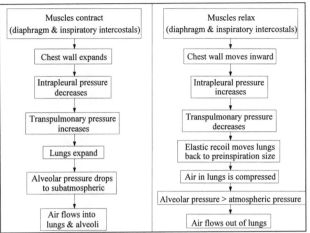

Figure 24-7. Flow chart of the events of tidal volume inspiration (left) and expiration (right).

SURFACTANT AND LUNG COMPLIANCE

Inspiration is produced by increasing the volume of alveoli, which, in turn, decreases alveolar pressure as predicted by Boyle's law. The increased alveolar volume, as described above, is produced by the negative intrapleural pressure surrounding the alveoli. When the volume of the lung is not changing, alveolar pressure is in equilibrium with the atmosphere. Using atmospheric pressure as a reference point, we say that alveolar pressure equals zero. Because the intrapleural pressure is less than atmospheric pressure, we say it is negative; and when pressure exceeds atmospheric pressure, we say it is positive. How much alveolar volume changes with a change in intrapleural pressure is dependent on the compliance of the lung (C_L). Lung compliance is defined as the volume of the lungs divided by transpulmonary pressure. Transpulmonary pressure is defined as the difference in pressure between the alveoli and pleural space (P_{alv} – P_{ip}). When alveolar pressure equals atmospheric pressure, transpulmonary pressure equals intrapleural pressure. The equation for lung compliance is $C_L = V/(P_{alv} - P_{ip})$. With low lung compliance (stiff lungs), a greater transpulmonary pressure must be generated by the muscles of inspiration, which means a greater muscular effort must be exerted to inspire a given volume. Compliance is decreased by alveolar edema, fibrosis, lack of inflation (atelectasis), and high surface tension (described below) in the alveoli. Because of the greater effort to stretch stiff lungs, more shallow, rapid breathing becomes energetically efficient. With excessively high lung compliance, the elastic recoil generated by

stretching the alveoli is lost. With normal expiration, the restoring force of the stretched alveoli is used to produce expiration. Therefore, diseases in which the lungs become too compliant result in difficulty in expiration. Compliance is increased in aging and emphysema.

Surface tension is a force across the surface of a liquid produced by the attraction of water molecules to each other by hydrogen bonds. This force is strong enough to allow insects to walk across water and to move water up 100-foot tall trees. Forces between adjacent molecules of water or other liquids are stronger than those between liquid and gas and cause bubbles to form. Wall tension is produced in bubbles by the hydrogen bonds between water molecules. According to the law of LaPlace, the smaller the bubble's radius, the greater the pressure inside ($P = 2\tau/r$). As a consequence of this prediction of the law of LaPlace, small bubbles will coalesce into large bubbles. The 300 million individual alveoli of the lungs can be considered as bubbles for the sake of this discussion. Inflation of the lungs must overcome the surface tension of the individual alveoli and, at the same time, stabilize the alveoli to prevent the collapse of smaller alveoli into larger alveoli. For many years, investigators tried to solve this problem. As predicted by the known effects of surface tension and the law of LaPlace, lungs inflated with saline were shown to have much greater compliance than lungs inflated with air because of the lack of a liquid-air interface and, therefore, a lack of surface tension. In 1957, it was observed that fluid draining from edematous lungs formed stable bubbles in contradiction with the law of LaPlace. Therefore, something in lungs must lower surface tension. This surface-active substance was given the

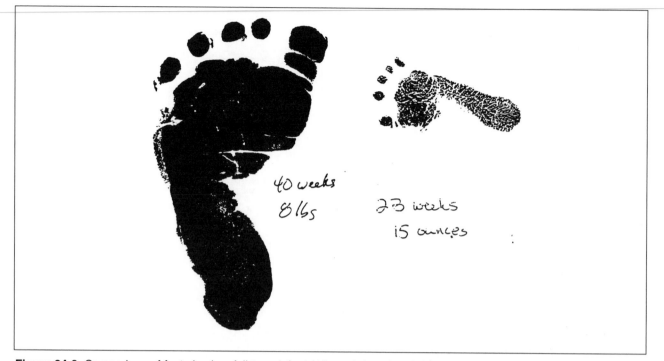

40 weeks
8 lbs

23 weeks
15 ounces

Figure 24-8. Comparison of foot size in a full-term infant (40 weeks) and an infant born prematurely (23 weeks). Although organs are formed by this time, tremendous growth and maturation continues. The lungs, in particular, are not mature at this time and are often not capable of producing surfactant, resulting in respiratory distress syndrome.

name surfactant. Since that time, it has been discovered that surfactant consists of a group of phospholipid molecules synthesized by type II cells.

Surfactant molecules have a hydrophilic and hydrophobic end. These surfactant molecules repel each other and dissolve between water molecules to diminish the attraction of water molecules for each other. Surfactant, by reducing surface tension, increases lung compliance (reduces the transpulmonary pressure required to attain a given lung volume), prevents collapse of alveoli into larger bubbles, and prevents movement of water into the alveoli from the interstitial space. Surfactant is produced shortly before birth and is synthesized rapidly upon initiation of breathing.

Lack of surfactant in premature infants produces respiratory distress syndrome (RDS). A child with RDS has stiff lungs, areas of atelectasis (partial collapse of the lung), and fluid in the alveoli as one would predict based on the roles of surfactant. The risk of RDS increases with the degree of prematurity. Normal gestation is 40 weeks. During the last trimester of gestation, fetal size more than doubles, and the ability to produce surfactant begins (Figure 24-8). A child born before 28 weeks of gestation is at very high risk of developing RDS. Respiratory distress syndrome was once almost uniformly fatal before the use of mechanical ventilators to support the neonate until adequate surfactant production

began, but even with ventilators, mortality was high. Today, the problem can be more directly solved by using surfactant replacement either from animal lung extracts or recombinant human surfactant.

Another form of respiratory distress is called adult or acute respiratory distress syndrome (ARDS). This disease process is much more complicated but has a similar result in which the lung loses its ability to produce surfactant and the lungs become stiff. The complexity of ARDS does not allow simple surfactant replacement alone to be an effective treatment. Today, the mortality of ARDS is about 50%.

LUNG MECHANICS

The breathing cycle, similar to the cardiac cycle, consists of pressure and volume changes that occur in a cycle, with a work period and a rest period. Inspiration, like systole, is approximately one-third of the respiratory cycle; and expiration, like diastole, is about two-thirds. Just as bulk flow of blood through the circulatory system can be described using Ohm's law, so can bulk flow of air through the airways as $Q = (P_{atm} - P_{alv})/R$. Alveolar pressure is altered according to Boyle's law, just as with intrapleural pressure. When the alveoli increase in size with the same number of air molecules within,

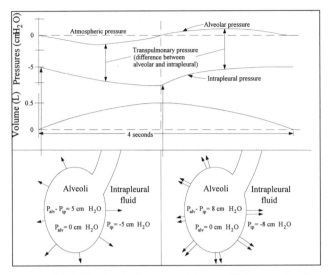

Figure 24-9. Mechanical events of the ventilatory cycle. The top panel depicts the pressure changes that result from contraction of muscles of inspiration to aid the outward movement of the chest wall. The changes in intrapleural and alveolar pressure and alveolar volume are also depicted in the top panel. In the lower left panel, resting alveolar conditions are depicted, and the change in alveolar pressure and dimensions is depicted in the lower right panel.

pressure falls. Alveolar pressure becomes subatmospheric, causing air to flow from the atmosphere into the alveoli. Expiration is a passive process. When respiratory muscles relax, the alveoli resume their resting size due to the elastic forces of the lungs and chest wall returning their equilibrium positions. When the muscles of inspiration relax, pressure within the alveoli increases according to the equation for compliance: $C_L = \Delta V / \Delta P_{transpulmonary}$. The energy provided by respiratory muscles to cause air to enter the lungs stretches alveoli and produces a restoring force that causes alveolar recoil and expiration until alveolar pressure again becomes equal to atmospheric pressure; at this time, outward flow ceases.

The change in the size of the alveoli during ventilation is determined by the transpulmonary pressure. At FRC, this difference in pressure is 5 cm H_2O. When the chest wall moves outward due to the pull of the muscles of inspiration, intrapleural pressure becomes more negative, becoming –9 cm H_2O with a normal inspiratory movement. As intrapleural pressure becomes more negative, the transpulmonary pressure forces the alveoli to become larger. As the alveoli enlarge, alveolar pressure becomes less than atmospheric in accordance with Boyle's law. The difference in pressure between the alveolus and atmosphere causes air to enter alveoli. Air continues to enter the alveoli until alveolar pressure returns to zero. The increased stretch on the alveolar wall

caused by inspiration increases the restoring force of the alveolus in proportion to the increased alveolar volume. The rate at which air enters or leaves the lungs, however, is dependent on the resistance of the airways as well as the difference in pressure.

As inspiration occurs, the flow of air into alveoli causes alveolar pressure to approach atmospheric pressure, and alveolar pressure during normal breathing does not become much greater than –1 cm H_2O. If the airways were occluded while the chest wall is pulled out, alveolar pressure would instead reach about –4 cm H_2O. Sudden release of the occlusion would cause rapid flow of air into the lungs. This can be demonstrated by attempting to inspire against a closed glottis. Take a deep breath with the glottis closed. You will feel your ribs moving outwardly but no flow of air. Open the glottis and air will rapidly fill the lungs. With normal breathing and an open glottis, the initiation of airflow as the intrapleural pressure becomes more negative prevents alveolar pressure from becoming more negative than –1 cm H_2O. At the end of inspiration, transpulmonary pressure is approximately 9 cm H_2O (4 cm H_2O greater than what exists at FRC) and does not return to 5 cm H_2O until the muscles of inspiration relax. At the end of inspiration, the alveoli have a restoring force, tending to collapse the alveoli equal to 9 cm H_2O, and the lung volume at end inspiration is equal to that which would be achieved by a positive pressure of 9 cm H_2O blowing air into the lungs. The restoring force of the alveoli, which is equal to 4 cm H_2O greater than that under resting conditions, becomes the driving force for expiration when the inspiratory muscles relax and intrapleural pressure returns toward –5 cm H_2O. Alveolar pressure becomes positive as the inspiratory muscles relax, and the restoring force of the stretched alveoli drives air from the alveoli into the atmosphere until resting conditions are restored such that the restoring force of the alveoli is equal and opposite to the intrapleural pressure (Figure 24-10).

Inspiration does not inflate the lungs equally but, in healthy lungs, produces greater ventilation of the dependent (lower) part of the lung. During standing, the apex of the lung is not ventilated as much as the base of the lung, and in supine, the anterior part of the lungs is not ventilated as well as the posterior of the lungs. Two reasons linked to the acceleration of gravity cause this phenomenon. Due to the weight of the lungs, the uppermost alveoli are stretched the most, and the lowermost alveoli are stretched the least. Many people have termed this the slinky effect because this phenomenon can be demonstrated by holding a slinky vertically. The uppermost turns of the coiled spring are stretched farther apart than the lower turns. Because of this effect,

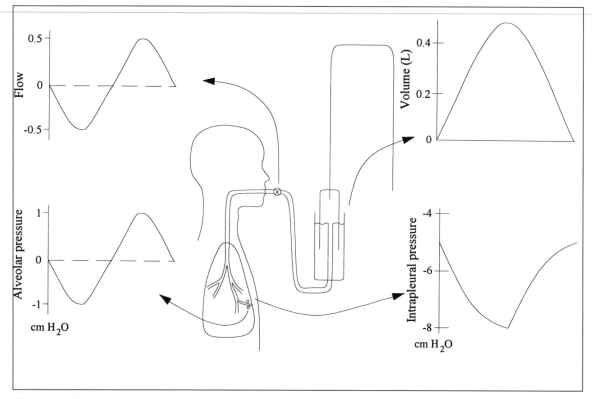

Figure 24-10. Mechanical events of the ventilatory cycle at the level of the whole lung. Changes in flow, alveolar pressure, lung volume, and intrapleural pressure are depicted.

the lower part of the lung is more compliant and can be stretched more by inspiration. Moreover, gravity causes a more negative intrapleural pressure at rest at the apex of the lung as the visceral pleura is pulled from the parietal pleura by the weight of the dependent part of the lungs, which also creates less compliant alveoli in the uppermost parts of the lung.

MECHANICAL VENTILATION

Forcing air into the lungs by producing a positive pressure outside the alveoli is called positive pressure ventilation. In terms of producing the difference in pressure needed for bulk flow of air, positive pressure ventilation is equivalent to producing a negative alveolar pressure and allowing atmospheric pressure to drive flow into the lungs. This is the method used by modern ventilators. The iron lung used commonly during the polio epidemic was a negative-pressure ventilator. An airtight chamber surrounding the thorax generated a subatmospheric pressure around the thorax that allows atmospheric pressure to drive airflow into the lungs. Negative-pressure ventilators are more difficult to manage than positive-pressure ventilators that can be hooked up to an

endotracheal tube. However, positive-pressure ventilators have disadvantages including damage produced by inserting an endotracheal tube and injury to the airways caused by the positive pressure, producing a condition called bronchopulmonary dysplasia.

Ventilators and modes of ventilation were designed to support breathing in a person with healthy lungs undergoing surgery or during paralysis. Ventilation of diseased lungs creates a vastly different interaction between airways and positive pressure. In lung disease, the dependent alveoli are collapsed by the weight of the lung tissue and the heart compressing the lungs against the posterior chest wall in the supine position, and atelectasis (partial collapse of the lung) results. Positive-pressure ventilation damages the dependent part of the lung by cyclic opening and closing of alveoli, which produces a shearing effect. In the upper part (anterior, in supine) of the lungs, the alveoli are distended by the weight of the lungs below. The high pressure exerted to open the dependent airways can damage alveoli that are already overdistended. Damage by positive pressure ventilation can be minimized by frequent position changes and adding continuous positive airway pressure (CPAP) to prevent collapse of dependent alveoli.

OBSTRUCTIVE AND RESTRICTIVE DISEASES

Breathing disorders are placed in two categories called obstructive and restrictive diseases. These diseases result from abnormal compliance of the lung or increased airway resistance. Lung volume for a given transpulmonary pressure is determined by lung compliance. With normal airway resistance, which is decreased by lateral traction during inspiration, a maximum pressure difference between the atmosphere and alveoli of only 1 to 2 cm H_2O is sufficient for ventilation. Decreased compliance requires greater muscular effort to establish normal transpulmonary pressure, which increases the work of breathing (WOB) and produces restrictive disease. However, a greater than normal compliance creates an equally serious problem. Because the elastic recoil of the lungs is used to drive flow out of the lungs during expiration, a normal tidal volume taken into lungs with high compliance results in a small restoring force in the alveolar walls that is inadequate for expiration. In emphysema, elastic fibers of the lungs are destroyed, resulting in lungs with high compliance. Functional residual capacity increases progressively as compliance increases in order to produce sufficient elastic recoil for expiration. Breathing disorders can also be caused by increased airway resistance. Increased airway resistance requires greater stretching of the alveoli to generate sufficient elastic recoil to produce adequate expiratory flow, which produces the same problem with breathing as emphysema. Therefore, both increased compliance and increased airway resistance produce obstructive disease.

Obstructive diseases are called such because they have characteristics associated with what would occur with physical obstruction of the airways. A greater difference between P_{alv} and P_{atm} is required to obtain the same expiratory airflow as a normal individual. Creating a more negative intrapleural pressure increases work of breathing. As disease progresses, the volume of air expired decreases until the lungs are stretched enough to produce sufficient elastic recoil to make inspiratory and expiratory volume equal. Loss of elastic recoil causes the outwardly directed chest wall elastic forces to overcome the weaker lung elastic forces, resulting in increased FRC and residual volume. A characteristic change in the shape of the chest (barrel-chest) results if the disease is severe enough. Obstructive disease may be caused by increased airway resistance or increased lung compliance, which decreases elastic recoil of the lungs. The lack of recoil to produce expiration requires a greater lung volume to produce sufficient flow during expiration. Obstructive diseases include asthma, bronchiectasis, chronic bronchitis, and emphysema. The first letters of these diseases, ABCE, can be used to remember what diseases belong in this category. Bronchiectasis is a condition in which airways (usually in the lower part of the lung) are plugged with mucus. A common cause of bronchiectasis is cystic fibrosis, a genetic disease in which the mucus of the lung becomes thick because of a defect in chloride ion active transport.

Restrictive diseases have characteristics associated with a physical restriction of chest wall movement, as if a wide belt were fastened around the entire chest. A person with restrictive disease requires greater effort for a given inspiratory flow rate but does not require a greater $P_{alv} - P_{atm}$ to drive inspiratory flow, unless the person also has an obstructive disease. In restrictive disease, the outwardly directed elastic force of the chest wall is overcome by increased inward elastic forces of the alveoli. A decrease occurs in FRC, residual volume, and all of the measured lung volumes. Restrictive disease may be caused by any factor that decreases lung compliance, such as edema, fibrosis, increased surface tension of the alveoli, or by any condition that impairs the ability to move the chest wall outward, such as weak inspiratory muscles, neurologic disease or injury, or deformities of the chest wall. Diseases include RDS, ARDS, neuromuscular diseases, chest wall deformities, and fibrosis caused by diseases, such as rheumatoid arthritis, systemic lupus erythematosus, and scleroderma. Pneumoconioses are caused by the chronic inflammation associated with exposure to coal dust, beryllium, silica, asbestosis, cotton, and other nondegradable substances. Pneumoconiosis causes fibrosis of the lungs and severe restrictive lung disease.

WORK OF BREATHING

Under normal circumstances, only a small fraction of the oxygen consumed is used to support the work of breathing. In a person with a breathing disorder, the fraction of oxygen consumed by ventilation can approach 50% or more. In restrictive disease, more muscular effort is required to produce a normal intrapleural pressure. In obstructive disease, work is increased by the need to create a more negative intrapleural pressure to generate airflow. Because alveolar ventilation can be generated by a combination of V_T and frequency, an optimal combination must be sought to minimize WOB. In lungs with normal compliance, a rate of breathing of 12 to 15 per minute at a V_T of 300 to 500 ml is optimal in terms of WOB. If lungs are stiff, a normal V_T requires too much work to be accomplished efficiently. As discussed previously with a stiff aorta, a faster rate and smaller volume is energetically more efficient. This can also be seen with maturation of the lungs. Compliance of the lungs increases as lung size increases with growth. Frequency is much higher in newborns and decreases with growth and development until adult size is reached. You will need to remember this difference in frequency and volume with age to pass your CPR exam. In lungs with high airway resistance, WOB is increased in opening airways to initiate inspiration. In this case, increased V_T with a lower frequency is more energetically efficient.

HYPOXIA

Four types of hypoxia have been described: hypoxic hypoxia, which is also called hypoxemia, anemic hypoxia, ischemic hypoxia, and histotoxic hypoxia. Hypoxic hypoxia is characterized by a low PO_2 of arterial blood and can be caused by breathing in a low atmospheric PO_2 (high altitude), breathing disorders, or abnormal circulation that causes deoxygenated blood to be returned to the systemic circulation. Anemic hypoxia is characterized by a normal PO_2 of the blood but a decreased O_2 content of blood. Anemic hypoxia can be caused by decreased hematocrit, decreased or abnormal hemoglobin, or by carbon monoxide poisoning. Hemoglobin has a much greater affinity for carbon monoxide than for oxygen; therefore, carbon monoxide decreases the oxygen-carrying capacity of blood. Ischemic hypoxia results from insufficient blood flow to carry oxygen to tissues in spite of normal PO_2 and O_2 content of the blood. Ischemic hypoxia is usually caused by arterial disease. Histotoxic hypoxia is the result of a derangement of mitochondrial function so that a normal amount of O_2 may reach the cells, but the cells are unable to use O_2. The derangement is usually caused by a poison, such as cyanide, that prevents use of O_2 by the cells. A given individual may experience more than one type of hypoxia simultaneously, resulting in severe tissue injury. For example, a person with existing coronary artery disease may suffer a myocardial infarction with superimposed anemia or hypoxemia.

SUMMARY

The muscles of ventilation include the diaphragm, external and internal intercostals, scalenes, and sternocleidomastoids. The diaphragm is the primary muscle of inspiration during rest. Intercostals stiffen the chest wall and aid in the upward and outward movement of the ribs. The scalenes and sternocleidomastoids become active during more vigorous breathing and in lung disease. Normal expiration is a passive process that uses the energy stored in the alveolar walls to drive air out. Abdominal muscles are used in forced expiration. Minute ventilation is the product of tidal volume and frequency. Tidal volume is the amount of air inspired or expired with a normal breath. Alveolar ventilation accounts for the ventilation of dead space. Hyperventilation, by definition, produces a reduction in arterial PCO_2, whereas hypoventilation produces an increased arterial PCO_2. The volume of air in the lungs following a normal expiration and with the muscles of ventilation at rest is called the functional residual capacity. Altering the lung volume from FRC requires expenditure of energy through muscle contraction. The volume of air that can be inspired above a normal inspiration is called the inspiratory reserve volume. The volume that can be forced out beyond a normal expiration is the expiratory reserve volume. The volume left in the lung after maximal expiration is the residual volume. Total lung capacity is the volume of gas present in the lung following maximal inspiration. Vital capacity is total lung capacity minus the residual volume and represents the maximal change in lung volume, usually measured as maximal expiration following a maximal inspiration. Ventilation is a product of tidal volume and frequency. Part of the tidal volume ventilates the anatomic dead space and is not effective in exchange of gases.

Very high frequencies of breathing, which may occur with panic, are associated with a shallow tidal volume that primarily ventilates the dead space and produces little exchange of gases between the blood and environment. FRC is determined by the opposite elastic forces present in the chest wall and alveoli. The tendencies of the alveoli to collapse and the chest wall to spring out pull the two layers of the pleura apart and generates a negative intrapleural pressure. This negative pressure produces equilibrium at the lung volume called FRC at which the elastic force of the chest wall is equal and opposite to the intrapleural pressure and the elastic force of the alveoli is also equal and opposite to the intrapleural pressure.

Muscles of inspiration assist the chest wall in moving outward against the elastic recoil of the lung to produce inspiration. Relaxation of the inspiratory muscles allows expiration to occur passively as the energy used to stretch the alveoli is used to drive air out. Compliance of the lung refers to the change in volume per difference in pressure between the alveoli and the intrapleural space. Low compliance requires a greater effort to produce inspiration; high compliance results in an insufficient elastic recoil to produce expiration. Surface tension results from the cohesion of water molecules at the air-liquid interface. Muscular force is required to pull the water molecules apart. Increased surface tension produces stiff lungs. Surfactant secreted by type II alveolar cells decreases the cohesive forces between water molecules and increases lung compliance. Decreased surfactant in either respiratory distress syndrome of the neonate (RDS) or adult (acute) respiratory distress syndrome produces a positive feedback cycle of decreased ventilation and increasing stiffness of the lungs.

Outward movement of the chest wall during inspiration creates a more negative intrapleural pressure as the two layers of pleura are pulled farther apart. The difference in pressure between the intrapleural space and alveoli (transpulmonary pressure) increases with outward movement of the chest wall, which increases alveolar volume and, therefore, decreases alveolar pressure. The negative pressure in the alveoli then generates the pressure difference necessary for flow of air into the alveoli from the atmosphere until enough air enters the lung to return alveolar pressure to atmospheric pressure. Relaxation of the inspiratory muscles approximates the two layers of pleura, causing the intrapleural pressure to return to its resting value. The elastic recoil of the alveoli then exceeds the intrapleural pressure, causing a positive transpulmonary pressure. The positive pressure in the alveoli drives air out of the lungs until FRC is attained.

Forced expiration causes a greater positive pressure on the alveoli and drives lung volume to a value less than FRC. Airway collapse due to positive pressure in the thorax limits the amount and the rate of forced expiration. Due to the weight of the lungs, the uppermost alveoli are stretched the most, and the lowermost alveoli, least (slinky effect). Obstructive disease causes an increase in residual volume and FRC to a value that produces sufficient driving force for expiration. Because of the difficulty in initiating expiration, a slow deep breathing pattern is more efficient. In restrictive disease, all lung volumes are decreased, but the rate of expiration can be greater due to increased lung recoil. Rapid, shallow breathing is more efficient when greater effort is required to produce transpulmonary pressure necessary for breathing. The greater the rate of ventilation relative to oxygen uptake, the closer the PO_2 of alveolar air comes to atmospheric air. PCO_2 decreases with increased ventilation. Four types of hypoxia are described. Hypoxic hypoxia is a decreased arterial PO_2. Anemic hypoxia is caused by a decreased oxygen-carrying capacity of the blood. Ischemic hypoxia is caused by insufficient blood flow to meet oxygen demands. Histotoxic hypoxia results from an inability of the tissues to use oxygen due to a metabolic derangement, usually cyanide poisoning.

BIBLIOGRAPHY

Hole JW Jr. *Essentials of Human Anatomy and Physiology.* 4th ed. Dubuque, Iowa: Wm. C. Brown Publishers; 1992.

Schauf C, Moffett D, Moffett S. *Human Physiology: Foundation and Frontiers.* St. Louis, Mo: Times Mirror/Mosby College Publishing; 1990.

Solomon EP, Davis PW. *Human Anatomy and Physiology.* Philadelphia, Pa: WB Saunders; 1983.

VanGolde LMG, Batenburg JJ, Robertson B. The pulmonary surfactant system. *News in Physiological Sciences.* 1994;9:13-20.

West JB. Respiratory *Physiology: The Essentials.* 4th ed. Baltimore, Md: Williams & Wilkins; 1990.

West JB, Mathieu-Costello O. Pulmonary blood-gas barrier: a physiological dilemma. *News in Physiological Sciences.* 1993;8:249-253.

STUDY QUESTIONS

1. What is the primary muscle of inspiration? What happens to the effectiveness of this muscle without the supporting roles of the abdominal muscles and intercostal muscles?

2. Describe the roles of the intercostal and abdominal muscles in inspiration.

3. How could an abdominal binder help breathing in a person with paralyzed abdominal muscles?

4. Draw a diagram showing residual volume, expiratory reserve volume, tidal volume, and inspiratory reserve volume. Draw another diagram showing functional residual capacity, tidal volume, and inspiratory reserve capacity. From a functional standpoint, how are these two diagrams related? What do we call the sum of expiratory reserve volume, tidal volume, and inspiratory reserve volume? What do we call the volume if we add residual volume?

5. What happens to the effectiveness of ventilation if a person's tidal volume in milliliters is approximately the same as the person's weight in pounds?

6. Explain the roles of surfactant. Why does a positive feedback of decreased lung compliance occur in adult respiratory distress syndrome?

7. Explain why alveolar pressure does not become more than -1 cm H_2O when intrapleural pressure becomes increasingly negative during inspiration. How can you demonstrate this effect?

8. In the healthy lung, what part receives the greatest ventilation? How is this different in lung disease?

9. How does residual volume change in restrictive disease? In obstructive disease?

10. What is the functional importance of an increased FRC in obstructive disease?

11. Explain how increased compliance and increased airway resistance produce a similar breathing problem.

12. Contrast the characteristics of the four types of hypoxia.

LABORATORY EXERCISE

LABORATORY EXERCISE 24-1

LUNG VOLUMES

Objective: Define and measure lung volumes.

A spirometer (respirometer) is used to measure lung volumes. Lung volumes of interest include: vital capacity (VC), tidal volume (VT), inspiratory reserve volume (IRV), expiratory reserve volume (ERV), functional residual volume (FRC), residual volume (RV), and sometimes inspiratory capacity (IC), which is equal to VT + IRV, and expiratory capacity (EC) which is equal to VT + ERV. The volume of the lungs at rest (no muscular contraction) is the FRC, which is equal to RV + ERV. Unfortunately RV cannot be measured directly but must be determined by helium dilution or nitrogen washout techniques. One may estimate RV of a normal, healthy individual based on a person's age and weight. RV changes with lung diseases, increasing with obstructive disease, and decreasing with restrictive disease.

The lung volumes are defined as follows:
VC: The maximum volume that can be expired after a maximum inspiration
V_T: Volume of air that is inspired in a normal breath (500 ml in a 70 kg adult)
IRV: The maximum volume that can be inspired beyond that of a normal breath
ERV: The maximum volume that can be expired after a normal expiration
FRC: The volume of the lungs when all ventilatory muscles are at rest; the volume produced by the passive forces tending to collapse the lungs opposed by the passive forces tending to move the chest wall out
RV: The volume that remains in the lung after maximum expiratory effort (1000 ml in a 70 kg adult)

FRC and RV cannot be recorded with a spirometer. A spirometer is only capable of measuring changes in volume that occur during inspiration and expiration. To obtain FRC and RV, dilution techniques involving helium or nitrogen may be used. The principle behind helium washout is that it is neither used nor generated by the body. Therefore, an amount of helium (concentration times volume) taken into the lungs does not change if the volume into which the gas is introduced changes, but the concentration will be diminished in a greater volume. A person expires to residual volume and then inspires from a tank containing a known volume and a known concentration of the inert gas. As helium is breathed back and forth the inert gas is diluted within the extra volume of the residual volume. The change in concentration of helium is used to compute the extra volume added to the system when the person began to breathe from residual volume. Mathematically: $C_1V_1 = C_2V_2$ in which C_1 and V_1 are the initial concentration of helium and the fixed volume of the gas system. C_2 is the final concentration after dilution within the residual volume and V_2 is the volume of the fixed system plus residual volume ($V_1 + RV$). By rearranging and substituting for V_2, we may then set up an equation to solve for residual volume as: $RV = (C_1V_1/C_2) - V_1$.

Evaluation of pulmonary function usually also includes measuring rates of air flow out of the lungs during expiration. Two important values are the forced vital capacity (FVC) and FEV_1. FVC is the volume of a rapid, maximum expiration following a maximum inspiration. FEV_1 is the volume of air that can be forcefully expired in one second. A decrease in the ratio of FEV_1/FVC is an indicator of obstructive lung disease. In restrictive disease, the ratio FEV_1/FVC may increase slightly as elastic recoil is greater than normal. Forced vital capacity may be lower than VC obtained at a slower rate of expiration because of earlier collapse of small airways.

LABORATORY EXERCISE

Materials:
Recording spirometer
Recording paper
Mouth pieces
Nose clips
Pulmonary function nomograms
Metric ruler

Methods:
1. Place a clean mouthpiece on the recording spirometer and noseclips on the subject.

2. Instruct the subject to take 8 to 10 normal breaths while recording at 1 mm/sec on the spirometer.

3. Instruct the subject to take a maximum inspiration, hold it for 1 second, then expire completely at a comfortable rate (at least 3 to 4 seconds) to obtain VC.

4. Repeat #3, instruct the subject to hold inspiration for at least 1 second before expiring as rapidly as possible to obtain forced vital capacity (FVC). Increase the speed of the recorder to 10 mm/sec so FEV_1 can be computed. Decrease the recorder speed back to 1 mm/sec as soon as the subject finishes complete expiration.

5. Using the first part of the record, measure VT, IRV, ERV, VC.

6. Using the second part of the record determine FEV_1/FVC as follows: FEV_1 is the volume of air expired after one second of FVC. Divide by the volume expired rapidly (FVC). Healthy adults should have a ratio of approximately 80%. A value of 60% or lower indicates significant obstructive disease. Restrictive disease tends to increase the ratio toward 90%, but the value of FVC is reduced markedly compared with a person without lung disease.

7. Compare values obtained for VC to the following equations after multiplying by 1.1 to correct for the water vapor content and the decreased volume of expired air as it cools in the room temperature spirometer. Check that FVC is within VC after 3 seconds of comfortable maximal expiration.

   For men, estimate VC = -3.18 + 0.136 x height (inches) - 0.22 x age (years)
   For women, multiply the result of the equation for men by 0.80 (80%)

TWENTY-FIVE

Transport of Gases

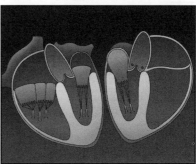

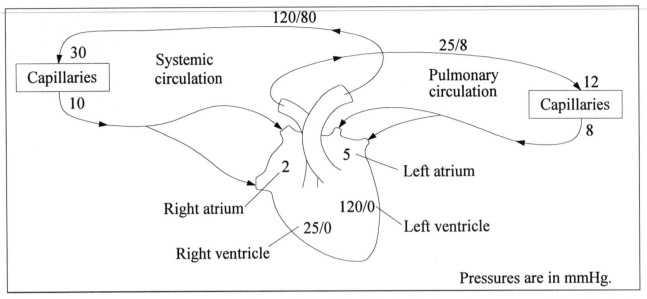

120/80

30
Capillaries
10

Systemic
circulation

25/8

Pulmonary
circulation

12
Capillaries
8

2

5

Left atrium

Right atrium

120/0

Left ventricle

25/0

Right ventricle

Pressures are in mmHg.

Figure 25-1. Comparison of the pulmonary and systemic circulation. Note the much greater pressures of the systemic circulation. The greater pressure allows for major adjustments in the distribution of blood flow to different organs in the systemic circulation in contrast to the more uniform distribution of the pulmonary circulation.

In a typical resting individual, 250 ml of O_2 are added to the blood, and 200 ml of CO_2 are eliminated to replace the O_2 consumed by tissues (VO_2) and CO_2 generated (VCO_2) each minute. This ratio of VO_2 to VCO_2 is called the respiratory quotient and varies under different conditions that will be described below. Blood flow through the lungs must take up as much O_2 from the alveoli as the tissues take up from the blood to maintain a steady state. To ensure exchange of O_2 from the alveolar air to the pulmonary capillaries, pulmonary blood flow must be adequate, alveolar ventilation must be adequate, and pulmonary capillary blood flow must be matched with alveolar ventilation (V_A). Of the 1050 ml of O_2 contained in the circulation, 25% needs to be replaced at rest. During heavy exercise, a greater amount of O_2 must be replenished. According to the Fick principle (VO_2 = CO x a-v O_2 difference), increased O_2 demand by tissues can be satisfied by either increased cardiac output or increased extraction of O_2 by the tissues (increased a-v O_2 difference). Both means require increased V_A to allow a slow blood flow past the alveoli to pick up a large amount of oxygen or a rapid blood flow past the alveoli to pick up a small amount of oxygen. Movement of gases across the alveoli occurs strictly by diffusion, with net movement from high to low PCO_2 and PO_2. In this chapter, the control of pulmonary blood flow, diffusion of gases, the matching of ventilation and perfusion (blood flow through the lung), and the transport of gases from the atmosphere to the tissues will be discussed.

PULMONARY BLOOD FLOW

The entire cardiac output of 5 to 6 L/min flows through the pulmonary circulation because the systemic and pulmonary circuits are in series. Total peripheral resistance of the systemic circulation is much greater than that of the pulmonary circulation because of the requirements of the systemic circulation to regulate blood flow to many different tissues that may vary in their individual needs from moment to moment. The pulmonary vessels are large, short, branch extensively, and do not need to redirect flow from one area to another to any large degree. Pulmonary pressures are very low compared to systemic pressure, with very little pressure decrease from arteries to arterioles to capillaries (Figure 25-1). The right heart with its thin wall is able to provide the pumping of blood through the circulation because of the low afterload.

The pulmonary circulation must be able to accept an increase in cardiac output caused by changes in the systemic circulation without a change in pulmonary pressure. This is accomplished because the pulmonary vessels respond differently to increased pressure than the systemic vessels (Figure 25-2). When pressure increases in the systemic arterioles, vasoconstriction occurs to maintain flow. This response is called pressure autoregulation. However, the response is just the opposite in the lungs. As pressure increases because of greater pumping of the right ventricle, pulmonary arteries and arterioles dilate to allow flow to increase without an

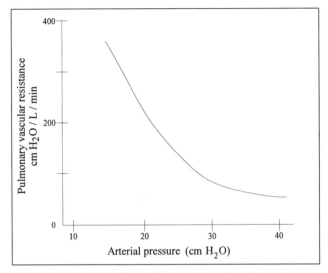

Figure 25-2. Effect of arterial pressure on pulmonary vascular resistance. In contrast to the systemic circulation, pulmonary arterial vessels dilate in response to increased pressure. This phenomenon allows pulmonary blood flow to increase with a relatively constant pulmonary pressure and avoids leakage of capillary fluid into the alveoli. In the systemic circulation, autoregulation provides a relatively constant flow in the face of changes in arterial pressure.

increase in pressure. Arterial pressure in the lungs must be regulated at a low value to prevent the filtration of fluid from capillaries into the interstitial space and alveoli. Pulmonary edema decreases the rate of diffusion of oxygen from the alveoli to the blood to a potentially life-threatening level.

Pulmonary arterial vessels also respond to oxygen in a manner opposite to that of most systemic vessels. In general, systemic vessels constrict in response to an elevated PO_2 and dilate as PO_2 falls, which acts to couple tissue metabolism and blood flow. The opposite response occurs in pulmonary vessels, which constrict in response to decreased PO_2. This vasoconstriction diverts blood flow from poorly ventilated areas of lungs to well-ventilated areas.

DIFFUSION OF OXYGEN FROM THE ALVEOLI TO THE BLOOD

Pulmonary capillaries branch so extensively over the surface of alveoli that they form a nearly continuous sheet of blood over the alveoli. At a resting cardiac output, the time spent by an individual red blood cell in the capillary is approximately 0.75 seconds. Under normal circumstances, this time is more than adequate; a normal red cell will equilibrate with the alveolar gas in 0.25 seconds. Even with a maximum cardiac output, the red

blood cell still has at least 0.25 seconds to load oxygen. Except in the most highly trained aerobic athletes, equilibrium occurs between the PO_2 of blood and alveolar gas. Therefore, the PO_2 of systemic arterial blood should be approximately equal to alveolar PO_2. In reality, a small difference exists that will be explained below. The time allowed for diffusion of oxygen across the alveoli may limit the ability to perform aerobic exercise, but only in individuals with extremely high aerobic capacities, perhaps two to 2.5 times that of an average person. In lung disease with diffusion impairment, red blood cells may be in capillaries long enough for equilibration with alveolar gas to occur at rest, but any increase in cardiac output occurring with increased activity level causes lack of equilibration and hypoxemia. As the lung disease progresses, equilibrium may not occur even at rest. In such cases, the individual will need to breathe air of a higher oxygen concentration than normal, usually through the use of a tank of compressed oxygen. The increased alveolar PO_2 is needed to produce enough diffusion to compensate for the increased barrier to diffusion. Oxygen from the tank is mixed with atmospheric air by changing the flow rate from the oxygen tank that is typically directed through a nasal cannula. Masks may also be used with a mixer valve to change the proportions of 100% oxygen and room air that enters the mask.

In the atmosphere with 760 mmHg pressure and 21% O_2, PO_2 is 160 mmHg, and PCO_2 is about 2 mmHg, while the alveolus maintains a PO_2 of approximately 105 mmHg and a PCO_2 of 40 mmHg. This discrepancy can be explained by two phenomena. First, inspired air is humidified to saturation with water vapor. The partial pressure of water at body temperature is 47 mmHg, reducing the partial pressure of other gases from 760 mmHg to 713 mmHg. Humidified air reaching the lungs has a PO_2 of 150 mmHg (21% of 713 = 150). Secondly, P_AO_2 is reduced by mixing of stale and fresh air. Removal of oxygen from the alveoli by the blood flowing past the alveoli reduces PO_2 of stale air. As oxygen is removed from the alveolar air, PO_2 falls and continues to fall until fresh air is brought to the alveoli by ventilation. The mixture of fresh air with a PO_2 of 150 with the stale air from the anatomic dead space and that remaining in the alveoli at the end of expiration (the functional residual capacity) produces an alveolar PO_2 at a value of about 105 mm Hg. The faster fresh air is brought into the alveoli to mix with stale air, the higher P_AO_2 will be. Also, because of the mixing of stale alveolar air with fresh air, alveolar PCO_2 is 40 mmHg compared to an atmospheric PCO_2 of 2 mmHg and a systemic venous PCO_2 of 45 mmHg. As discussed in the previous chapter, increasing the rate of ventilation relative to diffusion of oxygen from the alveoli into the pulmonary capillary blood will increase PO_2 and decrease PCO_2 of both the alveolar air and the systemic arterial blood to a maximum approaching 150 mmHg.

Under ideal conditions, alveolar PO_2 (P_AO_2) is nearly equal to arterial PO_2 (P_aO_2). However, the presence of physiological dead space complicates the exchange process. Some alveoli may be poorly ventilated, but are still perfused. The addition of blood with a low PO_2 to the systemic circulation causes a decrease in P_aO_2. The addition of poorly oxygenated blood draining areas of physiologic dead space is known as a shunt, because the effect of this blood flow is similar to what would happen if the blood were shunted directly from the systemic veins to the systemic arteries, bypassing the lungs (Figure 25-3).

Alveolar PO_2, which depends on the relative rates of ventilation and oxygen uptake from the blood by the tissues as discussed previously, is the physiological maximum for P_aO_2. How closely P_aO_2 approaches P_AO_2 is determined by matching of ventilation and perfusion of the lungs. Increased demand for blood flow at the local level causes a fall in total peripheral resistance, which is accompanied by an increased cardiac output to maintain arterial pressure. Increased cardiac output results in increased perfusion of the lung, which in turn causes greater uptake of oxygen from the alveoli. The greater removal of oxygen by pulmonary blood flow to replace the oxygen used by metabolically active tissue requires ventilation to be increased in proportion to the increase in cardiac output. Otherwise, the mismatch of alveolar ventilation and pulmonary blood flow will cause arterial PO_2 to fall. The ratio of ventilation to perfusion is used to discuss matching of pulmonary blood flow and ventilation and is called V/Q ratio. With a perfect V/Q ratio, arterial PO_2 would be nearly identical to alveolar PO_2 (105 mm Hg).

V/Q ratio can be understood by examining several simple examples (Figure 25-4). At one extreme, we have the situation in which V/Q = 0, meaning we have pulmonary blood flow, but no ventilation. Without ventilation to refresh alveolar gas, P_AO_2 would equilibrate rapidly with the partial pressure of the systemic venous blood. As metabolism continues to use more oxygen, venous PO_2 and P_AO_2 would continually decrease and P_ACO_2 would continually rise. At the other extreme, V/Q equals infinity, and we would have alveolar ventilation without any perfusion to carry oxygen away from the alveoli. In this condition, alveolar gas composition would become equal to 150 mmHg P_AO_2 and 2 mmHg P_ACO_2, and the stagnant blood in the capillaries would equilibrate to these values. Between these extremes, intermediate values result (as shown in Figure 25-4).

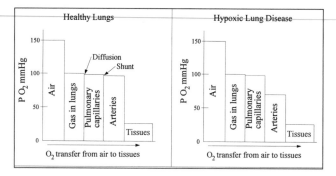

Figure 25-3. Gradients in PO_2 along the pathway of oxygen from the atmosphere to the tissues. The normal situation is shown on the left with a decrease in PO_2 between the atmosphere and alveoli due to the mixing of stale and fresh air, a small loss due to diffusion across the alveolar wall, and a small decrease due to a small V/Q mismatch. In the case of hypoxic lung disease, greater losses of PO_2 occur with a large loss due to V/Q mismatch.

Therefore, a low V/Q ratio causes P_aO_2 to fall, and a high ratio causes P_aO_2 to rise.

Some degree of shunting is unavoidable and is considered normal in the lung due to regional differences in ventilation and perfusion. Ventilation increases from the upper parts of the lung to the dependent part due to the "slinky" effect. Blood flow increases also from the upper to the dependent area due to the response of pulmonary arterial vessels to pressure. Due to the effects of gravity on a column of fluid, arterial pressure is least at the top of the lung and greatest at the lowermost part. Pulmonary arterial vessels respond to increased pressure by dilation to prevent an increase in pressure by allowing flow to increase. Therefore, the farther below the heart a pulmonary arterial vessel is, the greater the flow through it will be. Although the regional differences in ventilation and perfusion occur in the same direction, the change in perfusion due to position is greater than the change in ventilation. For this reason, ventilation is high relative to perfusion at the apex of the lung when upright and low relative to perfusion at the most dependent part of the lung. In terms of V/Q, V/Q is highest at the top and lowest in the dependent area of the lungs. As a consequence of the regional differences in V/Q, perfect matching of ventilation and perfusion is not possible, and P_aO_2 is less than P_AO_2. Lung diseases that affect either ventilation or perfusion of the lungs will alter blood gases to an even greater extent. As the ratio decreases below normal, alveolar air becomes more like systemic venous blood, resulting in hypoxemia. Arterial PO_2 is always less than alveolar PO_2, because areas with high V/Q cannot compensate for areas of low V/Q due to presence of Hb (the reason will be described below). Shunt results in decreased PO_2, but

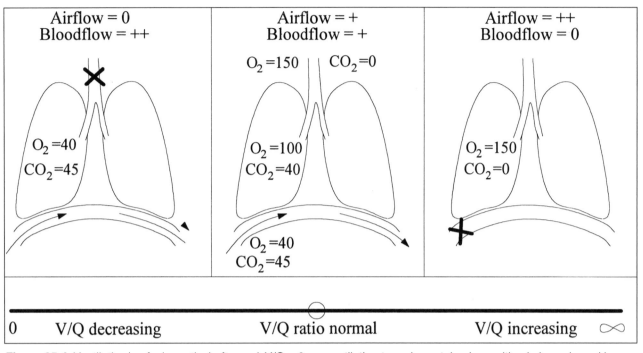

Figure 25-4. Ventilation/perfusion ratio. Left panel: V/Q = 0; no ventilation to replace stale air, resulting in hypoxia and hypercapnia. Middle panel: normal V/Q and arterial blood gases. Right panel: V/Q = ∞; no blood flow to pick up oxygen from the alveoli, blood gases are the same as atmospheric in the alveolar capillary blood, but no oxygen is available to tissues.

not increased PCO_2 because the CO_2 dissociation curve is linear and ventilation is controlled by P_aCO_2. Only if disease is severe will PCO_2 elevated.

Normal V/Q ratio is approximately 0.8 with an average V_A of 4 to 5 L/min and cardiac output of 5 to 6 L/min. Although the significance of V/Q ratio being less than 0.8 is clear in that it causes hypoxemia, why would a ratio higher than 0.8 be bad? As V/Q ratio increases, alveolar air becomes more like atmospheric air. Because of the way hemoglobin binds oxygen, large quantities of oxygen are loaded onto hemoglobin as PO_2 increases, but beyond 100 mmHg, very little increase in the quantity of oxygen present in the blood occurs. Therefore, increasing P_AO_2 above 105 mmHg has a negligible effect on the amount of O_2 carried by the blood. Increased ventilation that creates a P_AO_2 greater than 100 mmHg produces what is called "wasted ventilation." What is meant by the term wasted ventilation is that excess oxygen is consumed to create greater ventilation than what saturates hemoglobin. Therefore, creation of a high V/Q does not add a significant amount of oxygen to the blood, but causes more oxygen to be consumed to generate a given oxygen content of the blood. This potentially steals oxygen from other tissues that require oxygen. An analogy is depicted in Figure 25-5.

A common mistake is to think that arterial PO_2 is determined by either cardiac output or alveolar ventilation. To avoid this mistake, we need to distinguish between the processes of replenishing the oxygen content of the blood and supplying the demand for oxygen delivery by metabolically active tissue. The process of replenishing oxygen content of the blood is accomplished by matching ventilation and perfusion, whereas the process of supplying the demand for oxygen delivery depends on cardiac output to carry oxygen-rich blood to the tissues and oxygen-poor blood through the lungs to pick up oxygen. Sufficient alveolar ventilation is necessary to supply the pulmonary capillaries with oxygen. Although seeming counterintuitive, arterial PO_2 would be perfectly normal with a low pulmonary blood flow and low ventilation as long as they were matched. The arterial blood would be fully saturated with oxygen, but a low cardiac output would not carry sufficient oxygen to the tissues to support oxidative metabolism fully. Tissues would require anaerobic metabolism to supplement aerobic metabolism, leading to acidosis, multisystem organ failure, and, ultimately, death. The case of perfect V/Q matching at a low cardiac output would cause ischemic hypoxia, not hypoxemia.

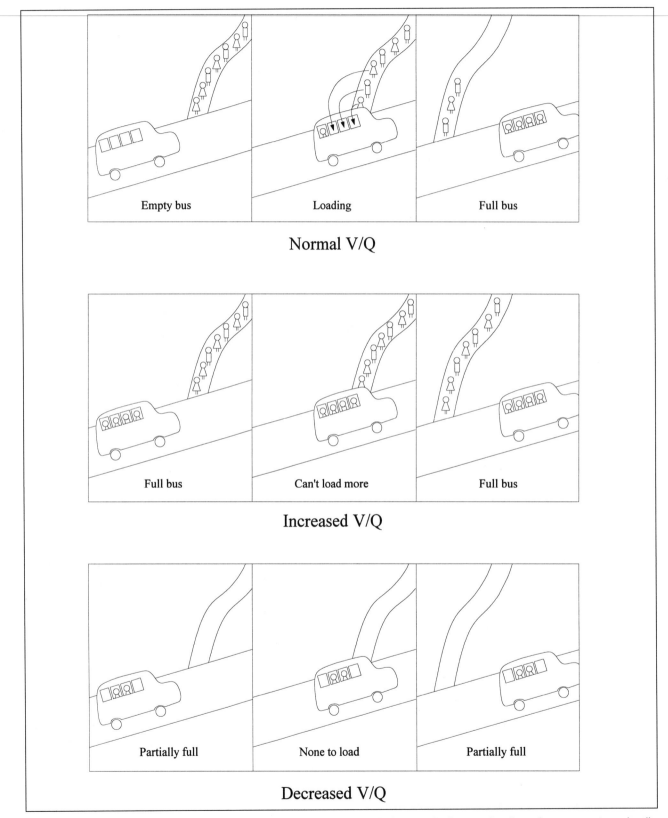

Figure 25-5. Bus analogy for V/Q. A high perfusion for a given ventilation results in poor loading of oxygen onto red cells and hypoxemia. A high ventilation for a given perfusion produces higher than normal PO_2, but because of saturation of hemoglobin, it provides slightly more oxygen content of the blood. The muscles of ventilation use more oxygen than needed, and, as such, a greater increase in oxygen consumption than oxygen uptake may occur.

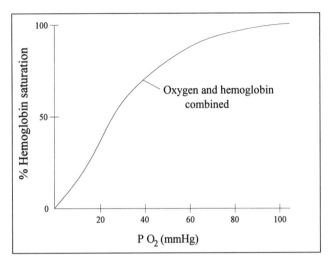

Figure 25-6. Oxyhemoglobin dissociation curve. A sigmoidal relationship exists between PO_2 of blood and the saturation of hemoglobin. Note that increasing PO_2 beyond normal provides little extra oxygen, which is dissolved in the blood.

REGULATION OF V/Q

Although V/Q is not regulated directly, two mechanisms act to minimize V/Q inequality. Pulmonary arterial PO_2 and airway PCO_2 modify perfusion and ventilation, respectively. Pulmonary arterioles constrict in the presence of low PO_2. During hypoventilation, a decreased V/Q ratio and P_aO_2 result. Vasoconstriction, as a response to hypoventilation, decreases pulmonary blood flow to bring perfusion back in line with ventilation, which equalizes V/Q ratio. Pulmonary vasoconstriction prevents the addition of low PO_2 blood to the systemic circulation by diverting blood flow to better ventilated alveoli. Unfortunately, long-term pulmonary disease associated with pulmonary vasoconstriction produces a condition called pulmonary hypertension, in which the pulmonary arterial pressure is increased. The increased afterload on the right ventricle can produce right heart failure, which inevitably leads to left heart failure.

To some extent, PCO_2 controls the resistance of airways. Hypoventilation results in increased alveolar PCO_2, which results in relaxation of bronchial smooth muscle. Improved ventilation results from decreased resistance and improves V/Q ratio.

OXYGEN CONTENT OF SYS-TEMIC ARTERIAL BLOOD

On average, each liter of arterial blood contains 200 ml of O_2. Oxygen is present in three forms: dissolved in plasma, dissolved within red cells, and bound to hemoglobin (Hb). By far, most of the O_2 carried in the blood is bound to Hb. At a PO_2 of 100 mmHg, each liter of arterial blood contains 3 ml of O_2 dissolved within the red cells and plasma and 197 ml bound to Hb. With 5 liters of blood, a total of about 1000 ml of O_2 is carried in the blood. Although only 1.5% of the O_2 content of blood at a PO_2 of 100 is carried dissolved in plasma, this quantity is critical because it determines plasma PO_2, which is the driving force for the diffusion of oxygen. The PO_2 within the red cell determines how much is carried by hemoglobin. Because oxygen is much more soluble in red cells because of hemoglobin, a small increase in plasma PO_2 causes a large increase in the quantity of oxygen carried in the blood. In the lung, O_2 diffuses from high PO_2 in the alveoli to a lower PO_2 in the plasma and into the red cells. The increased PO_2 inside red blood cells causes oxygen to bind to Hb. In tissue, Hb releases O_2 as O_2 diffuses out of the red cell, into the plasma, across the capillary endothelium, into the interstitial space, into the cell, through the intracellular space, then into the mitochondrion, again from high PO_2 to low PO_2.

The hemoglobin molecule has four binding sites for O_2. If all four sites on every hemoglobin (Hb) molecule bind O_2, Hb is 100% saturated (oxyhemoglobin). If, on average, three sites bind O_2, Hb is 75% saturated. Because there are many Hb molecules per red cell and billions of red cells, we can have a percent saturation of Hb between the 25% increments. Deoxyhemoglobin is the term given to Hb that is not saturated with O_2. Percent saturation is computed as the amount of O_2 bound to Hb divided by the maximum possible. Although binding of O_2 to Hb is dependent on the PO_2 inside red cells, the relationship between PO_2 and percent saturation is not linear, but is sigmoidal. The sigmoidal relationship occurs because the binding of O_2 to Hb is affected by the presence or absence of O_2 on the other three binding sites. If one site is already occupied, the second and third O_2 molecules bind readily to Hb, but if three sites are already bound, a greater increment in PO_2 is necessary to force Hb to bind the fourth molecule of oxygen. A graph of this relationship is called an oxyhemoglobin dissociation curve, implying the effect of PO_2 on the unloading of O_2 from Hb to the plasma and eventually into the mitochondria (Figure 25-6). We could just as accurately term the plot a deoxyhemoglobin association curve to describe how oxygen is loaded onto Hb in the lungs. Because saturation only falls to 75% under resting conditions, we have a reserve of oxygen in the blood; during exercise, more O_2 can be given up to tissue with a high metabolic rate.

EFFECT OF Hb ON O_2 DISTRIBUTION

The PO_2 of blood is determined by how much O_2 is dissolved in blood, which, in turn, is determined by the PO_2 of the gas with which blood is in equilibrium and the solubility of O_2 in blood. Solubility of oxygen in the blood is due almost exclusively to the presence of hemoglobin. For practical purposes, the content of O_2 in blood is determined by hemoglobin concentration and PO_2, which determines percent saturation of hemoglobin. A simple index of hemoglobin content of the blood is hematocrit, which can be obtained simply by centrifugation of a tube of blood.

The nonlinear shape of the O_2 dissociation curve complicates the mixing of blood with different PO_2. If the curve were linear instead, the resultant PO_2 from mixing equal volumes of blood would be the average of the PO_2 of the two volumes. Because of the shape of the upper part of the curve, we can see that increasing PO_2 of blood above 100 mmHg does not significantly increase the O_2 content of the blood. When blood with high and low PO_2 is mixed, the resultant mixture has a PO_2 closer to the value of the poorly oxygenated blood because the unsaturated Hb from the poorly oxygenated blood readily combines with the oxygen dissolved in the blood in which Hb is saturated. The binding of O_2 by the previously unsaturated Hb molecules removes large quantities of O_2 from the plasma, which then causes so much O_2 to be released from the previously saturated Hb molecules that the mixture has a low PO_2. For example, if two plasma solutions, one with a PO_2 of 50 and one of 150, are mixed, the resultant PO_2 is 100 mmHg. However, if blood with these values is mixed, the result is a PO_2 of 62 mmHg, not 100 mmHg. Moreover, it is not possible to compensate for the addition of low PO_2 blood from one area of the lungs by increased ventilation of other parts of the lungs. Increasing PO_2 above 100 mmHg provides an increase of only 3 ml of O_2 per liter of blood because hemoglobin is saturated, whereas 1 liter of blood with a PO_2 of 50 mmHg is capable of taking up approximately 50 more milliliters of O_2. To compensate for the low PO_2 of a volume of blood with a PO_2 of 50 ml, an equal volume with a PO_2 of 1770 mmHg would be necessary to bring the mixture to a PO_2 of 100.

As an example, we will say that one-half of the lungs are hypoventilated due to disease and the other half undergo compensatory hyperventilation to maintain arterial PCO_2. The O_2 content of blood when mixing can be computed easily using a diagram (see Figure 25-6), the solubility of oxygen in plasma of 3 ml/liter of blood per 100 mmHg, and an oxygen content of 208 ml of oxygen per liter of blood at 100% saturation. At a normal hemoglobin concentration, the O_2 content of blood with a PO_2 of 50 mmHg is 168 ml/liter and the O_2 content of blood with a PO_2 of 150 is 204 ml/liter (slightly less than 100% saturation). Combined, this solution has an O_2 content of 186 ml/liter when the blood mixes in the pulmonary veins. This oxygen content will result in a systemic arterial PO_2 of only 62 mmHg. Because almost all of the additional oxygen made available by hyperventilation is dissolved in plasma with near 100% saturation of Hb, increasing the PO_2 from 100 mmHg to 150 by hyperventilation adds only 1.5 ml of oxygen per liter of blood, which as we can see from the example cannot compensate for the hypoventilated region of the lungs. However, arterial PCO_2 will be close to its normal value.

TRANSPORT OF CO_2

CO_2 is carried in the blood in three forms: dissolved, bound to amino acids, and converted to H_2CO_3 by carbonic anhydrase and then to $HCO_3^- + H^+$. Carbon dioxide is much more soluble in water than O_2. This explains why so much CO_2 remains in arterial blood compared to oxygen. Dissolved CO_2 only accounts for 5% of CO_2 in blood; 90% of CO_2 in blood is in the form of HCO_3^- and 5% is bound to Hb (Figure 25-7). From aerobic metabolism, 40 ml of CO_2 is added to each liter of blood each minute. The CO_2 produced by metabolism is added to the blood as 10% (4 ml) dissolved in plasma, 60% is converted to bicarbonate (24 ml), and 30% is bound to Hb (12 ml). The presence of O_2 on Hb inhibits binding of CO_2 to Hb. As O_2 leaves Hb, CO_2 binds to Hb in venous blood. In pulmonary capillaries, dissolved CO_2 diffuses into alveoli, reversing the carbonic anhydrase reaction, and CO_2 is released from Hb.

TRANSPORT OF H^+

Hydrogen ions are produced in the reaction that generates bicarbonate ion and by other metabolism. Because the acid produced by carbon dioxide can be eliminated by ventilation, carbon dioxide is called a volatile acid. Other acids that must be eliminated by the kidney are called fixed acid. Control of pH will be described in the next chapter. Just as deoxyhemoglobin has a higher affinity for CO_2 than oxyhemoglobin, deoxyhemoglobin has a higher affinity for H^+ than oxyhemoglobin. Hemoglobin binds H^+ ions, thereby acting

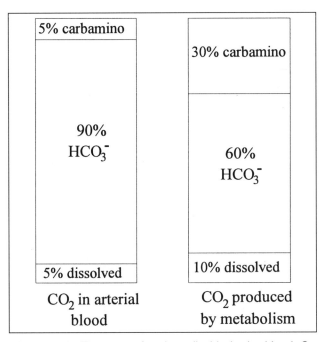

Figure 25-7. Transport of carbon dioxide in the blood. On the left: distribution of carbon dioxide in the arterial blood. On the right: destination of carbon dioxide produced by metabolism.

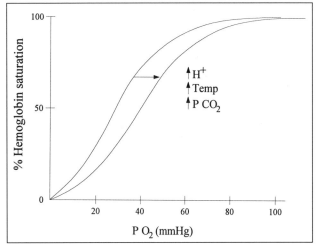

Figure 25-8. The Bohr effect. During exercise, production of carbon dioxide, acid, and heat decreases the ability of hemoglobin to bind oxygen. Metabolically active tissues receive more oxygen from the blood at a given tissue PO_2 during exercise due to the Bohr effect, which minimizes the fall in tissue PO_2 and potential hypoxic cell injury.

as a buffer. This buffering allows the pH of venous blood to be only slightly less than that of arterial blood. When the chemical reactions involving carbon dioxide are reversed in the lung, H^+ ions come off Hb molecules and combine with bicarbonate ions to form carbonic acid, which in turn, is converted to CO_2 and H_2O as CO_2 is expired. For this reason, hypoventilation decreases pH and hyperventilation increases pH.

FACTORS INFLUENCING BINDING OF O_2 BY Hb

For the same reasons that O_2 affects binding of CO_2 and H^+ by Hb, carbon dioxide and hydrogen ions decrease the ability of Hb to bind O_2. Carbon dioxide and H^+ alter the molecular conformation of Hb, which may be considered as an allosteric modulation of Hb's affinity for O_2. Most of the effect of CO_2 on oxygen binding to hemoglobin is due to production of H^+. Increased temperature also decreases the affinity of Hb for O_2. Another agent that affects hemoglobin's affinity for oxygen is a molecule called 2,3 diphosphoglycerate (2,3 DPG). Because red blood cells have no mitochondria, they use glycolysis for meeting their energy demands. The molecule called 2,3 DPG is a byproduct of glycolysis.

The change in the affinity of hemoglobin for oxygen during increased metabolic rate is called the Bohr effect. This effect was initially described by Christian Bohr in 1904. Briefly stated, increased metabolism promotes release of O_2 from Hb. With increased metabolism, increased PCO_2, increased H^+, and increased temperature occur, all of which decrease the affinity of Hb for O_2. At any given arterial PO_2, less O_2 will be bound to Hb, and more oxygen will be released into the plasma to maintain capillary PO_2 (Figure 25-8). The Bohr effect allows more O_2 to be available to the tissue rather than being bound to hemoglobin. The advantage of the Bohr effect is that, by releasing oxygen from hemoglobin at a higher PO_2, the difference in partial pressure of oxygen that drives diffusion of oxygen from the blood into the tissue is maintained during increased metabolic rate. Without the Bohr effect, the same quantity of oxygen diffusing from the plasma to the tissue would cause a greater decline in capillary PO_2, which would force tissue PO_2 to fall in order to maintain the same net transport of O_2 from blood to tissue that occurs with the Bohr effect. In the lungs with a lower PCO_2, a higher pH, and lower temperature than working muscle, the affinity of Hb for oxygen increases to help load oxygen onto Hb.

ADAPTATIONS TO ALTITUDE

At high altitude, atmospheric pressure is reduced, and, therefore, atmospheric PO_2 can be reduced sufficiently to cause hypoxemia. We compensate for this hypoxia in the short term by increasing ventilation and in the long term through physiologic adaptations that allow oxygen to be used more effectively. Alveolar ventilation, which at normal atmospheric pressure is regulated primarily by PCO_2, is stimulated by decreased arterial PO_2 secondary to decreased atmospheric pressure. Long-term adaptations include an increased O_2 content of the blood due to increased hematocrit and erythropoiesis. Increased 2,3 DPG provides rightward shift of oxyhemoglobin dissociation curve so that less O_2 is bound to Hb at a low PO_2, making more O_2 available to tissues as described above. Other adaptations include an increased ability to bring O_2 to tissues and to use O_2. An increased number of capillaries decreases diffusion distance for O_2, and an increased number of mitochondria are synthesized to use O_2 more readily. Increased concentration of the red pigment called myoglobin that solubilizes oxygen increases the solubility of O_2 in tissues, thereby increasing the rate of diffusion from the interstitial space into the cells.

SUMMARY

Pulmonary arterial pressure is 20% to 25% that of the systemic circulation. Arterial vessels in the lung respond differently to oxygen and pressure than systemic arterial vessels. Increases in both oxygen and pressure cause vasodilation in the lung. Vasoconstriction in response to low partial pressure of oxygen prevents the dumping of poorly oxygenated blood into the systemic circulation, which is called shunting. Vasodilation in response to increased pressure allows pulmonary blood flow to increase with increased systemic blood flow demands. Pulmonary arterial pressure must be regulated at a low value to prevent edema in the lungs that can interfere with diffusion of oxygen across the alveoli. Diffusion of oxygen from the alveoli into a red cell requires 0.25 seconds to complete. At rest, 0.75 seconds is available for diffusion to occur. During exercise, the normal individual has just enough time for equilibrium between the alveolar gas and the blood to occur.

Lung diseases that interfere with diffusion initially cause shortness of breath during exercise, progressing to SOB at rest. These diseases require the use of oxygen therapy. Partial pressure of alveolar gas is 105 mmHg compared to 150 mmHg in the airways because of the mixing of stale air already in the alveoli at the end of expiration when the lung is at function residual capacity

and the mixing of stale air from the anatomic dead space. A small decrease in PO_2 from the alveoli to the systemic arteries occurs because of ventilation/perfusion inequality. Shunt refers to blood flow through poorly ventilated alveoli, called physiologic dead space. The effect of shunt on PCO_2 can be compensated by increased ventilation because the relationship between PCO_2 and content of CO_2 in the blood is linear. PO_2 is decreased because the relationship is sigmoidal and because, under normal PO_2, hemoglobin is nearly saturated. Increasing PO_2 above 100 mmHg results in an insignificant quantity of oxygen added to the plasma and not to hemoglobin. V/Q is the ratio of alveolar ventilation to pulmonary blood flow (perfusion). The normal ratio is 0.8. Regional differences in ventilation and perfusion due to posture cause the V/Q ratio to change from the top of the lung to the bottom. Ventilation and perfusion both increase from top to bottom, but perfusion increases at a greater rate, so V/Q decreases from the top to the bottom of the lung. The oxyhemoglobin dissociation curve describes graphically the relationship between PO_2 and percent saturation. Saturation refers to hemoglobin's maximum occupancy by oxygen. Due to the effects of the presence of oxygen on one binding site on the others, the curve is not linear, but sigmoidal. The second and third oxygen molecules are more easily bound than the first, and the fourth is difficult to bind. Plasma will only hold 3 ml of oxygen for every liter per 100 mmHg of PO_2, whereas blood with a normal hematocrit holds a maximum of 200 ml of oxygen per liter of blood. The percent saturation is determined by PO_2.

Increased temperature, carbon dioxide, and hydrogen ion concentration decrease the affinity of hemoglobin for oxygen, allowing greater unloading of oxygen to the tissues during increased metabolic rate, according to the Bohr effect. Carbon dioxide is carried in the blood as dissolved CO_2 and bound to hemoglobin, but most is in the form of HCO_3^-, which acts as a buffer to prevent changes in blood pH. Hemoglobin also acts as a buffer by binding H^+. Expiration of CO_2 in the lungs reverses the carbonic anhydrase reaction and decreases the concentration of acid in the blood. At high altitudes, breathing is stimulated by low PO_2, which results in alkalosis. Long-term adaptations include increased 2,3 DPG to decrease the affinity of hemoglobin for oxygen, increased numbers of capillaries and mitochondria in the tissues, and increased myoglobin to enhance the transport of oxygen from the interstitial fluid into the cell.

BIBLIOGRAPHY

Branch AL, Denavit-Savbié M, Champagnat J. Central control of breathing mammals: neuronal circuitry, membrane properties, and neurotransmitters. *Physiological Reviews.* 1995;75:1-45.

Duffin J, Ezure K, Lipski J. Breathing rhythm generation: focus on the rostral ventrolateral medulla. *News in Physiological Sciences.* 1995;10:133-140.

Kubin L, Davies RO, Pack AI. Control of upper airway motor neurons during REM sleep. *News in Physiological Sciences.* 1998;13:91-97.

Orem J, Trotter RH. Behavioral control of breathing. *News in Physiological Sciences.* 1994;9:228-232.

West JB. *Respiratory Physiology: The Essentials.* 4th ed. Baltimore, MD: Williams & Wilkins; 1990.

STUDY QUESTIONS

1. Considering the structure of the right ventricle. Why must pulmonary arterial pressure be much lower than systemic arterial pressure? What would happen to the right ventricle if pulmonary arterial pressure increased substantially?

2. Contrast the response of systemic arterial vessels and pulmonary arterial vessels to increased pressure. What factor is maintained in systemic vessels? What factor is maintained in pulmonary vessels?

3. Contrast the response of systemic arterial vessels and pulmonary arterial vessels to PO_2. What benefit is derived from the systemic arterial response? What benefit is derived from the pulmonary arterial response?

4. Why is PO_2 in the airways only 105 mmHg instead of 21% of 760 mmHg = 160 mmHg?

5. How does breathing at a tidal volume near 150 ml affect PO_2 in the airways?

6. Explain why the ratio of oxygen consumption to alveolar ventilation determines alveolar PO_2.

7. What is the source of shunt in normal lungs? What is it in diseased lungs?

8. What mechanisms are available to minimize shunt in healthy lungs?

9. What are the consequences of long-term hypoxemia on pulmonary arteries, pulmonary arterial pressure, the right ventricle, and the left ventricle?

10. How does the shape of the oxyhemoglobin dissociation curve affect the ability of the lungs to compensate for areas of hypoventilation? Why can we compensate for CO_2, but not for O_2?

11. How does the Bohr effect benefit oxygen exchange from capillaries to tissues during exercise? What would happen to tissue PO_2 during exercise without the Bohr effect?

TWENTY-SIX

Control of Ventilation and pH

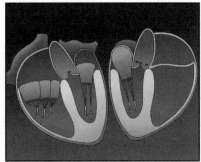

OBJECTIVES

1. Describe the effect of ventilation on acid-base status.

2. Define respiratory acidosis and alkalosis and metabolic acidosis and alkalosis.

3. Describe the central chemoreceptor mechanism controlling ventilation via PCO_2 and pH.

4. Describe the peripheral chemoreceptor mechanism involving PO_2.

As discussed in previous chapters, ventilation is controlled primarily to excrete volatile acid in the form of expired carbon dioxide. The loss of carbon dioxide from the lungs shifts the chemical reaction mediated by carbonic anhydrase toward production of carbon dioxide and water from carbonic acid, which, in turn, decreases the concentrations of bicarbonate and hydrogen ions in the arterial blood. The effects of ventilation on pH and the control of ventilation are described in this chapter. Although the level of oxygen in the blood is normally not a strong regulating variable, at low oxygen levels, it can be.

EFFECTORS INFLUENCING pH

The terms hyperventilation and hypoventilation usually convey the idea that a person is either breathing too much or not enough. The question is too much or too little in terms of what variable? If we look at the way ventilation is controlled, the answer becomes clear. The reference point for ventilation is maintaining a normal value of arterial PCO_2. Hypoventilation increases arterial PCO_2, which then results in decreased pH. Hyperventilation, on the other hand, decreases arterial PCO_2 and increases pH. This occurs because ventilation serves to eliminate volatile acid (CO_2), which increases plasma pH. Because acid can be lost by ventilation, the acid produced by carbon dioxide is called volatile acid. Acids generated by other metabolic pathways are called fixed acids and must be disposed by the kidneys. In the following discussion, it must be noted that the loss of either acid or base is equivalent to a gain of the other. Bicarbonate is the principal buffer in body fluids, so that loss of one bicarbonate ion frees one hydrogen ion, which lowers pH. The kidney is responsible for both retrieval of bicarbonate from the tubular fluid and active transport of hydrogen ions out of the blood and into the tubular fluid. Because the proximal tubule primarily removes bicarbonate from tubular fluid, the failure of the proximal tubule to perform this task is called proximal tubular acidosis. Failure of the distal tubule to actively transport hydrogen ions into the tubular fluid

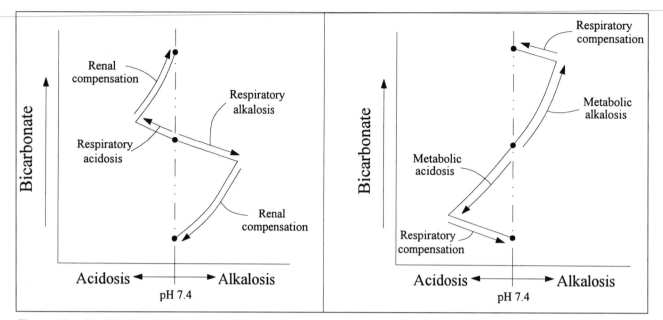

Figure 26-1. Modification of a Davenport diagram. The changes in pH and bicarbonate concentrations representative of pH changes and compensations can be graphically represented. Left: changes occurring with respiratory acidosis or alkalosis due to either hypo- or hyperventilation. The kidneys respond to respiratory alkalosis by allowing bicarbonate to be lost in the urine. In the case of respiratory acidosis, the kidneys respond by conserving and synthesizing more bicarbonate. Right: respiratory compensations for metabolic acidosis or alkalosis.

produces distal tubular acidosis. Fluid in the stomach is acidic, so loss of this fluid by vomiting produces an alkaline condition, whereas the fluid lost in diarrhea is alkaline and produces acidosis. In addition to the roles of the lungs and kidneys in maintaining pH, metabolism can generate large quantities of acid and, thereby, alter pH. Historically, the terms used to describe changes in pH are metabolic acidosis, metabolic alkalosis, respiratory acidosis, and respiratory alkalosis.

Metabolic acidosis is distinguished from respiratory acidosis because the increased $[H^+]$ is due to some cause other than an elevated PCO_2. Typical causes of metabolic acidosis are metabolic acid production, such as lactic acid from metabolism, or loss of alkali from diarrhea. Metabolic alkalosis is a decrease in $[H^+]$ not due to a decreased PCO_2, but due to a loss of acid, such as occurs with vomiting. Respiratory acidosis is a condition of elevated $[H^+]$ due to hypoventilation, and respiratory alkalosis is a decreased $[H^+]$ due to hyperventilation.

The respiratory and renal systems can influence the effect of the other on pH. Because of this, one type of acidosis or alkalosis can be compensated by other type of alkalosis or acidosis. The kidney compensates for respiratory acidosis by both increasing the reabsorption of bicarbonate from the tubular fluid and by synthesizing greater quantities of bicarbonate from the excess carbon dioxide while excreting the excess hydrogen ion. The

renal compensation returns pH toward 7.4 but results in an elevated bicarbonate concentration in addition to the elevated PCO_2. In respiratory alkalosis, the renal tubular cells decrease the rate of bicarbonate ion reabsorption with a net effect of normal pH, decreased bicarbonate concentration, and decreased PCO_2. Metabolic acidosis leads to a respiratory compensation of hyperventilation to return arterial pH toward 7.4 with a decreased PCO_2 and a decreased bicarbonate concentration. Metabolic alkalosis, which is characterized by an elevated pH but a normal PCO_2, results in a respiratory compensation of hypoventilation, which allows arterial PCO_2 to rise. Figure 26-1 shows normal arterial values of PCO_2 and bicarbonate ion concentration, how these two change with metabolic and respiratory alkalosis, metabolic and respiratory acidosis, and the renal and respiratory changes that produce a normal pH.

CONTROL OF VENTILATION

Ventilation is controlled primarily by central chemoreceptors; however, it is also under the control of peripheral chemoreceptors, reflexes, as well as voluntarily by higher centers of the brain. Involuntary breathing is controlled by centers in the medulla. These centers send bursts of action potentials to the phrenic nerve (diaphragm) and α motor neurons of other muscles of

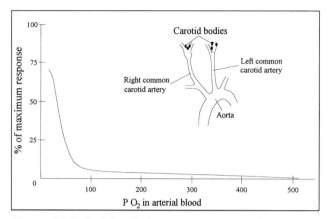

Figure 26-2. Peripheral chemoreceptor control of ventilation. Under normal circumstances, peripheral chemoreceptors for oxygen contribute little to ventilation. Under hypoxic conditions, especially chronic hypoventilation, low arterial PO_2 drives ventilation.

inspiration in a rhythmic pattern. The medullary respiratory centers are sensitive to depressants, such as alcohol, barbiturates, and morphine, which can produce hypoventilation or even death. These substances can also affect swallowing and lead to aspiration. Some reflexes that have been demonstrated in laboratory animals control ventilation. The Hering-Breuer reflex operates via pulmonary stretch receptors and terminates inspiration when V_T becomes extremely high, although its value to humans is not known. Peripheral chemoreceptors that influence breathing are found in areas called the aortic bodies and carotid bodies. These peripheral chemoreceptors are sensitive to decreased PO_2, increased $[H^+]$, and increased PCO_2, but are most responsive to decreased PO_2. The carotid bodies are located near the carotid sinus, the site of the major baroreceptors, and the aortic bodies are located in midarch of the aorta. However, PO_2 is not an important contributor to the control of ventilation until moderate to severe hypoxemia is present. Most of the drive for ventilation comes from the indirect effect of CO_2 on central chemoreceptors. PO_2 becomes important in cases of high altitude or severe pulmonary disease (Figure 26-2). After a long period of respiratory insufficiency, the effect of elevated CO_2 on the central chemoreceptors does not adequately drive ventilation. A steady state of ventilation that brings in sufficient oxygen and eliminates sufficient carbon dioxide results at a decreased arterial PO_2 from the combination of central and peripheral chemoreceptor stimulation. A person who has been in respiratory insufficiency for a long period becomes dependent on peripheral chemoreceptor stimulation to drive ventilation. Provision of supplemental oxygen needs to be carefully regulated to avoid hyper- or hypoventilation. Placing

such a person on 100% O_2 suddenly deprives the person of an adequate stimulus to breathe. This individual will slow breathing and allow CO_2 to accumulate. This person needs to be gradually given increasing concentrations of oxygen while the central chemoreceptors become more responsive.

Although hypoxemia stimulates peripheral chemoreceptors due to low PO_2, these receptors do not respond to low O_2 **content**. Therefore, hypoxia caused by anemia and carbon monoxide poisoning does not stimulate peripheral oxygen chemoreceptors, but may stimulate breathing due to decreased pH as a consequence of anaerobic metabolism. Central chemoreceptors will simply maintain arterial PCO_2 at approximately 40 mmHg without regard to the oxygen content of the blood.

CENTRAL CHEMORECEPTORS

Alveolar ventilation is proportional to PCO_2 in the arterial blood under normal circumstances. However, central chemoreceptors do not respond to arterial PCO_2 directly, but to the $[H^+]$ in the fluid surrounding the central chemoreceptors in the medulla. The link between hydrogen ions and carbon dioxide exists because hydrogen ions do not cross the blood-brain barrier to reach central chemoreceptors, but CO_2 can diffuse from blood to increase $[CO_2]$ of the extracellular fluid (ECF) and cerebrospinal fluid (CSF). By the carbonic anhydrase reaction, excess CO_2 leads to production of H^+ in the CSF and the interstitial fluid bathing the central chemoreceptors. Stimulation of the central chemoreceptors causes an increased alveolar ventilation, which, in turn, decreases arterial PCO_2 leading to decreased $[H^+]$ of the CSF and interstitial fluid of the medulla, completing negative feedback control of arterial PCO_2 (Figure 26-3).

VENTILATION DURING EXERCISE

The increased alveolar ventilation during exercise cannot be explained on the basis of any of the factors already discussed. Alveolar PO_2 and arterial PO_2 do not change with exercise, except at the highest levels of exercise in the most highly trained aerobic athletes, because the increased oxygen consumption is matched with increased alveolar ventilation. Even in the most well-trained athletes, this change is not sufficient to increase the ventilatory drive. During exercise, venous PO_2 does decrease, but peripheral chemoreceptors respond to changes in arterial, not venous, blood. In addition, alveolar PCO_2 and arterial PCO_2 do not increase with increased carbon dioxide production, and, with high levels of exercise approaching maximum oxygen consumption, arterial PCO_2 actually decreases due to hyperventilation. At lower exercise intensities, hyperpnea occurs. Hyperpnea implies increased breathing but does not indicate a change in PCO_2 accompanying the increased ventilation. Arterial [H+] does not change with low to moderate exercise, although alveolar ventilation is changing, but during strenuous exercise, production of lactic acid produces metabolic acidosis compensated by hyperventilation. This acidosis can partially explain high levels of ventilation (hyperventilation) that occur at maximal and supramaximal power outputs but not the matching of carbon dioxide production and alveolar ventilation.

Blood gases are unlikely to be related to the change in ventilation during exercise for another reason. Ventilation increases abruptly with the onset of exercise and decreases abruptly at the end of exercise. Neither event correlates with measured blood gas levels. After the initial increase, alveolar ventilation gradually reaches a steady state determined by the intensity of the exercise. Possible links between exercise intensity and alveolar ventilation are a conditioned response (learned behavior), oscillatory changes in PO_2, PCO_2, and [H+], rise in temperature, and the movement of limbs. The movement of limbs and activation of joint and muscle receptors appear to be responsible for a large component of the increased ventilation during exercise because the movement of denervated limbs does not increase ventilation, whereas passive movement in a pattern similar to exercise results in increased ventilation. Limb movement cannot explain the entire increase in ventilation, because ventilation remains elevated for some time after exercise has stopped.

SUMMARY

The respiratory and renal systems are responsible for maintaining arterial pH near a value of 7.4. The lungs excrete volatile acid in the form of carbon dioxide, and the kidneys remove fixed acids by reclaiming bicarbonate ions from the proximal tubule and secreting hydrogen ions into the distal tubule. A loss of a bicarbonate ion is equivalent to the gain of a hydrogen ion. Respiratory acidosis results in increased hydrogen ion concentration due to hypoventilation. Hyperventilation

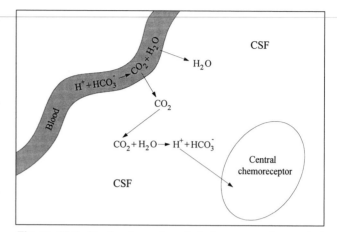

Figure 26-3. Mechanism of central chemoreceptor control of ventilation. Although ventilation is controlled in such a way to maintain arterial PCO_2, the direct stimulus is pH of the CSF surrounding chemoreceptive neurons in the brain stem. Under normal circumstances, arterial PCO_2 determines CSF pH, and, because CSF pH determines ventilation, ventilation is controlled to maintain arterial PCO_2.

causes respiratory alkalosis. Metabolic acidosis results from a cause other than increased PCO_2, such as loss of base or metabolic acid production or failure of the kidney to perform its role in pH regulation. Metabolic alkalosis results from a cause other than decreased PCO_2, such as loss of acid. Respiratory acidosis is compensated by an increase in bicarbonate concentration due to the kidneys. Respiratory alkalosis is compensated by a decrease in bicarbonate concentration due to the kidney reabsorbing less bicarbonate. Metabolic acidosis is compensated by hyperventilation, and metabolic alkalosis is compensated by hypoventilation. Peripheral chemoreceptors respond primarily to decreased arterial PO_2 but only very low levels. Central chemoreceptors act to maintain arterial PCO_2 by altering alveolar ventilation. The central chemoreceptors are indirectly stimulated by arterial PCO_2 by the effect on CSF and interstitial fluid pH. Ventilation during exercise cannot be explained based on blood gas changes during exercise. At an intensity of exercise approaching and exceeding maximum oxygen consumption, hyperventilation occurs as a response to metabolic acidosis. At lower levels of exercise, alveolar ventilation and carbon dioxide production are well matched to maintain arterial PCO_2. Movement of limbs and learning may be responsible for the changes in alveolar ventilation during exercise.

BIBLIOGRAPHY

Berne RM, Levy MN. *Physiology.* St. Louis, Mo: Mosby-Year Book; 1998.

Ganong WF. *Review of Medical Physiology.* Norwalk, Conn: Appleton & Lange; 1995.

Guyton AC, Hall JE, Schmitt W. *Human Physiology and Mechanisms of Disease.* Philadelphia, Pa: WB Saunders; 1997.

Hole JW Jr. *Essentials of Human Anatomy and Physiology.* 4th ed. Dubuque, Iowa: Wm. C. Brown Publishers; 1992.

Schauf C, Moffett D, Moffett S. *Human Physiology: Foundation and Frontiers.* St. Louis, Mo: Times Mirror/Mosby College Publishing; 1990.

Solomon EP, Davis PW. *Human Anatomy and Physiology.* Philadelphia, Pa: WB Saunders; 1983.

West JB. Respiratory *Physiology: The Essentials.* 4th ed. Baltimore, Md: Williams & Wilkins; 1990.

STUDY QUESTIONS

1. How does breathing affect pH? Why is carbon dioxide called a volatile acid?

2. Define hyper- and hypoventilation. Why do you think carbon dioxide is the reference point?

3. How does the kidney compensate for hyperventilation? For hypoventilation?

4. Why does CO_2 indirectly (not directly) control breathing?

5. If you were to hyperventilate voluntarily, what would happen to brain blood flow? What would happen to brain blood flow with hypoventilation?

6. Explain how voluntary hyperventilation in an attempt to swim underwater as long as possible can cause a person to lose consciousness underwater and drown.

7. Why cannot hyperpnea of exercise be explained on the basis of blood gases alone? On the basis of limb movement alone?

LABORATORY EXERCISE

LABORATORY EXERCISE 26-1

CONTROL OF VENTILATION

Objective: Describe how ventilation is influenced by carbon dioxide.

The strongest influence on ventilation within normal ranges of values is arterial PCO_2, which in turn alters ECF pH in brain stem respiratory centers. Although the respiratory system is controlled primarily to eliminate excess CO_2, severe hypoxia markedly increases ventilation.

Materials:
Nose clips
Physiograph
Impedance pneumograph coupler
Paper bags

1. Place the impedance pneumograph electrodes across the widest part of the thorax along the lateral aspects of the ribs. Balance the impedance pneumograph so that a recording of tidal volume can be centered. Instruct the subject to inspire maximally, hold it for one full second before expiring maximally. Adjust balance and gain of the impedance pneumograph so that the recordings can be observed. Run the paper at a speed of 2.5 mm/s to obtain resting respiratory rate and heart rate. Have the subject maintain the same posture throughout the experiments because changes in chest size with postural changes will affect the tracing. Carefully adjust the balance if necessary to keep the tracing on the paper. Do not allow the subject to watch the recorder. Visual feedback may influence the breathing pattern. Allow the subject to breathe normally for 2 to 3 minutes between experiments before proceeding.

Hypercapnia
1. While wearing noseclips, the subject will breathe into and out of a paper bag, thereby concentrating CO_2 within the gas that the subject breathes. Record ventilation and heart rate during rebreathing. Stop recording as soon as a marked change occurs or dyspnea ensues. A change should be observable within 2 to 3 minutes.

2. What was the effect of hypercapnia (rebreathing CO_2) on the respiratory rate? Compare both frequency and volume during rebreathing to the control measurements.

Hypocapnia
1. Wait 5 to 10 minutes for the subject to recover from the hypercapnia experiment before recording a baseline respiratory and heart rate. Make sure that both rates have returned to the previous baseline.

2. Hypocapnia is induced by voluntary hyperventilation for approximately 1 minute. Stop hyperventilation if the subject becomes very dizzy or lightheaded.

3. Upon completion of the hyperventilation, record respiratory and heart rate. It is not necessary to record respiratory rate during the hyperventilation, but immediately after hyperventilation.

LABORATORY EXERCISE

4. What was the effect of hypocapnia on the respiratory rate? Compare both frequency and volume during the post-hyperventilation period to the control measurements.

5. Recalling the effects of carbon dioxide on brain blood flow, what do you expect to happen during rebreathing and hyperventilation?

TWENTY-SEVEN

Cardiopulmonary Responses to Exercise

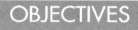

OBJECTIVES

1. Describe the changes in total peripheral resistance, cardiac output, and mean arterial pressure that occur during aerobic exercise.

2. Explain how the heart permits increased blood flow of skeletal muscle to occur and simultaneously maintain arterial pressure.

3. Describe the relationship between heart rate and stroke volume during exercise.

4. Describe how peripheral blood flow is redistributed during exercise.

5. Explain the potential conflict between temperature regulation and blood supply to working skeletal muscle during exercise and how heat exhaustion can result.

6. Describe the relationship between external work and oxygen consumption.

7. Describe how maximum oxygen consumption is measured in a laboratory.

8. Contrast the effect of body mass on oxygen consumption during treadmill walking and bicycle ergometry.

9. Describe the peripheral and central adaptations to aerobic exercise, and contrast their time courses.

10. Compare the heart rate and stroke volumes of fit and unfit people during aerobic exercise.

11. Explain the purpose of STPD.

12. Discuss means of analyzing body composition and their strengths and weaknesses.

Although skeletal muscle comprises 40% to 50% of body mass, it only receives about 15% of the cardiac output at rest. Aerobic exercise requires a large, steady supply of oxygen to the working muscles. During this type of exercise (large muscle group, moderate intensity, rhythmic work), local control produces vasodilation in the working muscle, increasing muscle blood flow as much as 10 times its resting value and creating a large decrease (50% or more) in total peripheral resistance (TPR). Cardiac output must, therefore, increase to maintain arterial pressure and supply working muscle. Cardiac output can increase from a resting value of 5 to 6 L/min up to 25 to 35 L/min in well-trained athletes. The increase in cardiac output is provided by increases in both heart rate and stroke volume, although the increase in heart rate is typically much greater than that in stroke volume. Heart rate may increase from 40 to 50 bpm at rest up to about 180 bpm. Maximum heart rate varies with age and can be estimated roughly as 220 minus age in years. Stroke volume, on the other hand, may increase only about 20%. In addition, changes in blood pressure are expected to occur. Typically, systolic pressure increases in proportion to the work load, and diastolic pressure decreases to a much lesser degree, with the result of a modest increase in mean arterial pressure. These changes in the circulation provide increased delivery of oxygen to working muscles to support increased aerobic metabolism.

CARDIOVASCULAR ADJUSTMENTS TO EXERCISE

The role of the heart during exercise is to maintain the relationships among mean arterial pressure, total peripheral resistance, and cardiac output. The active hyperemia produced in skeletal muscle during exercise progressively decreases total peripheral resistance with increasing intensity of work. For a given mean arterial pressure, decreasing TPR results in a greater flow of blood from the aorta back to the inferior and superior vena cava. As discussed in a previous chapter, if mean arterial pressure is regulated centrally, a change in conductance proportional to the increased needs of the tissue will provide adequate blood flow to the active tissue as well as maintain sufficient blood flow to all other tissues of the body. Therefore, the heart must pump out a volume of blood per minute equal to what the mean arterial pressure (MAP) and TPR cause to flow through the systemic circulation. Should pumping of the heart be inadequate to meet this demand for local blood flow, a new steady state will be reached at a lower MAP with less peripheral blood flow but at a cardiac output that

the heart can manage. A decrease in blood pressure with increasing intensity of exercise, therefore, should be interpreted as an inability of the heart to perform adequately for the exercise task, and exercise should be terminated.

A healthy heart will pump out the blood demanded by the peripheral circulation. This is accomplished by changes in both the heart and the peripheral circulation. The decreased TPR allows the heart to pump a greater volume of blood for a given systolic wall tension. Secondly, stimulation of β-adrenergic receptors by sympathetic nerves to the heart and circulating epinephrine cause heart rate to increase as described above and contractility of the ventricles to increase. A person with a transplanted heart has only circulating epinephrine to increase heart rate and contractility. As discussed in the chapter on control of the cardiovascular system, increases in cardiac output result in decreases in central venous pressure. Unless other interventions come into play, cardiac output and central venous pressure cannot change from their equilibrium values. The increased contractility produces a greater strength of ventricular contraction for a given preload. An increased heart rate produces more ejections of the heart per minute, and, as discussed above, the decreased peripheral resistance allows a greater volume of blood to be pumped out of the heart with each beat (Figure 27-1). Another factor that allows cardiac output to rise is the effect of sympathetic stimulation of the large central veins. Venoconstriction allows a greater volume of blood to be removed from the veins and placed into the arteries. By decreasing venous compliance, venous pressure is maintained in spite of a decrease in central venous volume. At the same time, the increased volume of blood on the arterial side of the circulation maintains arterial pressure in spite of a decreased TPR. Generalized constriction of arterioles in response to release of norepinephrine onto α-adrenergic receptors prevents TPR from falling as much as it would otherwise. This allows more of the cardiac output to be diverted to working muscles from tissues, such as the skin, kidneys, gastrointestinal tract, and fat (Figure 27-2). The heart and brain are spared from generalized vasoconstriction. Blood flow to the heart increases in proportion to the work performed by the heart, and blood flow increases to areas of the brain that are more active during exercise.

Although increasing heart rate results in a shortened time for ventricular filling, stroke volume remains elevated during exercise until near maximal levels. This is possible because very little of the filling of the ventricles occurs late in diastole. Secondly, with increased contractility, systole is shortened by the effects of increased cAMP. Cyclic AMP causes not only more calcium to

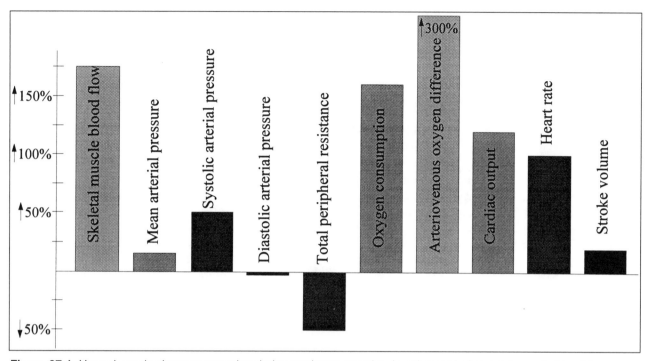

Figure 27-1. Hemodynamic changes occurring during moderate exercise. Local control of skeletal muscle blood flow causes dilation of skeletal muscle arterioles and a large decrease in TPR. The heart responds to the increased demand for peripheral blood flow by increases in both heart rate and stroke volume. The increased demand for oxygen by skeletal muscle blood flow is met by both increases in skeletal muscle blood flow and a-VO$_2$ difference.

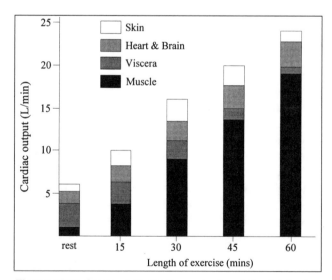

Figure 27-2. Changes in cardiac output and its distribution during a progressive exercise test in which intensity of exercise is increased every 3 minutes. Note the greatest change occurs in skeletal muscle blood flow. Also note that skin blood flow increases at every stage, except the last, which approaches maximum heart rate. Skin blood flow and, therefore, temperature regulation are decreased to maintain central hemodynamics.

enter the cell with each beat, but also increases the rate of cross-bridge cycling and the rate of uptake of calcium by the sarcoplasmic reticulum. When maximal aerobic intensity is approached, stroke volume levels off and begins to decrease with increasing intensity because decreased time for ventricular filling can no longer be compensated by shorter systole and increased contractility.

A potential conflict for the cardiovascular system is also caused by thermoregulation. During exercise, the heat generated by muscle activity must be dissipated to the environment to maintain body temperature at a reasonable value. Core temperature increases with the intensity of exercise approximately in proportion to the percentage of maximum oxygen consumption elicited by the work. A more aerobically fit individual experiences less of a rise in body temperature at a given intensity of exercise than a less fit individual. At high ambient temperatures, exercise may be limited by the competing demands for blood flow to the working muscles and to the skin to dissipate heat. Total peripheral resistance may fall to a level such that the heart cannot maintain its cardiac output high enough to prevent MAP from falling. Heavy sweating also depletes the blood volume and causes blood pressure to fall. Exercise in the heat, especially with high humidity, needs to be monitored carefully or avoided until the physiologic adaptations described in the chapter on thermoregulation occur. A decrease in arterial pressure caused by exercise in the heat is called heat exhaustion.

Within narrow limits, a given external workload requires the same energy production by the working muscles by different individuals and from one time to another. This allows us to predict oxygen consumption (VO_2) for a given work load. If one can estimate the power output of the activity accurately, an accurate estimate of VO_2 can be made. Devices such as treadmills, bicycle ergometers, and rowing ergometers are often used because the power output of the person exercising can be determined accurately. Unfortunately, many activities do not lend themselves to accurate measurement of the power output. These activities include most sports, which have intermittent periods of activity or fluctuations in activity levels. Measurements taken from subjects on treadmills or bicycle ergometers have demonstrated a linear relationship between power output (or workload) and oxygen consumption. Therefore, knowledge of the workload performed by an individual allows us to predict the subject's VO_2 accurately. Oxygen consumption can be estimated during exercise as VO_2 (ml/min) $= 300 + 12 \times W$, where W is the power output in watts and 300 is the resting metabolic rate.

Because of this relationship between workload and oxygen consumption, the most objective and reliable measurement to predict an individual's capacity for sustained work (or exercise) is determination of maximum oxygen consumption (VO_2 max). This is typically performed by measuring oxygen consumption while walking on a treadmill. Oxygen consumption is measured after 3 minutes of exercise at a given treadmill speed and elevation. Either speed or elevation is increased, and VO_2 is measured again after 3 minutes at the new workload. Workload on a treadmill is directly related to the weight of the subject walking on the treadmill. Thus, a given workload is determined by treadmill speed, elevation, and weight of the subject and requires a given number of ml of oxygen per minute per kilogram of body mass (ml $\times$ min^{-1} $\times$ kg^{-1}). The workload is increased until maximum oxygen consumption is reached. This is determined by the lack of an increase (or an increase of less than 1 ml $\times$ min^{-1} $\times$ kg^{-1}) of body weight with an increase in workload.

Measurement of oxygen consumption in the laboratory requires collection of expired gas, measurement of the volume of the gas, and the fraction of the expired gas consisting of oxygen and carbon dioxide. The temperature of the expired gas is measured, and the volume is corrected to STPD (standard temperature and pressure, dry) to take into account the differences in tem-

perature of the collected gas, barometric pressure, and the presence of water vapor in the collected sample. The difference in fraction of inspired oxygen (assumed to be 20.93%) and that in the collected gases is computed and multiplied by the volume of air inspired. Usually, the volume of inspired air is not measured; the volume of expired air is. The volume of carbon dioxide generated and volume of oxygen consumed may not be equal depending on the mixture of fuels used to regenerate ATP. At low metabolic rates, less carbon dioxide is generated for the amount of oxygen used because fat is the primary substrate for energy production. As more carbohydrate is used for metabolism, the ratio (respiratory quotient) approaches unity. At a metabolic rate that exceeds maximum oxygen consumption, the ratio exceeds 1.0 because of hyperventilation. The volume of inspired air is computed based on the idea that the quantity of nitrogen inspired equals the quantity of nitrogen expired. Therefore, by adding the fractions of expired oxygen and carbon dioxide, we can compute the fraction of expired nitrogen. Comparing the ratio of expired nitrogen to inspired nitrogen we get the ratio of inspired gas to expired gas. We then multiply the difference in fraction of inspired and expired oxygen by inspired volume to compute oxygen consumption. The intensity of work is increased until a person cannot continue or oxygen consumption reaches a plateau value. Usually, a sharp increase in respiratory quotient occurs when maximum oxygen consumption is exceeded.

Maximum oxygen consumption is generally expressed relative to body size in units of ml $\times$ min^{-1} $\times$ kg^{-1}. This takes into account the ability of the person to perform activities, such as locomotion, in which the load is determined by the person's own body weight. Treadmill locomotion lends itself directly to this type of prediction, because the subject is moving his or her own body weight. Aerobic fitness is easily predicted by the treadmill speed and elevation without having to consider body weight. The person who can continue to walk at faster treadmill speeds or higher elevations is obviously the most fit. In contrast, bicycle or rowing ergometry requires movement of an external object (the flywheel) against a resistance. Oxygen consumption in ml/min is directly related to workload, which is generally expressed in watts. A prediction of aerobic fitness in ml $\times$ min^{-1} $\times$ kg^{-1} is then obtained by measuring VO_2 in ml/min during work and dividing by body mass.

Aerobic training produces an increased maximum intensity of aerobic activity (Figure 27-3). This results from adaptations in the heart, the blood vessels of the muscle, and in the muscle tissue itself. The heart hypertrophies with an increased wall thickness. This increased thickness places more cross bridges in parallel, which

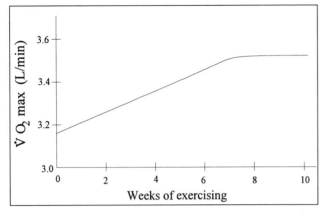

Figure 27-3. Changes in maximum oxygen consumption with aerobic training. Note the plateau—in this case, at 7 weeks.

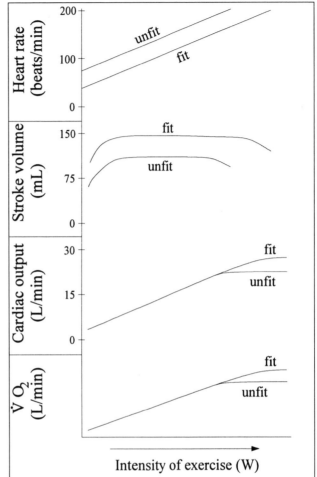

Figure 27-4. Hemodynamic changes during exercise in fit and unfit individuals. Whether fit or unfit, a given intensity of exercise demands a similar oxygen consumption and cardiac output. The fit person continues to experience an increase in oxygen consumption and cardiac output after a plateau is reached by the unfit individual. Also note that for any given intensity of exercise, the fit person has a greater stroke volume and, therefore, lower heart rate. A simple index of fitness is to measure heart rate at a standardized intensity of exercise.

increases the strength of the heart. Because of the increased myocardial strength, the heart can produce a greater stroke volume for a given cardiac output with training. Therefore, heart rate in a trained individual is less at any given intensity of exercise (Figure 27-4). Increased vascular conductance of the trained muscles produces a greater maximum blood flow to the muscle, which allows a greater convective transport of oxygen and other nutrients to the muscle during work. Within the muscle itself, an increase in the number of capillaries surrounding the muscle cells, an increase in the number of mitochondria within each muscle cell, and an increase in the quantity of myoglobin, an oxygen binding pigment, occur with training. Endurance-type training, in addition to the changes described above, produces biochemical changes that allow the muscle to use less glycogen and more fatty acids, which prolongs the availability of glycogen within the muscle cell itself and liver glycogen for the entire body. Muscle cells and the liver can also store more glycogen as a result of endurance training.

The type of training responses are specific to the type of training performed. Athletes training for high-intensity aerobic activity have a greater increase in maximum oxygen consumption and a higher muscle blood flow during exercise. Those training for less intense, longer-lasting activity experience greater metabolic changes and lesser cardiovascular changes. Endurance athletes can perform at moderately high intensity levels for a long time, whereas high-intensity aerobic athletes must sustain a very high aerobic activity for a shorter period, in the range of 4 to 15 minutes. Athletes engaged in activities that require bursts of activity that greatly exceed the energy supplied at maximum oxygen consumption develop characteristics that enhance glycolytic metabolism and the ability to withstand heavy

acid production. Anaerobic training results in an increased buffering capacity of the muscle cells for acid. This training allows some individuals to run at near full speed for up to 44 seconds; the world record for the 400-meter dash is only slightly more than four times that of the 100-meter dash.

The sequence in which adaptations to aerobic activity occur is determined by the complexity of "construction." Changes in the oxidative capacity of skeletal muscle cells by increasing the number of mitochondria and oxidative enzymes occur rapidly (time frame of days) and result in greater endurance. These adaptations can be elicited most efficiently by large numbers of exercise bouts of increasing intensity and duration. Deconditioned patients respond more favorably to a progression of many short exercise sessions working toward longer, more intense, and fewer sessions. Cardiovascular changes occur over a period of weeks and require more extensive changes, including the production of more blood vessels to carry nutrients to the muscle cells. Increased delivery of nutrients and oxygen to the exercising muscles produce a greater maximum intensity of sustained work, which we can assess by measuring maximum oxygen consumption. Therefore, endurance increases rapidly, and intensity increases slowly with the initiation of training. With cessation of training, endurance decreases more rapidly, and maximum intensity decreases more slowly.

Several ways of assessing a person's ability to tolerate sustained activity are available. The heart rate response to a given intensity of exercise will be used in the laboratory exercise for this chapter. Its basis lies in the proportionality of fitness and stroke volume. In addition to requiring a given quantity of oxygen consumption for a given intensity of exercise, a proportional increase from resting cardiac output is required to deliver the oxygen needed by working muscles. Because of the larger stroke volume available to the more fit individual, this person can perform a higher intensity of sustained work, and, at any given workload, the more fit individual has a lower heart rate.

Because of this relationship, we may assess fitness by measuring heart rate at a given external workload. We can predict maximum oxygen consumption in L/min while the subject pedals a bicycle ergometer by measuring heart rate at a given power output. Some older bicycle ergometers will not be calibrated in watts but may be in units of kpm. Three hundred kpm/min equals approximately 50 watts. The unit kpm/min is an archaic term that is not based on standard scientific units. Dividing estimated VO_2 max by body weight provides an accurate estimate of aerobic capacity. An average VO_2 max is 30 to 40 ml $\times$ min^{-1} $\times$ kg^{-1}, whereas a successful participant in aerobic athletic events may have a VO_2 max of 80 ml $\times$ min^{-1} $\times$ kg^{-1} or more. At any given workload, a person with a higher maximum oxygen consumption will have a lower heart rate, and, as workload increases, heart rate increases proportionally. Based on these relationships and the research of Astrand (1960), for men with heart rates between 120 and 170 at workloads between 50 and 250 W, maximum oxygen consumption can be estimated by the formula $VO2$ max (ml $\times$ min^{-1} $\times$ min^{-1}) = 6.5 − 0.04 $\times$ HR + 0.02 $\times$ W, where HR is heart rate (beats/min) and W is workload in watts.

Wellness

The concepts of wellness are among the most important in helping others attain maximal health. Unfortunately, the concepts of wellness have been embraced by pseudoscientific groups resulting in dismissal by many people in mainstream health care professions. The purpose of wellness is to maintain or improve overall health or "wellness" with a major emphasis on active participation of the individual. Typically, six components of health have been described and are addressed in wellness programs. These components are physical, social, psychological, intellectual, environmental, and spiritual health. A concept related to wellness is that of health promotion in which all health care providers should be active. Health promotion is a major component of the field of health education and consists of both education and organizational, economic, and environmental support for behaviors conducive to health.

Aspects of wellness include lifestyle choices, physical fitness, nutrition, psychological wellbeing, and stress management. Examples of lifestyle choices include smoking, inappropriate use of drugs and other substances, and engaging in unsafe behaviors. Certainly, it is easy to see how poor lifestyle choices impact negatively on the physical aspect of health as well as the other aspects of health listed above. Self-efficacy or the willingness of individuals to empower themselves in lifestyle and other health-related decisions is probably the most important aspect of wellness. A person who takes control of his or her own life and understands the reasons for healthy behaviors and consequences of unhealthy behaviors is more likely to adhere to a plan of care developed by the health care provider and challenge the health care provider to establish an optimal plan. Related to self-efficacy is self-confidence, another issue important to the person staying with an optimal plan for health.

Psychological wellbeing and stress management are taught in most health care professional programs. Certainly, more severe problems need to be referred to mental health experts. Biofeedback and relaxation techniques are employed by several health care disciplines. Nutritional aspects of health are the specialty of dieticians; however, other health care providers may be involved at a more rudimentary level as well as designing programs that address body composition, including exercise training, to promote a healthy body composition.

Dieting alone results in loss of lean body mass in addition to fat and results in less than optimum improvements in health. Exercise preserves lean body mass and requires less of a decrease in caloric intake to produce weight loss. Resistance training increases bone density and reduces the risk of osteoporosis later in life.

Some simple guidelines to effective weight loss include:
- Do not markedly restrict caloric intake
- Do not completely restrict food types
- Do not decrease weight by more than 1 to 2 pounds per week
- Reduce portions, decrease fat intake (eg, 2% milk instead of whole milk)
- Increase exercise
- Avoid daily weighings

Daily weighings have two possible negative consequences. Those who do not lose weight quickly may become demoralized and give up. Others may take up an unhealthy diet in an effort to see the scale decrease every day. Various diets do provide rapid weight loss in the determined individual. Unfortunately, rapid weight loss leads to rapid weight gain (plus interest) once the weight loss goal is reached, especially in those who deprive themselves completely of one type of food that the person enjoys. Body composition is the relative portions of lean body mass and fat, usually expressed as percent body fat. Body composition is implicated in many diseases: cardiovascular disease, type 2 diabetes mellitus, several forms of cancer, and hypertension.

The components of physical fitness include aerobic fitness, strength, muscular endurance, flexibility, and body composition (addressed above).

Aerobic fitness involves the use of large muscle groups in continuous, rhythmic activity for an extended period, usually at least 15 minutes. Examples of aerobic exercise include running, swimming (if skill permits), and bicycling. The author's own experience with swimming is that, with practice, swimming can be converted from an anaerobic activity that can be sustained for only 2 to 3 minutes to an aerobic one that can be enjoyed for more than an hour. Benefits of aerobic fitness include improved cardiovascular health with improved cardiac function, improved vascular supply, increased glucose uptake, reduced body fat, and reduced risk of cardiovascular disease. Intermittent activities, including most games such as basketball, do not provide aerobic training because the intensity is not sustained for a long enough time without rest for aerobic conditioning to occur. Unfortunately, many of the general public perceive these games to be aerobic. Although intermittent activities, such as games, do not provide as great an aerobic benefit, they are enjoyable to those who participate, and participants are more likely to continue to be active doing what they enjoy, rather than being bored by strict aerobic exercise.

Muscular fitness is defined in terms of strength and endurance of muscles. Strength is the ability to generate a maximum force over a short duration (single lift of weight, isokinetic device, etc). Endurance is the ability to perform repeated movements or how many times a fixed or relative weight (often body weight) can be lifted.

The component termed flexibility actually contains some controversial concepts. The name is one of them. As typically measured, flexibility is really a measure of how well we can extend soft tissues of the trunk and limbs. Therefore, many prefer the term extensibility. The second issue is whether we consider flexibility (or extensibility) as the end range of motion involving one or more nonpathological joints and determined by soft tissue length, or if we consider the presence of pathologic joints to be a limiting factor in flexibility. The sit and reach test, in which the person sits in front of a box with a tape measure and reaches as far past the feet as possible, is a screening tool for flexibility promoted by several organizations involved in fitness. Unfortunately, this test cannot distinguish between low back and hamstring flexibility. Many tests are available for testing flexibility of different body parts.

SPECIFICITY OF TRAINING

Adaptations that occur with training are specific to the type of training, and, as such, training programs should be prescribed with specific goals of the individual training in mind. Aerobic training leads to increased maximum oxygen consumption, increased muscle blood flow, increased oxidative capacity of muscle tissue (mitochondrial and oxidative enzymes), and the ability to move oneself for an extended period (eg, middle distance, long distance). Resistance training leads to an increased ability to generate torque at specific joints produced by hypertrophy of muscle and motor learning (eg, weightlifting).

Anaerobic training improves the ability to sustain a very high level of metabolism, beyond maximum oxygen consumption, by improved buffering of generated acid (eg, 400-meter run). Each training regimen contains some unique combination of each type of training effect. Every training program, regardless of how unbalanced it may be, probably improves, at least to a small degree, each aspect of fitness. However, if a person wishes to improve all aspects of physical fitness, all aspects need to be addressed in training.

Wellness in *The Guide to Physical Therapist Practice* (November 1997 issue of *Physical Therapy*) is addressed most specifically in cardiopulmonary practice pattern A, which describes patients/clients with decreased maximum aerobic capacity who are at risk for developing cardiac disease, pulmonary disease, or both. This practice pattern is based on well-accepted risk factor profiles that have been published in the literature. These risk factors include diabetes mellitus, family history of heart disease, hypercholesterolemia, hypertension, obesity, and smoking. Tests and measures typically used to measure fitness include aerobic capacity and endurance, anthropometric measurements, and muscle performance tests. The guide suggests that, within one to six visits, the patient/client will demonstrate independence in an aerobic exercise program and be able to identify personal risk factors for cardiopulmonary disease and methods he or she will use to reduce risk. Some of the most commonly used interventions included in cardiopulmonary practice pattern A are aerobic endurance exercise, aquatic exercise, body mechanics and ergonomics training, breathing exercise, strengthening, and stretching. The interventions' expected outcomes include safe performance of self-care and home management performed efficiently and at a maximal level of independence with or without devices and equipment, enhancement of health-related quality of life, maintenance of optimal role function, an understanding of personal and environmental factors that promote optimal health status, and an understanding of prevention strategies. Thus, the American Physical Therapy Association is suggesting a major role to be played beyond providing interventions that allow discrete physical functions to be performed, but also to make the patient/client responsible for future health.

Screening for Participation in Exercise Programs

Health screens, using tools such as the PAR-Q (Physical Activity Readiness Questionnaire), are used to clear presumably healthy individuals for involvement in fitness programs. The PAR-Q is a simple questionnaire used to screen for risk factors for vigorous activity (exercise) in a general population. It consists of seven questions related to the possibility of cardiovascular disease, orthopedic conditions, or unspecified other causes.

Red flags from screening include angina, shortness of breath, dyspnea on exertion, dizziness/syncope, orthopnea, peripheral edema, arrhythmias, peripheral vascular disease, murmur. Other risk factors for coronary artery disease include age older than 45 for men and 50 for women, family history of heart disease, cigarette smoking, hypertension, hypercholesterolemia, diabetes mellitus, and sedentary lifestyle. Any of these red flags should be a part of a verbal or written medical history that is taken before clearing a person to engage in a physical fitness program.

The concept of risk stratification is different from screening. Screening is done for those presumed to be healthy. Risk stratification is done with those who have known disease. Based on several criteria, such as the presence of angina, the maximum exercise capacity from an exercise test, and presence of arrhythmias, a patient is placed into either a low-risk, moderate-risk, or high-risk category. A person in the high-risk category is monitored more carefully and undergoes a more conservative exercise program than a person in the low-risk category.

For those without a known history of heart disease, screening is followed by placing the person into either a group with minimal risk or a group with risk of untoward events, requiring different levels of monitoring. This is based on specific criteria. Individuals may be classified as apparently healthy if they are asymptomatic with no more than one major risk factor described above, such as smoking or sedentary lifestyle; these individuals are suitable for moderate-intensity exercise. The category of increased risk includes individuals with signs or symptoms of possible disease and/or two or more risk factors. These individuals need to be cleared by a physician before starting an exercise program. They may require a graded exercise test. Patients/clients with known disease and requiring stratification as described above need to be in a formal cardiac rehab program. They almost always have a graded exercise test done.

The American College of Sports Medicine recommends exercise testing prior to exercise participation for certain individuals. Before beginning an exercise program, a graded exercise test with a physician present is recommended for those who have known disease and have increased risk of cardiovascular disease with symptoms. In addition, a test is recommended if a person wishes to begin a vigorous exercise program, but has increased risk of disease without symptoms or is apparently healthy but older. Older in this recommendation is defined as 40 years of age and older for men and 50 and older for women.

PHYSICAL FITNESS TESTING FOR THE APPARENTLY HEALTHY

Fitness tests, included graded exercise tests, may be performed on healthy individuals. The purpose of fitness testing is to accumulate data for basing an exercise prescription, evaluating progress in an exercise program, setting goals to motivate individuals, and education.

BODY COMPOSITION

Several methods are used for determining body composition. These include hydrostatic weighing, skin fold calipers, anthropometric methods, bioelectric impedance, and body mass index. Hydrostatic weighing is based on Archimedes' principle. Body density can be determined by determining the volume of water displaced. The water produces a buoyant force equal to the volume of water displaced. By weighing on land and in the water, the buoyant force produced by the water is determined. By knowing the density of water, the volume of water displaced is determined. The volume of the water displaced is the volume of the person. Knowing the mass of the person and the volume of the person allows computation of the person's density. Percent body fat is then determined by a regression formula from the person's density. Skin fold measurements are simply a convenient but less accurate and reliable means of determining percent body fat. Anthropometric method is the measurement of certain aspects of an individual that are convenient but not as accurate as hydrostatic weighing or skin-fold measurements. Body mass index is a ratio of mass in kilograms to the square of height in meters. Example: A person weighs 165 lbs (75 kg) and is 6'1" tall (1.85 m) BMI = (75 kg/1.85 m x 1.85 m) = 18.75, which indicates a relatively thin individual. Waist-to-hip ratio indicates the pattern of fat distribution on the body. A greater amount of fat on the trunk is associated with several diseases. The waist is measured at the smallest circumference between the ribs and hips. The hips are measured at the largest circumference, including the buttocks. Bioelectrical impedance analysis uses an electric current to determine the relative proportions of fat (poor conductor) and lean body mass (good conductor). Percent body fat is overestimated in lean individuals and underestimated in obese individuals. It is also influenced by degree of hydration.

AEROBIC FITNESS

A graded exercise test may be maximal in which the workload is increased until the client cannot continue or it may be submaximal, in which the test is stopped when a certain criterion is reached. Maximal testing is necessary to determine maximum oxygen consumption, but submaximal testing can be used to estimate it. There is an increased risk of untoward events with maximal testing, but maximal tests are more likely to find coronary artery disease if it exists. Graded exercise tests may also be arranged to be either discontinuous, in which the person is allowed a rest period between each incremental work bout, or continuous, in which the workload is incremented every 2 to 3 minutes without a rest break. Discontinuous tests alternate rest periods with exercise; therefore, there is **less probability of local fatigue limiting the testing procedure**, but discontinuous protocols take much longer to complete and are not used a great deal.

DESIGNING A FITNESS PROGRAM

During the beginning phase, there is rapid improvement, but potential for injury, soreness, and boredom. A major part of the improvement comes from motor learning (ie, learning efficient movement patterns of sequencing agonist, antagonist, and synergist). During the progression phase, there is continued improvement more limited to strength and endurance. During the maintenance (plateau) phase, there is little improvement over a short timeframe. Those seeking to maintain a healthy fitness level will continue for an extended time with a similar intensity of exercise with this understanding. Those who fail to grasp the concept of the plateau phase may become frustrated and either injure themselves or quit exercising.

Exercise Prescription

An exercise prescription must address the type of exercise, the intensity and duration of exercise, and how frequently exercise is performed. Aerobic activities include walking, running, cycling, swimming, skating, aerobics, rowing, cross country skiing, and stepping. Less aerobic activities include games with intermittent running. Resistance activities include weightlifting, isokinetic devices, medicine balls, and exercises involving movement of body weight at a mechanical disadvantage. These activities can be incorporated into the exercise prescription of a healthy person. A person with known cardiovascular disease may or may not be appropriate for heavy resistance exercise. Several organizations have provided guidelines on the appropriate use of resistance exercise for those with known cardiovascular disease. Certainly, we cannot escape the periodic need to move heavy objects in our lives. On the other hand, we need to be prudent in prescribing heavy-resistance activities. Current research indicates that we have been too conservative in the use of resistance exercise for those with cardiovascular disease. Typically, individuals use a weight that can be lifted about 10 to 15 times for three sets and progress to a greater weight when a greater number of repetitions can be accomplished. Multiple and various protocols can be incorporated in terms of repetitions, sets, and resistance and can be found in both scientific and popular literature.

Frequency

Through the years, the number three has become the magic number for exercise frequency. The rule of thumb of three sessions of aerobic activity at least 20 minutes long each week at the proper intensity has been shown to reduce the risk of cardiovascular disease. However, a person could exercise every day. If a person is exercising to control blood glucose, it makes sense to have the same "dose" of exercise every day. Heavy resistance exercise is usually limited to every other day to avoid muscle soreness or injury. Many individuals will alternate upper and lower body workouts each day.

Intensity

A decreased risk of cardiovascular disease in the general population exists with a mild intensity of walking. A conservative intensity of exercise is 40% of the heart rate reserve (HRR). Heart rate reserve is the difference between maximum and resting heart rate. Maximum heart rate can be determined in the lab or estimated. The usual equation for estimating maximal heart rate (HR_{max}) is 220 minus age in years. This formula underestimates HR_{max} in the elderly, making the exercise prescription more conservative. An example is, for a 50-year-old, $HR_{max} = 220 - 50 = 170$, resting HR = 70, HRR = 170 − 70 = 100, 40% of HRR = 100 x 0.40 = 40, added to resting = 70 + 40 = 110. A more liberal limit is 70% of HRR, which, for the same example, would be 140.

Duration

A duration of at least 20 minutes at the appropriate intensity and frequency has been shown to decrease the risk of cardiovascular disease. More recent studies have indicated that any level or duration of activity is beneficial.

As seen from the description above, wellness is a complex concept with many facets easily dismissed. However, addressing each of the components is more likely to produce a good outcome from our intervention than simply focusing on "where it hurts."

SUMMARY

Blood flow increases markedly to skeletal muscle during exercise, requiring compensations in the central circulation to maintain arterial pressure as TPR falls. Sympathetic stimulation of the heart and blood vessels increases contractility and heart rate to increase the cardiac output for a given preload, constrict central veins to maintain preload on the heart, and distribute blood flow away from less active tissues during exercise. Stroke volume increases with increasing intensity of exercise in spite of a gradual decrease in the time available for ventricular filling. Stroke volume decreases at a very high intensity of exercise. A conflict between thermoregulation and supplying blood flow to active muscles can result, especially in a hot environment, and heat may limit the potential for exercise or cause heat exhaustion. External work, such as treadmill walking or bicycle ergometry, requires approximately the same oxygen consumption for all individuals. The intensity of external work that can be sustained for more than 3 minutes is limited by the maximum oxygen consumption that can be generated due to peripheral and cardiovascular characteristics of the individual. Maximum oxygen consumption is used as an index of aerobic fitness. Those with a greater maximum oxygen consumption can sustain a higher intensity of exercise and have a higher stroke volume and lower heart rate as well as a lower core temperature at any given intensity of exercise proportional to body size. Treadmill walking takes body size directly into consideration, because part of the load is the person's body weight, whereas body weight is supported in bicycle ergometry. Aerobic training results in a greater density of mitochondria and oxidative enzymes within a few days and rapidly increases a person's endurance. Increased delivery of oxygen to working muscles limits intensity and requires much longer aerobic training to improve. Adaptations resulting from exercise are specific to the type of training in terms of intensity, duration, aerobic, and anaerobic. Metabolic rate and oxygen consumption can be estimated for a given intensity of external work using formulas presented.

BIBLIOGRAPHY

Astrand I. Aerobic work capacity in men and women with special reference to age. *Acta Physiologica Scandinavica*. 1960;49(Suppl):45-60.

Berne RM, Levy MN. *Physiology*. St. Louis, Mo: Mosby-Year Book; 1998.

Ganong WF. *Review of Medical Physiology*. 17th ed. Norwalk, Conn: Appleton & Lange; 1995.

Guyton AC, Hall JE, Schmitt W. *Human Physiology and Mechanisms of Disease*. Philadelphia, Pa: WB Saunders; 1997.

Kenney WL (ed). *ACSM's Guidelines for Exercise Testing and Prescription*. Baltimore, Md: Williams & Wilkins; 1995.

Kisner C, Colby LA. *Therapeutic Exercise Foundation and Techniques*. 2nd ed. Philadelphia, Pa: FA Davis; 1990.

O'Sullivan SB, Thomas JS. *Physical Rehabilitation Assessment and Treatment*. 3rd ed. Philadelphia, Pa: FA Davis; 1994.

Roitman JL (ed). *ACSM's Resource Manual*. Baltimore, Md: Williams & Wilkins; 1998.

Schauf C, Moffett D, Moffett S. *Human Physiology: Foundation and Frontiers*. St. Louis, Mo: Times Mirror/Mosby College Publishing; 1990.

STUDY QUESTIONS

1. What is the predicted maximum heart rate of a 20-year-old? A 50-year-old?

2. How can arterial pressure be maintained with the substantial decrease in TPR that occurs during exercise?

3. Explain how constriction of arterioles in tissues other than working muscle reduces the work of the heart.

4. Describe how stroke volume changes as the intensity of exercise increases. How does heart rate affect stroke volume?

5. Describe the role of the sympathetic nervous system in allowing us to sustain a high intensity of exercise. How do you think exercise tolerance is affected in people taking β-adrenergic blocking drugs?

6. Explain the dangers of exercising in a hot environment.

7. Why is maximum oxygen consumption considered the "gold standard" for aerobic fitness? How might the relationship between external work and oxygen consumption change in a person with neurologic deficits or musculoskeletal injury?

8. Why are stages of exercise tests usually 2 to 3 minutes in duration?

9. Why is the volume of air inspired per minute not equal to the volume expired during exercise? If conservation of mass exists, where do the extra molecules go?

10. Why does hyperventilation occur during very intense exercise?

11. Compare the timeframe of adaptations resulting in improved endurance and increased intensity of exercise tolerated.

12. Explain the basis of the submaximal bicycle test for estimating maximum oxygen consumption. Why do we need to correct the result for body mass?

LABORATORY EXERCISES

LABORATORY EXERCISE 27-1

SUBMAXIMAL BICYCLE TEST OF FITNESS

Objectives:
1.   Examine the relationships between exercise and heart rate and blood pressure.

2.   Estimate aerobic fitness by a bicycle ergometer test.

Materials:
Bicycle ergometer
Impedance pneumograph
Calculator

Methods:
1.   Prepare the subject for recording of the EKG with the impedance pneumograph. Place electrodes across the widest part of the chest. Balance the impedance pneumograph to obtain a record of chest movement. From this record both respiratory and heart rate can be determined while the subject sits on the bicycle ergometer.

2.   Have the subject pedal the bicycle ergometer without any load and determine heart rate and respiratory rate.

3.   Begin test at 50 W. Allow the subject to pedal at least 3 minutes before recording EKG. If heart rate does not fall between 120 and 170 bpm, increase workload by another 50 W for males, 25 W for females. Continue to increase workload until heart rate exceeds 170 bpm or the subject cannot continue due to local muscle fatigue.

4.   Use the formula for predicted VO_2 max (L/min) = 6.5 - .04 x HR + .02 x W

5.   Correct VO_2 max for body mass (ml x min^{-1} x kg^{-1}). One kg = 2.2 lb. Repeat with as many subjects as time allows. Normal VO_2 max = 35 to 40 ml x min^{-1} x kg^{-1}, 60 to 80 for well-trained aerobic athletes.

Questions:
1.   What factors determine VO_2 max? Why is this the single best predictor of fitness?

2.   Why do we correct VO_2 max for body weight?

3.   What are the differences between determining maximum capacity for work on a treadmill compared with a bicycle ergometer?

4.   How would you predict the following types of athletes would rank in terms of VO_2 max: tennis player, hockey player, miler, marathon runner, cross-country skier? State your reasons.

5.   How can elite athletes benefit from blood doping (artificially increasing hematocrit)? What does this say about factors that limit exercise performance? If a hematocrit of 60% is better than 45% during maximal exercise, what do you speculate is the adaptive significance of our species having such a low hematocrit?

LABORATORY EXERCISES

LABORATORY EXERCISE 27-2

BODY COMPOSITION

Objective: Demonstrate the use of skinfold calipers in assessment of body composition.

Materials: Skinfold calipers

Assessment of body composition is a nice way of saying determination of percent body fat. Fitness is inversely correlated with fatness. Not only are aerobic activities, which require movement of body weight, hampered by excess weight, but obesity is a major health risk factor. Obesity is generally defined as a percentage of body fat of >20% in males and >30% in females. The average American male under 30 years old is approximately 20% body fat and the average female is 24.8%. A healthy acceptable level of body fat is about 15% for males and 20% for females, although athletes successful in events that require movement of their own body weight may have a percentage body fat of 5% to 10% in males and 10% to 15% in females. Weight for height charts are not good predictors of ideal body weight, for lean body mass (weight other than fat) may vary greatly among individuals of the same height.

There are several good methods for determining percent body fat, but most require extensive and expensive equipment that is not portable. One of the most accepted methods is that of hydrostatic or underwater weighing, in which the person's weight is measured on a scale and then again while submerged in water. Using Archimedes principle, which states that when an object is immersed in a fluid, the fluid exerts an upward force on the body equal to the weight of the fluid displaced by the object, one can then compute the volume of the subject, and then the subject's body density. A somewhat less reliable, but certainly less expensive and more portable, method is the skinfold caliper. The thickness of subcutaneous fat is measured at standardized sites on the body. The numbers are then put into a regression equation to estimate percent body fat.

Methods:

1. Read instructions for use of the skin fold calipers, including the sites of measurements and formulas for determining body density from the skin fold measurements and converting body density to percent body fat.

2. Locate the sites shown in the manual. When you take a skin fold, avoid grasping underlying muscle, which increases the measurement—measure only the skin. Grasp a fold of skin and roll it between the fingers to ensure only skin and subcutaneous fat is present. If unsure, ask your partner to contract the underlying muscle. Skin fold measurement accuracy is highly dependent on the skill of the person making the measurements and requires practice!

3. Compare results obtained from different formulas in the manual and simple graphic means if they appear in the manual.

4. An individual weighs 70 kg. He has a percent body fat of 30%. Say that ideal percent body fat is 15%. What is his present lean body mass? _____kg. What is his fat weight? _____ kg. Assume that this person will only lose fat. Lean body mass will not change. Only total weight and fat weight will change. How much would he weigh if he loses enough fat to become 15% body fat? _____ kg. How much weight does he need to lose? _____ kg.

LABORATORY EXERCISES

LABORATORY EXERCISE 27-3

METABOLIC RATE DURING EXERCISE

Materials:
Respirometer with soda-like canister
Bicycle ergometer
EKG or EMG electrodes
Physiological recorder

Objectives:
1. Demonstrate the effects of aerobic training on heart rate, metabolic rate, and temperature during exercise.

2. Compute volume corrected to standard temperature and pressure, dry (STPD).

3. Describe the relationship between external work and metabolic rate.

Two individuals of approximate size will exercise at the same intensity on a bicycle ergometer. One person will be a sedentary individual and the other will be an individual of the same gender who trains aerobically on a regular basis. If a gas collection system and gas analyzers are not available, a spirometer can be used to measure oxygen consumption. The spirometer is filled with 100% oxygen. If the carbon dioxide produced during metabolism is absorbed by a soda lime canister in the spirometer circuit, the decrease in the volume of the spirometer tank as oxygen is removed from it per minute allows measurement of oxygen consumption in L/min. The rate of work performed by the subject allows us to predict the subject's oxygen consumption. Compare the predicted value with the measured value. Also measure heart rate and temperature of the gas in the spirometer at each intensity of work.

Because the volume of air and the partial pressure of water in the air varies with temperature and humidification by the airways, we will need to correct the volume of oxygen consumed to a standard volume called STPD. This standard refers to the number of oxygen molecules occupied per liter when pressure equals 760 mmHg, temperature is 273°K (0°C), and the air is dry. Volume is corrected for STPD by taking into account the water vapor pressure (which is dependent on temperature), the atmospheric pressure, and the temperature of the gas. Volume at STPD = $(P_{atm} - P_{H_2O})/760 \times (273/T_{gas})$. Temperature of the gas is given in Kelvin degrees. To convert to Kelvin, add 273 to the number of Celsius degrees. Water vapor pressure is computed as WVP = $(RH/100 \times 10^{(.0275 \times T + .6985)})$, where WVP is water vapor pressure, RH is relative humidity, and T is the temperature of expired gas.

The volume of oxygen consumed in L/min is converted to units of kcal/hr by multiplying by 289.5 (1 L/min = 4.825 kcal/min). Metabolic rate is then standardized based on body surface area (BSA). Body surface is the most accurate means of allowing for body size. The DuBois formula for body surface area predicts BSA for a given height and weight according to the formula BSA (m^2) = $wt^{0.425} \times ht^{0.725} \times 0.007184$, where weight is in units of kilograms and height is in centimeters. An individual who weighs 155 lbs and is 6'1" tall has a BSA of 1.985 m^2. For the average adult, resting metabolic rate is about 40 kcal/(m^2x hr) for men and about 36 kcal/(m^2x hr) in women. We can then compute the subject's mechanical efficiency by converting the workload in watts to kcal/hr by multiplying the number of watts by 3.5 and dividing by metabolic rate.

LABORATORY EXERCISES

Methods:

1. Two subjects of the same size, one of whom trains regularly and one of whom is sedentary, will breathe into the spirometer to measure oxygen consumption at rest and at two intensities of aerobic exercise.

2. Attach three EMG electrodes on the subjects and to the EMG cable. Attach the cable to the cardiac coupler to measure heart rate. Attach the electrodes firmly over well-prepared skin and tape a loop of the electrode leads to the skin to prevent pulling on the electrode during movement.

3. Fill the spirometer with 100% oxygen. At rest, allow the subject 2 to 5 minutes to utilize a quantity of oxygen in the spirometer. Measure heart rate, the decrease in volume per time of the spirometer, and the temperature of the expired gas.

4. Repeat during exercise at 50 W and 100 W, but only breathe into the spirometer for 15 to 20 seconds.

5. Convert volumes of gas to STPD by the formula: Volume (STPD) = $(P_{atm} - P_{H_2O})/760$ x $(273/T_{tank})$. Obtain water vapor pressure from the formula given above.

6. Determine the metabolic rate required for the workload as 1 W = 3.5 kcal/hr and predicted oxygen consumption (ml/min) = 300 ml/min + 12 x W.

7. Compare the two values obtained in #6 by converting oxygen consumption in L/min x 289.5.

UNIT VI

Other Systems

Smooth muscle is used to control diameters of hollow organs in blood vessels, gastrointestinal system, and multiple other systems. Basic principles of the gastrointestinal system, which provides nutrients other than oxygen, and certain aspects of the gastrointestinal system that impact directly on patient/client care are presented in Chapter Twenty-Eight. The reproductive system is necessary for procreation but is also important in the rehabilitation professional's body of knowledge for three major reasons: First, changes that occur as a consequence of reproduction result in neuromuscular, integumentary, musculoskeletal, and cardiopulmonary problems addressed by rehabilitation professionals. Second, an understanding of how changes occur with pregnancy aids in the prevention of impairments, functional limitations, and disability. Third, changes in the reproductive systems with age and menopause in particular have profound effects on the musculoskeletal and cardiopulmonary systems.

TWENTY-EIGHT

Smooth Muscle and Gastrointestinal System

OBJECTIVES

1. Contrast the structure and locations of smooth muscle and skeletal muscle.

2. Describe the possible inputs for smooth muscle.

3. Describe tonic and phasic contraction of smooth muscle.

4. Contrast single-unit and multi-unit smooth muscle.

5. Describe excitation-contraction coupling in smooth muscle, and contrast it with skeletal muscle.

6. Describe the four processes of the digestive system and how they interact.

7. Describe the structure of the villus and its functions.

8. Describe the receptors and effectors of negative feedback mechanisms of the digestive system.

9. List the stimuli for release and actions of gastrin, cholecystokinin, and secretin.

10. Describe the process of swallowing and the need for upper and lower esophageal sphincters.

11. Discuss briefly the roles of the stomach and small and large intestine in the digestive process.

12. Describe the functions of the gall bladder and bile.

13. Describe the rectosphincteric reflex and its role in defecation.

Smooth muscle, in contrast to skeletal muscle, is a type of muscle over which we have little or no voluntary control. The neural input to smooth muscle comes from the three divisions of the autonomic nervous system. The gastrointestinal tract has its own intrinsic nervous system, the enteric division of the autonomic nervous system, which can be influenced by both the sympathetic and parasympathetic divisions of the autonomic nervous system. Smooth muscle is found in walls of hollow organs, such as blood vessels, the uterus, ureters, bladder, gastrointestinal (GI) tract, and airways, and many other types of structures. Smooth muscle is different from skeletal muscle in its structure. The most obvious differences are the cell size and appearance with light microscopy. Smooth muscle cells are not striated because they are not organized into sarcomeres and they are much smaller than skeletal muscle cells. In addition to the differences in size, smooth muscle cells are more energy efficient than skeletal muscle.

STRUCTURAL ORGANIZATION OF SMOOTH MUSCLE

Smooth muscle is not organized into detectable sarcomeres but does have contractile proteins similar to those found in skeletal muscle, differing in arrangement and amount. Smooth muscle has no troponin, the thick filaments are longer, and thin filaments insert into dense bodies, rather than into Z lines that can be pulled together in a linear fashion. Contraction of smooth muscle cells changes the shape of the cell from a spindle to a rounded shape (Figure 28-1). Compared with skeletal muscle, smooth muscle has more actin and less myosin. It has no t-tubular system, but a t-tubular system is not necessary because of the smaller diameter of smooth muscle (5 to 10 μm compared with 20 to 100 μm in skeletal muscle) and because the rate of contraction is much slower in smooth muscle. Smooth muscle does have a sarcoplasmic reticulum that qualitatively performs the same functions as those in skeletal muscle, although calcium flux is handled differently in smooth muscle.

Smooth muscle physiology is much more complex than skeletal muscle, and a diversity of characteristics among smooth muscle tissues exists, which complicates the discussion of smooth muscle even more. Smooth muscle performs different jobs in different tissues, and it behaves and is controlled in many different ways. A brief description of some of the physiology of smooth muscle is presented in this chapter. Smooth muscle has multiple inputs, not just a single motor nerve as exists in skeletal muscle. However, a factor common to all smooth mus-

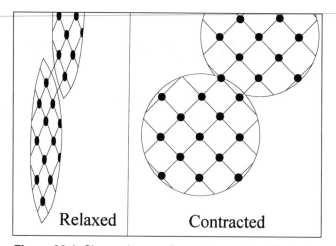

Figure 28-1. Shape change of smooth muscle cells during contraction. At rest, smooth muscle cells have a spindle shape and become rounder with increased excitation of the cells.

cle cells is that the intracellular Ca^{++} level determines the force of contraction.

INNERVATION AND CONTROL OF SMOOTH MUSCLE

Whereas skeletal muscle is controlled strictly by the somatic nervous system, smooth muscle can be controlled by many of the signaling mechanisms described in Chapter Five. Examples include nervous system control over large blood vessels, endocrine control (such as the effects of oxytocin on the uterus and cholecystokinin on the gall bladder), paracrine control of blood vessel diameter by endothelial derived relaxing factor (NO), various metabolites, prostacyclin, intrinsic control called myogenic control as in peristalsis in the GI tract), and autoregulation of blood flow by arterioles.

MECHANICAL PROPERTIES OF SMOOTH MUSCLE

Smooth muscle produces two types of contractions called phasic and tonic contractions. Phasic contractions are similar to the twitch of skeletal muscle but are much slower. Tonic contractions are sustained contractions. This maintained level of contractile activity of smooth muscle is called smooth muscle tone. The role of smooth muscle in many cases is to vary its tone to allow volume, pressure, and compliance of hollow organs to be adjusted. An example of this was discussed previously with the bladder in which the smooth muscle relaxes

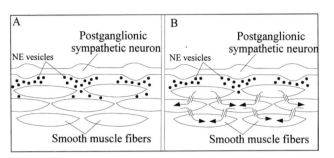

Figure 28-2. Nondirected synapses typical of those innervating smooth muscle. Release of norepinephrine depolarizes adjacent smooth muscle cells. Current generated by the depolarized cells depolarizes neighboring cells through gap junctions to propagate contraction of the muscle cells as a sheet.

as the bladder fills. Changes in neural, hormonal, or paracrine input in addition to myogenic properties make possible an increased or decreased smooth muscle tone. In contrast, skeletal muscle remains in a relaxed state unless motor neurons signal excitation-contraction coupling to occur.

Smooth muscle displays a length-tension relationship similar to skeletal muscle but, due to the way that thick and thin filaments are arranged in smooth muscle, these cells can produce force over a much greater range of cell length. This property allows for tremendous volume changes in hollow organs. For example, the uterus can produce forceful contractions even though it has increased tremendously in size during pregnancy. Although the strength of smooth muscle is similar to skeletal muscle with a maximum contractility of about 3 kg/cm^2, smooth muscle contracts much more slowly than skeletal muscle, has a much lower rate of ATP utilization, and can maintain tone without a high rate of ATP regeneration.

TYPES OF SMOOTH MUSCLE

For convenience of discussion, smooth muscle can be categorized as either multiunit or single-unit smooth muscle. In multiunit smooth muscle, the individual cells act independently of each other. Examples of multiunit smooth muscle are found in the airways, intrinsic eye muscles, and large blood vessels. Multiunit smooth muscle does not display spontaneous activity or tone but usually requires neuronal input similar to skeletal muscle with directed synapses for each cell. The firing rate of the sympathetic or parasympathetic nerves synapsing with these cells determines the rate at which neurotransmitter is released, which produces varying degrees of tone. Examples include the ciliary muscles that

change the shape of the lens. These muscles reflexively change tone to focus on nearby objects and hold the lens in its new shape until focus is shifted. The muscles that control the size of the pupils function in the same way. A simple demonstration of the speed at which multiunit smooth muscle tone changes is the consensual light reflex. Look in the mirror and cover one eye. The uncovered pupil dilates as less light enters the eye (both are dilating, you can only see the uncovered eye). Uncover the eye, and watch how slowly, compared with skeletal muscle, the iris constricts as more light enters the eye. The pupil size in response to light can also be demonstrated with the direct light reflex with a flashlight. Responses of the pupils to light are used for testing the integrity of cranial nerves and brain stem function.

In contrast to multiunit smooth muscle, sheets or tubes of single-unit smooth muscle cells act as one contractile mass. Single-unit smooth muscle is found in the GI tract, ureters, and other tracts displaying coordinated motor activity, and in the uterus. Multiunit smooth muscles have few, if any, gap junctions, whereas single-unit smooth muscle uses gap junctions to spread electrical activity throughout multiple cells. Single-unit smooth muscle functions well with nondirected synapses over the surface of the tissue and gap junctions. Because signaling can be carried out by gap junctions in single-unit smooth muscle, they contract slowly, and they act in unison. Many examples of single-unit smooth muscle display a background tone on which waves of greater tone are superimposed, producing a rhythmic contraction. This occurs because of spontaneous fluctuations in resting potentials called slow waves, or a basic electrical rhythm (Figure 28-3). In different organs, the amplitude of this rhythm can vary from being constantly present, fluctuating with changes in conditions, or increased force may occur only under specific stimuli. Whether a stronger contraction occurs at these peaks of depolarization is determined by signals that further depolarize the smooth muscle cell membrane. The exact shape of smooth muscle contractile rhythm depends on both the basic electrical rhythm and input from other sources. The basic electric rhythm determines the frequency at which superimposed, stronger mechanical events can occur, and local, neural, and hormonal stimuli determine the force of contraction.

One input to single-unit smooth muscle is stretch. The myogenic response refers to the way smooth muscle responds to stretch. In general, single-unit smooth muscle responds with a sustained contraction to oppose a rapid stretch, but responds to slow stretch with an initial contraction followed by decreased tone called stress relaxation. This property is responsible for the ability of the bladder to accommodate increases in volume with little increase in pressure at volumes less than about 400 ml.

ACTIVATION OF THE CONTRACTILE PROCESS

Excitation-contraction coupling in smooth muscle involves release of calcium from the sarcoplasmic reticulum, but the process is much more complex than that of skeletal muscle. Moreover, smooth muscle can be stimulated to contract or change its tone by processes that do not involve a change in the membrane potential as occurs in excitation-contraction coupling. The use of ligand to cause a change in smooth muscle contractile state is called pharmacomechanical coupling. In either case, an elevated intracellular calcium ion concentration is required to alter the contractile state of smooth muscle. In contrast to skeletal muscle in which the control over cross-bridge cycling resides on the thin filament through calcium ion binding to troponin, regulation in smooth muscle occurs on the thick filament due to covalent modulation of myosin. Elevated levels of the second messenger, calcium, lead to phosphorylation of myosin. As the level of calcium increases, more molecules of myosin are phosphorylated and become capable of interacting with actin to produce contractile activity. Contraction is initiated and maintained as long as intracellular calcium ion concentration remains elevated. Removal of calcium allows inactivation of myosin and produces relaxation.

In skeletal muscle, the sarcoplasmic reticulum is the sole source of the calcium necessary for cross-bridge cycling to occur. In smooth muscle, calcium comes from both the sarcoplasmic reticulum and the interstitial fluid. Calcium can enter the smooth muscle cell through voltage-operated channels that open when the membrane is depolarized beyond a threshold membrane potential, or it may enter via receptor-operated channels that open when a specific ligand binds to a surface receptor. Electromechanical coupling of smooth muscle requires a change in membrane potential to produce a change in contractile state, but this change does not need to be an action potential. In some tissues, one or several action potentials can occur at the peak depolarization of the basic electrical rhythm and cause a greater influx of calcium, but in other tissues, calcium concentration can change sufficiently without action potentials by what is called a graded depolarization. In contrast to skeletal muscle, the sarcoplasmic reticulum of smooth

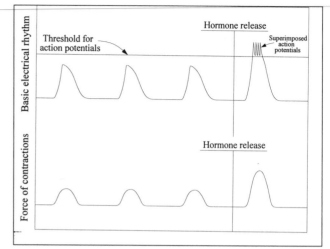

Figure 28-3. Electrical and mechanical activity of typical smooth muscle cells. A basic electrical rhythm exists with the potential for superimposed electrical activity caused by hormones, neurotransmitters, and other chemical signals. The basic electrical rhythm determines when contractions can occur; the other inputs determine the force of the contractions.

muscle does not store sufficient quantities of calcium to produce a maximum contraction and takes up calcium very slowly. Moreover, relaxation depends on active transport of Ca^{++} out of the cell, either by a primary mechanism that directly uses ATP or by secondary active transport by exchange for sodium ions.

In pharmacomechanical coupling, tension is changed by a signal other than a change in membrane potential. The ligand may cause an increased contractile state by opening of calcium ion channels or by release of calcium from the sarcoplasmic reticulum by second messengers, including IP_3. Ligands, especially those that bind to β-adrenergic receptors and generate cAMP, cause decreased tone (relaxation) by increasing the transport of calcium out of the intracellular space. Many of these controls may operate simultaneously. For example, a basic electric rhythm can cause waves of smooth muscle contractions to occur. Some neurotransmitters or hormones may cause greater intracellular calcium ion concentration to increase the force of contraction, whereas others may cause calcium to be removed from the intracellular space to diminish or even prevent the waves of smooth muscle contraction. In certain situations, several different, even conflicting, signals may converge at once on the smooth muscle to produce a given level of smooth muscle tone. Many drugs are designed specifically to alter smooth muscle contractile activity, such as bronchodilators for treating asthma and antispasmodics for treating diarrhea.

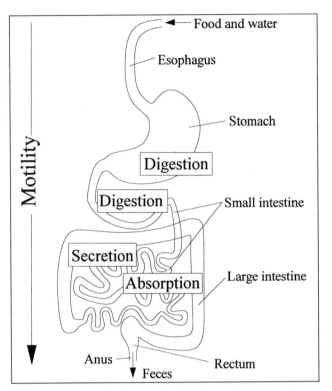

Figure 28-4. Basic processes of the gastrointestinal system.

THE DIGESTIVE SYSTEM

The role of the digestive system is to transfer material (nutrients and water) from the external environment to the internal environment so it can be distributed by the circulatory system. The gastrointestinal system is largely a part of the external environment, and, as such, perforation of the GI tract can result in life-threatening sepsis. The system consists of the tract, with its muscular walls for mechanically reducing food size and net propulsion through the tract, and several glands that secrete digestive enzymes and hormones to aid in digestion and control of the system. The liver assists the digestive system by producing bile and processing materials after they are absorbed.

The result of the processes of the digestive system is the absorption of nutrients. Three additional processes are necessary for absorption to occur. These are digestion, secretion, and motility (Figure 28-4).

Digestion is the mechanical and chemical degradation of ingested materials into molecules that can be absorbed. Digestion begins in the mouth and is completed largely in the proximal small intestine. Secretion of enzymes into the GI tract permits the breakdown of macromolecules, such as starch, fat, and protein, into simpler molecules, such as monosaccharides, free fatty acids and glycerol, and amino acids that can be absorbed in the small intestine. Motility is the rhythmic contraction of smooth muscle in the GI tract. Two forms of motility are segmentation and peristalsis. Segmentation is a type of contraction that produces mechanical digestion by physically squeezing the contents of the tract locally. Peristalsis is an organized wave of contraction that propels the contents through the tract. Most of the intestinal motility consists of segmentation. Periodic peristalsis sweeps processed material, called chyme in the small intestine and feces in the large intestine, through the bowels. The digestive system, for the most part, does not regulate the amount absorbed or the concentration of substances in body. Important exceptions are absorption of calcium and magnesium ions, which are controlled by vitamin D, and absorption of iron.

The waste product of the digestive system, feces, is composed of mainly of bacteria and nonabsorbable material, including cellulose and nonfood items that children, especially, may swallow. Metabolic waste products are, for the most part, excreted by the kidneys, although lungs excrete carbon dioxide; and bilirubin, a product of hemoglobin breakdown, is excreted in the bile and through the intestine. A few other products of metabolism are also excreted in the bile. Urobilinogen, which colors urine and feces, is generated by bacteria in the intestines from bilirubin and is partially absorbed from the intestine and excreted in the urine.

ABSORPTION

Water-soluble substances are absorbed into blood circulating through the small intestine and are carried in the venous blood draining the intestine into the portal circulation to the liver, where the liver can process these solutes. Fat-soluble substances are absorbed by lacteals, part of lymphatic system within the tips of the villi of the intestine. Villi are projections from the wall of the intestine that increase surface area available for absorption (Figure 28-5). Active transport of solutes is performed when necessary by epithelial cells covering the villi. These cells last approximately 5 days, as new cells migrate from base to tip of villus to replace about 17 billion cells shed into the intestine each day. These cells are among the most rapidly reproducing cells in the body. Chemotherapy for treating cancer often leads to digestive problems when drugs that preferentially affect rapidly dividing cells are used.

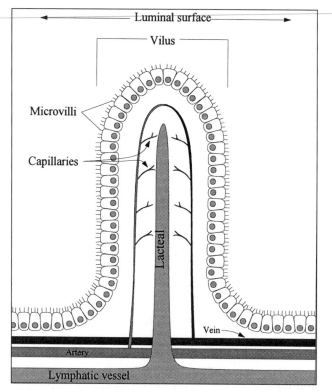

Figure 28-5. Anatomy of an intestinal villus. Villi increase the surface area available for absorption of nutrients, electrolytes, and water. Fatty acids are absorbed by specialized lymphatic vessels called lacteals, whereas water-soluble substances are absorbed in the capillaries of the villus.

GI REGULATION

Several components of gastrointestinal regulation exist, as the discussion of smooth muscle above suggests. Only a few general aspects will be described here. Some important negative feedback mechanisms involve neural and hormonal control with systems consisting of mechano-, osmo-, and chemoreceptors to detect conditions of the gastrointestinal tract. Effectors include the enteric, sympathetic, and parasympathetic divisions of the autonomic nervous system, endocrine cells within the gastrointestinal tract and its accessory organs, smooth muscle, and exocrine glands. Integration of input occurs both locally within the enteric division and within the central nervous system. Neural regulation consists of long reflexes that involve the central nervous system (CNS) and may originate with senses and emotion. Short reflexes do not involve the CNS, but occur within the nervous plexuses within the walls of the gastrointestinal tract (Figure 28-6).

HORMONAL REGULATION

Many hormones are involved in control of the digestive system, and some substances act as both neurotransmitters and hormones. The list of chemical messengers found in the gastrointestinal tract grows annually. Many of the same substances are also found in the central nervous system. Three important hormones that account for much of the behavior of the digestive system and have historical significance as well are gastrin, cholecystokinin, and secretin. Gastrin, as the name implies, is secreted by cells in the stomach in response to amino acids. Although it has many other functions, its major function is to stimulate acid production by the stomach and to stimulate contractile activity of the stomach. Gastrin secretion is inhibited by increased acidity of the stomach.

Cholecystokinin (CCK) secretion is stimulated by the presence of free fatty acids and amino acids in the intestine and stimulates secretion of digestive enzymes by the pancreas, contraction of the gall bladder, and relaxation of sphincter of Oddi. The functions of CCK promote digestion of fat by release of lipase, release of bile by contraction of the smooth muscle of the gall bladder, and relaxation of the sphincter of Oddi. Relaxation of the sphincter of Oddi allows bile from the common bile duct and enzymes from the pancreatic duct to enter the duodenum.

Secretin secretion is stimulated by acidity of the intestine. Secretin produces secretion of HCO_3^- by ductal cells of the pancreas and inhibits release of acid by the stomach. Thus, secretin acts in a negative feedback mechanism to prevent the intestine from becoming too acidic. Excessive acid from the stomach decreases the effectiveness of the digestive enzymes released from the pancreas. Secretin also decreases the emptying of the stomach by decreasing the contractile state of the stomach.

SALIVATION

Salivation and chewing are the first acts of the digestive system. Saliva is produced by three sets of glands:

- The parotid glands, which are found near the ear in each cheek
- The submandibular glands, which are located below the mouth along both sides of the mandible
- The sublingual glands, which are located below the tongue and under the mouth

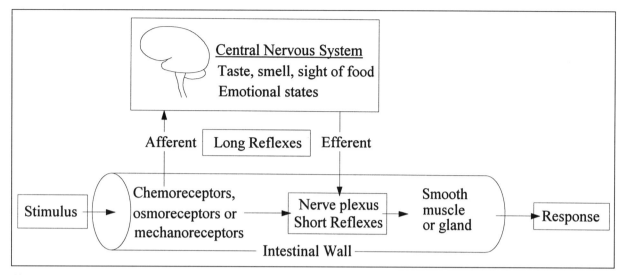

Figure 28-6. Reflexes of the gastrointestinal system.

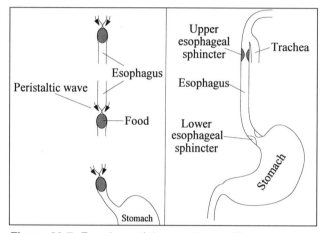

Figure 28-7. Functions of the esophagus. The esophagus propels food and fluid toward the stomach by peristalsis. Because the esophagus exists inside the thorax and is surrounded by a negative pressure, sufficient upper and lower esophageal sphincters are needed to protect the esophagus from either swallowing air from above or from damage from stomach acid from below.

Saliva produced by the three different types of glands has different properties and constituents. In addition to lubricating the food, saliva contains salivary amylase, which begins the digestive process for starches. If starch is allowed to remain in the mouth long enough, it begins to taste sweet because of the breakdown of starch to sugar within the mouth by salivary amylase. Salivation is stimulated both by mechanoreceptors in the mouth and through integration of senses, especially smell, or even by thinking of food. Control of salivation is mostly through the parasympathetic division using muscarinic receptors. Therefore, atropine and other anticholinergic drugs cause the mouth to become dry.

ESOPHAGUS

Swallowing is a coordinated muscle response to food, which is integrated by the swallowing center in the CNS. Swallowing requires careful timing to be successful, because not only the muscle of the esophagus but also the muscles involved in covering the airways to prevent aspiration, must be controlled. Alcohol intoxication can lead to choking, and alcoholism is associated with a high risk of pneumonia and development of lung abscesses from aspiration of infectious material. Ironically, cocktail weenies and meatballs, which can obstruct airways, are often served at gatherings along with alcohol. Cerebrovascular accidents (strokes) often affect the ability to sense the presence of food in the mouth and to swallow effectively. Therefore, especially after meals, the health care professional should check for food remaining in one side of the mouth that may be a choking hazard and should be up-to-date on CPR, including management of the choking victim.

Because the esophagus is located in the thorax, surrounded by the lungs, pressure surrounding the esophagus is lower than pressure in the mouth or in the abdomen. This difference in pressure requires the presence of both upper and lower esophageal sphincters that must be coordinated with swallowing (Figure 28-7). Without sphincters to protect the esophagus from the pressure difference, air would be taken into the esophagus from the atmosphere, but, more importantly, the acidic gastric contents would be displaced into the esophagus. The stomach wall is protected by its mucus lining, but the esophagus and pharynx can be severely damaged by frequent exposure to gastric contents as occurs in bulimia. Acid reflux has been associated with

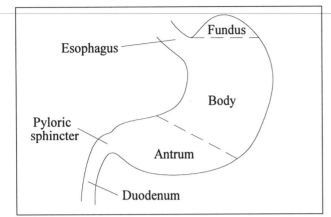

Figure 28-8. Functional regions of the stomach.

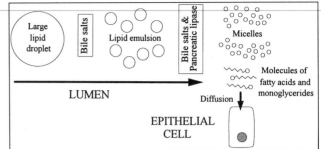

Figure 28-9. Functions of bile salt in digestion of lipid.

asthma and with esophageal cancer. Pregnancy and stomach and abdominal distention can cause reflux into the esophagus. Individuals with scleroderma, a disease affecting connective tissue (especially the hands and face), often have a dysfunctional lower esophageal sphincter and gastric reflux. Anyone with gastric reflux will not tolerate horizontal positioning (supine or prone) well and should be positioned with the head up during therapeutic activities.

STOMACH

The stomach produces much of the mechanical digestion of food in general and some chemical digestion of proteins, specifically. During digestion, the stomach empties liquid, not solids. Therefore, the primary function of the stomach is to liquefy food and move the liquefied material, now called chyme, in a controlled manner into the first part of the small intestine, the duodenum. As described above under hormonal control, the stomach releases acid, which aids in digestion of proteins and has some protective effect against ingested pathogens. It should also be pointed out that stomach acid breaks down the cysts of some protozoa, allowing them to infect the bowels. Histamine stimulates acid release via H_2 receptors. These receptors are different from those that mediate allergic responses and, therefore, respond to different drugs. Several H_2 blocker drugs have been developed in recent years to treat ulcers and are now sold over-the-counter for treatment of "heartburn" (esophageal reflux). The stomach undergoes churning types of contractions, as shown in Figure 28-8, that propel the contents toward the pyloric valve but does not allow solids through the valve into the duodenum. The strength of contraction is greater from the body of the stomach toward the antrum (distal part

of stomach). Thus, the food is progressively propelled and compressed until it is liquefied and it passes into the duodenum. The fundus of the stomach is the uppermost part of the stomach, located above the esophagus. It regulates pressure within the stomach through changes in its tone. As the stomach fills with food, the fundus relaxes to prevent an increase in the stomach pressure, and, as the stomach empties, the tone of the fundus increases to maintain pressure in the stomach.

GALL BLADDER

The gall bladder is a sac located on the inferior surface of the liver that functions to concentrate and intermittently release the bile synthesized by the liver. Bile is continuously synthesized by the liver but is only needed intermittently for digestion. When the sphincter of Oddi is closed, the bile produced by the liver drains into the gall bladder where the bile is concentrated. During digestion and under control of CCK, the gall bladder contracts and the sphincter of Oddi relaxes, allowing the concentrated bile to empty into the duodenum. Bile functions with intestinal motility to emulsify fat from large chunks into small droplets. Bile also solubilizes fat to provide an aqueous interface at which water-soluble lipases can function to digest free fatty acids, and other fat-soluble substances to improve their absorption. These functions are summarized in Figure 28-9. The gall bladder allows large quantities of ingested fat to be nearly completely absorbed. In the absence of the gall bladder, large meals containing fat would result in steatorrhea, the passing of fat in the stool. In cystic fibrosis, the pancreatic ducts become occluded and prevent the pancreatic enzymes from reaching the duodenum. Fat, in particular, is poorly digested, resulting in malabsorption and steatorrhea.

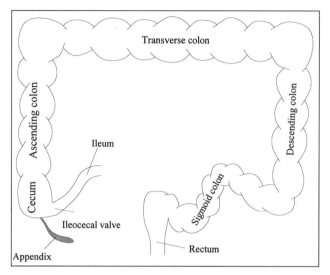

Figure 28-10. Regions of the large intestine.

INTESTINES

Most of the motility of the small intestine produces mixing, rather than net propulsion. Mixing is needed to increase the surface area of the chyme exposed to enzymes and bile. Most of the absorption of digestible material occurs early in the small intestine, although active transport mechanisms for certain materials are found in specific regions of the small intestine. Periodic peristalsis produces net movement of material through the small intestine toward the large intestine. A decrease in the basic electrical rhythm from the duodenum to the jejunum and to the ileum produces net movement.

Nondigestible material is moved out of the stomach and through the intestines by a complex, coordinated type of motility called the migrating motor complex, which includes the stomach. The migrating motor complex produces net movement of indigestible materials and only occurs when digestion is not occurring.

LARGE INTESTINE

The large intestine functions (Figure 28-10) principally as an organ of convenience that allows emptying of waste at a convenient time. In addition, the large intestine allows absorption of water, K^+, and vitamins synthesized by bacteria (B_{12}, K). Mass movement propels material long distances through the large intestine three to four times per day, usually following a meal. Mass movement is produced by the gastroileal reflex, which opens the ileocecal valve and produces peristalsis through the large intestine to the rectum. Emptying of fecal material is largely the result of the rectosphincteric reflex. This reflex is produced by distention of the rec-

tum and results in relaxation of the internal anal sphincter. Because the external anal sphincter is under voluntary control, it can be contracted to prevent defecation. Similar to what occurs in the bladder, the rectosphincteric reflex can be extinguished until the rectum is stretched again. The rectosphincteric reflex can also be elicited by increased abdominal pressure or by stretching the rectum digitally or with a special device. The rectosphincteric reflex does not require input from higher centers so that this reflex can be used to elicit defecation in people with spinal cord injuries. Although bile salts are largely absorbed, bile that passes in the stool is very acidic and can damage the skin. Breakdown of skin due to fecal material is called "stool burn." This can occur if feces are allowed to remain in a child's diaper. Potentially more serious is the case of the individual with decreased cognition and mobility who also has fecal incontinence. The combination of these can lead to serious open wounds that might be prevented by prompt cleaning. Urine, too, is acidic, but this problem can be avoided by inserting a Foley catheter through the urethra into the bladder. Sometimes, a fecal collection system is used in the form of a bag, pouch, or tube. While moving a person with these in place, one must be careful not to dislodge the catheter(s). In particular, fecal bags are often applied with adhesive, and pulling these off can damage the skin. Many hospitalized patients remain in bed for several days and do not pass stool due to horizontal positioning. Health care professionals need to be aware that sudden vertical positioning may provide a strong stimulus to empty the bowels.

SUMMARY

Smooth muscle provides contractile activity in tissues not under voluntary control and is innervated by the autonomic nervous system. Its activity is also influenced by hormones and paracrine signals, as well as its own inherent responses to stretch and cyclic changes in membrane potential. Smooth muscle can perform phasic contractions similar to skeletal muscle or tonic contractions that allow the volume, pressure, and compliance of hollow structures to be controlled. Single-unit smooth muscle acts as a unit, is connected by gap junctions, and often shows cyclic changes in membrane potential and contractile activity. Multiunit smooth muscle usually requires neuronal input and does not have gap junctions.

Excitation-contraction coupling may take the forms of electromechanical coupling in which the membrane is depolarized to signal contraction or pharmacomechanical contraction, in which binding of a ligand to a receptor causes a change in tone. Contraction is dependent on the intracellular calcium level but does not use troponin. Calcium acts as a second messenger, resulting in the covalent modulation of myosin. The sarcoplasmic reticulum of smooth muscle is very slow and does not store sufficient calcium to produce a maximal contraction. Contraction is slow and usually requires calcium to enter through calcium channels. Relaxation is also slow and usually requires active transport of calcium out of the cell.

The digestive system has four processes of digestion, secretion, motility, and absorption. Digestion is the chemical and mechanical breakdown of food, which is aided by secretion of acid, bile, and digestive enzymes and by motility of the gastrointestinal tract. Water-soluble substances are absorbed into the blood and are routed to the liver via the portal circulation. Fat-soluble substances are taken up by lymphatic vessels, called lacteals, within the villus. Three major hormones participate in the digestive process. Gastrin causes secretion of acid and increased stomach motility, CCK causes release of bile and digestive enzymes, and secretin prevents excessive acid from entering the duodenum.

Swallowing is a complex sequence of motor activity of the esophagus and the pharynx coordinated by a swallowing center. The gall bladder stores and concentrates bile, which is released during digestion to emulsify and solubilize fat and fat-soluble components of a meal. Mass movement of the large intestine propels material through the large intestine, usually following a meal. Mass movement can stimulate defecation by stretching the rectum via the rectosphincteric reflex.

BIBLIOGRAPHY

Allen A, Flemström G. Gastroduodenal mucosal protection. *Physiological Reviews.* 1993;73:823-857.

Hersey SJ, Sachs G. Gastric acid secretion. *Physiological Reviews.* 1995;75:155-189.

Horowitz A, Menice CB, Laporte R, Morgan KG. Mechanism of smooth muscle contraction. *Physiological Reviews.* 1996;76:967-1003.

Kuriyama H, Kitamura K, Itoh T, Inove R. Physiological features of visceral smooth muscle cells, with special reference to receptors and ion channels. *Physiological Reviews.* 1998;78:811-920.

O'Donnell ME, Owen NE. Regulation of ion pumps and carriers vascular smooth muscle. *Physiological Reviews.* 1994;74:683-721.

Owens GK. Regulation of differentiation of vascular smooth muscle cells. *Physiological Reviews.* 1995;75:487-517.

Quayle JM, Nelson MT, Standen NB. ATP-Sensitive and inward rectifying potassium channels in smooth muscle. *Physiological Reviews.* 1997;77:1165-1232.

Rehfeld JF. The new biology of gastrointestinal hormones. *Physiological Reviews.* 1998;78:1087-1108.

Sims SM, Janssen LJ. Cholinergic excitation of smooth muscle. *News in Physiological Sciences.* 1993;8:207-212.

STUDY QUESTIONS

1. Why is it important after a meal to check the mouth of a person who has had a stroke?

2. Why do alcohol and cocktail weenies not mix?

3. Why do individuals with cystic fibrosis (CF), thought of as a lung disease, so often appear malnourished? How can nutrition be improved in CF?

4. In terms of the time of day, why are individuals most likely to defecate after a meal?

5. Why is it important to clean fecal material promptly from children and people who are incontinent of bowel?

6. Why is bile important? What happens if a person without a gall bladder eats a large, fatty meal?

7. What is the major form of motility in the intestines? How does it complement the role of secretion?

8. Where in the alimentary canal does digestion begin? Where does absorption end?

9. Why should you be careful in positioning a pregnant person with the head down? Who else might have a problem with head-down positioning due to the gastrointestinal system?

10. What determines the frequency of peristalsis? What determines the force of peristalsis?

11. Contrast the motor activity of the intrinsic eye muscles and intestine. What properties of smooth muscle produce these differences?

TWENTY-NINE

Reproductive System

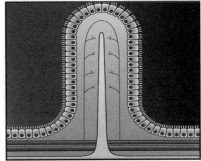

OBJECTIVES

1. Describe the embryologic development of the male and female reproductive systems.

2. Describe the functions of the Sertoli cells, Leydig cells, granulosa cells, and theca cells.

3. Describe the functions of gonadotropin-releasing hormone, luteinizing hormone, and follicle stimulating hormone.

4. Describe the functions of testosterone, estrogen, and progesterone.

5. Describe the process of erection, including stimuli, innervation, and vascular changes.

6. Describe the process of emission and ejaculation, including the stimuli, innervation, muscles, and accessory organs involved.

7. Describe the changes in hormone secretion that account for puberty and the menstrual cycle.

8. Describe the changes in hormone secretion that accompany pregnancy, lactation, and menopause.

The reproductive system is obviously responsible for the persistence of our species, but, in terms of physiology for health care professionals, a number of specific issues have greater importance. Rather than an exhaustive description of reproduction, these specific issues will be discussed. Changes in the reproductive system due to injury, disease, pregnancy, and menopause are also accompanied by needs for both medical treatment and therapy. Spinal cord injury may interfere with the ability of a man to reproduce, and, while not preventing pregnancy in the woman, it may render vaginal delivery dif-

ficult. Many diseases, especially those affecting the nervous system or vascular system, can produce the same effects as spinal cord injury. Pregnancy brings with it enormous hormonal changes, cardiovascular changes, and musculoskeletal changes with a tremendous shift of the center of gravity and production of hormones that affect ligamentous stability. Changes that occur with birth and the responsibilities of child rearing and the hormonal changes that accompany menopause may also require therapeutic intervention.

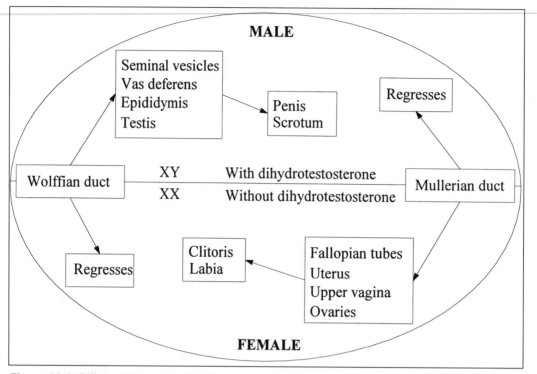

Figure 29-1. Differentiation of the Wolffian and Mullerian ducts into either male or female reproductive structures.

EMBRYOLOGIC DEVELOPMENT OF THE REPRODUCTIVE SYSTEM

Initial development of the male and female reproductive systems are identical, but, at approximately 10 weeks, they begin to develop separately with appropriate influences of the Y chromosome and male and female hormones. The Wolffian duct and Muellerian ducts give rise to the male and female reproductive structures, respectively, with differential development of the existing structures into either a clitoris or penis, labial folds or scrotum, and ovaries or testes as shown in Figure 29-1.

CELLS OF THE REPRODUCTIVE SYSTEM

As the gonads develop, two major types of cells develop that are necessary for gamete development and function. The testis develops the medullary portion of the gonad into seminiferous tubules (Figure 29-2), whereas in the ovary, the medullary portion regresses as the cortical portion develops as the major functional part of the ovary.

Four major types of cells perform vital functions of the testes and ovaries, including the Sertoli and Leydig cells of the testis and the granulosa cells and theca cells of the ovary. The Sertoli cells and granulosa cells have supportive functions for the developing spermatozoa and ova, respectively. These cells provide nutritional support, hormones, and enzymes necessary for maturation of the gametes. Sertoli cells are located in the walls of the seminiferous tubules, in which the primitive germ cells called spermatogonia develop, whereas granulosa cells form a layer around oocytes (Figure 29-3).

The interstitial cells of the ovary, called theca cells, create a layer around the granulosa cells, and, together, this structure is termed a follicle. In the testis, the interstitial cells, called Leydig cells, are found in the spaces between seminiferous tubules. Both interstitial cell types are endocrine cells of the gonads, producing androgens. In the male, testosterone is the primary androgen. In females, androgens are converted to estrogens by the granulosa cells. The primary estrogen in humans is called estradiol. Androgens, or male sex hormones, are also secreted by the adrenal glands. Secretion of androgens by Leydig and theca cells is stimulated by luteinizing hormone from the anterior pituitary. Conversion of androgens to estradiol by granulosa cells is stimulated by follicle-stimulating hormone also from the anterior pituitary.

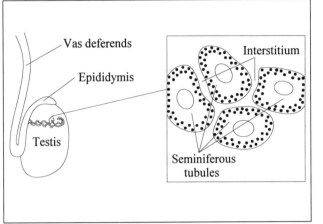

Figure 29-2. Tubular structures of the testes.

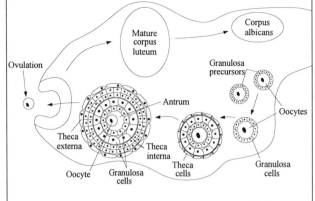

Figure 29-3. Development of follicles within the ovary, culminating in ovulation and development of the corpus luteum.

HORMONES OF THE HYPOTHALAMUS AND ANTERIOR PITUITARY

The functional cells of the gonads require stimulation of luteinizing hormone (LH) and follicle-stimulating hormone (FSH). In addition, the release of the gonadotrophic hormones (LH and FSH) is under the control of the hypothalamic hormone, gonadotropin-releasing hormone (GnRH). As discussed in Chapter Five, many anterior pituitary hormones are controlled by releasing hormones from the hypothalamus. GnRH is secreted in a pulsatile fashion from the hypothalamus for several minutes every 1 to 3 hours during the day. When the role of this hormone was discovered, gynecologists hoping to increase fertility soon found that typical types of drug administration would not produce the desired effect. Continuous infusion was not effective either. To be effective, GnRH needs to be infused in a pulsatile manner similar to its natural release pattern. Special pumps have now been designed for this purpose. Pulsatile release of GnRH produces a pulsatile release of luteinizing hormone (Figure 29-4) and follicle-stimulating hormone in women after puberty.

Follicle-stimulating hormone stimulates the Sertoli cells of the testis to produce maturation of spermatozoa in the male and maturation of the follicle in the female, thus the name follicle-stimulating hormone. FSH stimulates the production of estradiol by follicles in the ovary, and a burst of FSH activity initiates the positive feedback mechanism that leads to ovulation.

In addition to the role of LH in stimulating androgen production by the interstitial cells, LH is also responsible for ovulation and, following ovulation, for the maturation of the follicle into the corpus luteum, thus the name luteinizing hormone. Production of androgens by the theca cells is necessary for the production of estradiol by the granulosa cells. LH also stimulates progesterone production by the granulosa cells. At low levels prior to ovulation and at high levels following ovulation, estradiol inhibits release of GnRH, FSH, and LH in a negative feedback mechanism, but at high levels that occur prior to ovulation, estradiol increases the release of GnRH, LH, and FSH as a positive feedback cycle develops in which estradiol release is stimulated by LH and FSH, and LH and FSH are stimulated by estradiol. The estradiol plasma concentration rises rapidly over the course of approximately 1 week preceding ovulation, triggering the surges in GnRH, LH, and FSH that lead to ovulation. What changes the control of estradiol and gonadotropin release from a negative to a positive feedback mechanism is not understood well at this time.

FUNCTIONS OF THE SEX HORMONES

Sex hormones are steroids that bind to internal receptors within target cells. The hormone/receptor complex alters synthesis of proteins within the target cell. Gene expression can be either enhanced or suppressed, leading to increases or decreases of specific proteins.

Estrogens are secreted at low levels in childhood and increase approximately 20 times following puberty. Estrogen causes fat deposition in the breasts and other

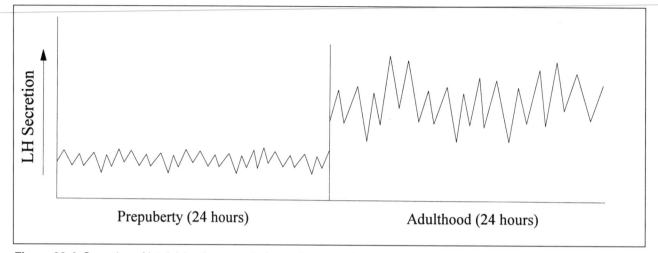

Figure 29-4. Secretion of luteinizing hormone before puberty and in adulthood.

body regions, producing the characteristic female body shape, and is responsible for the greater deposition, on average, of adipose tissue in females. Estrogen also stimulates production of the ductal structures in the breast, but not the lobules and alveoli of the breast. Bone growth is stimulated by the effect of estrogen on osteoblastic activity. Height increases rapidly at the onset of puberty, but estrogen also closes the epiphyseal plates. Epiphyseal plates are more sensitive to estrogen than testosterone, causing earlier closure and causing average height to be less in women than in men. Following puberty, estrogen inhibits bone reabsorption. Loss of estrogen at menopause leads to osteoporosis. Uterine growth is stimulated by estrogen, especially the proliferation of the endometrium in preparation for ovulation during each menstrual cycle. In addition, estrogens stimulate growth of other reproductive structures. With menopause, atrophy of the breasts and genitalia occur. Atrophy of the genitalia can cause vaginal dryness and itching and painful intercourse. This can be treated locally with topically applied estrogen. Bladder infection and weakness of the pelvic floor muscles can lead to urinary incontinence, which was discussed in Chapter Six. Atrophy of the glandular portion of the breast causes sagging that should be taken into account when using a gait belt. Other effects of estrogen include increased sodium reabsorption, leading to fluid retention, and a protective effect against coronary artery disease. Before menopause, women are at a much lower risk than men are but, following menopause, risk of coronary artery disease becomes similar in men and women. Just as younger men may suffer from coronary artery disease, premenopausal women may have significant disease. Coronary artery disease may go undetected in younger

women partially because of the belief that premenopausal women are not at risk.

Progesterone has several functions that serve to promote gestation, thus the name. Progesterone stimulates tubal and endometrial glands of the uterus to secrete nutrients for the zygote, maintains the uterine lining, and inhibits uterine contractions. Progesterone also inhibits smooth muscle elsewhere, including gastrointestinal and vascular smooth muscle. Progesterone also stimulates the development of the lobules and alveoli of the breast and the ability of the maternal breast to produce milk. Progesterone is also used to synthesize cortisol and aldosterone by the fetus, which lacks the ability to synthesize these steroid hormones. Progesterone also increases body temperature, causing a 0.5°C increase that occurs shortly after ovulation. This increase in body temperature is often used as a sign of ovulation to increase the likelihood of conception.

Testosterone may produce direct effects, but many of the effects are due to dihydrotestosterone or estradiol produced from testosterone. Androgens are responsible for differentiation of the male sex structures during development and descent of the testes into the scrotum during the last 2 months of gestation. Muscle mass is increased greatly following puberty so that men, on average, have 50% more muscle mass than women. Blood cell mass also is stimulated by testosterone, which may account for the greater hematocrit of men compared with women. During puberty, testosterone produces the secondary sex characteristics, stimulates sperm production, and, interacting with a genetic predisposition, may be responsible for male pattern baldness. Similar to estrogens, testosterone stimulates bone growth and closure of the epiphyseal plates.

MALE REPRODUCTIVE FUNCTION

Successful reproduction by the male usually depends on the three processes of erection, emission, and ejaculation. Erection is a function of the parasympathetic division of the autonomic nervous system, whereas emission and ejaculation are controlled by the sympathetic division. It is, therefore, possible for ejaculation to occur without erection and for erection to occur in an individual incapable of ejaculation due to disease or injury.

Sacral nerves of the parasympathetic system innervate the penis as well as corresponding structures of the female. Acetylcholine released by these nerves causes arteriolar dilation, which results in filling of venous sinuses within the erectile tissue. High pressure within the erectile tissue compresses veins, which aids the erectile process. In a condition called priapism, erection is prolonged to the extent that tissue injury and necrosis of the penis can occur and must be treated medically. Erection can be stimulated reflexively by tactile stimulation or by neurons from the brain due to psychologic stimulation. In the usual case, both local stimulation and central stimulation are required. However, one input, if strong enough, can be sufficient. Erection occurs periodically during sleep when no local stimulation is present. Erection can be achieved without conscious perception of touch if the sensory neurons and the parasympathetic neurons creating the reflex are intact. Damage to either the sensory neurons of the penis or damage to the descending pathways to the parasympathetic neurons does not preclude erection, but requires a greater synaptic input to the parasympathetic neurons to achieve erection if one of the two inputs is removed. Loss of the parasympathetic neurons or loss of both inputs to these neurons will prevent erection. Fertility is not lost with inability to achieve erection, but the ability to inseminate a partner naturally is greatly diminished. The parasympathetic nerves also stimulate the secretion of mucus by urethral glands and the bulbourethral glands. In women, parasympathetic stimulation produces engorgement of the clitoris and erectile tissue surrounding the vagina and lubrication of the vagina.

Emission and ejaculation are the result of summation of synaptic potentials on sympathetic neurons in the lumbar spinal cord, producing the male orgasm. Both tactile stimulation of the penis and surrounding structures and excitation from higher centers in the brain produce excitatory postsynaptic potentials on the sympathetic neurons and somatic motor neurons innervating associated skeletal muscle. As in erection, conscious perception of tactile stimulation is not required but summates with the descending stimulatory input. Strong descending excitation without sensory input to the spinal cord or strong local sensory input in the absence of descending excitatory information can result in emission and ejaculation. Loss of the sympathetic nerves or both local and descending excitatory pathways results in the loss of voluntary ejaculation. Ejaculation can be caused artificially by electrical stimulation. At present, sperm quality is usually too poor to achieve fertilization. This appears to be the result of the lack of ejaculation causing old spermatozoa to fill the epididymis. Recently, higher success rates of fertilization are being achieved as research on rehabilitation of spinal cord injuries continues.

Emission includes the process of contractions of the various ducts to move spermatozoa and secretions from the seminal vesicles and prostate into the urethra to mix with the fluid already secreted by the bulbourethral glands to form semen. Emission then stimulates rhythmic contractions of the ischiocavernosus and bulbocavernosus muscles, internal ducts, and even larger skeletal muscles in the pelvic region, resulting in ejaculation. The 3 to 4 ml of semen ejaculated contain many substances in addition to approximately 300 million spermatozoa, including a number of nutrients, hormones, enzymes, and prostaglandins. The ejaculated prostaglandins are believed to enhance contractions of the uterus and fallopian tubes, causing the spermatozoa to travel at a rate greater than they can propel themselves. This is one possible explanation for the higher success rate of natural insemination over artificial insemination.

Spermatozoa have a lifespan of about 2 days in the female genital tract. They cannot fertilize an ovum within the first 4 to 6 hours, requiring a process called capacitation. The composition of the sperm membrane is altered in this process, and motility is enhanced. These changes also allow enzymes from the spermatozoa to break down the membrane of the ovum to allow penetration of one spermatozoon to release its genetic material. Of these 300 million spermatozoa ejaculated, only 1 in 100,000 ever reach the ovum.

PUBERTY

Female puberty (Figure 29-5) is initiated with an increase in gonadotropin secretion at 10 to 12 years of age. The underlying cause is presently unknown. Increasing breast size with increasing plasma levels of estradiol is the first sign of puberty. Menstrual cycles do not begin until approximately 2 years after breast enlargement begins. Ovulation usually does not occur

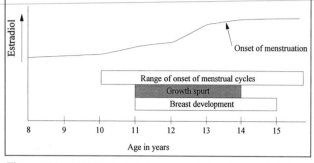

Figure 29-5. Hormonal changes and developmental characteristics of female puberty.

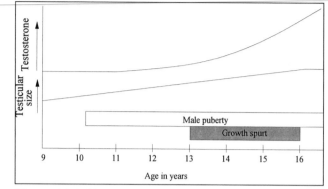

Figure 29-6. Hormonal changes and developmental characteristics of male puberty.

until after several cycles have occurred and a positive feedback between estradiol and gonadotropins begins. With puberty, a growth spurt due to estrogen occurs, and the increase in height is halted about 1 to 2 years following the onset of menses.

Puberty begins at an average of 2 years later in boys (Figure 29-6). During this time, boys develop the ability to reproduce, develop the required number of Leydig cells, and reach the adult plasma testosterone concentration. Enlargement of the testes, similar to enlargement of the breasts in girls, is the first sign of puberty. An increase in seminiferous tubule size caused by a rise in FSH accounts for much of the increased testicular size. Rapid increases in muscular strength and skeletal development during puberty increase the risk of several musculoskeletal disorders including Osgoode-Schlatter's disease, which affects the insertion of the patellar tendon at the tibial tuberosity. The use of systemic corticosteroids to treat systemic lupus erythematosus in pubescent girls can cause aseptic necrosis of the head of the femur, in particular.

THE MENSTRUAL CYCLE

The menstrual cycle is divided into three phases: the follicular phase, the ovulatory phase, and the luteal phase (Figure 29-7). The follicular phase begins with shedding of the endometrium built up in the previous cycle (menses). This phase is the most variable in length and averages 15 days. The ovulatory phase occurs with the gonadotropin surge, lasts 2 to 3 days, and ends in ovulation. The luteal phase is the most consistent phase and lasts 13 days. During the luteal phase, the corpus luteum releases large quantities of estrogens and progesterone until either it regresses into the corpus albicans or the corpus luteum is stimulated by human chorionic gonadotropin (HCG) following fertilization. The menstrual cycle lasts 21 to 35 days, with its overall length being determined primarily by the variation in the follicular phase.

During each cycle, approximately 20 follicles are recruited for maturation in both ovaries by an unknown mechanism. These follicles are then called primary follicles. FSH stimulates growth of granulosa cells to produce estrogen from androgens produced by the theca cells of the follicles. Estradiol production by the developing follicles initiates a positive feedback mechanism that causes estradiol levels, which rise slowly at the beginning of the follicular phase, to rise rapidly by the end of the follicular phase.

FSH during the follicular phase stimulates the granulosa cells to produce a number of molecules that assist in development of a mature oocyte, including growth factors. By day 5 to 7 of the follicular phase, one follicle has increased from 2 to 4 mm to about 11 mm. This follicle, called the dominant follicle, has advanced farther in the positive feedback cycle. The dominant follicle then inhibits development of the other primary follicles and may reach a size greater than 20 mm (almost 1 inch in diameter). Under normal circumstances, only one follicle has the opportunity to ovulate. However, the use of fertility drugs has allowed many women to develop multiple viable follicles, which has resulted in a recent explosion in the number of multiple births.

A shift from negative feedback to positive feedback is culminated as the rapidly rising estradiol production of the dominant follicle triggers the surges of GnRH, LH, and FSH that produce ovulation. Stimulation of progesterone leads to the biochemical events necessary for rupture of the follicle and ovarian wall. Some women can feel this phenomenon occur with each cycle and, therefore, know when ovulation is occurring. The ruptured follicle, now called the corpus luteum, is stimulated to produce estrogens and progesterone by LH. Following ovulation, control shifts back to negative

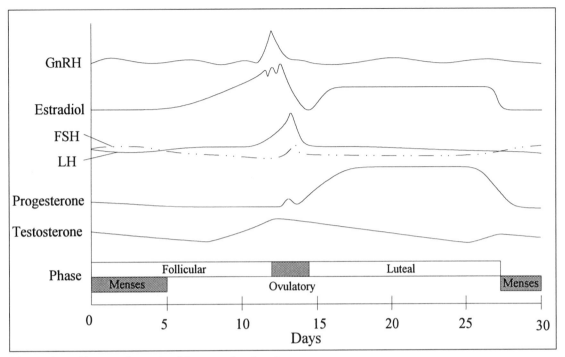

Figure 29-7. Hormonal events of the menstrual cycle.

feedback, and rising levels of progesterone and estradiol produced by the corpus luteum cause decreases in LH and FSH. The corpus luteum requires hormonal stimulation to maintain estrogen and progesterone production beyond 10 days. Unless pregnancy occurs and a new hormone (human chorionic gonadotropin) is produced to stimulate the corpus luteum, estrogen and progesterone levels begin to fall. Production of estrogen and progesterone by the corpus luteum ceases by day 14 if fertilization does not occur. By 12 days after ovulation, progesterone and estrogen levels fall far enough to remove the negative feedback inhibition of FSH, and a new menstrual cycle begins. The cycle returns to the point that has been arbitrarily designated as the beginning as progesterone decreases to a level too low to sustain the endometrium and menstruation occurs.

PREGNANCY

As discussed in the introduction to the chapter, pregnancy is accompanied by a multitude of changes, including hormonal, musculoskeletal, cardiovascular, respiratory, and renal changes. Several of these changes are discussed below, beginning with hormonal changes.

To maintain the changes in the endometrium that occur in preparation of pregnancy, secretion of estrogen and progesterone must continue. As the placenta develops, it will become the chief source of these required hormones (Figure 29-8). Until that point, maternal cells are needed to perform this function. As the follicle ages at the end of the luteal phase, it stops becoming a source of these hormones, as stimulation by GnRH, FSH, and LH stop. Without fertilization, the endometrium is sloughed off in the process of menstruation. The luteal phase typically lasts 12 days; before this time, another source of stimulation must be present to prevent the corpus luteum from degenerating. HCG secreted by the trophoblastic cells (interfacing cells between the endometrium and the cells that will develop into an embryo) begins within 10 days of conception. This hormone shows a rapid rise and peaks between the eighth and 10th weeks of pregnancy and leads to secretion of progesterone and estrogens at higher levels than those of the luteal phase. The level of this hormone decreases and plateaus at about 24 weeks of gestation. By 11 weeks of gestation, the placenta can produce sufficient estrogen and progesterone.

During pregnancy, estrogens are produced by the placenta, resulting in a level up to 30 times that before pregnancy. It has the same effects during pregnancy that were described above, such as increasing the size of the uterus, the breasts, and other reproductive structures, but to a greater degree. The uterus increases in size from 60 g to 1 kg, and each breast may increase by 500 g (about 1 pound). In addition, an increased pigmentation of the areola, increased nipple size, and stretch marks (striae gravidarum) may be observed. Estrogen also has a relaxing effect on ligaments of pelvis and sacroiliac joint.

Another hormone called relaxin also affects ligaments during pregnancy. It is secreted by the corpus luteum when it is stimulated by HCG. Relaxin reaches a peak level in the first trimester and remains elevated until a few days after delivery. Relaxin relaxes ligaments of the pelvis, inhibits uterine contraction, and softens the cervix. In addition to the effects of estrogen and relaxin on pelvic ligaments, the increased weight of the uterus during pregnancy places more stress on joints of the pelvis and lumbar spine. Sacroiliac joints widen 2 to 3 mm, and the pubic symphysis widens an average of 5 mm. These changes in the pelvic ring, coupled with increased mass of the uterus, amniotic fluid, and fetus, cause low back pain in most pregnancies. Many of these problems are caused by movement of one sacroiliac joint that is highly treatable. Unfortunately, low back pain during pregnancy is usually accepted as part of pregnancy even though appropriate therapeutic intervention is available.

Progesterone causes generalized smooth muscle relaxation, including the uterus and gastrointestinal tract. Decreased motility of the gastrointestinal tract often results in constipation and, combined with venous dilation and obstruction of the iliac veins by the enlarged uterus, increases the risk of varicose veins, including hemorrhoids. Because of hormonal changes increasing blood flow to the reproductive structures, the external genitalia and perineum become edematous and uncomfortable. Because progesterone increases sensitivity to carbon dioxide, a phenomenon called hyperventilation of pregnancy occurs. Progesterone also increases the set point of central thermoregulation to increase temperature an average of 1°C during pregnancy.

Cortisol is elevated in the first trimester and continues to rise throughout pregnancy to levels considered pathologic (similar to Cushing's syndrome). No signs of Cushing's syndrome are present, possibly because of competing hormones, such as progesterone. Cortisol may be responsible for the stretch marks that occur during pregnancy that resemble those seen in Cushing's syndrome. The high level of cortisol has an inhibitory effect on the immune system and calms autoimmune diseases. Immediately following delivery, cortisol levels fall dramatically, and autoimmune diseases may either flare up or may first become evident.

The abdominal wall and pelvic floor muscles are stretched by increased uterine size during the first pregnancy but usually resolves to a large degree. However, multiparous women may have a significant decrease in abdominal and pelvic floor tone allowing the uterus,

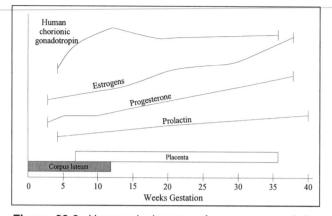

Figure 29-8. Hormonal changes of pregnancy and the structures responsible for hormone synthesis. Note early hormone synthesis from the corpus luteum and later from the placenta.

bladder, and rectum to sag. Downward displacement of these organs is called prolapse. Urinary and fecal incontinence may result from prolapse, which may need to be treated surgically. In many pregnancies, diastasis recti occurs. This is a separation of the rectus muscles at the midline. Stretching of ligaments of the uterus may cause low abdominal or low back pain in some women. This pain can be decreased by back extension to release some tension on the ligaments.

Posture is affected tremendously by pregnancy and is characterized by lumbar lordosis caused by increased uterine size shifting the center of gravity forward. Rounded shoulders and protracted scapulae with internal rotation of upper extremities occur due to increased breast size. A forward head compensates for shoulder alignment. In addition, compensatory thoracic kyphosis can cause thoracic outlet syndrome in which the brachial plexus is compressed as it exits the neck and enters the upper extremity. This is sometimes confused with carpal tunnel syndrome, which can also occur during pregnancy. Carpal tunnel syndrome occurs due to swelling of the hands and wrist compressing the median nerve as it enters the hand from the wrist. It can be distinguished from thoracic outlet syndrome because it only affects the sensory distribution of the median nerve in half of the palm and causes weakness of hand muscles, whereas thoracic outlet syndrome would typically involve both the median and ulnar nerve distribution, including structures proximal to the wrist.

An average weight gain during pregnancy is 20 to 30 lbs, although some women may experience little weight gain and others may increase as much as 100 lbs. Approximately half of the normal weight gain includes the fetus, placenta, and amniotic fluid, 25% uterus and breasts, and about 25% maternal body fluids (Figure 29-9).

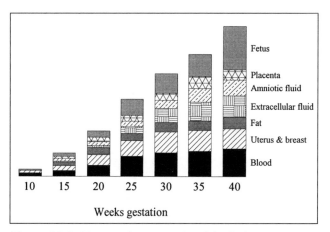

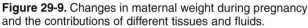

Figure 29-9. Changes in maternal weight during pregnancy and the contributions of different tissues and fluids.

Increased pigmentation on the face in a mask-like distribution, areolae, and linea alba occur during pregnancy. Striae caused by breakdown of subcutaneous tissue with rupture of elastic fibers called striae gravidarum or stretch marks are also commonly observed. These marks appear pink, red, or purple during pregnancy and become white after delivery. Areas typically affected are the abdomen, thighs, iliac crest, and breasts.

CARDIOVASCULAR CHANGES DURING PREGNANCY

Due to increased metabolic demands, both maternal and fetal, maternal cardiac output increases 20% to 50% during pregnancy. Most of the increase occurs in first 8 to 10 weeks. Heart rate increases progressively throughout pregnancy to an increase of about 15 bpm at term (20%), and stroke volume increases about 25%. Arterial blood pressure decreases early in the first trimester, with greater decrease in diastolic pressure. Blood pressure is lowest at midpregnancy, gradually rising to prepregnant levels about 6 weeks before delivery. Most of the increase in cardiac output is accounted for by a decrease in total peripheral resistance, which decreases by the same percentage as cardiac output increases, except during the blood pressure decrease during the mid-second trimester. Additional vascular beds through the placenta, increased uterine blood flow, and generalized decreased vascular tone due to progesterone account for the decreased peripheral resistance.

Venous pressure is not significantly affected in the upper extremities, but increases markedly in the lower extremities in the upright position but not in the horizontal position. Due to mechanical pressure by the weight of the uterus causing obstruction of the iliac veins and inferior vena cava, varicose veins in the lower extremities and hemorrhoids are common. Varicose veins may become worse or first appear during pregnancy. During the third trimester, the supine position (lying on the back) may cause occlusion of the inferior vena cava due to a posterior shift of the uterus onto the vertebral column. Elevation of the right side by 30° avoids compression.

Because blood volume cannot keep pace with the increased vascular volume initially, blood vessels are relatively unfilled, thereby stimulating retention of fluid, especially during the third trimester. Compression palsies including carpal tunnel syndrome, ulnar nerve, and posterior tibial nerve compression can occur. Swollen feet and ankles are very common, especially late in pregnancy. Although both plasma volume and red cell mass increase, plasma volume increases more than red cell volume, resulting in a decreased hematocrit. Plasma volume increases 50%, and red cell volume increases 18% in women not given iron supplements and by 30% in women receiving supplementation.

RESPIRATORY SYSTEM

Basal metabolic rate and oxygen consumption are increased 20% during pregnancy. Hyperventilation due to the effect of progesterone on the respiration center reduces PCO_2 by 25% and increases PO_2 slightly. Increased breathing is primarily due to an increase in tidal volume, not frequency. Functional residual capacity and residual volume decrease due to elevation of the diaphragm. Dyspnea may occur with mild exercise as early as 20 weeks into pregnancy.

RENAL SYSTEM

Progesterone causes relaxation of the smooth muscle of the bladder, and estrogen causes hyperplasia and hypertrophy of the internal sphincter of the bladder. The bladder is displaced anteriorly and superiorly by the enlarging uterus, resulting in a decreased ability to empty the bladder completely, which carries an increased risk of urinary tract infection. Frequent urination occurs due to pressure of the uterus on the bladder. Following delivery, the stretching of the muscles of the pelvic floor, especially the levator ani, decreases the ability of the new mother to control micturition and causing stress incontinence. Stimuli, such as sneezing, coughing, or heavy exercise, can cause urine to leak.

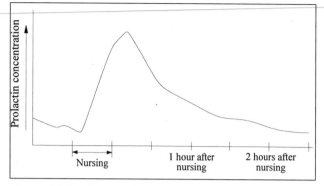

Figure 29-10. Control of plasma prolactin by suckling.

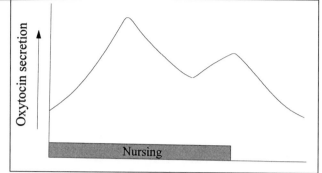

Figure 29-11. Control of plasma oxytocin by suckling.

LACTATION

Prolactin secretion from the anterior pituitary rises linearly throughout pregnancy to eight to 10 times non-pregnant levels. Prolactin is necessary for the effects of estrogen and progesterone on the breast to stimulate milk production. Prolactin stimulates the lactogenic apparatus, whereas the other hormones increase size and cause development of the physical structure. Some milk is produced within the first 5 months, but because estrogen and progesterone inhibit milk synthesis, milk production does not increase to a sufficient level until after delivery with a great decrease in estrogen and progesterone concentrations. During the first 4 to 8 weeks, prolactin concentration in the blood decreases but increases during breastfeeding or pumping (Figure 29-10). Breastfeeding also stimulates oxytocin secretion from the posterior pituitary via stimulation of mechanoreceptors of the nipple. Synthesis is also stimulated, causing a peak plasma concentration about 5 minutes after initiation of suckling (Figure 29-11). Oxytocin produces contraction of the myoepithelial cells of the alveoli of the breast, causing milk to be ejected into the ducts (milk is "let down"). Although changes in oxytocin during delivery cannot explain the birthing process, its effect of initiating and strengthening uterine contractions can be used to induce labor therapeutically. Breast engorgement, cracked nipples, and mastitis are common problems associated with breastfeeding. The combination of engorgement and cracked nipples can permit bacteria access to milk within the ducts. Plugging of the ducts exacerbates the situation because the bacteria are not flushed out, but multiply in a suitable environment. Infection of the breast, called mastitis, can cause large abscesses to develop and may lead to systemic infection. Engorgement can be decreased by packing ice around the breasts and wrapping with a compression bandage.

MENOPAUSE

At an average age of 50 and preceded usually by several years of irregularity of the menstrual cycle, menopause occurs. Irregular peaks of estradiol and insufficient secretion of progesterone due to diminishing numbers of follicles precede menopause. With no follicles remaining, ovarian secretion of estrogens ceases. Low levels of estrogens, now primarily estrone rather than estradiol, are produced by enzymes in peripheral tissues from androgens produced by the adrenal glands. After menopause, a loss of negative feedback from estradiol causes gonadotropin levels to increase to four to 10 times that of the follicular phase. Cycles of gonadotropin secretion are lost, but the pulsatile pattern of secretion remains. With low levels of estrogens, bone reabsorption is not inhibited as much, genitalia and breasts atrophy, and the risk of coronary vascular disease increases. During the first few years of menopause, vascular flushing and hot flashes may occur with LH pulses. Because adipose tissue contains the enzyme that converts androgens to estrogens, obese individuals may exhibit fewer effects of decreased estrogen levels.

SUMMARY

The male and female reproductive structures develop from common embryologic structures under the influence of genetic and hormonal differences. Corresponding male and female cells are responsive to the same hormones and serve similar functions. The interstitial cells of the male and female are called Leydig cells and theca cells, respectively. Both respond to luteinizing hormone and produce androgens. The Sertoli cells of the male and granulosa cells of the female have nurturing roles for the gametes and respond to follicle-stimulating hormone. Granulosa cells also convert androgens into estrogens and synthesize progesterone. Release of LH and FSH from the anterior pituitary is controlled by a hypothalamic-releasing hormone called gonadotropin-releasing hormone (GnRH). In adults, GnRH is released in pulses, resulting in pulsatile release of LH and FSH. FSH stimulates Sertoli cells and granulosa cells to produce maturation of the gametes and becomes involved in the positive feedback mechanism that leads to ovulation. Luteinizing hormone stimulates androgen production, causes ovulation, and stimulates the corpus luteum to produce estrogen and progesterone. Sex hormones alter gene expression on target cells and stimulate or inhibit production of specific proteins in target cells. Testosterone causes development of male structures in the embryo and descent of the testes, increases muscle and red blood cell mass, stimulates bone growth and closure of the epiphyseal plates, and produces the secondary sex characteristics of males. Estrogen causes changes in the female body proportions, stimulates breast and genitalia growth, bone growth, closure of the epiphyseal plates, and sodium reabsorption. Estrogen also has a protective effect against coronary artery disease. Progesterone functions to promote gestation by stimulating tubal and endometrial gland secretions, maintaining the endometrium, inhibiting uterine contraction and causing generalized smooth muscle relaxation, stimulating development of the milk apparatus, and causing increased body temperature and hyperventilation.

Erection is produced by parasympathetic stimulation via reflexes from mechanoreceptors of the genitalia and descending stimulation from the brain. Emission and ejaculation are produced by sympathetic stimulation resulting from tactile stimulation and descending stimulation from the brain. The ability to achieve erection and ejaculation are independent events but require similar excitatory input from tactile simulation or higher centers of the central nervous system.

Puberty is stimulated by a yet unknown mechanism that stimulates gonadotropin secretion. In girls, breast enlargement stimulated by estrogen and in boys, testicular enlargement stimulated by testosterone mark the beginning of puberty. The menstrual cycle begins about 2 years after breast enlargement begins. The cycle is divided into a follicular phase beginning with menstruation and is characterized by a positive feedback mechanism of estrogen to produce a surge in GnRH, FSH, and LH—the mark of the beginning of the ovulatory phase. The ovulatory phase ends with rupture of the follicle and development of the corpus luteum, which produces large quantities of estrogen and progesterone to support implantation of a fertilized ovum. The luteal phase lasts 13 days, ending with either degeneration of the corpus luteum and precipitous declines in estrogen and progesterone that lead to menstruation, or the corpus luteum is stimulated by human chorionic gonadotropin produced by the trophoblastic cells after fertilization.

During pregnancy, estrogen and progesterone are produced by the placenta. Estrogen increases the size of the breasts and uterus, and progesterone produces a generalized smooth muscle relaxation and causes hyperventilation and increased body temperature. Relaxin produced by the corpus luteum causes relaxation and softening of ligaments of the pelvis. The breast requires prolactin for milk production. The ability to produce milk is stimulated by prolactin but is inhibited by estrogen and progesterone, so that, after delivery, milk production markedly increases. Oxytocin causes contraction of myoepithelial cells to release milk into the ducts to be available by suckling. Suckling stimulates secretion of both prolactin and oxytocin.

Menopause is caused by depletion of follicles and a loss of the ability to synthesize androgens to produce estrogen by the ovary at an average age of 50. Menopause often causes osteoporosis, increases the risk of coronary artery disease, causes atrophy of the genitalia and breasts, and, in many women, causes vascular flushing and "hot flashes" with LH pulses. In men, testosterone production is well maintained until 70 to 80 years of age.

BIBLIOGRAPHY

Berne RM, Levy MN. *Physiology*. St. Louis, Mo: Mosby-Year Book; 1998.

Ganong WF. *Review of Medical Physiology*. Norwalk, Conn: Appleton & Lange; 1995.

Guyton AC, Hall JE, Schmitt W. *Human Physiology and Mechanisms of Disease*. Philadelphia, Pa: WB Saunders; 1997.

Hole JW Jr. *Essentials of Human Anatomy and Physiology*. 4th ed. Dubuque, Iowa: Wm. C. Brown Publishers; 1992.

Schauf C, Moffett D, Moffett S. *Human Physiology: Foundation and Frontiers*. St. Louis, Mo: Times Mirror/Mosby College Publishing; 1990.

Solomon EP, Davis PW. *Human Anatomy and Physiology*. Philadelphia, Pa: WB Saunders; 1983.

STUDY QUESTIONS

1. List some reasons for urinary incontinence following childbirth and with menopause.

2. Contrast the increase in height of boys and girls.

3. How can the symptoms of genital atrophy be treated in menopausal women without systemic estrogen replacement?

4. Why do women experience anemia during pregnancy? Name one simple way of increasing hematocrit.

5. Why is low back pain so common in pregnancy?

6. Why does thoracic outlet syndrome occur in pregnancy? Why does carpal tunnel syndrome occur? How can one distinguish between these two conditions?

7. List some health problems associated with menopause.

INDEX

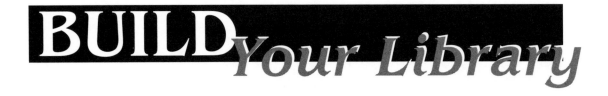